Basic Mechanisms of Physiologic and Aberrant Lymphoproliferation in the Skin

NATO ASI Series

Advanced Science Institutes Series

A series presenting the results of activities sponsored by the NATO Science Committee, which aims at the dissemination of advanced scientific and technological knowledge, with a view to strengthening links between scientific communities.

The series is published by an international board of publishers in conjunction with the NATO Scientific Affairs Division

A	Life Sciences	Plenum Publishing Corporation
B	Physics	New York and London
C	Mathematical and Physical Sciences	Kluwer Academic Publishers
D	Behavioral and Social Sciences	Dordrecht, Boston, and London
E	Applied Sciences	
F	Computer and Systems Sciences	Springer-Verlag
G	Ecological Sciences	Berlin, Heidelberg, New York, London,
H	Cell Biology	Paris, Tokyo, Hong Kong, and Barcelona
I	Global Environmental Change	

Recent Volumes in this Series

Volume 265 — Basic Mechanisms of Physiologic and Aberrant Lymphoproliferation
in the Skin
edited by W. Clark Lambert, Benvenuto Giannotti, and
Willem A. van Vloten

Volume 266 — Esterases, Lipases, and Phospholipases: From Structure to
Clinical Significance
edited by M.I. Mackness and M. Clerc

Volume 267 — Bioelectrochemistry IV: Nerve Muscle Function—
Bioelectrochemistry, Mechanisms, Bioenergetics, and Control
edited by Bruno Andrea Melandri, Giulio Milazzo, and Martin Blank

Volume 268 — Advances in Molecular Plant Nematology
edited by F. Lamberti, C. De Giorgi, and D. McK. Bird

Volume 269 — Ascomycete Systematics: Problems and Perspectives in
the Nineties
edited by David L. Hawksworth

Volume 270 — Standardization of Epidemiologic Studies of Host Susceptibility
edited by Janice Dorman

Volume 271 — Oscillatory Event-Related Brain Dynamics
edited by Christo Pantev, Thomas Elbert, and Bernd Lütkenhöner

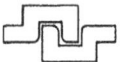

Series A: Life Sciences

Basic Mechanisms of Physiologic and Aberrant Lymphoproliferation in the Skin

Edited by

W. Clark Lambert

UMD–New Jersey Medical School
Newark, New Jersey

Benvenuto Giannotti

University of Florence
Florence, Italy

and

Willem A. van Vloten

University Hospital, Utrecht
Utrecht, The Netherlands

Springer Science+Business Media, LLC

Proceedings of a NATO Advanced Research Workshop on
Basic Mechanisms of Physiologic and Aberrant Lymphoproliferation in the Skin,
held October 1–6, 1991,
in San Miniato, Pisa, Italy

NATO-PCO-DATA BASE

The electronic index to the NATO ASI Series provides full bibliographical references (with keywords and/or abstracts) to more than 30,000 contributions from international scientists published in all sections of the NATO ASI Series. Access to the NATO-PCO-DATA BASE is possible in two ways:

—via online FILE 128 (NATO-PCO-DATA BASE) hosted by ESRIN, Via Galileo Galilei, I-00044 Frascati, Italy

—via CD-ROM "NATO Science and Technology Disk" with user-friendly retrieval software in English, French, and German (©WTV GmbH and DATAWARE Technologies, Inc. 1989). The CD-ROM also contains the AGARD Aerospace Database.

The CD-ROM can be ordered through any member of the Board of Publishers or through NATO-PCO, Overijse, Belgium.

Library of Congress Cataloging-in-Publication Data

Basic mechanisms of physiologic and aberrant lymphoproliferation in
  the skin / edited by W. Clark Lambert, Benvenuto Giannotti, and
  Willem A. van Vloten.
       p.   cm. -- (NATO ASI series. Series A, Life sciences ; v.
  265)
     "Proceedings of a NATO Advanced Research Workshop on Basic
  Mechanisms of Physiologic and Aberrant Lymphoproliferation in the
  Skin, held October 1-6, 1991, in San Miniato, Pisa, Italy"--T.p.
  verso.
     "Published in cooperation with NATO Scientific Affairs Division."
     Includes bibliographical references and index.
     ISBN 978-0-306-44736-5   ISBN 978-1-4615-1861-7 (eBook)
     DOI 10.1007/978-1-4615-1861-7
     1. Lymphomas--Congresses. 2. Skin--Cancer--Congresses.
  3. Lymphoproliferative disorders--Congresses. I. Lambert, W.
  Clark. II. Giannotti, B. III. Vloten, W. A. van. IV. North
  Atlantic Treaty Organization. Scientific Affairs Division. V. NATO
  Advanced Research Workshop on Basic Mechanisms of Physiologic and
  Aberrant Lymphoproliferation in the Skin (1991 : San Miniato, Italy)
  VI. Series.
     [DNLM: 1. Lymphoma, T-Cell, Cutaneous--congresses. 2. T
  -Lymphocytes--immunology--congresses. 3. Skin Neoplasms-
  -congresses.   WR 500 B311 1994]
  RC280.L9B37 1994
  616.99'442--dc20
  DNLM/DLC
  for Library of Congress   94-34190
                                                                 CIP

©1994 Springer Science+Business Media New York
Originally published by Plenum Press in 1994

Participants in the NATO Advanced Studies Workshop:
BASIC MECHANISMS OF PHYSIOLOGIC AND ABERRANT LYMPHOPROLIFERATION IN THE SKIN

Bagot, M (France)

Bakels, V (Netherlands)

Bernengo, M (Italy)

Berti, E (Italy)

Borst, J (Netherlands)

Burg, G (Switzeland)

Busschots, AM (Belgium)

Cerroni, L (Austria)

Chementi, G (Italy)

Cooper, K (USA)

Crosti, L (Italy)

D'Incan, M (France)

Dummer, R (Switzerland)

Edelson, RL (USA)

Geerts, ML (Belgium)

Giannotti, B (Italy)

Hartfield, PJ (England)

Kadin, M (USA)

Kaltoft, M (Denmark)

Kaudewitz, P (Germany)

Kerl, H (Austria)

Lambert, MW (USA)

Lambert, WC (USA)

Laroche, L (France)

Lawley, Th (USA)

Luger, Th (Germany)

MacDonald, DM (England)

Manzari, V (Italy)

Melief, C (Netherlands)

Meyer, CJLM (Netherlands)

Mielke, V (Germany)

Nestle, F (Switzerland)

Nickoloff, B (USA)

Oostveen, H van (Netherlands)

Pimpinelli, N (Italy

Preesman, AH (Netherlands)

Ralfkiaer, E (Denmark)

Ramsay, D (USA)

Rijlaarsdam, U (Netherlands)

Santucci,M (Italy)

Schwarz, Th (Germany)

Smith, N (England

Souteyrand, P (France)

Sterry, W (Germany)

Stingl, G (Austria)

Thestrup Pedersen, K (Denmark)

Tigelaar, R (USA)

Veelken, H (USA)

Vloten, WA van (Netherlands)

Vonderheid, E (USA)

Whittaker, S (England)

Willemze, R (Netherlands)

PREFACE

This book is based upon a series of papers originally presented at a NATO Advanced Studies Workshop of the same title held at the study Center "I Cappuccini," a converted monastery in San Miniato, a small village located between Pisa and Florence, Italy, in October 1991. Authors were asked to submit their completed chapters by the following February; these were then scanned onto computer disks, edited and returned to the authors for final revision, and updating, with a final deadline of February 1993. The authors were encouraged to make whatever modifications they wanted, especially regarding updating their chapters, with an eye to making the final product both comprehensive and current. In this we succeeded beyond our expectations, with most chapters extensively altered and many completely re-written and significantly expanded. Thus, although the original meeting was held in 1991, the chapters in this volume may be regarded as current from at least February, 1993, with some of the final updated revisions received as late as July, 1993.

This book, as agreed in our original contract, has been delivered to the publisher "camera-ready." This means that all of the scanning, editing, proofing and typesetting were done here, by the office of the Department of Dermatology at the New Jersey Medical School. We essentially produced the book, which the publisher, for the most part, then photocopied. This has been an enormous burden, borne mainly by my colleague in this division, Robert A. Schwartz, M.D., and especially by our hardworking secretary, Mrs. Valeria R. Carter. For many months, Bob has cheerfully tolerated ridiculous shortfalls in his secretarial support, whereas Mrs. Carter has undauntingly accomplished seemingly impossible tasks, not only mastering the complexities of scanning computer technology and correlating text to its original, but also assisting me in editing out awkward, often ambiguous and sometimes even downright wrong English usage in many of these papers. We have been assisted in this endeavor by a series of dermatopathology residents, Drs. David Arbesfeld, Stephen Nychay and Philip J. Cohen, and particularly by Hon-Reen Kuo, Ph.D., a post-doctoral fellow in my laboratory who spent many hours assisting us in the final editing phases. We also are grateful for the critical support of the Computing Center at the New Jersey Medical School, at which the chapters were scanned and this book was produced in its present form.

Although the task of editing this volume has fallen primarily on me and those unfortunate enough to be closely associated with me, I have been greatly assisted in this endeavor by Dr. Willem A. van Vloten, who also took the primary role in designing the meeting, and Dr.

Benvenuto Giannotti, who, along with his hardworking associate, Dr. Nicola Pimpinelli, was also responsible for the arrangements for the meeting, itself. We were also greatly assisted by an Organizing Committee made up of Drs. Richard Edelson, New Haven, CT, U.S.A., Chairman, Günter Burg, Zurich, Switzerland, Donald M. MacDonald, London, U.K., and Pierre Souteyrand, Clermont Ferrand, France, as well as by Dr. Robert A. Tigelaar, New Haven, CT, who presented a summary on the last day of the meeting.

We are also grateful to the Scientific Branch of the North American Treaty Organization for the financial support which made this meeting possible and to the Cassa [Bank] di Risparmio di San Miniato for the use of their splendid meeting facility in San Miniato, as well as to Lederle, Hoffman La Roche and Wellcome Laboratories for their support of this meeting. I am also grateful for the enormous support and advice given by the Plenum Publishing corporation, who guided us through the complexities associated with preparation of this book, and who will, happily for us, take over from this point on in its completion.

The magnificent evenings in the hills of Tuscany are memories now, as are the intensive scientific, as well as social interactions that greatly enriched all who were fortunate enough to take part in this meeting. A conference of this type is far different from the more usual busy congress, in which one barely feels he or she has time to think, much less reflect and discuss science in depth. Thus this gathering was especially important, because it allowed, even forced us to think about what we do and think and why we do it, and because there have been too few meetings of this type in this field; it is clearly apparent that more are needed. The other editors, together with the authors of this book and myself, have endeavored to capture what we could of the flavor of this meeting in these pages. We sincerely hope that the reader will find our efforts to have been fruitful.

Newark, New Jersey   W. Clark Lambert, M.D., Ph.D.
September 30, 1993   For the editors

CONTENTS

SECTION I : CELL BIOLOGY

SECTION II : LYMPHOCYTE HOMING

SECTION III : VIRUSES

SECTION IV : HISTOLOGY

SECTION V : GENOTYPING

SECTION VI : IMMUNOMODULATION AND TUMOR PROGRESSION

γδ T LYMPHOCYTES IN MICE AND MAN: A REVIEW

Jannie Borst
Lex Bakker
Ferry Ossendorp

Division of Immunology
The Netherlands Cancer Institute
Amsterdam, The Netherlands

Correspondence to: Dr. J. Borst, Ned. Kanker Instituut,
Plesmanlaan 121,
1066 CX, Amsterdam, The Netherlands

ABSTRACT

With the discovery of a second type of T cells, those expressing T cell receptor (TCR) γδ, the question has arisen: "What contribution do these cells make to the immune system?" We review here how TCR diversity is generated at the molecular level and what this means for the capability of TCR αβ and TCR γδ to recognize a variety of antigenic peptides in the context of conventional and alternative presenting molecules. We will discuss how tissue distribution and repertoire selection of γδ T cells are in part developmentally regulated and how the repertoire may be further shaped by antigenic stimulation. Critical investigation of the causes and consequences of γδ T cell proliferation in human disease situations will hopefully provide insight into the normal functions of this elusive T cell population.

INTRODUCTION

Until recently, all T cell receptors were considered to be heterodimers composed of polymorphic α and β glycoproteins. During the search for the TCR α and β genes, a third gene

Basic Mechanisms of Physiologic and Aberrant Lymphoproliferation in the Skin
Edited by W.C. Lambert *et al.*, Plenum Press, New York, 1994

1

was found that specifically rearranges in T lymphocytes (Saito et al., 1984). Subsequent studies revealed that this gene encodes the γ chain, one subunit of a new type of TCR (Lew et al., 1986). Its partner chain turned out to be the product of a fourth rearranging gene, TCR γ (Chien et al., 1987). With that finding, TCR $\gamma\delta$, a heterodimer different from TCR $\alpha\beta$, was molecularly defined.

After a few fruitful years of research regarding, particularly, the molecular biology and biochemistry of TCR $\gamma\delta$, the question remains: "What contribution do $\gamma\delta$ T cells make to the immune system?" Two major issues must be elucidated. First, is there an overlap in antigenic specificities between $\alpha\beta$ and $\gamma\delta$ T cells, or are $\gamma\delta$ T cells designed to recognize different antigens? Second, do $\gamma\delta$ T cells display the same functional activities as $\alpha\beta$ T cells, or do they exert other functions, possibly at specific sites of action?

T CELL RECEPTOR (TCR) $\gamma\delta$ STRUCTURE

Analogous to the immunoglobulin genes (Tonegawa, 1983), the TCR loci contain variable (V), diversity (D), joining (J) and constant (C) gene segments that undergo somatic rearrangement during T cell differentiation to generate functional TCR genes. In this process, V, D (in TCR β and δ genes), and J segments are joined to encode the variable domain of a given TCR chain, while the C segment encodes the constant domain. The variable domains of the two TCR chains together form the binding site for antigenic peptides and for the MHC class I or MHC class II molecules by which they are presented (Davis and Bjorkman, 1988).

The human TCR β locus lies on chromosome 7, band q35 (Rabbitts et al., 1985). It contains more than 70 Vβ gene segments and 2 Cβ gene segments, with each Cβ gene segment preceded by 1 Dβ and 6, or 7, Jβ segments (Toyonaga and Mak, 1987; Wilson et al., 1988; Figure 1). The TCR γ gene is also located on chromosome 7, but at a different site (bands p14-p15; Murre et al., 1985). It contains 8 functional and 7 non-functional Vγ segments, and 2 Cγ segments, with each Cγ segment preceded by 2 or 3 Jγ gene segments (Huck et al., 1988). Surprisingly, the α and δ genes are found in the same locus, on chromosome 14, band q11 (Caccia et al., 1985; Boehm et al., 1988). The Cδ gene segment lies between the Vα and Jα segments. It is preceded by 3 Dδ and 3 Jδ segments, and by about 6 Vδ gene segments, all of which are exclusively used in conjunction with Cδ (Satyanarayana et al., 1988; Takihara et al., 1989; Hata et al., 1989). There are more than 50 different Vα segments, some of which may also be used in conjunction with Cδ, and should therefore be termed Vα/δ segments. More than 50 Jα segments are spread out over the more than 85 kb distance to the single Cα segment (Toyonaga and Mak, 1987; Wilson et al., 1988) (Figure 1).

Overall, the murine TCR genes have an organization similar to that of their human counterparts. Since the murine TCR γ gene is somewhat differently organized, however, it is also shown in Figure 1. The locus contains 4 Jγ-Cδ gene segment tandems, one of which, the

2

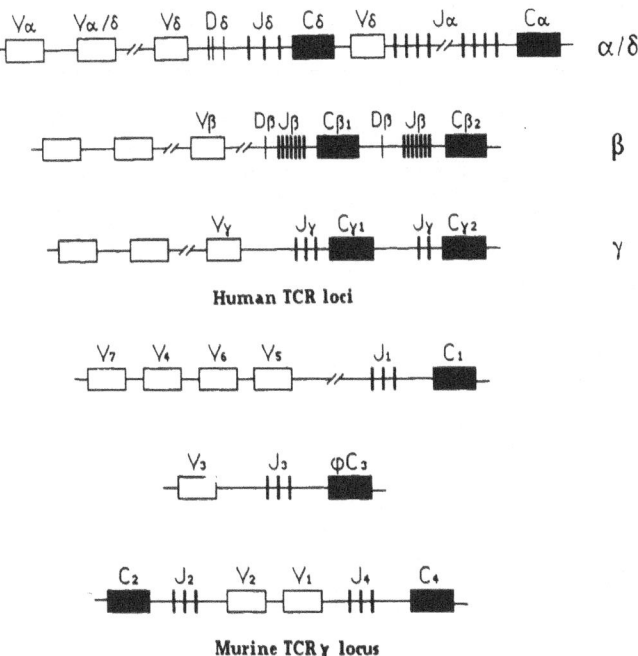

Figure 1. Organization of TCR genes. Top three lines, human TCR loci, type as indicated on right. Bottom three lines, murine TCR δ locus.

Jγ3-Cγ tandem, does not give rise to a functional TCR γ protein. Vγ7, Vγ4, Vγ6 and Vγ5 can rearrange to align with Jγl-Cγl, Vγ2 to align with Jγ2-Cγ2 and Vγl to align with Jγ4-Cγ4 (Raulet, 1989a).

It is important to understand the genomic organization of the TCR genes, since it allows an estimation of the potential TCR repertoire (i.e., range of antigens recognized), and with this, of the capability of an organism to see variety of antigens. The repertoire is determined by three factors: i) the germline diversity, determined by the number of different gene segments, ii) the combinatorial diversity, resulting from combination of the gene segments and the pairing of the two receptor chains, and iii) the junctional diversity. The junctional diversity is a consequence of the way the recombination machinery works. In the excision and subsequent joining of DNA fragments, random modification of the termini of the recombining V, D and J gene segments occurs. Exonucleases may remove nucleotides from these ends and transferases (perhaps terminal deoxynucleotidyl transferase TdT; Alt and Baltimore, 1982) may add what are termed "N-nucleotides" at the junctions, independent of a template (Tonegawa, 1983). This leads to additional diversity in the variable domains of the TCR chains.

As shown in Table 1, the TCRγ and δ loci contain fewer V and J gene segments than are contained in the TCR α and β loci. However, the potential junctional diversity in TCR δ chains

Table 1. Estimation of the potential primary repertoire of human TcR molecules

Source of diversity	TcR-$\alpha\beta$ molecules		TcR-$\gamma\delta$ molecules	
	TcR-α	TcR-β	TcR-γ	TcR-δ
Germline diversity; number of genes				
V genes	>50	>70	8	$\geq$6
D genes	—	2	—	3
J genes	about 55	13	5	3
Combinatorial diversity				
per chain	>2750	>1820	40	>75
per complete molecules	> 5 x 10^6		>3000	
Junctional diversity				
number of joining sites	1	1	1	1-4
N region insertion	+	+ +	+ +	+ + + +
estimated degree of increase in diversity	x 10^2	x 10^4	x 10^3	x 10^9
Estimation of total primary receptor repertoire	x 10^{12}		x 10^{15}	

is significantly larger than in any of the other TCR chains. This is due to the fact that a rearranged TCR δ gene may include up to three Dδ elements (Elliot et al., 1988). Each additional joining event, accompanied by trimming of the gene segment termini and inclusion of N-nucleotides, increases the diversity in this part of the TCR δ protein.

The three dimensional structure of the TCR molecule is not yet known. However, the TCR shares important features with immunoglobulin, the structure of which has been resolved by X--ray diffraction of protein crystals (Alzari et al., 1988). A possible three dimensional structure of the TCR has been proposed, based on these data (Chotia et al., 1988; Davis and Bjorkman, 1988). Hypervariable portions within the receptor have been deduced from comparison of cDNA sequences, and these sites have been projected in the model. Three hypervariable portions can be identified, provisionally termed complementarity-determining regions (CDR) 1,

2 and 3, that together would form a relatively flat surface that could interact with the peptide/MHC complex. The V gene segment of TCR α or δ would contribute to CDRl, the V gene segment of TCR β or γ to CDR2, and the combined D-J gene segments of TCR α and β or of TCR γ and δ would form CDR3. Since the D-J junction contains the greatest diversity, CDR3 would be the most variable.

Davis and Bjorkman (1988) and Chotia et al. (1988) have proposed that the most variable part of the TCR would make contact primarily with the most variable part of the antigen/MHC complex, that is, with the peptide. The CDRl and CDR2, contributed by the V domains, would fit over the two α-helices of the MHC molecule. If, indeed, the junctional regions are the parts of the TCR involved in the recognition of antigenic peptides, the capacity of TCR $\gamma\delta$ to recognize a variety of antigens may be very large and may even exceed that of TCR $\alpha\beta$, even though only a small number of V and J gene segments are available in the γ and δ loci. The diversity of the TCR would be primarily located in the CDR3 region, however, which may have consequences for MHC restriction. In the recognition of superantigens, it appears that CDR3 does not play a role. There is, however a requirement for the use of particular Vβ gene segments. This is consistent with the proposed model, since classical superantigens, such as staphylococcal enterotoxins (Marrack and Kappler, 1990), are thought to bind to the MHC class II molecules outside the groove and may interact directly with the CDR portion contributed by the TCR β chain (Dellabona, et al., 1990).

$\gamma\delta$ T CELL DIFFERENTIATION

In the fetal thymus of the mouse, $\gamma\delta$ T cells are the first TCR bearing cells to appear. Until about day 17 of gestation, $\gamma\delta$ T cells comprise the majority of thymocytes, but thereafter their relative numbers decrease to only about 1% of total thymocytes. This is due to a large increase in absolute numbers of thymocytes which express TCR $\alpha\beta$ (Havran and Allison, 1988). Based on these observations, a model has been proposed for the developmental relationship of TCR $\gamma\delta$ and TCR $\alpha\delta$ bearing cells. According to this model, in fetal thymocytes, TCR δ and γ genes rearrange first. In each thymocyte destined to undergo differentiation as a $\gamma\delta$ T cell, successful rearrangement arrests differentiation to yield a $\gamma\delta$ T cell. Unproductive rearrangement, however, is followed by TCR β and α gene rearrangement, which may produce an $\alpha\beta$ T cell (Pardoll et al., 1987).

Studies in TCR transgenic mice, however, have unambiguously shown that $\gamma\delta$ T cells and $\alpha\beta$ T cells are of independent lineages. Introduction of functionally rearranged γ and δ transgenes into the germline does not inhibit TCR α and β gene rearrangement. Only a small proportion of T cells, apparently predestined to become the $\gamma\delta$ T cell subset, express the transgenic receptor, while the majority of T cells express endogenous TCR $\alpha\beta$ (Bonneville et al., 1990). The separation of $\gamma\delta$ and $\alpha\beta$ T cell lineages is most likely regulated by δ- and α-enhancer activities (De Villartay and Cohen, 1990). According to this hypothesis, in precursor T cells predestined to become $\alpha\beta$ T cells, transcriptional activity may make the TCR α locus accessible for rearrangement. An early rearrangement event, involving a V-like segment and a pseudo-Jα segment, eliminates the δ gene that lies in between, thus cutting off the γδ T cell differentiation pathway. In γδ T cells, transcription of the TCR α locus would be putatively inhibited by a specific silencer.

In murine fetal thymocytes, Vγ gene expression seems to be regulated. During development, cells expressing different γδ TCR appear in partially overlapping waves. The first γδ T cells express Vγ5; the next wave expresses Vγ6; followed by γδ T cells expressing Vγ4. In the newborn thymus, γδ T cells express predominantly Vγ4 and Vγ7 segments (Ito et al., 1989). A look at the organization of the murine γ locus (Figure 1) makes it tempting to speculate that sequential rearrangements occur, during development, progressing from the Vγ segments most proximal to the Cγ1 segment to the Vγ segments located further upstream from it and that these sequential rearrangements determine the sequence of Vδ gene expression, but this is by no means proven (Carding et al., 1990).

The earliest murine Vδ gene segment to be expressed is Vδ1 (Ito et al., 1989). While adult γδ TCR often use more than one Dδ element and contain extensively modified gene segment termini, the fetal γδ TCR, in which the Vγ5 and Vδ6 segments are used in conjunction with Vδ1, have no junctional diversity and, therefore, are essentially monomorphic (Allison and Havran, 1990). Lack of TdT activity early in development might explain the absence of N-nucleotides. Although it is not clear to what extent T cell selection plays a role in the formation of the γδ T cell repertoire, it is clear that the mechanism of γδ TCR gene rearrangement at least in part determines the γδ TCR repertoire generated at different time points in development.

It has recently been demonstrated that in human T cell development, also, TCR γ and δ loci may be rearranged and expressed in an ordered fashion (Krangel et al., 1990). As in the murine locus, the Vγ segments more proximal to the Cγ gene recombine first. The repertoire in early fetal thymocytes is dominated by Vγ9/Jγ1/Cγ1-Vδ[+] cells. This is in contrast to the situation later in development, where more upstream Vγ's of the Vγ1 subfamily, joined to Jγ2/Cγ1, are used in combination with the Vδl segment located further upstream. Also, as in the murine system, the γδ TCR of early fetal thymocytes has little junctional diversity. There is no time point in human T cell development at which the thymus harbors only γδ T cells and no αβ T cells (Campana et al., 1989), however. This is in striking contrast with the situation in the mouse, and correlates with differences in the tissue distribution of γδ T cells between mouse and man.

TISSUE DISTRIBUTION OF γδ T CELLS

In the mouse, γδ T cells are very abundant in the epidermis where they form 95% of the total T cell population (Stingl et al., 1987). These γδ T cells have a highly dendritic morphology (they are also known as dendritic epidermal cells, DEC). They possess a monomorphic TCR in which Vγ5 and Vδ1 gene segments are used (Allison and Havran, 1990). In the epithelia of female reproductive organs and of the tongue, γδ T cells are also the major T cell population. Similar to epidermal γδ T cells, these γδ T cells also possess a monomorphic TCR, but one in which the Vδ6 gene segment, rather than the Vδ5 gene segment, is used with the Vδ1 gene segment (Itohara et al., 1990).

The epithelium of the intestine harbors a major γδ T cell population as well (Goodman and Lefrancois, 1988). While the majority of intestinal αβ T cells are located in the lamina propria, γδ T cells are mainly found in between the villous epithelial cells. In contrast to the two γδ T cell subsets mentioned above, intestinal γδ T cells possess highly polymorphic TCR, using mainly Vγ7 and a variety of Vδ gene segments in which considerable junctional diversity exists in both γ and δ chains (Asarnow et al., 1989).

Due to their specific localization in certain murine epithelia, it has been hypothesized that γδ T cells have a special role in continuous immunosurveillance of epithelia (Janeway et al., 1988). It has been proposed that they may monitor epithelial cells by recognizing a specific change induced by infection or transformation. Since the skin and reproductive organ γδ T cells have a monomorphic receptor, such a change would not involve expression of a variety of novel antigens, introduced by an infectious agent, but rather induction of one particular autologous antigenic determinant. Heat shock proteins are candidates for such target antigens (Raulet, 1989b). Analysis of γδ T cell tissue distribution in the human system, however, suggests that such epithelial surveillance cannot be a general feature of γδ T cells. In the human epidermis, the absolute number of T cells is much lower than in the murine epidermis. Also, γδ T cells clearly constitute a minority of total T cells at this site, and their morphology is not comparable to that of the highly dendritic murine epidermal γδ T cells (Groh et al., 1989; Bos et al., 1990). Thus, the human system lacks the equivalent of the murine Vγ5/Vδ1+ T cell. Scrutiny of epithelial layers in a great variety of normal human tissues, including the respiratory tract, digestive tract and reproductive organs (Groh et al. 1989; Vroom et al., 1991), has revealed that the human equivalent of the murine Vγ6/Vδ1+ T cell is also lacking. γδ T cells constitute a small minority (< 5%) of total T cells in all epithelia, with one clear exception, the intestinal epithelium. In the human small and large intestine, 10-40% of total intra-epithelial T cells express TCR γδ (Halstensen et al., 1989; Deusch et al., 1991). As in the mouse, γδ T cells are rarely detected in the lamina propria, where significant numbers of αβ T cells are found.

The γδ T cell subsets in murine epidermis and reproductive organ/tongue epithelium are most likely derived from the first two waves of γδ T cells that dominate the fetal thymus (Allison and Havran, 1990). In the human thymus, an early γδ T cell type, expressing Vγ9 and Vδ2 gene segments, is recognizable, but it always forms a small minority of total TCR bearing thymocytes. Homing capacities of the murine thymus-derived γδ T cells are not determined by their TCR, itself, since studies in transgenic mice have revealed that γδ T cells bearing other types of TCR can also colonize these epithelia (Bonneville et al., 1989). Perhaps specific homing receptors that are expressed at the time points in development when these cells are generated determine the tissue localization of these two γδ T cell subsets in mice. The absence of these γδ T cells in human epidermis and reproductive organ epithelium may thus be explained by the lack of expression of such homing receptors, or their ligands. Another possibility is that the γδ T cells undergo replication, and thus expand their numbers, in the murine thymus and in the two murine epithelial sites due to specific stimulation, and that this specific stimulation, or something like it, may not occur in human tissues.

The intra-epithelial γδ T cell type found in the murine intestine is now thought to develop extrathymically. It is present in nude mice (De Geus et al., 1990) and in thymectomized animals (Lefrancois et al., 1990). In mice, these γδ T cells preferentially use the Vγ7 gene segment (Asarnow et al.,1989; Carding et al., 1990). In humans, these γδ T cells predominantly express the Vδ1 gene segment (Halstensen et al., 1989; Deusch et al., 1991). This V gene segment use may be developmentally regulated, but it may also be the result of specific antigenic stimulation and/or interaction with autologous proteins at this site (Lefrancois et al., 1990). The preferential intra-epithelial localization of γδ T cells in the intestine is conserved in all species investigated and may therefore provide a clue for the specific function of this γδ T cell subset. As stated above, these γδ T cells have the potential to recognize a wide variety of antigens, primarily due to their extensive junctional diversity. A possible specialized function we would like to propose is regulation of the development of IgA$^+$ B lymphocytes in the intestinal mucosa.

In human peripheral blood and lymphoid organs, γδ T cells constitute < 1-15% of the total T cell population (Borst et al., 1988; Groh et al., 1989). Again, these cells are characterized by specific Vγ and Vδ gene usage. In most healthy individuals, over 80% of peripheral γδ T cells express the Vγ9 gene segment in combination with the Vδ2 gene segment (Triebel et al., 1988a;b; Borst et al., 1989). These receptors have extensive junctional diversity. Whereas the γδ T cell repertoire in newborns is dominated by cells expressing Vδ1, during the first few years after birth Vδ2 and Vγ9 expression increase (Borst and Van Dongen, 1990; Parker et al., 1990). Thymic selection most likely does not play a role in the repertoire change, since it has also been observed in a patient with complete DiGeorge anomaly, characterized by a virtual absence of thymic epithelial mass (Borst and Van Dongen, 1990). Rather, the change is due to an increase in asolute numbers of Vγ9/Vδ2$^+$ cells. Cells in this γδ T cell subset, in contrast to the Vδ1$^+$ cells, express the CD45RO epitope, a hallmark of previously activated, or "memory" cells (Parker et al., 1990). Therefore, it has been postulated that this subset enlarges as a result of stimulation by an undefined antigen. If so, this should be classified as a superantigen, since it expands all cells that use Vγ9 and Vδ2 gene segments, independent of diversity in the CDR3 region. The expansion is not induced by recognition of an autologous determinant, since identical twins may have different γδ T cell repertoires (Parker et al., 1990). In individuals that have a peripheral γδ T cell repertoire dominated by Vγ9/Vδ2$^+$ cells, intraepithelial intestinal cells may preferentially express the Vδ1 gene segment in combination with Vγ's other than Vγ9 (Deusch et al., 1991). This indicates that intestinal γδ T cells are resident cells that are not directly connected to the circulating T cell pool.

$\gamma\delta$ T CELL FUNCTION

Activated proliferating $\gamma\delta$ T cell clones are rather similar to $\alpha\beta$ T cells with respect to their ability to produce a variety of biologically active cytokines. After stimulation with anti-CD3 antibody or concanavalin A, $\gamma\delta$ T cells can produce IL-2, IL-4, IL-5, TNFα, GM-CSF and IFNγ (Patel et al., 1989; Krangel et al., 1990). However, the possibility that certain $\gamma\delta$ T cell clones can synthesize unique, yet to be defined cytokines that endow them with a unique functional activity cannot be ruled out.

Another important function of $\gamma\delta$ T cells, demonstrated in vitro, is their cytolytic activity. $\gamma\delta$ T cell clones, cultured in vitro, may develop cytolytic granules, containing pore-forming protein or perforin and serine esterases, such as are found in NK cells and activated, cytolytic $\alpha\beta$ T cells. Triggering of the $\gamma\delta$ TCR by specific antigen (Spits et al., 1990), or triggering of CD16, an Fc receptor for IgG expressed on a fraction of $\gamma\delta$ T cells (Van de Griend et al., 1987), induces granule exocytosis and target cell killing. In addition, similar to NK cells, but unlike most $\alpha\beta$ T cells, $\gamma\delta$ T cells can easily be induced to mediate MHC non-restricted cytolysis of tumor cell lines by in vitro culture with IL-2 (Borst et al., 1987; Moingeon et al., 1987). This MHC non-restricted lymphokine activated killer (LAK) activity of $\gamma\delta$ T cells is not mediated via their TCR (Borst et al., 1988) and does not involve granule exocytosis (Spits et al., 1990). The mechanism of LAK activity must therefore involve mediators other than those contained in cytolytic granules. These mediators remain to be defined. In contrast to freshly isolated NK cells, freshly isolated $\gamma\delta$ T cells are resting T cells that have no cytolytic granules (Borst et al., 1988) and are unable to bring about target cell lysis.

$\gamma\delta$ T CELL INTERACTION WITH MHC MOLECULES AND ANTIGEN

The structure of the $\gamma\delta$ TCR suggests that it can mediate antigen specific recognition in a manner analogous to the $\alpha\beta$ TCR, i.e., by interaction with processed peptides of foreign antigens bound to MHC molecules. There is not one example in the literature of antigen recognition by $\gamma\delta$ T cells, however, in which the peptide as well as the restriction element has been defined.

$\gamma\delta$ T cell specificity for allo-MHC class I (Spits et al., 1990) and class II molecules (Kozbor et al., 1989) has been demonstrated. Although these results show that $\gamma\delta$ T cells are able to interact with conventional MHC molecules, the question remains whether these generally serve as the antigen presenting elements for $\gamma\delta$ T cells. The majority of $\gamma\delta$ T cells lack expression of CD4 and CD8 molecules that make an essential contribution in TCR $\alpha\beta$-MHC interactions by associating with nonpolymorphic portions of MHC class II or class I molecules, respectively. In human peripheral blood, on average 88% of $\gamma\delta$ T cells have the CD4$^-$ CD8$^-$ phenotype; 2% express CD4 and 10% CD8 (Borst et al., 1988; Groh et al., 1989). In intestinal epithelium, the majority express CD8 (Deusch et al., 1991). The independence of CD4 and CD8 molecules in antigen/MHC interactions may imply that TCR $\gamma\delta$ interacts with conventional MHC molecules with high affinity, without the need for accessory molecules, or uses accessory molecules other than CD4 or CD8. Alternatively, $\gamma\delta$ T cells may interact with antigen presenting molecules other than MHC class I or class II.

Potential candidates for these other presenting molecules are the MHC class I related proteins Qa, TL and CD1 (Strominger, 1989). Qa and TL have only been described in the mouse system. CD1 is a family of molecules, consisting of CD1a, -b, -c, -d, and -e in humans, of which CD1e has not yet been defined at the protein level. These molecules display differential tissue distributions. CD1a is well known for its expression on epidermal Langerhans cells. CD1d appears to be present on intestinal epithelial cells (Balk et al., 1991). In the mouse, two CD1 genes have been defined, one of which is also expressed on intestinal epithelial cells (Bleieher et al., 1990). Human $\gamma\delta$ T cells reactive with CD1 molecules have been described (Porcelli et al., 1991), but $\alpha\beta$ T cells can also display such reactivity (Porcelli et al., 1991; Balk et al., 1991).

Thus, although it is an attractive possibility, it remains to be proven to what extent CD1 molecules are preferred restriction elements for $\gamma\delta$ T cells. Evidence for antigen presentation by CD1b has been reported by Porcelli et al. (1992). Qa, TL and CD1 all associate with $\beta2$ microglobulin, like MHC class I. However, $\beta2$-microglobulin-negative transgenic mice harbor very small numbers of CD8$^+$ $\alpha\beta$ T cells, but have normal numbers of circulating $\gamma\delta$ T cells (Zijlstra et al., 1990). This may imply that MHC class I or MHC class I-like molecules are not the dominant presenting elements for $\gamma\delta$ T cells, or that, unlike $\alpha\beta$ T cells, $\gamma\delta$ T cells are not subject to positive selection. Recently, a new molecule has been identified, T-cell target 1 (TCT.1), which is encoded by an Ig superfamily gene in the CD1 region of human chromosome 1 (Del Porto et al., 1991). Antibodies to TCT.1 can selectively inhibit MHC non-restricted cytotoxicity of certain $\gamma\delta$ T cells.

When we look for molecularly defined antigens that are recognized by $\gamma\delta$ T cells, few examples can be found. In one case, $\gamma\delta$ T cells have been isolated from a hyperimmunized individual that specifically responded to purified tetanus toxoid (Kozbor et al., 1989). Autologous HLA-DR4$^+$ antigen-presenting cells were necessary to induce this response. In another case, murine TCR $\gamma\delta^+$ hybridomas recognized mycobacterial heat shock protein (HSP) 65. The specificity was mapped to a peptide fragment of HSP 65, but the antigen-presenting molecule could not be determined (Born et al., 1990).

The Vγ9/Vδ2$^+$ $\gamma\delta$ T cell subset in human peripheral blood is interesting in that it strongly proliferates in response to crude bacterial preparations. This response was originally found with <u>Mycobacterium tuberculosis</u>, but could be extended to a great variety of bacteria (Abo et al., 1990). It is not directed to HSP 65, which elicits a strong $\alpha\beta$ T cell response (Kabelitz et al., 1990). It is tempting to speculate that the in vivo expansion of the peripheral Vγ9/Vδ2$^+$ T cells is induced by a similar bacterial challenge. As yet, it has not been proven that antigen recognition by the Vγ9/Vδ2 receptor triggers the proliferation. Indeed, TCR negative natural killer cells also respond to this type of bacterial stimulation (Abo et al., 1990). If specific recognition by TCR $\gamma\delta$ takes place, the antigen must behave like a superantigen, since the responding population has extensive junctional diversity. The nature of the putative (super)antigen remains unknown. Human $\gamma\delta$ T cells can react to a well defined superantigen, staphylococcal enterotoxin A (Rust et al., 1990). Here, the cells responded not by proliferation, but with cytotoxicity. These responses are dependent on the expression of MHC class II molecules on target cells and on the presence of the Vγ9 region in the $\gamma\delta$ TCR.

$\gamma\delta$ T CELL FUNCTION IN VIVO

Expansion of $\gamma\delta$ T cells in response to antigenic stimulation in vivo has been observed, but in none of these cases, in humans or in other species, has binding of a specific antigen to TCR $\gamma\delta$ been implicated in the initiation of such $\gamma\delta$ T cell proliferation.

One of the first examples of $\gamma\delta$ T cell expansion in vivo came from the analysis of reversal reactions in the skin of leprosy patients (Modlin et al., 1989). In vitro, $\gamma\delta$ T cells derived from these skin biopsies proliferated in response to mycobacterial antigens, but did not respond to recombinant mycobacterial HSP 65 or to tetanus toxoid. Supernatant fluids of these cultures contained lymphokines that caused macrophage adhesion, aggregation and proliferation, suggesting that the activated $\gamma\delta$ T cells stimulated the granuloma formation observed in vivo.

$\gamma\delta$ T cell clones derived from the synovial fluid of a rheumatoid arthritis patient responded to Mycobacterium tuberculosis preparations without the need for presentation by syngeneic MHC molecules (Holoshitz et al., 1989). The antigen recognized by these clones remains to be molecularly defined.

Intraperitoneal immunization of rats with syngeneic W439 lymphoma cells induced expansion of $\gamma\delta$ T cells that displayed specific anti-tumor cytotoxicity (Ericsson et al., 1991). Specificity was lost upon $\gamma\delta$ T cell cloning, however. We had a similar experience in our laboratory, when attempts were made to generate antigen specific $\gamma\delta$ T cells to adenovirus-transformed mouse cells. Immunization of C57/BL6 mice with syngeneic mouse embryo cells, expressing the adenovirus nucleoprotein, E1A, induces a strong $\alpha\beta$ T cell response that is directed at a well defined nucleoprotein peptide, presented in the context of H2-D^b. $\gamma\delta$ T cells, purified to homogeneity from such immunized mice, showed an adenovirus-specific response in bulk culture that was lost upon cloning.

In another mouse model, using influenza virus, $\gamma\delta$ T cells expanded late in the course of the inflammatory process in the lung, after an $\alpha\beta$ T cell response had taken place and the infectious virus had been eliminated (Eichelberger et al., 1991). Virus-specificity of $\gamma\delta$ T cells could not be demonstrated.

The above are just some examples from the literature that illustrate how difficult it is to determine what contribution $\gamma\delta$ T cells make to the immune system. Perhaps the $\gamma\delta$ T cells that have been found to expand in vivo upon immunization with bacteria, viruses or tumor cells do not contribute to an antigen-specific cellular response, but are recruited by the TCR $\alpha\beta^+$ effector cells or other cells which appear at the site of action early after infection. The obvious question remains, why do $\gamma\delta$ T cells bear such an intricate antigen receptor? Experiments in genetically manipulated mice, in which differentiation of either $\gamma\delta$ T cells or $\alpha\beta$ T cells has been completely blocked by elimination of TCR genes from the germline, are expected to bring a breakthrough in this field.

REFERENCES

Abo T, S Sugawara, S Seki, M Fujii, H Rikiishi, K Takeda and K Kumagai, 1990. Induction of human TCR$\gamma\delta$+ and TCR$\gamma\delta$- CD2+CD3- double negative lymphocytes by bacterial stimulation. **Int. Immunol.**, 2:775.

Allison JP and WL Havran, 1990. The immunobiology of T cells with invariant $\gamma\delta$ antigen receptors. **Ann. Rev. Immunol.**, 9:679.

Alt FW and D Baltimore, 1982. Joining of immunoglobulin heavy chain gene segments: Implications from a chromosome with evidence of three D-JH fusions. **Proc. Natl. Acad. Sci.** U.S.A., 79:4118.

Alzari PM, M-B Lascombe and RJ Poljak, 1988. Three-dimensional structure of antibodies. **Ann. Rev. Immunol.**, 6:555.

Asarnow D, T Goodman, L Lefrancois and JP Allison, 1989. Distinct antigen receptor repertories of two classes of murine epithelium associated T cells. **Nature**, 341:60.

Balk S, EC Ebert, RL Blumenthal, FV McDermott, KW Wucherpfennig, SB Landau and RS Blumberg, 1991. Oligoclonal expansion and CD1 recognition by human intestinal intraepithelial lymphocytes. **Science**, 253:1411.

Bleicher PA, SP Balk, SJ Hagen, RS Blumberg, TJ Flotte and C Terhorst, 1990. Expression of murine CD1 on gastrointestinal epithelium. **Science,** 250:679.

Boehm T, R Baer, I Lavenir, A Forster, JJ Waters, E Nacheva and TH Rabbitts, 1988. The mechanism of chromosomal translocation t (11; 14) involving the T cell receptor Cδ locus on human chromosome 14q11 and a transcribed region of chromosome 11p15. **EMBO. J.,** 7:385.

Bonneville M, S Itohara, EG Krecko, P Mombaerts, I Ishida, M Katsuki, A Berns, A G Farr, CA Janeway and S Tonegawa, 1990. Transgenic mice demonstrate that epithelial homing of $\gamma\delta$ T cells is determined by cell lineages independent of T cell receptor specificity. **J. Exp. Med.,** 171:1015.

Born W, L Hall, A Dallas, J Boymel, T Shinnick, D Young, P Brennan and R O'Brien, 1990. Recognition of a peptide antigen by heat shock reactive $\gamma\delta$ T lymphocytes. **Science,** 249:67.

Borst J, RJ van de Griend, JW van Oostveen, S-L Ang, CJM Melief, JG Seidman and RLH Bolhuis, 1987. A T cell receptor γ/CD3 complex found on cloned functional lymphocytes. **Nature,** 325:683.

Borst J, JJM van Dongen, RLH Bolhuis, PJ Peters, DA Hafler, E de Vries and RJ van de Griend, 1988. Distinct molecular forms of human T cell receptor γ/δ detected on viable T cells by a monoclonal antibody. **J. Exp. Med.**, 167:1625.

Borst J, A Wicherink, JJM van Dongen, E de Vries, W M ComansBitter, F Wassenaar and P van den Elsen, 1989. Non-random expression of T cell receptor γ and δ variable gene segments in functional T lymphocyte clones from human peripheral blood. **Eur. J. Immunol.**, 19:1559.

Borst J and JJM van Dongen, 1990. Repertoire selection of human $\gamma\delta$ T cells. **Res. Immunol.**, 141:663.

Bos JD, MBM Teunissen, I Cairo, SR Krieg, ML Kapsenberg, PK Das and J Borst, 1990. T-cell receptor $\gamma\delta$ bearing cells in normal human skin. **J. Invest. Dermatol.**, 94:37.

Caccia N, GAP Bruns, IR Kirsch, GF Hollis, V Bertness and TW Mak, 1985. T cell receptor α chain genes are located on chromosome 14 at 14q11-14q12 in humans. **J. Exp. Med.**, 161:1255.

Campana D, G Janossy, E Coustan-Smith, PL Amlot, W-T Tian, S Ip and L Wong, 1989. The expression of T cell receptor-associated proteins during T cell ontogeny in man. **J. Immunol.**, 142:57.

Carding SR, S Kyes, EJ Jenkinson, R Kingston, K Bottomly, JT Owen and AC Hayday, 1990. Developmentally regulated fetal thymic and extrathymic T-cell receptor $\gamma\delta$ gene expression. **Genes & Development**, 4:1304.

Chien Y, M Iwashima, KB Kaplan, JF Elliott and MM Davis, 1987. A new T-cell receptor gene located within the alpha locus and expressed early in T-cell differentiation. **Nature**, 312:455.

Chotia C, DR Boswell and AM Lesk, 1988. The outline structure of the T-cell $\alpha\beta$ receptor. **EMBO J.**, 7:3745.

Davis MM and PJ Bjorkman, 1988. T cell antigen receptor genes and T cell recognition. **Nature**, 334:395.

De Geus B, M van den Enden, C Coolen, L Nagelkerken, P van der Heyden and J Rozing, 1990. Phenotype of intraepithelial lymphocytes in euthymic and athymic mice: Implications for differentiation of cells bearing a CD3-associated $\gamma\delta$ T cell receptor. **Eur. J. Immunol.**, 20:291.

Dellabona P, J Peccoud, J Kappler, P Marrack, C Benoist and D Mathis, 1990. Superantigens interact with MHC class II molecules outside of the antigen groove. **Cell**, 62: 1115.

Del Porto P, F Mami-Chouaib, J-M Bruneau, S Jitsukawa, J Dumas, M Harnois and T Hercend, 1991. TCT.1, a target molecule for $\gamma\delta$ T cells, is encoded by an immunoglobulin superfamily gene (Blast-1) located in the CD1 region of human chromosome 1. **J. Exp. Med.**, 173:1339.

Deusch K, F Luling, K Reich, M Classen, H Wagner and K Pfeffer, 1991. A major fraction of human intraepithelial lymphocytes simultaneously expresses the γ/δ T cell receptor, the CD8 accessory molecule and preferentially uses the Vδ1 gene segment. **Eur. J. Immunol.**, 21: 1053.

De Villartay J-P and DI Cohen, 1990. Gene regulation within the TCR α/β locus by specific deletion of the δ cluster. **Res. Immunol.**, 141:618.

Echelberger M, W Allan, SR Carding, K Bottomly and PC Doherty, 1991. Activation status of the CD4-CD8- $\gamma\delta$ T cells recovered from mice with influenza pneumonia. **J. Immunol.**, 147:2069.

Elliott JF, EP Rock, PA Patton, MM Davis and Y Chien, 1988. The adult T cell receptor δ-chain is diverse and distinct from that of fetal thymocytes. **Nature**, 331:627.

Ericsson PO, J Hansson, B Widegren, M Dohlsten, H-O Sjogren and G Hedlund, 1991. In vivo induction of $\gamma\delta$ T cells with highly potent and selective anti-tumor cytotoxicity. **Eur. J. Immunol.**, 21:2797.

Goodman T and L Lefrancois, 1988. Expression of γ-δ T-cell receptor on intestinal CD8+ intraepithelial lymphocytes. **Nature**, 333:855.

Groh V, S Porcelli, M Fabbi, LL Lanier, LJ Picker, T Anderson, RA Warnke, AK Bhan, JL Strominger and MB Brenner, 1989. Human lymphocytes bearing T cell receptor $\gamma\delta$ are phenotypically diverse and evenly distributed throughout the lymphoid system. **J. Exp. Med.**, 169: 1277.

Halstensen TS, H Scott and P Brandtzaeg, 1989. Intraepithelial T cells of the TCR γ/δ+CD8- and Vδ1/Jδ1+ phenotypes are increased in coeliac disease. **Scand. J. Immunol.**, 30:665.

Hata S, M Clabby, P Devlin, H Spits, JE de Vries and MS Krangel, 1989. Diversity and organization of human T cell receptor variable gene segments. **J. Exp. Med.**, 169:41.

Havran W L and J P Allison, 1988. Developmentally ordered appearance of thymocytes expressing different T cell antigen receptors. **Nature**, 335:443.

Holoshitz J, F Koning, J E Coligan, J De Bruyn and S Strober, 1989. Isolation of CD4-CD8- mycobacteria-reactive T lymphocyte clones from rheumatoid arthritis synovial fluid. **Nature**, 339:226.

Huck S, P Dariavach and M-P Lefranc, 1988. Variable region genes in the human T-cell rearranging gamma (TRG) locus: V-J junction and homology with the mouse genes. **EMBO J.**, 7:719.

Ito K, M Bonneville, Y Takagaki, N Nakanishi, O Kanagawa, EG Krecko and S Tonegawa, 1989. Different $\gamma\delta$ T-cell receptors are expressed on thymocytes at different stages of development. **Proc. Natl. Acad. Sci. U.S.A.**, 86:631.

Itohara S, AG Farr, JJ Lafaille, M Bonneville, Y Takagaki, W Haas and S Tonegawa, 1990. Homing of a $\gamma\delta$ thymocyte subset with homogenous T cell receptors to mucosal epithelia. **Nature**, 343:754.

Janeway CA, B Jones and A Hayday, 1988. Specificity and function of T cells bearing $\gamma\delta$ receptors. **Immunol. Today**, 9:73.

Kabelitz D, A Bender, S Schondelmaier, B Schoel and SHE Kaufmann, 1990. A large fraction of human peripheral blood γ/δ+ T cells is activated by Mycobacterium tuberculosis but not by its 65-kD heat shock protein. **J. Exp. Med.**, 171:667.

Kozbor D, G Trinchieri, DS Monos, M Isobe, G Russo, JA Haney, C Zmijewski and CM

Croce, 1989. Human TCR-γ+/δ+, CD8+ T lymphocytes recognize tetanus toxoid in an MHC-restricted fashion. **J. Exp. Med.**, 169:1847.

Krangel MS, H Yssel, C Brocklehurst and H Spits, 1990. A distinct wave of human T cell receptor γ/δ lymphocytes in the early fetal thymus: Evidence for controlled gene rearrangement and cytokine production. **J. Exp. Med.**, 172:847.

Lefrancois L, R LeCorre, J Mayo, JA Bluestone and T Goodman, 1990. Extrathymic selection of TCR γδ+ T cells by class II major histocompatibility complex molecules. **Cell**, 63:333.

Lew AM, DM Pardoll, WL Maloy, BJ Fowlkes, A Kruisbeek, S-F Cheng, RN Germain, JA Bluestone, RH Schwartz and JE Coligan, 1986. Characterization of T cell receptor gamma chain expression in a subset of murine thymocytes. **Science**, 234:1401.

Marrack P and J Kappler, 1990. The staphylococcal enterotoxins and their relatives. **Science**, 248:705.

Modlin RL, C Pirmez, FM Hofman, V Torigian, K Kyemura, TH Rea, BR Bloom and MB Brenner, 1989. Lymphocytes bearing antigen specific γδ T cell receptors accumulate in human infectious disease lesions. **Nature**, 339:544.

Moingeon P, S Jitsukawa, F Faure, F Troalen, F Triebel, M Graziani, F Forrestier, D Bellet, C Bohuon and T Hercend, 1987. A γ chain complex forms a functional receptor on cloned human lymphocytes with natural killer-like activity. **Nature**, 325:723.

Murre C, RA Waldmann, CC Morton, KF Bongiovanni, TA Waldmann, TB Shows and JG Seidman, 1985. Human γ-chain genes are rearranged in leukaemic T cells and map to the short arm of chromosome 7. **Nature**, 316:549.

Pardoll DM, BJ Fowlkes, JA Bluestone, AM Kruisbeek, WL Maloy, JE Coligan and RH Schwartz, 1987. Differential expression of two distinct T-cell receptors during thymocyte development. **Nature**, 326:79.

Parker CM, V Groh, H Band, SA Porcelli, C Morita, M Fabbi, D Glass, JL Strominger and M B Brenner, 1990. Evidence for extrathymic changes in the T-cell receptor γ/δ repertoire. **J. Exp. Med.**, 171:1597.

Patel SS, MC Wacholtz, AD Duby, DL Thiele and PE Lipsky, 1989. Analysis of the functional capabilities of CD3+CD4-CD8- and CD3+CD4+CD8+ human T cell clones. **J. Immunol.**, 143:1108.

Porcelli S, MB Brenner and H Band, 1991. Biology of the human T-cell receptor. **Immunol. Rev.**, 120:137.

Porcelli S, CT Morita and MB Brenner, 1992. CD1b restricts the response of human CD4-8- T lymphocytes to a microbial antigen. **Nature**, 360:593.

Rabbitts TH, MP Lefranc, MA Stinson, JE Sims, J Schroder, M Steinmetz, NL Spurr, E Solomon and PN Goodfellow, 1985. The chromosomal location of T cell receptor genes and a T cell rearranging gene: Possible correlation with specific translocations in human T cell leukaemia. **EMBO J.**, 4:1461.

Raulet DH, 1989a. The structure, function and molecular genetics of the γδ T cell receptor. **Ann. Rev. Immunol.**, 7:175.

Raulet DH, 1989b. Antigens for γ/δ T cells. **Nature**, 339:342.

Rust CJJ, F Verreck, H Vietor and F Koning, 1990. Specific recognition of staphylococcal enterotoxin A by human T cells bearing receptors with the Vγ9 region. **Nature**, 346:572.

Saito H, DM Kranz, Y Takagaki, AC Hayday, HN Eisen and S Tonegawa, 1984. Complete primary structure of a heterodimer T-cell receptor deduced from cDNA sequences. **Nature**, 309:757.

Satyanarayana K, S Hata, P Devlin, MG Roncarolo, JE de Vries, H Spits, JL Strominger and MS Krangel, 1988. Genomic organization of the human T cell antigen-receptor α/δ locus. **Proc. Natl. Acad. Sci. U.S.A.**, 85:8170.

Spits H, X Paliard, VH Engelhard and JE de Vries, 1990. Cytotoxic activity and lymphokine production of T cell receptor TCR-αβ+ and TCR-γδ+ cytotoxic T lymphocyte (CTL) clones recognizing HLA-A2 and HLA-A2 mutants. Recognition of TCR-γδ+ CTL clones is affected by mutations at positions 152 and 156. **J. Immunol.**, 144:4156.

Stingl G, F Koning, H Yamada, WM Yokoyama, E Tschacler, JA Bluestone, G Steiner, LE Samelson, AM Lew, JE Coligan and E Scevach, 1987. Thy-1+ dendritic epidermal cells express T3 antigen and the T-cell receptor γ chain. **Proc. Natl. Acad. Sci. U.S.A.**, 84:4586.

Strominger JL, 1989. The γδ T cell receptor and class Ib MHC-related proteins: Enigmatic molecules of immune recognition. **Cell**, 57:895.

Takihara Y, J Reimann, E Michalopoulos, E Ciccone, L Moretta and TW Mak, 1989. Diversity and structure of human T cell receptor δ chain genes in peripheral blood γ/δ bearing T lymphocytes. **J. Exp. Med.**, 169:393.

Tonegawa S, 1983. Somatic generation of antibody diversity. **Nature**, 302:575.

Toyonaga B and TW Mak. Genes of the T-cell antigen receptor in normal and malignant T cells, 1987. **Ann. Rev. Immunol.**, 5:585.

Triebel F, F Faure, M Graziani, S Jitsukawa, M-P Lefranc and T Hercend, 1988a. A unique V-J-C rearranged gene encodes a y protein expressed on the majority of CD3 + T cell receptor α/β circulating lymphocytes. **J. Exp. Med.**, 167:694.

Triebel F, F Faure, F Mami-Chouaib, S Jitsukawa, A Griscelli, C Genevee, S Roman-Roman and T Hercend, 1988b. A novel human Vδ gene expressed predominantly in the TiγA fraction of γ/δ peripheral lymphocytes. **Eur. J. Immunol.**, 18:2021.

Van de Griend, RJ, WJM Tax, BA van Krimpen, RJ Vreugdenhil, CPM Ronteltap and RLH Bolhuis, 1987. Lysis of tumor cells by CD3+4-8-16+ T cell receptor αβ- clones regulated via CD3 and CD16 activation sites, recombinant interleukin 2 and interferon β. **J. Immunol.**, 138:1627.

Vroom T M, G Scholte, F Ossendorp and J Borst, 1991. Tissue distribution of human γδ T cells: No evidence for a general epithelial tropism. **J. Clin. Pathol.**, 44:1012.

Wilson RK, E Lai, P Concannon, RK Barth and LE Hood, 1988. Structure, organization and polymorphism of murine and human T-cell receptor α and β gene families. **Immunol. Rev.**, 101:149.

Zijlstra M, M Bix, ME Simister, JM Loring, DH Raulet and R Jaenisch, 1990. β2 microglobulin deficient mice lack CD4+8+ cytolytic T cells. **Nature**, 344:742.

ONTOGENY, FEATURES AND FUNCTIONS OF EPIDERMAL T LYMPHOCYTES

Georg Stingl
Elisabeth Payer
Adelheid Elbe

Division of Immunology, Allergy and Infections Diseases
Department of Dermatology
University of Vienna Medical School
Vienna International Research Cooperation Center (VIRCC)
Vienna, Austria

Correspondence to: Dr. G. Stingl, Department of Dermatology I,
University Hospital, Brunner Strasse 59,
A-1235 Vienna, Austria

INTRODUCTION

In the past decade, it has become increasingly clear that the mammalian skin harbors an indigenous population of lymphocytes, almost all of which belong to the T cell system (Stingl et al., 1989). In man, the majority of cutaneous T lymphocytes are found in the dermis, where they are preferentially clustered around postcapillary venules and around the appendages (Bos et al., 1987). Intraepidermal T cells account for only $\leq$ 10% of all T cells within human skin. In mice, the epidermis contains a regular network of T cells (Tschachler et al., 1983). Because of their characteristic morphology, they are referred to as Thy-1[+] dendritic epidermal cells (Thy-1[+] DEC) or, more recently, as dendritic epidermal T cells (DETC; Stingl et al., 1989).

MURINE DENDRITIC EPIDERMAL T CELLS

Discovery and phenotype

In 1983, we and others simultaneously encountered a previously unrecognized Thy-1[+],

Basic Mechanisms of Physiologic and Aberrant Lymphoproliferation in the Skin
Edited by W.C. Lambert *et al.*, Plenum Press, New York, 1994

17

Ia⁻, dendritic cell population within the murine epidermis (Tschachler et al., 1983; Bergstresser et al., 1983). Interest in these cells increased considerably when it was found that Thy-1⁺ dendritic cells originate from bone marrow-derived precursor cells, as evidenced by the demonstration of CLA/T200 antigens on these cells, and by the use of Thy-1-disparate bone marrow chimeras (Bergstresser et al., 1985; Breathnach and Katz, 1984; Romani et al., 1985b; Tschachler et al., 1983). Due to the expression of asialo GM1 (Romani et al., 1985 a;b) and the absence of CD5, CD4 and CD8 antigens (Steiner et al., 1988; Tschachler et al., 1983), it was originally believed that these cells belong to the natural killer (NK)-cell system. The demonstration of T cell receptor (TCR) gene transcripts within these cells, and, subsequently, the precipitation of the CD3/TCR complex from the surface of Thy-1⁺ DEC and Thy-1⁺ DEC-derived cell lines, however, clearly demonstrated their T cell nature (Steiner et al., 1988; Stingl et al., 1987a;b). While most peripheral T cells express a CD3 complex associated with a TCR α/β heterodimer, almost all DETC express a TCR γ/δ (Havran et al., 1989; Steiner et al., 1988). Most interestingly, this TCR on DETC is nearly exclusively encoded for by Vγ3/Vδ1 genes (Asarnow et al., 1988; 1989), a TCR type which is not detectable in other lymphoid organs of adult mice (Havran et al., 1989).

Ontogeny

Several observations have indicated that the perinatal period is of critical importance for both maturation and expansion of the DETC population. DETC first appear during the last days of gestation and reach their mature phenotype, and their full numerical density, within the first few weeks of the postnatal period (Elbe et al., 1989; Romani et al., 1986). Moreover, depletion of the DETC population of adult animals by physicochemical agents is not followed by its reappearance (Aberer et al., 1986).

Furthermore, we found that reconstitution of adult γ-irradiated thymus-containing AKR/0La or B6PL-Thy-1a mice (both of which express the Thy-1.1 allele), with T-cell depleted C3H/He/Han or C57BL/6 bone marrow (BM) cells (both of which express the Thy-1.2 allele) resulted in the appearance of round Thy-1.2⁺ cells in the epidermis which remained CD3⁻ over the course of several months. In contrast, lymph nodes and spleens of chimeric mice were colonized by large numbers of Thy-1.2⁺/CD3⁺ lymphocytes (Honjo et al., 1990). The possibility that the phenomenon observed was due to an adverse effect of γ-irradiation on the capacity of the epidermal symbiants to induce CD3/TCR expression in DETC-precursors was ruled out in experiments in which newborn skin was transplanted onto chimeric animals. Again, Thy-1.2⁺ cells immigrating into the transplant did not acquire CD3 antigens (E. Payer, unpublished observation).

While all of these findings support the contention that DETC maturation happens early in life, rather than in the adult animal, the important question remains whether this event occurs in a thymus-dependent or in a thymus-independent fashion. At first glance, the finding of predominantly round Thy-1$^+$/CD3$^+$ cells, but not of dendritic Thy-1$^+$/CD3$^+$ cells, in the epidermis of athymic mice (Nixon-Fulton et al., 1988) could be taken as a strong argument for the thymus-dependence of DETC. On the other hand, the skin of athymic mice (nu/nu) is grossly abnormal and may not be able to provide the appropriate microenvironment for DETC maturation.

The hypothesis that DETC originate from fetal thymocytes was originally put forward by Havran and Allison (1988) when they found that a monoclonal antibody (mAb) against the TCR Vγ3 determinant reacts with both the first CD3-bearing fetal thymocytes (day 14 - day 18 of gestation) and with the DETC population of adult animals. The similarity between these two cell systems was further supported by the observation that -- with a few notable exceptions (McConnell et al., 1989) -- the entire TCR configuration of these early fetal thymocytes is essentially indistinguishable from that expressed by freshly isolated DETC and DETC-derived clones/hybridomas, respectively (Asarnow et al., 1988; 1989; Lafaille et al., 1989). To test the assumption that these TCR Vγ3$^+$ fetal thymocytes are the actual DETC precursors, we injected day 16 and day 19 fetal, as well as adult, thymocytes into either syngeneic (C3H, BALB/c) or Thy-1-disparate (B6PL-Thy-1a in C57BL/6 nu/nu) athymic nude mice, the epidermis of which is reportedly devoid of CD3/TCR-bearing lymphocytes (Nixon-Fulton et al., 1988). Results obtained showed that the injection of day 16 fetal thymocytes resulted regularly (as did the injection of day 19 fetal thymocytes in most instances) in the appearance of distinct clusters of donor-type CD3$^+$/TCR Vγ3$^+$ dendritic epidermal cells. When examined from two to 12 weeks after cell transfer, the cell density within a given cluster showed a continuous and dramatic increase. This suggests that DETC derived from day 16 fetal thymocytes undergo vigorous proliferation within the epidermis. By contrast, the injection of adult thymocytes was not followed by the emergence of the DETC population (Payer et al., 1991). The presence of CD3$^+$/TCR Vγ3$^+$ cells in day 16 and day 19 fetal, but not in adult, thymocyte populations, together with the failure to detect DETC after transfer of Thy1$^+$/CD3$^-$ fetal thymocytes, strongly suggests that, under the experimental conditions chosen, CD3$^+$/TCR Vγ3$^+$ thymocytes are the DETC precursors. Similar results were obtained by Havran and Allison (1990), who found that implantation of day 14 fetal thymic lobes, but not of day 2 postpartum thymic lobes, from euthymic mice into either syngeneic athymic nude mice or Thy-1-disparate euthymic newborn mice results in the appearance of TCR Vγ3$^+$ DETC. These two reports lend strong support to the concept that CD3$^+$/TCR Vγ3$^+$ fetal thymocytes are the actual precursors of DETC.

The above findings do not exclude the possibility that the microenvironment of the fetal skin/epidermis can provide T cell-educating stimuli similar to those of the fetal thymic epithelium. Following this reasoning, we have hypothesized that the CD45$^+$/Thy-1$^+$/CD3$^-$ cells present within day 17 fetal epidermis (Elbe et al., 1989) could represent the target for these putative stimuli. As a consequence, these cells would mature into DETC and, thus, should not be detectable in adult murine epidermis. In fact, this appears to be the case, as we have failed to detect appreciable numbers of such Thy-1$^+$/CD3$^-$ epidermal lymphocytes in the adult animal (A. Elbe and E. Payer, unpublished observations). To see whether the CD45$^+$/Thy-1$^+$/CD3$^-$

fetal skin cells can indeed qualify as DETC precursors, we transplanted day 16 fetal skin from C57BL/6 mice (expressing Thy-1.2) onto adult B6PL-Thy-1a mice (expressing Thy-1.1). While the C57BL/6 skin contained only very few round $CD45^+$/Thy-1.2^+ cells and no $CD3^+$ cells at the time point of grafting, the number of Thy-1^+ cells increased steadily during the following weeks. An ever increasing number of the Thy-1.2^+ cells gained a dendritic shape and CD3/TCR Vγ expression, and 10 weeks after grafting > 95% of all $CD45^+$/Thy-1.2^+ cells qualified as DETC (Elbe et al., 1992). Being aware of the possibility that the day 16 fetal skin may contain a few TCR V$\gamma3^+$ cells that might have escaped detection by in situ immunofluorescence analysis, we (i) performed FACS analysis of day 16 fetal skin single cell suspensions and (ii) tried to establish T cell lines from the fetal skin. However, we never detected TCR V$\gamma3^+$ cells, even when 50,000 $CD45^+$ cells were recorded, and all of the generated T cell lineage commited (truncated TCR messages) cell lines were $CD3^-$ (Elbe et al., 1992). Although these data strongly argue against the presence of TCR V$\gamma3^+$ cells in the day 16 fetal skin, the PCR amplification of TCR V$\gamma3$/C$\gamma1$ cDNA from some, but not all, day 16 fetal skin RNA preparations could be taken as an argument for the presence of minute numbers of "contaminating" fetal thymocytes. Since (i) we have never observed cluster formation of TCR V$\gamma3^+$ cells cells in the grafts (one would expect to see growing clusters of TCR V$\gamma3^+$ cells if a minute number of "contaminating" TCR V$\gamma3^+$ cells were to expand), and (ii) the number of "contaminating" TCR V$\gamma3^+$ cells could by no means suffice to explain the kinetics of the DETC density encountered in the fetal skin grafts, our data are most compatible with the view that fetal skin harbors CD3/TCR V$\gamma3^-$ precursors and that the fetal epidermis can provide stiumli promoting the expression of CD3/TCR genes in these cells.

With respect to the apparently conflicting results showing (i) that fetal thymocytes are DETC precursors, and (ii) that Thy1^+ $CD3^-$ precursor cells can mature intraepidermally into DETC, one should keep in mind that both results are obtained in experimental systems. It remains to be shown if one or both of these pathways to generate DETC are operative in the physiologic development of the animals.

As already mentioned, Nixon-Fulton et al. (1988) reported that the epidermis of athymic nude mice is devoid of TCR-bearing lymphocytes. We have recently reinvestigated this topic using another mouse strain (C57BL/6 nu/nu vs. BALB/c nu/nu). We confirmed that the overall majority of Thy-1^+ cells in the epidermis of nude mice are $CD3^-$. Upon careful examination, however, we detected a small population of Thy-1^+/$CD3^+$ cells, comprising 0.06% of Thy-1^+ cells, in 6 week old C57BL/6 nu/nu mice. With advancing age of these animals, the absolute numbers of $CD3^+$ cells, as well as their percentage among Thy-1^+ cells, continuously increased. In 12 month old nude animals, up to 3% of all Thy-1^+ cells reacted with the anti-CD3 mAb. Phenotypic examination of $CD3^+$ epidermal cells of athymic mice, as well as of lines derived from these cells, indicated that the nude mouse epidermal T cells are similar to DETC in that they are Thy-1^+, $CD45^+$, asialo $GM1^+$, $CD5^-$, $CD4^-$ and predominantly $CD8^-$. We further observed that 85% of the nude mouse epidermal T cells bear TCR γ/δ receptors while the remaining 15% express TCR α/β. The majority of TCR γ/δ^+ cells were found to express V$\gamma2$

and Vδ4 specificities, whereas Vγ3$^+$ cells were barely detectable. RNA from the epidermis of 10 month old C57BL/6 nu/nu mice further revealed the presence of very abundant messages for Cα, Cδ, Vγ2, Vγ4, Vγ5 and Cγ1, while message for Vγ3 was hardly detectable and messages for Vγ1 (Vγ1.1 and Vγ1.2) and Cγ4 were absent (Payer et al., 1992). It is so far not clear whether these cells mature within the epidermis of athymic mice, or whether TCR-bearing lymphocytes present in other organs migrate to the epidermis. It is clear, however, that they mature without the influence of a thymus and, most probably, also without the influence of a fetal skin milieu as most of the cells are only detected in older mice.

Summarizing our current knowledge about the ontogeny of murine epidermal T cells, one has to postulate the existence of two different types of cells. One population is found, in very limited numbers, in athymic nude mice as well as euthymic mice (Itohara et al., 1990; Ota et al., 1992; R. Strohal, unpublished observation), is composed of cells with different TCR specificities and, at least in the nude mouse, matures thymus-independently. The other population, i.e., TCR Vγ3/Vδ1$^+$ DETC, is only found in euthymic mice and requires the fetal thymic or skin microenvironment for maturation.

Function

The functional role of DETC is presently unknown. Some evidence exists that TCR γ/δ are putative receptors for first line defense (e.g., enterotoxins, heat shock proteins); that they function as adhesion molecules (homing receptors); that they recognize MHC or MHC-like molecules (MHC class I and class II, Qa and TL in mouse, CD1 in humans); that they recognize antigen in conjunction with MHC or MHC-like structures; and that they behave as anti-self receptors, thereby regulating ontogeny and response of TCR α/β-bearing cells (Ferrick et al., 1989). In the case of DETC, Havran et al. (1991) have recently found that freshly isolated DETC, as well as long term DETC lines, can be stimulated to IL-2 production by irradiated keratinocytes but not by irradiated fibroblasts. Additional experiments by Lewis and Tigelaar (1991) showed that DETC lines respond to heat shocked, but not to untreated, keratinocytes. Taking the results of these two groups together, it appears that the TCR Vγ3 recognizes a protein which is solely expressed on stressed/damaged keratinocytes. It remains to be seen whether this phenomenon can be correlated with the in vivo observation that antigen presented in the context of DETC leads to the activation of suppressor cell circuits (Sullivan et al., 1986; Welsh and Kripke, 1990) and with the hypothesis that DETC can protect the murine epidermis from a T cell-mediated attack (Shiohara et al., 1990).

HUMAN EPIDERMAL T CELLS

In contrast to the detailed characterization of murine DETC, there exists only little information about lymphocytes of human skin. Similar to the mouse system, human skin lymphocytes belong almost exclusively to the T cell lineage. Approximately 80% of them are located around the postcapillary venules of the dermis, some are scattered throughout the dermis, and only 5-10% are found within the epidermis, mainly in the basal layer (Bos et al., 1987; Foster et al., 1990). T cells, as defined by their CD3/TCR expression, comprise 0.5 - 1 % of all human epidermal cells as determined by immunostaining of single epidermal cell smears. In sharp contrast to the mouse system, the vast majority of human epidermal T cells bear TCR α/β, rather than TCR γ/δ (Bos et al., 1990; Dupuy et al., 1990; Foster et al., 1990; Groh et al., 1989b). Further phenotypic analysis of human epidermal T cells revealed that most, if not all of them express CD2 and CD5 antigens (Foster et al., 1990), that CD8[+] cells outnumber CD4 bearing cells (Foster et al., 1990; Groh et al., 1989b) and that some CD3[+] cells, mostly of the TCR α/β type, are CD4/CD8-double negative (Groh et al., 1989a).

To date, little is known about the TCR diversity of human epidermal T cells. Using PCR technology, we have attempted to define their Vγ repertoire and found it to be rather diverse (R. Strohal, J. Friedl, L. Paucz, H. Pehamberger, and G. Stingl, manuscript in preparation). In order to understand the functional role of these polyclonal human epidermal T cells in the immune response, it was important to define their state of sensitization. In 1990, Foster et al. (1990) reported that the vast majority of intraepidermal T cells of adult humans react with the anti-CD45RO mAb UCHL-1, which implies that they are memory cells. Theoretically, they could have been generated by Langerhans cell-mediated antigenic stimulation of naïve T cells indigenously residing within the epidermis. Alternatively, they could have entered the skin/epidermis in an already sensitized state. The observation that approximately 20% of CD3[+] cells within the normal human epidermis of adults belong to the CD45RA[+] subset (Foster et al., 1990) is in keeping with the former concept and it may well be that this particular subset predominates in newborns and young children. The second theory gains support from studies using the mAb HECA-452. This antibody reacts with 10-20% of peripheral blood T cells and to 85% of lymphocytes in inflammatory skin lesions (Picker et al., 1990). HECA-452-reactive cells have the CD45RA[low], CD44[high] phenotype and, thus, qualify as memory cells. Cell attachment experiments have shown that memory cells, but not resting T cells, adhere to cells expressing endothelial lymphocyte adhesion molecule-1 (ELAM-1; Shimiza et al., 1991) and that the HECA-452[+] T cell subset is the predominant ELAM-1-binding population among circulating lymphocytes (Picker et al., 1991). Furthermore, it has been shown that ELAM-1 is preferentially expressed in endothelial cells of venules within inflammatory skin lesions and that these venules are associated with a predominantly HECA-452[+] T cell infiltrate (Picker et al., 1991). These data strongly suggest that the interaction between HECA-452-reactive molecules and ELAM-1 mediates the adhesion of memory T cells to the endothelial cells of the dermal microvasculature and, thus, promotes the migration of memory T cells into the dermis. The further migration of these cells into the epidermis involves various cytokines, chemotactic factors and adhesion molecules. Primarily on the basis of in vitro studies, one would assume that IL-1 (Sauder et al., 1985) and IL-8 (Larson et al., 1989) as well as the IFN-γ-induced peptide 10 (IP-10; Luster and Ravetch, 1987) are the most important keratinocyte-derived T cell chemotactic signals. In vitro, IFN-γ and TNF-α are capable of inducing IP-10 and IL-8 production by keratinocytes (Barker et al., 1990; Luster et al., 1987) and, thus, presumably play an important role in T cell recruitment to the epidermis. Additionally, these cytokines trigger the expression of the intercellular adhesion molecule-1 (ICAM-1) by keratinocytes (Barker et al., 1990; Dustin et al., 1988) rendering these cells capable of binding lymphocyte function--associated antigen 1 (LFA-1)-bearing T cells (Marlin and Springer, 1987). These data support the concept that the epidermotropic migration of dermal T cells is initiated by certain keratino-cyte-derived cytokines (the production of which can also be induced or enhanced by secretory products of activated T cells, themselves, e.g., IFN-γ) and that their attachment to, and, finally, their entrance into the epidermis can be mediated by the LFA-1/ICAM-1 interaction (Nickoloff et al., 1988; Shiohara and Nagashima, 1988; Shiohara et al., 1989).

In summary, we favor the concept that the vast majority of human epidermal T cells are not the descendants of naïve, resting T cells indigenously residing in the epidermis, but rather represent the progeny of activated T cells which had entered the skin/epidermis in the course of an inflammatory reaction.

Thus, the epidermis, or, for that matter, even the skin should not be regarded as a closed and self-sustaining immunological circuit, but rather as an initiation and target site for immune reactions that is functionally linked to peripheral lymphoid organs. This reemphasizes the validity of the SALT (skin-associated lymphoid tissues) concept originally introduced by Streilein (1983). According to this concept, exogenous (e.g. haptens, microorganisms) or endogenous (e.g., neoantigens) antigens are captured by epidermal Langerhans cells, which then migrate across the dermal-epidermal junction and travel through the lymph to the parafollicular cortex of draining nodes. At this site, they activate naïve, antigen specific T cells, and the effector lymphocytes thus generated disseminate through the blood to enter the skin at the site of a local (e.g., antigenic) stimulus. After encounter with the antigen, the sensitized effector T cells undergo clonal proliferation (expansion) and trigger a mediator cascade which results in the clinical expression of the immune response.

ACKNOWLEDGEMENTS

We thank Mrs. Sabine Seizov and Mrs. Renate Kosma for their help in the preparation of this manuscript.

REFERENCES

Aberer W, N Romani, A Elbe and G Stingl, 1986. Effects of physicochemical agents on murine epidermal Langerhans cells and Thy-1-positive dendritic epidermal cells. **J. Immunol.**, 136:1210-1216.

Asarnow DM, WA Kuziel, M Bonyhadi, RE Tigelaar, PW Tucker and JP Allison, 1988. Limited diversity of γδ antigen receptor genes of Thy-1+ dendritic epidermal cells. **Cell**, 55:837-847.

Asarnow DM, T Goodmann, L LeFrancois and JP Allison, 1989. Distinct antigen receptor repertoires of two classes of murine epithelium-associated T cells. **Nature**, 341:60-62.

Barker JNWN, V Sarma, RS Mitra, VM Dixit and J Nickoloff, 1990. Marked synergism between tumor necrosis factor-α and interferon-γ in regulation of keratinocyte-derived adhesion molecules and chemotactic factors. **J. Clin. Invest.**, 85:605-608.

Bergstresser PR, RE Tigelaar, JH Dees and JW Streilein, 1983. Thy-1 antigen-bearing dendritic cells populate murine epidermis. **J. Invest. Dermatol.**, 81:286-288.

Bergstresser PR, S Sullivan, JW Streilein and RE Tigelaar, 1985. Origin and function of Thy-1+ dendritic epidermal cells in mice. **J. Invest. Dermatol.**, 85: 85S-90S.

Bos JD, I Zonneveld, PK Das, SR Krieg, CM van der Loos and ML Kapsenberg, 1987. The skin immune system (SIS): Distribution and immunophenotype of lymphocyte subpopulations in normal human skin. **J. Invest. Dermatol.**, 88:569-573.

Bos JD, MBM Teunissen, I Cairo, SR Krieg, ML Kapsenberg, PK Das and J Borst, 1990. T-cell receptor γδ bearing cells in normal human skin. **J. Invest. Dermatol.**, 94:37-42.

Breathnach SM and SI Katz, 1984. Thy-1+ dendritic cells in murine epidermis are bone marrow-derived. **J. Invest. Dermatol.**, 83:74-77.

Dupuy P, M Heslan, S Fraitag, T Hercend, L Dubertret and M Bagot, 1990. T-cell receptor-γ/δ bearing lymphocytes in normal and inflammatory human skin. **J. Invest. Dermatol.**, 94:764-768.

Dustin ML, KH Singer, DT Tuck and TA Springer, 1988. Adhesion of T lymphoblasts to epidermal keratinocytes is regulated by interferon-γ and is mediated by intercellular adhesion molecule 1 (ICAM-1). **J. Exp. Med.**, 167:1323-1340.

Elbe A, E Tschachler, G Steiner, A Binder, K Wolff and G Stingl, 1989. Maturational steps of bone marrow-derived dendritic murine epidermal cells. Phenotypic and functional studies on Langerhans cells and Thy-1+ dendritic epidermal cells in the perinatal period. **J. Immunol.**, 143:2431-2438.

Elbe A, O Kilgus, R Strohal, E Payer, S Schreiber, R. Fritsche and G Stingl 1992. Fetal skin: A site of epidermal T cell development. **J. Immunol.**, 1491694-1701.

Ferrick DA, PS Ohashi, V Wallace, M Schilham and TW Mak, 1989. Thymic ontogeny and selection of B and T cells. **Immunol. Today**, 10:403-407.

Foster CA, H Yokozeki, K Rappersberg, F Koning, B Volc-Platzor, A Rieger, JE Coligan, K Wolff and G Stingl, 1990. Human epidermal T cells predominately belong to the lineage expressing α/β T cell receptor. **J. Exp. Med.**, 171:997-1013.

Groh V, M Fabbi, F Hochstenbach, RT Maziarz and JL Strominger, 1989a. Double-negative (CD4- CD8-) lymphocytes bearing T-cell receptor α and β chains in normal human skin. **Proc. Natl. Acad. Sci. USA**, 86:5059-5063.

Groh V, S Porcelli, M Fabbi, LL Lanier, LJ Picker, T Anderson, RA Warnke, AK Bhan, JL Strominger and MB Brenner, 1989b. Human lymphocytes bearing T cell receptor γ/δ are phenotypically diverse and evenly distributed throughout the lymphoid system. **J. Exp. Med.**, 169:1277-1294.

Havran WL and JP Allison, 1988. Developmentally ordered appearance of thymocytes expressing different T-cell antigen receptors. **Nature**, 335:443-445.

Havran WL and JP Allison, 1990. Origin of Thy-1+ dendritic epidermal cells of adult mice from fetal thymic precursors. **Nature**, 344:68-70.

Havran WL, YH Chien and JP Allison, 1991. Recognition of self antigens by skin-derived T cells with invariant γδ antigen receptors. **Science**, 252:1430-1432.

Havran WL, S Grell, G Duwe, J Kimura, A Wilson, AM Kruisbeek, RL O'Brien, W Born, RE Tigelaar and JP Allison, 1989. Limited diversity of T-cell receptor γ-chain expression of murine Thy-1+ dendritic epidermal cells revealed by Vγ3-specific monoclonal antibody. **Proc. Natl. Acad. Sci. USA**, 86:4185-4189.

Honjo M, A Elbe, G Steiner, I Assmann, K Wolff and G Stingl, 1990. Thymus-independent generation of Thy-1+ epidermal cells from a pool of Thy-1 bone marrow precursors. **J. Invest. Dermatol.**, 95:562-567.

Itohara S, AG Farr, JJ Lafaille, M Bonneville, Y Takagaki, W Haas and S Tonegawa, 1990. Homing of a γδ thymocyte subset with homogeneous T-cell receptors to mucosal epithelia. **Nature**, 343:754-757.

Lafaille JJ, A DeCloux, M Bonneville, Y Takagaki and S Tonegawa, 1989. Junctional sequences of T cell receptor γδ genes: Implications for γδ T cell lineages and for a novel intermediate of V-(D)-J joining. **Cell**, 59:859-870.

Larsen CG, AO Anderson, E Appella, JJ Oppenheim and K Matsushima, 1989. The neutrophil-activating protein (NAP-1) is also chemotactic for T lymphocytes. **Science**, 243:1464-1466.

Lewis JM and RE Tigelaar, 1991. Recognition of an epidermal stress antigen by murine γ/δ dendritic epidermal T cells (DETC). **J. Invest. Dermatol.**, 96:538A. (Abstract).

Luster AD and V Ravetch, 1987. Biochemical characterization of a γ interferon-inducible cytokine (IP-10). **J. Exp. Med.**, 166:1084-1097.

Marlin SD and TA Springer, 1987. Purified intercellular adhesion molecule-1 (ICAM-1) is a ligand for lymphocyte function-associated antigen 1 (LFA-1). **Cell**, 51:813-819.

McConnell TJ, WM Yokoyama, GE Kikuchi, GP Einhorn, G Stingl, EM Shevach and JE Coligan, 1989. δ-chains of dendritic epidermal T cell receptors are diverse but pair with γ-chains in a restricted manner. **J. Immunol.**, 142:2924-2931.

Nickoloff BJ, DM Lewinsohn, EC Butcher, AM Krensky and C Clayberger, 1988. Recombinant gamma interferon increases the binding of peripheral blood mononuclear leukocytes and a Leu3+ T lymphocyte clone to cultured keratinocytes and to a malignant cutaneous squamous carcinoma cell line that is blocked by antibody against the LFA-1 molecule. **J. Invest. Dermatol.**, 90:17-22.

Nixon-Fulton JL, WA Kuziel, B Santerse, PR Bergstresser, PW Tucker and RE Tigelaar, 1988. Thy-1+ epidermal cells in nude mice are distinct from their counterparts in thymus-bearing mice. A study of morphology, function, and T cell receptor expression. **J. Immunol.**, 141:1897-1903.

Ota Y, T Kobata, M Seki, H Yagita, S Shimada, Y Huang, Y Takagaki and K Okumura, 1992. Extrathymic origin of Vγ1/Vδ T cells in the skin. **Eur. J. Immunol.**, 22:595-598.

Payer E, A Elbe and G Stingl, 1991. Circulating CD3+/T cell receptor Vγ3+ fetal murine thymocytes home to the skin and give rise to proliferating dendritic epidermal T cells. **J. Immunol.**, 146:2536-2543.

Payer E, R Strohal, R Kutil, A Elbe and G Stingl, 1992. Demonstration of a lymphocyte subset in the epidermis of athymic nude mice. Evidence for T cell receptor diversity. **J. Immunol.**, 149:413-420.

Picker LJ, SA Michie, LS Rott and EC Butcher, 1990. A unique phenotype of skin-associated lymphocytes in humans. Preferential expression of the HECA-452 epitope by benign and malignant T cells at cutaneous sites. **Am. J. Pathol.**, 136:1053-1068.

Picker LJ, TK Kishimoto, CW Smith, RA Warnock and EC Butcher, 1991. ELAM-1 is an adhesion molecule for skin-homing T cells. **Nature.**, 349:796-799.

Romani N, G Stingl, E Tschachler, MD Witmer, RM Steinman, EM Shevach and G Schuler, 1985a. The Thy-1-bearing cell of murine epidermis. A distinctive leukocyte perhaps related to natural killer cells. **J. Exp. Med.**, 161:1368-1383.

Romani N, E Tschachler, G Schuler, W Aberer, R Ceredig, A Elbe, K Wolff, PO Fritsch and G Stingl, 1985b. Morphological and phenotypical characterization of bone marrow-derived dendritic Thy-1-positive epidermal cells of the mouse. **J. Invest. Dermatol.**, 85:91S-95S.

Romani N, G Schuler and P Fritsch, 1986. Ontogeny of Ia-positive and Thy-1-positive leukocytes of murine epidermis. **J. Invest. Dermatol.**, 86:129-133.

Sauder DN, MM Monick and GW Hunninghake, 1985. Epidermal cell derived thymocyte activating factor (ETAF) is a potent T-cell chemoattractant. **J. Invest. Dermatol.**, 85:431-433.

Shimizu Y, S Shaw, N Graber, TV Gopal, KJ Horgan, GA Van Seventer and W Newman, 1991. Activation independent binding of human memory T cells to adhesion molecule ELAM-1. **Nature**, 349:799-802. 1991.

Shiohara T and M Nagashima, 1988. Monoclonal antibody (MAb) to lymphocyte function associated antigen -1 (LFA-1) inhibits epidermotropic migration of T cells in vitro and in vivo. **J. Invest. Dermatol.**, 90:608A.

Shiohara T, N Moriya, C Gotoh, J Hayakawa, K Saizawa, H Yagita and M Nagashima, 1989. Differential expression of lymphocyte function-associated antigen 1 (LFA-1) on epidermotropic and non-epidermotropic T-cell clones. **J. Invest. Dermatol.**, 93:804-808.

Shiohara T, N Moriya, C Gotoh, J Hayakawa, M Nagashima, K Saizawa and H Ishikawa, 1990. Loss of epidermal integrity by T cell-mediated attack induces long-term local resistance to subsequent attack. I. Induction of resistance correlates with increases in Thy-1+ epidermal cell numbers. **J. Exp. Med.**, 171:1027-1041.

Steiner G, F Koning, A Elbe, E Tschachler, WM Yokoyama, EM Shevach, G Stingl and JE Coligan, 1988. Characterization of T cell receptors on resident murine dendritic epidermal T cells. **Eur. J. Immunol.**, 18:1323-1328.

Stingl G, KC Gunter, E Tschachler, H Yamada, RI Lechler, WM Yokoyama, G Steiner, RN Germain and EM Shevach, 1987a. Thy-1+ dendritic epidermal cells belong to the T-cell lineage. **Proc. Natl. Acad. Sci. USA**, 84:2430-2434.

Stingl G, F Koning, H Yamada, WM Yokoyama, E Tschachler, JA Bluestone, G Steiner, LE Samelson, AM Lew, JE Coligan and EM Shevach, 1987b. Thy-1+ dendritic epidermal cells express T3 antigen and the T cell receptor γ chain. **Proc. Natl. Acad. Sci. USA**, 84:4586-4590.

Stingl G, C Hauser, E Tschachler, V Groh and K Wolff, 1989. The immune functions of epidermal cells. In: D. A. Norris, Ed.: **Immune mechanisms in cutaneous disease.** Marcel Dekker. Inc. New York and Basel. pp. 3-72, 1989.

Streilein JW, 1983. Skin-associated lymphoid tissues (SALT): Origins and functions. **J. Invest. Dermatol.**, 80:12S-17S.

Sullivan S, PR Bergstresser, RE Tigelaar and JW Streilein, 1986. Induction and regulation of contact hypersensitivity by resident, bone marrow-derived, dendritic epidermal cells: Langerhans cells and Thy-1+ epidermal cells. **J. Immunol.**, 137:2460-2467.

Tschachler E, G Schuler, J Hutterer, H Leibl, R Wolff and G Stingl, 1983. Expression of Thy-1 antigen by murine epidermal cells. **J. Invest. Dermatol.**, 81: 282-285.

Welsh EA and ML Kripke, 1990. Murine Thy-1+ dendritic epidermal cells induce immunologic tolerance in vivo. **J. Immunol.**, 144:883-891.

ACTIVATION OF REACTIVE VERSUS MALIGNANT T CELLS IN CUTANEOUS T CELL LYMPHOMA: ROLE OF ABNORMAL ANTIGEN PRESENTING CELLS AND T CELL ACTIVATING MOLECULES

Kevin D. Cooper*†
Laurent Meunier*[1]
Vincent Ho*[2]
Ole Baadsgaard*‡
May-Sen Lee*
Erik Hansen*‡
Steen Lisby‡
Darius Mehregen*
Ed Allen†
Gunhild Lange Vejlsgaard‡
J.T. Elder*†

* Immunodermatology Unit
  Department of Dermatology
  University of Michigan
  Ann Arbor, Michigan

‡ University of Copenhagen
  Copenhagen, Denmark

† Ann Arbor Veterans Administration Hospital
  Ann Arbor, Michigan

Correspondence to: Dr. K. D. Cooper, Department of Dermatology,
University of Michigan School of Medicine, R5538 Kresge I, Box 0530,
Ann Arbor, MI 48109, U.S.A.

1 Current address: Hopital St. Charles, Montpellier, France
2 Current address: University of British Columbia, Vancouver, B.C., Canada

Basic Mechanisms of Physiologic and Aberrant Lymphoproliferation in the Skin
Edited by W.C. Lambert *et al.*, Plenum Press, New York, 1994

29

ABSTRACT

We review our data suggesting that interactions between reactive and malignant T cells in lesions of cutaneous T cell lymphoma (CTCL) may play a role in the biology of CTCL. T cell receptor gene rearrangement (TCRGR) analysis allows the identification of the malignant clone on the basis of the unique size of the TCR gene fragments after enzyme digestion. We identified the malignant clone by TCRGR analysis of DNA extracts from lesional skin of patients with CTCL, mycosis fungoides type, and compared the TCRGR pattern to that of T cell clones established from lesional skin of the same patients. We found that each clone demonstrated a TCRGR pattern unique from the others and different from that of the malignant clone identified in the lesion. These data established that a polyclonal population of tumor infiltrating lymphocytes (TIL) are present in the lesion (and potentially regulating the malignant clone), and also suggest that the malignant clone and the TIL's may have different activation requirements. Intralesional activation of malignant or TIL clones may be induced by abnormal antigen presenting cells (APC's) in the lesion. We showed that lesional $CD1a^+$ cells (Langerhans cells;LC), purified on immunomagnetic beads, demonstrated ultrastructural abnormalities such as hyperconvoluted nuclei and significant melanophagocytosis. In addition, these LC demonstrated strong expression of CD36, CD11c and CD1c, markers normally more highly expressed on dermal perivascular dendritic cells, in addition to expression of molecules present on normal LC, such as HLA-DR and CD1a. Although these modulated LC are hyperstimulatory for autologous T cells, it is not yet clear whether they are stimulating the malignant clone or the TIL's in the lesion. The balance between progression versus indolence may be related to complex interactions between the cells of the malignant clone, TIL's , and APC's.

INTRODUCTION

Several observations regarding the mycosis fungoides form of cutaneous T cell lymphoma (MF-CTCL) suggest that complex immunoregulatory events occur within the cutaneous lesions and/or the regional lymph nodes. Clinical recognition of lesional features such as annularity, atrophy, and postinflammatory hypo- and hyperpigmentation may be taken as evidence for a dynamic balance between tumor cell growth and tumor cell regulation in the lesional tissue. The protracted and indolent course of the typical mycosis fungoides type of CTCL, and the efficacy of extracorporeal photochemotherapy (Edelson et al., 1987), also suggest that knowledge of immunoregulatory mechanisms may be important for understanding CTCL biology and for designing new treatments.

Histologically, it has been observed that reactive-appearing lymphocytes are intermixed among the lymphocytes demonstrating clear atypia, but the distinction between activated T cells and the T cells of mycosis fungoides is not absolute (Vonderheid et al., 1981). T cell marker staining has provided additional support for the concept that both cells of malignant phenotype ($CD3^+$ $CD4^+$ $CD7^-$ with CD2 or CD5 loss) (Vonderheid, 1989) as well as cells of a phenotype typical of skin infiltrating lymphocytes ($CD3^+$ $CD4^+$ $CD7^+$ $CD2^+$ $CD5^+$) are present in the lesion. However, CD4$^+$ CD7$^-$ T cells represent a subset normally present in peripheral blood and benign dermatoses, and therefore cannot be used to definitively mark the malignant population. Because of the inherent limitations of surface marker analysis, a clear demonstration that "malignant" and "reactive" T cells are present has not been accomplished with this approach.

METHODS AND RESULTS

Demonstration of Reactive Tumor Infiltrating Lymphocytes in CTCL by Southern Blot Analysis

A definitive demonstration that the malignant T cell clone is accompanied by a polyclonal population of T lymphocytes distinct from the malignant clone required us to assess skin infiltrating T cell receptor gene rearrangements at the individual clone level (Ho et al., 1990a). The ability to uniquely identify each T cell and its clonal progeny by its characteristic pattern of rearranged components of the gene encoding the T cell receptor provides a way to uniquely identify the predominating clone in the skin and/or blood (Waldmann et al., 1985; Weiss et al., 1989; Weiss et al., 1985). This clonal population is operationally defined as the malignant population.

To identify cells of reactive and clonal origin in CTCL skin, we obtained punch biopsies of patch stage and erythrodermic skin of untreated patients with CTCL and treated them in two ways. One piece was digested and the DNA extracted, subjected to restriction enzyme digestion, and electrophoresed on agarose gels. The DNA fragments, separated by size, were transferred and immobilized on nylon (Southern Blot) and hybridized with a ^{32}P labeled oligonucleotide DNA probe that binds to the constant region of the beta chain of the T cell receptor (C beta). After washing away free oligonucleotide probe, autoradiography then allowed visualization of the T cell receptor gene fragments encoding portions of the C beta chain. Bands distinct from the bands characteristic of the unrearranged, or germ line, configuration of the gene identified the clonal population that was expanded sufficiently to reach the level of detection by this method (Figure 1, T$_{M1}$) (Ho et al., 1990b). The unique position and pattern of the band also provided a "fingerprint" of the malignant clone for future comparisons.

The other piece of tissue was diced into 1 mm^3 pieces of epidermis plus papillary dermis, and placed in organ culture with interleukin 2 (IL-2). Skin infiltrating lymphocytes were then cloned by limiting dilution and expanded by stimulation with the nonspecific mitogen, phytohemaglutinin (PHA), every two weeks. When at least 5 x 10^6 cells of a particular clone could be obtained, DNA extraction and Southern blot analysis with the C beta-specific probe was performed as above.

The data clearly demonstrated the existence of a number of T cell populations of distinct clonal lineage. Not only were most of the skin infiltrating T cell clones distinct from each other

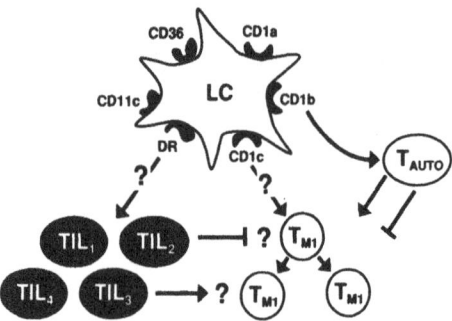

Figure 1. Potential interrelationships among malignant T lymphocytes (T_{m1}), multiple clones of reactive T lymphocytes (tumor infiltrating lymphocytes or TIL_{1-4}) and abnormal antigen presenting cells such as Langerhans cells (LC) in lesions of MF-CTCL.

(unique bands), they were also distinct from the malignant clone that dominated the lesion in vivo (Ho et al., 1990a). We were not able to provide culture conditions sufficient for the long term growth of the malignant clone, however, despite extensive manipulation of cytokines, mitogens, and accessory cells in the culture milieu. In lines not subjected to cloning, the malignant clone could be observed to gradually be replaced by other clones (Hansen et al., 1988).

These data indicated several points. One, the malignant clone appears to have very fastidious and somewhat variable culture requirements (Abrams et al., 1991b; Abrams et al., 1991a). Two, a variety of reactive T cells of distinct clonal lineages are definitively demonstrable in the lesion. These can be termed tumor infiltrating lymphocytes (TIL's) (Figure 1, TIL 1-4). Third, the inability to grow the malignant clone may be due to down regulatory influences or cytoxicity by the TIL's. Because we have been unable to grow the malignant clone in our laboratory, however, we do not have any type of direct evidence for such a negative interaction. Thus, it remains entirely possible that the TIL's may provide signals that favor the expansion of the malignant clone (Figure 1, TIL - T_{M1} interactions).

Activation of TIL's and the Malignant Clone

Identification of the signals responsible for intralesional expansion or activation of the malignant clone and TIL's may provide new avenues for therapeutic intervention. That intralesional T cell activation is ongoing is supported by the finding of HLA-DR expression on keratinocytes (Tjernlund, 1978), which has so far only been inducible by the T cell lymphokine, gamma interferon (gamma IFN) (Basham et al., 1984). Whether the gamma interferon is released by the TIL's or the malignant clone in most cases is unknown. In a case of Sézary syndrome that we studied in detail, however, the malignant clone was unable to produce gamma IFN in response to mitogens, despite the fact that activation occurred, as evidenced by increased IL-2 receptor release (Nickoloff et al., 1989). The fact that this patient exhibited HLA-DR expression by keratinocytes, however, indicated that the TIL's were the likely source of gamma IFN, and that, by inference, they were undergoing intralesional activation.

How might TIL's or malignant clones undergo intralesional activation? Dendritic antigen presenting cells are potent providers of T cell receptor-mediated signalling as well as co-stimulatory accessory molecule signalling (Steinman et al., 1980). Langerhans cells (LC) have been observed in the clusters of lymphocytes within Pautrier microabscesses, and CD1a$^+$ cells are also present in the dermis in apposition to clusters of lymphocytes (Wood et al., 1982). These and other observations have led investigators to postulate that Langerhans cells may be involved in providing signals that promote the expansion of malignant cells (Figure 1, LC-T$_{MI}$). On the other hand, the malignant clone may grow autonomously, and the TIL's may receive their stimulatory signal through the APC's (Figure 1, LC-TIL). The stimulatory signal could include antigenic peptides derived from the malignant clone.

CD36$^+$ LC with Convoluted Nuclei

We have found increasing evidence that Langerhans cells in the lesions of mycosis fungoides-type CTCL have acquired a modified phenotype and functional program. Initially, Lisby noted that lesional Langerhans cells could express an aberrant phenotype and described the abnormal expression of CD36 on CD1a$^+$ cells within epidermal cell suspensions (Lisby et al., 1988). Because CD36 also demonstrates increased expression on lesional keratinocytes, it was important to verify that the CD36 was also expressed on bone marrow derived cells, such as HLe1$^+$ or CD1a$^+$ cells in the epidermal suspension. To further verify the identity of the cells expressing CD36, we labeled lesional epidermal cells with anti CD1a, anti CD36, or an IgG1 isotype control antibody. Immunomagnetic beads coated with goat anti-mouse IgG were used to specifically absorb the positively labeled cells onto the beads. The beads and cells were fixed and examined under transmission electron microscopy. In contrast to the isotype control-stained cells that bound to beads, which were all keratinocytes, the CD1a$^+$ and CD36$^+$ cell populations that were bound to beads contained typical Langerhans cells (with Birbeck granules, dense intermediate filaments, and an active cytoplasm with rare lysosomes), as well as indeterminate cells (like LC, but without Birbeck granules) and macrophagic cells (containing phagolysosomes) (Lisby et al., 1990). Of great interest, cells in the latter two subsets exhibited hyperconvoluted nuclei. CD36 was not co-expressed by intraepidermal T cells. These data suggest that lesional DR$^+$ macrophages and indeterminate cells (putative APC's) undergo nuclear morphologic changes similar to those of atypical T lymphocytes in CTCL, and confirm ultrastructural observations by Braverman et al., that MF-CTCL skin relapsing from electron beam therapy contains macrophage-like cells with convoluted nuclei (Braverman et al., 1987).

Loss of Anatomic Compartmentalization of Dendritic Cell Markers in Lesional Skin

In normal skin, CD1a is expressed on epidermal Langerhans cells, whereas CD1b (Koller et al., 1987; Cattoretti et al., 1987) and CD36 (Weiss et al., 1988) are expressed on dermal perivascular cells, some of which exhibit a somewhat dendritic morphology. The expression of CD1c by the CD1b perivascular subset as well as by LC has led us to postulate that these subsets share a common lineage. Indeed, using a monoclonal antibody now known to bind CD1c, Murphy et al., demonstrated that CD1c⁺ dermal cells exhibit features of indeterminate-type Langerhans cells (Murphy et al., 1985).

In lesional mycosis fungoides type CTCL, there is a loss of the normally compartmental-ized expression of CD1a by epidermal Langerhans cells, and expression of CD1b by dermal indeterminate perivascular dendritic cells. Using dual color immunofluorescence on cryostat skin sections, we quantified the percentage of CD1a⁺ cells that also expressed DR, CD1b, and CD36. The results demonstrated that CD1b and CD36 are abnormally expressed on a significant percentage of intraepidermal CD1a⁺ Langerhans cells.

Flow Cytometric Analysis with Three Color Staining

Although dual color immunofluorescence gives valuable insights into molecule co-expression, complex and precise relationships can better be approached through simultaneous triple marker flow cytometry. Lesional epidermal cells were prepared in a suspension and

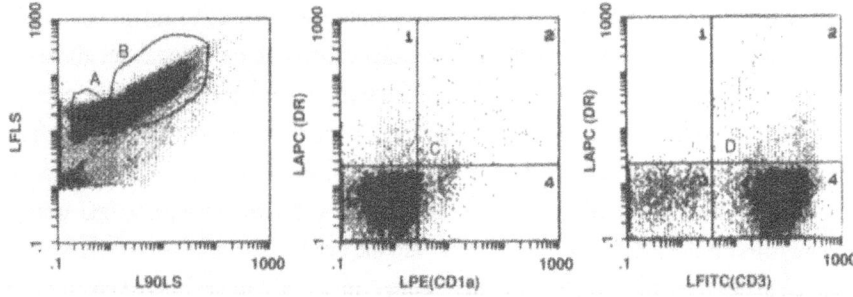

Figure 2. Flow cytometry of lesional MF-CTCL epidermal cells to allow electronic isolation of CD3⁺ T lymphocytes ("A") from keratinocytes and APC's ("B") by light scatter, Left panel: Forward (LFLS) versus side scatter (L9OLS) of incident light defines two populations. Middle and right panels: The smaller, less granular population ("A") is comprised mostly of T lymphocytes that stain with anti-CD3, but not with anti DR or CD1a.

stained with anti HLA-DR, anti CD1a, anti CD11c, anti CD1c, and anti CD3, and compared to isotype controls. Forward (LFLS) and side (L9OLS) light scatter analysis allows separation of lymphocytes (Figure 2, left panel, "A") containing mainly CD3⁺ T lymphocytes from the larger, more granular keratinocytes and Langerhans cells (Figure 2, left panel, "B"). Thus, the smaller epidermal population "A" contains few CD1a⁺ or DR⁺ cells (Figure 2, middle panel) but many CD3⁺ T lymphocytes (Figure 2, right panel).

We then restricted our analysis to the DR⁺ cells contained in the larger, more granular epidermal cell population (Figure 2, left panel, population "B", and Figure 3, upper left panel).

Analysis of DR⁺ cells (Figure 3, upper middle panel, LAPC > 40), demonstrates that they exhibited moderate IgG binding, consistent with avid FcIgGRII expression (Figure 3, upper right panel, lower middle sector). Replacement of the IgG2b isotype control antibody with anti CD1a markedly increased their PE fluorescence and replacement of the IgG1 isotype antibody with anti CD1c increased the level of green fluorescence (from the lower middle sector of the upper right panel, to the upper right-most sector of the lower left panel), confirming the impression from light microscopy that expression of CD1c was high on MF-CTCL Langerhans cells. If IgG2b is replaced with anti CD11c, and IgG1 with an IgG1 anti CD1a, it is clear that virtually all the DR⁺ cells also express bright CD11c, with the majority expressing bright CD1a (Figure 3, lower middle panel, upper right sector). Bright (> 100) CD11c and CD1c were also mainly co-expressed (Figure 3, lower right panel, upper right sector), but there is also a population of cells with lower levels of CD11c and CD1c (Figure 3, lower right panel, PE CD11c intensity between 20 and 100). Anti CD3 did not increase the green fluorescence of the larger DR⁺ cells (not

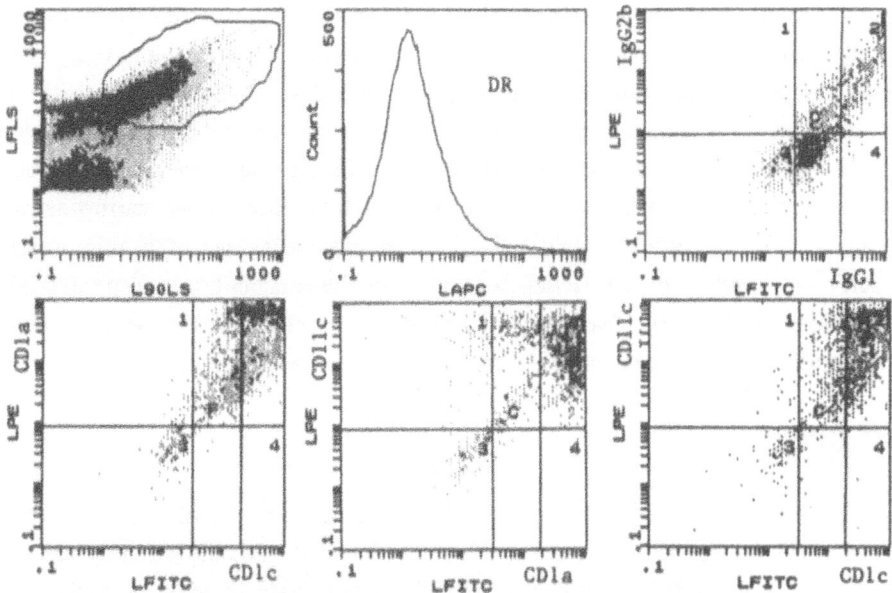

Figure 3. Triple color flow cytometric analysis of lesional MF-CTCL epidermal cells.

shown). Thus, by flow cytometric analysis, the majority of DR⁺ cells in lesional epidermis was CD1a$^{+bright}$, CD1c$^{+bright}$, CD11c$^{+bright}$, CD3⁻, whereas another subset appears to be DR⁺, CD1a$^{+bright}$, CD1c^{+dim}, CD11c^{+dim}, CD3⁻. CD36 and CD1b appear to have been expressed on a portion of both subsets, based on dual color experiments in tissue sections (not shown). Epidermotropic T lymphocytes were excluded by analyzing only the larger (high LFLS) more granular (high L9OLS) cells (Figure 3, upper left panel). The majority of keratinocytes and melanocytes were excluded by analyzing only DR⁺ cells stained brightly (> 40) with the far red fluorescing dye, APC (Figure 3, upper middle panel). The remaining panels of Figure 3 represent analyses of only the DR⁺ cells. Staining with phycoerythrin (PE) and FITC labeled isotype control antibodies reveals the majority of DR⁺ cells to lie within the lower middle sector of the upper right panel. Anti CD1a (PE on the lower left panel and FITC on the lower middle panel) results in a clear increase in fluorescence intensity such that CD1a$^+$ cell intensity was >300. Similarly, anti CD1c (FITC fluorescence on the lower left panel) results in movement of the DR$^+$ CD1a$^+$ cells from a FITC intensity contained in the middle sector to an intensity in the right-most sector (Figure 3, lower left panel). Anti CD11c (PE fluorescence on the lower middle panel) reveals that the majority population expresses both CD1a and abundant CD11c (upper right sector). There appears, however, to be two sub-subsets of CD11c$^+$ subsets, most evident in Figure 3, lower right panel, one with high CD11c and CD1c expression and one with lower CD11c and CD1c expression.

Hyperstimulatory Function of Phenotypically Abnormal CTCL LC

The phenotype of CTCL LC resembles in several ways the phenotype of LC in lesional epidermis of atopic dermatitis, but is distinct from that of psoriasis. In atopic dermatitis, CD1a$^+$ epidermal cells also coexpress CD1b and CD36, and demonstrate a hyperstimulatory capacity to activate autologous T lymphocytes in the absence of added antigens (Taylor et al., 1991). Similarly, we showed that lesional mycosis fungoides-type CTCL epidermal cells share with atopic dermatitis epidermal cells the abnormal capacity to activate autologous resting blood CD4$^+$ T lymphocytes in the absence of added antigens (Hansen et al., 1990). The activating capacity was critically dependent on the presence of CD1a$^+$, HLe1$^+$ (bone marrow-derived) cells, and partially dependent on CD36$^+$ cells. Purified cells bearing each of the prior markers were sufficiently capable on their own to activate T cells, ruling out critical co-dependent APC activity (Hansen et al., 1990). These data indicate that LC in lesional CTCL epidermis are not only abnormal in phenotype, but have also acquired enhanced APC activity.

CONCLUSIONS

The nature of the T cells undergoing activation and their functional relationship to the malignant clone and the TIL's is unclear at this point (Figure 1). Because we and others have shown that the malignant clone appears to be difficult to activate (Baadsgaard et al., 1988; Nickoloff et al., 1989) the resting blood T cells activated in our system (experiments were performed in non-Sézary patients) may model the interactions among lesional APC's with freshly recruited TIL's into the skin. Thus, these "autoreactive" T cells (Figure 1, T auto) may exert regulatory influences over the malignant clone [either positive or negative (Figure 1)], and may represent the TIL response. Alternatively, these cells may be providing direct hyperstimulatory signals to the malignant population.

REFERENCES

Abrams JT, S Lessin, Sk Ghosh, et al., 1991a. A clonal CD4- positive T-cell line established from the blood of a patient with Sézary syndrome. **J. Invest. Dermatol.**, 96:31-37.

Abrams JT, SR Lessin, SK Ghosh, et al., 1991b. Malignant and nonmalignant T cell lines from human T cell lymphotropic virus type I-negative patients with Sezary syndrome. **J. Immunol.**, 146:1455-1462.

Baadsgaard O, ER Hansen, V Ho, et al., 1988. Activation of T cells from Sezary patients can occur through both antigen dependent and independent pathways. **J. Invest. Dermatol.**, 91:386.

Basham TY, BJ Nickoloff, TC Merigan and VB Morhenn, 1984. Recombinant gamma interferon induces HLA-DR expression on cultured keratinocytes. **J. Invest. Dermatol.**, 83:88-90.

Braverman IM, S Klein and A Grant, 1987. Electron microscopic and immunolabeling studies of the lesional and normal skin of patients with mycosis fungoides treated by total body electron beam irradiation. **J. Am. Acad. Dermatol.**, 16:61-74.

Cattoretti G, E Berti, A Mancuso et al., 1987. An MHC class I related family of antigens with widespread distribution on resting and activated cells. In: AJ McMichael, PCL Beverley, W Gilks et al., Eds., **Leucocyte Typing III. White Cell Differentiation Antigens**, Oxford, Oxford University Press, pp. 89-91.

Edelson R, C Berger, F Gasparro, et al., 1987. Treatment of cutaneous T-cell lymphoma by extracorporeal photochemotherapy. Preliminary results. **N. Engl. J. Med.**, 316:297-303.

Hansen ER, O Baadsgaard, S Lisby, KD Cooper, K Thomsen and GL Wantzin, 1988. Epidermal cells from mycosis fungoides demonstrate MHC-Class II dependent activation of the CD4+CD8- lymphocyte subset. **J. Invest. Dermatol.**, 91:386A.(Abstract)

Hansen ER, O Baadsgaard, S Lisby, KD Cooper, K Thomsen and GL Vejlsgaard, 1990. Cutaneous T-cell lymphoma lesional epidermal cells activate autologous CD4+ T lymphocytes: Involvement of both CD1+OKM5+ and CD1+OKM5- antigen-presenting cells. **J. Invest. Dermatol.**, 94:485-491.

Ho VC, O Baadsgaard, JT Elder, et al., 1990a. Geno-typic analysis of T-cell clones derived from cutaneous T-cell lymphoma lesions demonstrates selective growth of tumor infil-trating lymphocytes. **J. Invest. Dermatol.**, 95:4-8.

Ho VC, ER Hansen, JT Elder, et al., 1990b. T cell receptor beta-chain gene rearrangement without gamma-chain gene rearrangement in cutaneous T cell lymphoma: An unusual finding. **Clin. Immunol. Immunopathol.**, 54:354-360.

Koller U, V Groh, O Majdic, H Stockinger and W Knapp, 1987. Subclustering of CD1 antibodies on the basis of their reaction pattern with different types of dendritic cells. In: AJ McMichael, PCL Beverley, W Gilks et al., Eds., **Leucocyte Typing III. White Cell Differentiation Antigens**, Oxford, Oxford University Press, pp. 85-86.

Lisby S, O Baadsgaard, KD Cooper, K Thomsen and GRL Wantzin, 1988. Expression of OKM5 antigen on epidermal cells in mycosis fungoides plaque stage. **J. Invest. Dermatol.**, 90:716-719.

Lisby S, O Baadsgaard, KD Cooper, et al., 1990. Phenotype, ultrastructure, and function of CD1+DR+ epidermal cells that express CD36 (OKM5) in cutaneous T cell lymphoma. **Scand. J. Immunol.**, 32:111-119.

Murphy GF, BR Bronstein, RW Knowles and AK Bhan, 1985. Ultrastructural documentation of M241 glycoprotein on dendritic and endothelial cells in normal human skin. **Lab. Invest.**, 52:264-269.

Nickoloff BJ, CEM Griffiths, O Baadsgaard, JJ Voorhees, CA Hanson and KD Cooper, 1989. Markedly diminished epidermal keratinocyte expression of intercellular adhesion molecule-1 (ICAM-1) in Sézary syndrome. **JAMA**, 261:2217-2221.

Steinman RM and MC Nussenzweig, 1980. Dendritic cells: features and functions. **Immunol. Rev.**, 53:127-147.

Taylor RS, O Baadsgaard, C Hammerberg and KD Cooper, 1991. Hyperstimulatory CD1a+CD1b+CD36+ Langerhans cells are responsible for increased autologous T lymphocyte reactivity to lesional epidermal cells of patients with atopic dermatitis. **J. Immunol.**, 147:3794-3802.

Tjernlund UM, 1978. Epidermal expression of HLA-DR antigens in mycosis fungoides. **Arch. Dermatol. Res.**, 261:81-86.

Vonderheid E, 1989. Diagnostic Methods for Cutaneous T-Cell Lymphoma. In: SA Muller, Ed., **Parapsoriasis**, Rochester, Mayo Foundation, p. 83-94.

Vonderheid EC, DW Tam, WC Johnson, EJ Van Scott and PE Wallner, 1981. Prognostic significance of cytomorphology in the cutaneous T-cell lymphomas. **Cancer**, 47:119-125.

Waldmann TA, MM Davis, KF Bongiovanni and SKJ Korsmeyer, 1985. Rearrangements of genes for the antigen receptor on T cells as markers of lineage and clonality in human lymphoid neoplasms. **N. Engl. J. Med.**, 313:776-783.

Weiss JS, WD James and KD Cooper, 1988. Melanophages in inflammatory skin disease demonstrate the surface phenotype of OKM5+ antigen-presenting cells and activated macrophages. **J. Am. Acad. Dermatol.**, 19:633-641.

Weiss LM, E Hu, GS Wood, et al., 1985. Clonal re-arrangements of T-cell receptor genes in mycosis fungoides and dermatopathic lymphadenopathy. **N. Engl. J. Med.**, 313:539-544.

Weiss LM, GS Wood, E Hu, EA Abel, RT Hoppe and J Sklar, 1989. Detection of clonal T-cell receptor gene rearrangements in the peripheral blood of patients with mycosis fungoides/Sézary syndrome. **J. Invest. Dermatol.**, 92:601-604.

Wood GS, DG Deneau, RA Miller, R Levy, RT Hoppe, and RA Warnke, 1982. Subtypes of cutaneous T-cell lymphoma defined by expression of leu-1 and Ia. **Blood**, 59:876-882.

FACTORS INVOLVED IN THE LOCALIZATION AND ACTIVATION OF MURINE γδ POSITIVE DENDRITIC EPIDERMAL T CELLS

Robert E. Tigelaar*

Julia M. Lewis†

* Department of Dermatology

† Department of Immunobiology

Yale University School of Medicine

New Haven, CT

Correspondence to: Dr. R. E. Tigelaar, Department of Dermatology,

Yale University School of Medicine, 333 Cedar Street,

New Haven, CT 06510, U.S.A.

ABSTRACT

The vast majority of dendritic epidermal T cells (DETC) in normal mice express a monomorphic γδ-type T cell receptor (TCR) (V5J1Cγ1 and V1D2J2Cδ coding segments, totally lacking junctional diversity). Cells with identical TCRs are also found in the early fetal thymus, but are not found in newborn or adult thymus, in peripheral lymphoid tissues or in other epithelial sites known to be populated by γδ cells expressing distinct receptors (e.g., in the gastrointestinal tract or in the reproductive tract). Early fetal thymocytes can serve as precursors for the DETC that populate adult skin; our recent adoptive transfer studies indicate an important role for cycling hair follicles in the localization and/or in situ proliferation of such precursors. The restricted tissue distribution and TCR homogeneity of DETC has suggested the possibility that the physiologic ligand for the DETC TCR is a common self-antigen expressed by keratinocytes or by other cells in their immediate microenvironment under a variety of potentially harmful circumstances (i.e., a stress protein). Recent in vitro data are consistent with this hypothesis: a DETC line was activated by exposure to stressed epidermal cells. Furthermore, increases in the densities of Vγ5/Vδ1[+] DETC in spontaneously depigmenting C57BL/6 vit/vit

Basic Mechanisms of Physiologic and Aberrant Lymphoproliferation in the Skin
Edited by W.C. Lambert *et al.*, Plenum Press, New York, 1994

39

mice, in mice undergoing contact dermatitis reactions, and in normal mice during the neonatal period, all are consistent with the in situ activation/proliferation of DETC in response to a variety of pathologic and physiologic stimuli. It is now clear that human skin does not harbor a precise morphologic equivalent of mouse DETC. A number of persistent gaps in our knowledge about mouse DETC must be filled (including more precise identification of their physiologic ligand and their relevant functional roles in vivo), however, before we can really understand the relevance of mouse DETC to human cutaneous immunity and immunopathology.

INTRODUCTION

In 1983, previously unrecognized cells, now accepted as constituents of skin associated lymphoid tissue (SALT), were identified in normal mouse epidermis (Bergstresser et al., 1983; Tschachler et al., 1983). These cells were initially called Thy-1$^+$ dendritic epidermal cells because of their characteristic expression of the Thy-1 alloantigen and formation of a conspicuous dendritic network among basal layer keratinocytes. Renamed dendritic epidermal T cells (DETC) following the demonstration that the overwhelming majority of these cells express the $\gamma\delta$ form of the CD3-associated T cell receptor (TCR; Stingl et al., 1987; Kuziel et al., 1987; Bonyhadi et al., 1987), DETC have generated extraordinary interest among investigators in a variety of disciplines. With this intensive research interest has come the realization that murine DETC have several unique features which distinguish them both from $\alpha\beta$ T cells and from other $\gamma\delta$ T cells. The purpose of this review is not only to highlight our current state of understanding of $\gamma\delta$ cells in the mouse, but also to emphasize several persistent gaps in that understanding, such as the relationship of mouse DETC to $\gamma\delta$ cells identified in human skin and the normal physiologic and pathologic role(s) of these cells.

PHENOTYPIC AND FUNCTIONAL CHARACTERISTICS OF MURINE DETC

DETC have been found in all strains of normal mice; however there is significant variation in DETC density, both at a given anatomic location (e.g., flank skin) between different inbred mouse strains and between different anatomic locations in the same animal (Bergstresser et al., 1985). Phenotypic analyses of resting DETC from normal mice have shown that these cells are Thy-1$^+$, Ia$^-$, CD45$^+$, Ly-5$^+$, asialo GM1$^+$, NK-1$^-$, CD4$^-$, CD8$^-$, CD3$^+$, and that they express TCRs which, on the overwhelming majority of cells, are of the $\gamma\delta$ type (Bergstresser et al., 1983; Tschachler et al., 1983; Romani et al., 1985; Stingl et al., 1987; Steiner et al., 1988; Kuziel et al., 1987; Bonyhadi et al., 1987). The epidermis of *scid* mice is essentially devoid of Thy-1$^+$ DETC (Nixon-Fulton et al., 1987), and while young (6-8 week old) nu/nu epidermis contains readily detectable Thy-1$^+$ cells, such cells are almost invariably CD3$^-$ and TCR$^-$ (Nixon-Fulton et al., 1988). Before antibodies to the CD3/TCR complex were available, the most compelling data suggesting that Thy-1$^+$ dendritic epidermal cells are in the T cell lineage were those showing that these cells can display several of the in vitro functional activities of conventional T cells, including Con A-stimulated proliferation, IL-2 secretion, and IL-2-dependent cell growth (Nixon-Fulton et al., 1986; Caughman et al., 1986). Further examination of IL-2 dependent DETC lines and clones has shown that they can exhibit major histocompatibility complex (MHC) non-restricted cytotoxicity, which can be antibody dependent (ADCC), (LAK)-like, or natural killer cell (NK)-like (Nixon-Fulton et al., 1988; Takashima et al., 1988; Havran et al., 1989; Kuziel et al., 1991). While DETC freshly isolated from normal skin, as well as many long-term DETC lines and clones, are CD4⁻ and CD8⁻, some long-term clones (especially ones with high cytotoxic activity) display variable but unequivocal staining with anti-CD8 (Takashima et al., 1988); more recently, it has been shown that the CD8 expressed on such DETC is a homodimer of the CD8 α chain (M. Tutt, personal communication). While such CD8 α-α homodimers have been reported on some $\alpha\beta$ and $\gamma\delta$ cells isolated from the intestinal epithelium, the CD8 expressed by most conventional T cells is a heterodimer of CD8α and CD8β (Guy-Grand et al., 1991; Rocha et al., 1991). The functional significance of this alternate form of CD8 expressed on some DETC remains to be established. DETC can be activated in response to either immobilized anti-CD3 or anti-$\gamma\delta$ TCR antibodies to proliferate and secrete lymphokines (such as IL-2, IFN-γ, and IL-3) (Havran et al., 1989; Lewis & Tigelaar, 1991). At present, however, we do not know whether the range of functional activities and profiles of lymphokine secretion by DETC will prove to be comparable to those of conventional $\alpha\beta$ T cells (e.g., whether, under appropriate conditions, activated DETC can secrete "T$_{H2}$-type" lymphokines such as IL-4 and IL-5 (Mosmann & Coffman, 1989; Rocken et al., 1991)).

LACK OF TCR HETEROGENEITY IN THE DETC OF NORMAL ADULT MICE

While cells bearing $\gamma\delta$ TCRs constitute only a very minor subset of T cells recirculating in the blood and peripheral tissues of mice and humans, studies in mice have demonstrated not only that various epithelia which are in contact with the external environment (e.g., skin, reproductive tract, GI tract) are populated preferentially by $\gamma\delta^+$ T cells, but also that the $\gamma\delta$ TCRs expressed in a particular epithelium are characteristic, and in some cases unique, to that site. The first suggestion that DETC TCR expression is not heterogeneous was the observation by Kuziel et al. (1987) that five independently derived, long-term DETC lines, or clones, from AKR/J mice express the same Vγ gene segment, Vγ5. On further analysis of these same cells, Asarnow et al. (1988) unexpectedly found they each use identical γ and δ coding segments (V5J1Cγ1 and V1D2J2Cδ). Furthermore, each clone had identical γ junctional sequences and identical δ junctional sequences which were conspicuous for their total lack of both nongermline encoded (N) nucleotide additions and exonucleolytic nibbling, two of the mechanisms most widely used by conventional T cells for generating TCR diversity (Asarnow et al., 1988). The issue of whether the demonstration of such monomorphic TCRs on DETC clones propagated in vitro has relevance in vivo has been addressed in several ways. FACS analysis of freshly prepared epidermal suspensions showed that virtually all CD3$^+$ cells (i.e., TCR$^+$) also stain with an antibody specific for Vγ5$^+$ TCRs (Havran et al., 1989). Most convincingly, utilizing double staining of epidermal sheets from various strains of mice with both anti-CD3 and a monoclonal antibody (named 17D1) specific for Vγ5/Vδ1-containing TCRs, we have found that >95% of DETC in situ are Vγ5/Vδ1$^+$ (Tigelaar et al., 1990; Lewis & Tigelaar, 1989). Furthermore,

PCR analysis of freshly isolated DETC has confirmed that the vast majority of Vγ5 and Vδ1 sequences are devoid of junctional diversity (Asarnow et al., 1989). Collectively these results indicate that the TCR repertoire of DETC is essentially monomorphic.

At least in adult mice, T cells with this particular Vγ5/Vδ1 TCR are apparently restricted to the skin (and possibly the epidermis), since this is the only site reliably shown to contain γδ cells with this specific receptor. Such cells have not been isolated from lymphoid tissues such as spleen, lymph nodes, or adult thymus (Havran et al., 1989). Cells expressing DETC-type TCRs also have not been isolated from other epithelial sites known to be populated with γδ cells bearing TCRs distinct from those on DETC (but also characteristic for that particular epithelium). For example, the TCR repertoire of the γδ cells in the gut epithelium is strongly biased toward selective expression of Vγ7-containing TCRs; however, unlike DETC TCRs, there is apparently no preferential pairing with a specific δ chain, and the Vγ7 coding sequences show considerable junctional diversity (Bonneville et al., 1988; Takagaka et al., 1989; Kyes et al., 1989). The TCR homogeneity and tissue restriction of DETC has recently been shown to be mimicked by the γδ cells in vaginal and uterine epithelium. These cells, like DETC, express a TCR which is essentially monomorphic and totally lacking in junctional diversity, and the δ chain is identical to that on DETC (V1D2J2Cδ); however, the γ chain is distinct (V6 instead of V5) (Itohara et al., 1990).

EARLY FETAL THYMOCYTES CAN ACT AS DETC PRECURSORS

While few, if any, T cells outside the epidermis of adult mice express DETC-type TCRs (V5J1Cγ1 and V1D2J2Cδ coding segments lack junctional diversity), identical TCRs are seen on the earliest fetal thymocytes to express a CD3/TCR complex (gestation day 13), and such Vγ5/Vδ1[+] cells are the predominant CD3[+] thymocytes until about day 17 (Garman et al., 1986; Chien et al., 1987; Havran and Allison, 1988; Ito, et al., 1989, Lafaille et al., 1989). After day 17, the proportion of CD3[+] fetal thymocytes expressing the DETC-type TCR drops rather abruptly, coincident both with the rapid accumulation of αβ[+] cells and with a second, also transient, "wave" of γδ cells with receptors identical to those expressed by the T cells in reproductive epithelia (Havran & Allison, 1988; Ito et al., 1989). After birth, expression of either the DETC-type or reproductive-type γ or δ coding segments is rarely seen (Elliott et al., 1988; Lafaille et al., 1989).

Such identity between the TCRs on adult DETC and early fetal thymocytes suggested the obvious possibility that early fetal thymocytes could serve as DETC precursors; three different laboratories have generated data consistent with this possibility. Adoptive transfer of either unfractionated or FACS-sorted CD3[+] or 17D1[+] (Vγ5/Vδ1[+]) day 16-17 fetal thymocytes into either young nu/nu or Thy-1 congenic recipients results in the gradual appearance in recipient epidermis of dendritic cells which are CD3[+] and Vγ5/Vδ1[+] (Lewis & Tigelaar, 1989; Havran & Allison, 1990; Payer et al., 1991). Furthermore, kinetic studies of both the morphology and numbers of CD3[+] cells in the epidermis have strongly suggested rather vigorous proliferation in situ. By contrast, transfer of neither sorted CD3⁻ nor Vγ5/Vδ1⁻ fetal thymocytes resulted in repopulation of recipient epidermis with CD3⁺ Vγ5/Vδ1⁺ DETC (Lewis & Tigelaar, 1989; Payer et al., 1991), indicating that fetal thymocyte precursors of DETC rearrange and express their TCR genes before they enter the epidermis. These data also indicate that nude mouse epidermis, despite its obvious abnormality, can receive DETC precursors and permit their post-thymic expansion. Collectively, these results are consistent with the hypotheses that some, if not all, the DETC found in normal mice are (fetal) thymic dependent, and that the absence of Vγ5/Vδ1⁺ DETC in young nu/nu mice is secondary to their lack of a thymus.

INFLUENCE OF STATE OF HAIR GROWTH ON LOCALIZATION AND/OR PROLIFERATION OF EARLY FETAL THYMOCYTES IN THE SKIN

In our studies of the skin of adult BALB/c nu/nu recipients of day 16 fetal thymocytes, 8-12 weeks after reconstitution, the distribution of CD3⁺ Vγ5/Vδ1⁺ DETC was never uniform throughout body wall epidermis; some areas of skin had relatively normal densities, but large areas were devoid of any Vγ5/Vδ1⁺ DETC. Furthermore, ear epidermis of adult nude recipients of day 16 fetal thymocytes never contained detectable Vγ5Vδ1⁺ DETC. On the other hand, when day 16 fetal thymocytes were injected into newborn nu/nu recipients and the skin analyzed 8-12 weeks later, Vγ5Vδ1⁺ DETC were always found in sheets of ear epidermis and were much more consistently found in epidermis obtained from body wall skin.

Several observations influenced our decision to examine the role of hair follicle cycling in the above distributions of DETC in recipients of early fetal thymocytes. The first relates to the fact that there is conspicuous regional variation in DETC density (i.e., different anatomic sites on the same animal) which may relate to hair follicles/hair growth. For example, normal footpad epidermis has an extremely low density of DETC (Shiohara et al., 1990a). Further-more, in several mouse strains, DETC density in ear epidermis is considerably lower (4-20 fold) than it is in trunk skin epidermis from the same animal (Bergstresser et al., 1985). While the reasons for such regional variability are not known, they may relate to the facts that footpad skin lacks hair follicles and that hair follicle cycling patterns may be distinctly different for body wall skin than for skin on the crown of the head (and most likely also ear skin).

Although follicular keratinization is abnormal in nude mice, hair follicles are present in normal numbers and do undergo normal follicle cycling (Rigdon & Packchanian, 1974; Eaton, 1977). Hair follicle cycling in mice is markedly different from the basically random cycling pattern which occurs in man. In mice, entry into anagen is synchronized and occurs in one contiguous region after another, producing "waves" of hair growth which move in predictable, head-to-tail patterns (Dry, 1926; Chase & Eaton, 1959; Eaton, 1977). In nude mice these waves are visible as areas of obviously thickened skin (secondary to expanding follicles in the dermis) with barely visible hairs broken off near the skin surface. Newborn mice are hairless, but the initial wave of anagen begins very shortly after birth and rapidly progresses over virtually the entire skin surface, including the crown of the head and ear buds (Chase, 1954). This initial anagen cycle is then followed (at several week intervals) by slower, periodic head-to-tail waves; thus it is likely that, in adult mice, the follicles in some portion of the skin will be in anagen at any given time. In adult mice, however, two factors substantially increase the probability that the region of skin in anagen will be on the trunk rather than the ears. The first is a simple size consideration, the ears being small compared to the entire trunk. Second, in the subsequent waves of hair growth that follow the initial neonatal total body anagen cycle, "lag areas" occur, i.e., regions that skip a wave. Common lag areas are the tail and the crown of the head (very possibly including the ears) (Chase & Eaton, 1959).

Thus, the observed distributions of DETC in newborn and adult nude recipients of fetal thymocytes could be explained if factors relating to active hair growth were involved in the localization and/or proliferation of fetal thymocytes in the skin. The probability of both ear and trunk skin being in anagen at or near the time of injection of fetal thymocytes would be much greater in newborn recipients than in adult recipients. To test this hypothesis, regions of trunk skin of adult nude mice which were obviously in anagen were outlined with a permanent marker immediately prior to injection of fetal thymocytes. Eight weeks later epidermal sheets were prepared from skin which had either been in or out of active hair growth at the time of injection. $V\gamma5V\delta1^+$ DETC were found exclusively in skin sites which had been in anagen at the time of injection. These results are consistent with an important role for cycling hair follicles in determining the density of $\gamma\delta^+$ DETC in adult mouse skin.

The mechanisms by which cycling follicles contribute to the adult DETC density remains to be determined. Conceivably they could participate by affecting the initial localization of fetal thymocyte precursors and/or their subsequent in situ proliferation. Initial localization in regions of active hair growth could be simply the consequence of the obviously increased blood flow through skin containing anagen hair bulbs surrounded by a rich vascular network. We increased blood flow in ear and trunk skin (both in inactive and active hair growth at the time) by epicutaneous application of an irritating concentration of the contact sensitizer, dinitrofluorbenzene. Twenty-four hours later, when the ears were obviously erythematous, day 16 fetal thymocytes were injected. Analysis of DETC density 8 weeks later again revealed that DETC localized exclusively in trunk skin where follicles had been in anagen at the time of injection; no DETC were found in the ear or in trunk skin sites of DNFB-induced hyperemia which were not in anagen at the time of injection; i.e., simple hyperemia did not increase localization of DETC precursors. By analogy with other models of selective lymphocyte migration/recirculation, however, it is still possible that fetal thymocyte precursors of DETC have a special affinity for anagen follicle endothelial cells on the basis of a reciprocal expression of appropriate "homing receptors" on the DETC precursors and "addressins" on those particular endothelial cells.

Alternatively, following the arrival of small numbers of fetal thymocytes in the skin, factor(s) expressed within the microenvironment of anagen hair follicles may stimulate the in situ proliferation of $V\gamma5/V\delta1^+$ DETC. Such factors could be antigen (and TCR) independent, i.e., cytokine growth factors. A more intriguing possibility, however, is that such in situ proliferation is the result of localized, transient expression of the physiologic ligand (antigen) for the Vγ5/Vδ1$^+$ TCR selectively expressed by DETC.

Preliminary studies comparing the densities of Vγ5/Vδ1$^+$ and/or CD3$^+$ DETC in normal mice at different times after birth have provided data consistent with the above possibility. In the newborn epidermis, the density of CD3$^+$ cells (i.e., all T cells, irrespective of the specific TCR they also express) is very low, but increases dramatically during the first few weeks of life (Elbe et al., 1989). We found the density of CD3$^+$ cells in newborn C57BL/6 ear epidermis to be only 10% of that seen in 8 week old mice. While >98% of the CD3$^+$ cells in adult epidermis also stained with the monoclonal antibody, 17D1 (i.e., were Vγ5/Vδ1$^+$), only approximately 50% of the CD3$^+$ T cells in one day old epidermis expressed the DETC-type TCR. By one week, CD3$^+$ cell density was 25% of adult levels, and 80% of these cells were also Vγ5/Vδ1$^+$. By three weeks, CD3$^+$ densities were equivalent to those in adult mice, and 95% of the CD3$^+$ cells were Vγ5/Vδ1$^+$. These results not only reiterate the fact that the density of intraepidermal T cells increases dramatically during the neonatal period, but suggest that there is preferential proliferation of CD3$^+$ cells expressing the DETC-type TCR. Analysis of the densities of CD3$^+$ Vγ5/Vδ1$^+$ (prototypic DETC TCR) and CD3$^+$ Vγ5/Vδ1$^-$ ("atypical" DETC TCR) at various ages reveals that while there is a striking increase in density of cells with prototypic DETC TCRs, the density of CD3$^+$ Vγ5/Vδ1$^-$ cells remains essentially constant with time. Such results are consistent with the possibility that the density and TCR homogeneity of the DETC present in normal adult skin are a result, at least in part, of preferential proliferation of Vγ5/Vδ1$^+$ DETC in response to expression of the physiologic ligand for this TCR in the microenvironment of anagen hair follicles.

RESPONSE OF DETC TO STRESSED EPIDERMAL CELLS

The unique properties of $\gamma\delta$ T cells such as DETC have raised the possibility that these cells play distinctive roles in host immunity and/or immunopathology compared to conventional $\alpha\beta$ T cells. One of the most conspicuous features of conventional recirculating $\alpha\beta$ T cells, as well as of the typically minor subset of $\gamma\delta^+$ T cells found in the blood or peripheral lymphoid tissues of mice and humans, is their collective TCR heterogeneity. Such heterogeneity is presumably reflective of their (collective) abilities to recognize the myriad of distinct antigenic specificities to which the host may be exposed. Furthermore, the ready capacity of these cells to recirculate throughout the body maximizes the opportunities for a particular T cell bearing a particular TCR to confront its physiologic antigen. By contrast, DETC, given their apparent restriction in adult mice to the epidermis, do not have this opportunity, but rather are likely to contact only those cells in their immediate microenvironment. In addition, the virtually complete homogeneity of the TCRs expressed by adult DETC effectively limits the range of antigens recognizable by DETC to a single ligand.

These properties led to the hypothesis that $\gamma\delta$ cells such as DETC participate in immune surveillance by recognizing a common self-antigen expressed by keratinocytes or other cells in their immediate microenvironment under a variety of potentially harmful conditions (Asarnow et al., 1988; Janeway et al., 1988). A prime candidate for such a self-antigen is a member of one of the families of stress-induced proteins, otherwise known as heat shock proteins (HSPs). HSPs are among the most highly conserved families of proteins known, being present in all prokaryotic and eukaryotic cells examined, where they perform a variety of as yet incompletely understood, but vital, functions, including assisting in protein folding and transport between intracellular compartments (Lindquist & Craig, 1988; Young, 1990; Kaufmann, 1990). Normally, HSPs are present at undetectable or relatively low levels, but, in response to potentially damaging stimuli, they accumulate rapidly. Stresses inducing HSP synthesis include heat shock, nutrient deprivation, infection with intracellular pathogens, oxidizing agents, heavy metal ions, and malignant transformation (Kaufmann, 1990). DETC are ideally positioned to respond to self-HSPs on stressed/altered epidermal cells. Furthermore, several HSP families have been shown to be major targets in immune responses to bacteria, protozoa, and helminths (Kaufmann, 1990; Kaufmann et al., 1991). Because of the high degree of evolutionary conservation among HSPs, DETC might also recognize homologs of self-HSPs expressed by invading organisms. Indeed, recent data examining the antigenic specificity of another distinct subset of mouse $\gamma\delta$ cells (present in newborn thymus and adult peripheral lymphoid tissues and expressing junctionally diverse Vγ1/Vδ6 TCRs) has recently been shown to be stimulated by a member of the 60 kilodalton (kDa) family of HSPs which is present both on autologous cells and in purified fractions from mycobacterial extracts (O'Brien et al., 1989; Born et al., 1990).

To test the above hypothesis, we recently tested the capacity of a Vγ5/Vδ1$^+$ DETC line (established by stimulation with immobilized anti-CD3 and maintained in vitro with IL-2) to respond to heat shocked or nutrient deprived epidermal cells (Lewis & Tigelaar, 1989). Exposure of this line to syngeneic epidermal cells pretreated by brief heat shock (42°C for 2 hours) or nutrient deprivation (culture for 48 hours in medium devoid of keratinocyte growth factors) resulted in brisk proliferation and secretion of IL-2. Equivalent results were obtained using stressed epidermal cells depleted of both Langerhans cells and DETC, suggesting that stressed keratinocytes express the stimulatory antigen and that conventional antigen presenting cells are not required for recognition/stimulation. Obviously, these results do not exclude the possibility that other stressed epidermal cells, including melanocytes, Langerhans cells or DETC themselves, cannot also activate DETC. That DETC recognition of stressed keratinocytes occurs via the TCR is strongly suggested by the capacity of Fab fragments of monoclonal antibody 17D1 (specific for Vγ5/Vδ1$^+$ cells) to block completely the responses of the DETC line to stressed epidermal cells. That the ligand for the DETC TCR is distinct from the 60 kDa HSP which triggers another subset of murine $\gamma\delta$ cells (Vγ1/Vδ6$^+$) is suggested by the failure of DETC to respond to either tuberculin purified protein derivative (PPD) or crude mycobacterial extracts, even in the presence of added epidermal or splenic antigen presenting cells.

Given the restricted tissue distribution of DETC, one might expect the antigen recognized by DETC (and/or the restricting element on which the ligand is presented, if such restricting elements are required) to be similarly confined to the epidermis. Indeed, studies to date have shown that DETC which proliferate in response to stressed epidermal cells do not respond to either stressed splenic adherent cells or to stressed dermal fibroblasts; however, more stringent tests of the site restriction of antigen/restricting element expression, such as other stressed epithelial cells (e.g., from the gastrointestinal or reproductive tracts), have yet to be performed.

Finally, the equivalent stimulatory capacities of stressed syngeneic or stressed allogeneic epidermal cells strongly suggest that, if the DETC ligand is presented on a restricting molecule, then this restricting element is not likely to be a conventional member of the polymorphic class I or class II MHC families, the presenting molecules for most $\alpha\beta$ T cells. Theoretically attractive alternative restricting element(s) for DETC (and other subsets of epitheliotropic $\gamma\delta$ cells) are the genetically much less polymorphic class Ib molecules (e.g., CD1 and TL), so named because of their genetic and structural similarities with conventional class I MHC molecules, including their similar association with $\beta2$ microglobulin (Strominger, 1989). Some of this theoretical appeal lies in the fact that expression of class Ib is both tissue specific and dependent on the state of activation or differentiation of a cell (Bonneville et al., 1989). Not only have several reports shown that some $\gamma\delta$ cells recognize and/or are restricted by class Ib molecules (Bonneville et al., 1989; Vidovic et al., 1989; Porcelli et al., 1989), but more recent data has shown that particular mouse TL genes are expressed in some epithelia (i.e., intestinal), but not in others (i.e, skin) (Wu et al., 1991).

EFFECTS OF IN SITU STRESSES ON DETC

Prompted by the responses of our DETC line to epidermal cells stressed in vitro, we investigated the effect of in situ perturbations of the skin on DETC. Within one week of epicutaneous application of the primary irritant, croton oil, or the contact sensitizer, DNFB, striking alterations were noted in both the density and morphology of $V\gamma5/V\delta1^+$ DETC. The density was increased 2-3 fold over controls, and the proportion of $V\gamma5/V\delta1^+$ cells which were round rather than dendritic was increased, including pairs of round cells, suggesting in situ proliferation of DETC in response to these stresses (Miyauchi & Hashimoto, 1989). The facts that these increases in $V\gamma5/V\delta1^+$ density were totally unaffected by prior adult thymectomy, but were blocked by X-irradiation immediately prior to skin painting, are both consistent with this possibility. In addition, epidermal cells from sites painted with croton oil 16 hours earlier were able to stimulate brisk in vitro proliferation of the DETC line with any additional pretreatment, while epidermal cells from untreated mice only stimulated proliferation after in vitro heat shock or nutrient deprivation.

We have also examined $V\gamma5/V\delta1^+$ DETC densities in the skin of C57BL6 vit/vit mice, a spontaneous mutant strain which exhibits relatively normally pigmentation at birth (except for a piebald patch of variable size), but which at approximately two months begins to undergo progressive graying (with loss of melanocytes) with each successive wave of active hair growth (Rheins et al., 1986; Lerner et al., 1986). As in human vitiligo, it is not certain whether the melanocyte loss represents a primary melanocyte defect or a primary autoimmune disease.

Nevertheless, it is clear that the skin of these mice is significantly perturbed during this process. We found that ageing vit/vit mice had densities of Vγ5/Vδ1$^+$ DETC approximately twice those seen in age-matched normal C57BL/6 mice, and, similar to skin sites undergoing contact dermatitis, many of these cells were round and pairs of round cells were readily found. These studies confirm and extend those of Amornsiripanitch et al. (1988), who first reported an increase in density of Thy-1$^+$ cells (not further phenotyped) in ageing vit/vit mice. While the above alterations in DETC are very consistent with their recognition of, and activation by, a stress-associated molecule expressed in the environment of depigmenting skin, further studies are required to determine whether the melanocytes, themselves, express the DETC ligand, or whether the loss of melanocytes is a consequence of this recognition.

Collectively, the above results are consistent with the hypothesis that the physiologic antigen for Vγ5/Vδ1$^+$ DETC is a stress-associated ligand which is expressed by keratinocytes and perhaps other epidermal cells in their immediate microenvironment after a variety of stimuli. While these stimuli may commonly be associated with pathologic processes, expression of the identical ligand may also be up-regulated during physiological processes (e.g., active hair growth).

RELATIONSHIP(S) OF MURINE DETC TO γδ CELL IN HUMAN SKIN

It is clear that the precise human equivalent of mouse DETC i.e., a readily detectable network of γδ cells with a strikingly monomorphic TCR identical to those expressed on the first "wave" of early fetal thymocytes, does not exist. The resident population of CD3$^+$ T cells (either γδ or αβ) in normal human epidermis is small and not strikingly dendritic (Groh et al., 1989; Bucy et al., 1989; Bos et al., 1989; Foster et al., 1990; Dupuy et al., 1990). Also, while a greater proportion of CD3$^+$ cells in the epidermis express γδ TCRs than in the dermis (indicating a modest preferential epidermotropism), γδ cells are significantly outnumbered in both sites by αβ cells (Bos et al., 1989; Dupuy et al., 1990; Foster et al., 1990). Furthermore, recent PCR analysis of the TCR γδ repertoire in normal human skin revealed relatively polymorphic receptors with no preferential utilization (compared to blood) of particular Vδ gene segments and considerable junctional diversity (Modlin et al., 1991).

In lepromin skin test sites, the overlying epidermis is significantly enriched (compared to the dermis) for γδ cells expressing the Vδ1-Jδ1 coding segments, suggesting preferential migration into, retention in, or in situ proliferation of this subset in the epidermis (Modlin et al., 1991); however, such sites still contained a relatively low density of γδ cells compared to that seen in normal mouse epidermis. Furthermore, while PCR analysis of TCR gene utilization in such lepromin skin test sites revealed limited heterogeneity (Modlin *et al.*, 1991), this oligoclonality had the features of antigen-driven selective proliferation of specific cells from a heterogeneous pool, rather than the in situ proliferation of a resident population of cells with homogeneous TCRs.

The reason(s) for such species differences in intraepidermal $\gamma\delta$ cells remain poorly understood. One potential explanation for the lack of a regular network of $\gamma\delta$ DETC in humans could relate to the significant differences in early fetal thymic development in mice and humans. In mice, the fetal thymocytes which express TCRs identical to those on DETC, which clearly can act as DETC precursors, and which are not found in the blood in significant numbers in adult mice, are the first TCR-bearing thymocytes to appear in the fetal thymus, preceding by several days the appearance of significant numbers of other $\gamma\delta$ or $\alpha\beta$ cells. By contrast, during human early fetal thymic ontogeny, $\alpha\beta$ cells apparently outnumber $\gamma\delta$ cells at all times (Haynes et al., 1988).

Furthermore, while the earliest population of human $\gamma\delta$ thymocytes does have limited TCR heterogeneity and junctional diversity, this same subset re-emerges as the major population of $\gamma\delta$ cells recirculating in adult peripheral blood (Krangel et al., 1990; McVay et al., 1991; Parker et al., 1990). Another potential factor to explain these differences may involve differential expression in mice and humans of those intraepidermal ligands which are ultimately responsible for positioning of mouse DETC within the basal layer of keratinocytes; however, those factors must first be characterized in mice, then human epidermis can be probed for the presence or absence of similar ligands. The role of hair follicle cycling in the localization and in situ proliferation of intraepidermal $\gamma\delta$ cells has just begun to be examined; it is possible that factors related to the obvious differences in body hair between mice and humans account for the differences in density of $\gamma\delta$ cells in mouse and human epidermis.

Finally, the absence of a precise morphologic homolog of murine DETC in human epidermis does not speak to the ultimately more relevant, but currently unanswered question of whether humans have a biologically relevant equivalent to this unusual subset of mouse T cells, i.e., cells that can carry out similar physiologic and/or pathologic roles in vivo. In other words, it is conceivable that the biologic roles of a sessile, nonrecirculating intraepidermal network of $\gamma\delta$ cells with monomorphic TCRs in mice have been assumed by some other, perhaps recirculating cell(s) in humans, e.g., the oligoclonal $\gamma\delta$ cells present in lepromin skin test sites (Modlin et al., 1991). It is obvious, however, that to answer this question, one must first understand the physiologic and/or pathologic roles of mouse DETC. Unfortunately, as is the case for all $\gamma\delta$ cells studied to date, whether in mice, humans or any other species, these roles are not yet known.

To date, interpretations of available data have centered around the possibility that DETC represent a rapid, first line of local defense called into play in a broad variety of situations which, if unchecked, would compromise the skin's functions (e.g., as a barrier). The hypothesis has been forwarded that mouse DETC function in immune surveillance through recognition of a common self-antigen expressed by cells in their immediate microenvironment under a variety of potentially harmful situations. Such a role might well involve recognizing, and then effecting the removal, either directly or indirectly, of damaged, altered or transformed keratinocytes, melanocytes, etc. On the other hand, it is equally possible that DETC function to downregulate intracutaneous responses mediated by conventional $\alpha\beta$ (or $\gamma\delta$) T cells and which, if unchecked, would compromise the skin's functional integrity. A rather substantial body of data has been generated which is consistent with such a suppressor role for DETC (Sullivan et al., 1986; Amornsiripanitch et al., 1988; Bigby et al., 1989; Cruz et al., 1989; Shiohara et al., 1990a; 1990b). Still another potential role for DETC or other $\gamma\delta$ cells expressing TCRs which may recognize self antigens involves their participating as aggressor (effector) cells in autoimmune diseases.

The absence of a precise morphologic homolog of murine DETC in human skin has opened the door to whispers (whispers so as not to hurt the feelings of individuals studying mouse DETC!) that further detailed examination of mouse DETC is irrelevant to human biology. It is clearly premature to adopt such a stance. For until the murine DETC ligand has been definitively identified and cloned and its potential homolog sought in human skin, and until, in a variety of experimental models, the consequences of the selective depletion from and/or addition to otherwise normal mice of DETC are known, we cannot rationally address the issue of the potential relevance of this unique constituent of SALT in mice to human cutaneous immunity and immunopathology.

ACKNOWLEDGEMENT

This investigation was supported by the National Institutes of Health Grant AI 27404 awarded to R.E.T.

REFERENCES

Amornsiripanitch S, LM Barnes, JJ Nordlund, LS Trinkle and LA Rheins, 1988. Immune studies in the depigmenting C57BL/Ler-vit/vit mice: An apparent isolated loss of contact hypersensitivity. **J. Immunol.**, 140:3438.

Asarnow DM, T Goodman, L Lefrancois and JP Allison, 1989. Distinct antigen receptor repertoires of two classes of murine epithelium-associated T cells. **Nature**, 341:60.

Asarnow DM, WA Kuziel, M Bonyhadi, RE Tigelaar, PW Tucker and JP Allison, 1988. Limited diversity of antigen receptor genes of Thy-1+ dendritic epidermal cells. **Cell**, 55:837.

Bergstresser PR, S Sullivan, JW Streilein and RE Tigelaar, 1985. Origin and function of Thy-1+ dendritic epidermal cells in mice. **J. Invest. Dermatol.**, 85:85S.

Bergstresser PR, RE Tigelaar, JH Dees and JW Streilein, 1983. Thy-1 antigen-bearing dendritic cells populate murine epidermis. **J. Invest. Dermatol.**, 81:286.

Bigby M, R Vargas and M-S Sy, 1989. Production of hapten-specific T cell hybridomas and their use to study the effect of ultraviolet B irradiation on the development of contact hypersensitivity. **J. Immunol.**, 143:3867.

Bonneville M, K Ito, EG Krecko, S Itohara, D Kappes, I Ishida, O Kanagawa, CA Janeway Jr, DB Murphy and S Tonegawa, 1989. Recognition of a self major histocompatibility complex TL region product by $\gamma\delta$ T-cell receptors. **Proc. Natl. Acad. Sci. USA,** 86:5928.

Bonneville M, CA Janeway, K Ito, W Haser, I Ishida, N Nakanishi and S Tonegawa, 1988. Intestinal intraepithelial lymphocytes are a distinct set of $\gamma\delta$ T cells. **Nature,** 336:479.

Bonyhadi M, A Weiss, PW Tucker, RE Tigelaar and JP Allison, 1987. Delta is the C_x-gene product in the γ/δ antigen receptor of dendritic epidermal cells. **Nature,** 330:574.

Born W, L Hall, A Dallas, J Boymel, T Shinnick, D Young, P Brennan and R O'Brien, 1990. Recognition of a peptide antigen by heat shock-reactive $\gamma\delta$ T lymphocytes. **Science,** 249:67.

Bos JD, MBM Teunissen, I Cairo, SR Krieg, ML Kapsenberg, PK Das and J Borst, 1989. Expression of TCR $\gamma\delta$ and TCR $\alpha\beta$ in normal human skin. **J. Invest. Dermatol.,** 93:296(A).

Bucy RP, C-LH Chen and MD Cooper, 1989. Tissue localization and CD8 accessory molecule expression of T$\gamma\delta$ cells in humans. **J. Immunol.,** 142:3045.

Caughman SW, SM Breathnach, SO Sharrow, DA Stephany and SI Katz, 1986. Culture and characterization of murine dendritic Thy-1 epidermal cells. **J. Invest. Dermatol.,** 86:615.

Chase HB, 1954. Growth of the hair. **Physiol. Rev.,** 34:113.

Chase HB and GJ Eaton, 1959. The growth of hair follicles in waves. **Ann. NY Acad. Sci.,** 83:365.

Chien Y-H, M Iwashima, DA Wettstein, KB Kaplan, JF Elliott, W Born and MM Davis, 1987. T-cell receptor δ gene rearrangements in early thymocytes. **Nature,** 330:722.

Cruz PD, Jr, J Nixon-Fulton, RE Tigelaar and PR Bergstresser, 1989. Disparate effects of in vitro low-dose UVB irradiation on intravenous immunization with purified epidermal cell subpopulations for the induction of contact hypersensitivity. **J. Invest. Dermatol.,** 92:160.

Dry FW, 1926. Coat of the mouse *(Mus musculus)*. **J. Genet.,** 16:87.

Dupuy P, M Heslan, S Fraitag, T Hercend, L Dubertret and M Bagot, 1990. T-cell receptor-γ/δ bearing lymphocytes in normal and inflammatory human skin. **J. Invest. Dermatol.,** 94:764.

Eaton GJ, 1977. Hair growth waves and cycles in nude mice. In: **Proceedings of the Second International Workshop on Nude Mice,** University of Tokyo Press/Gustav Fischer Verlag, Stuttgart, p. 89-93.

Elbe A, E Tschachler, G Steiner, A Binder, K Wolff and G Stingl, 1989. Maturational steps of bone marrow derived dendritic murine epidermal cells: Phenotypic and functional studies on Langerhans cells and Thy-1 dendritic epidermal cells in the perinatal period. **J. Immunol.,** 143:2431.

Elliott JF, EP Rock, PA Patten, MM Davis, and Y-H Chien, 1988. The adult T-cell receptor δ-chain is diverse and distinct from that of fetal thymocytes. **Nature,** 331:627.

Foster CA, H Yokozeki, K Rappersberger, F Koning, B Volc-Platzer, A Rieger, JE Coligan, K Wolff, and G Stingl, 1990. Human epidermal T cells predominately belong to the lineage expressing α/β T cell receptor. **J. Exp. Med.**, 171:997.

Garman RD, PJ Doherty and DH Raulet, 1986. Diversity, rearrangement and expression of murine T cell gamma genes. **Cell**, 45:733.

Groh V, S Porcelli, M Fabbi, LL Lanier, LJ Picker, T Anderson, RA Warnke, AK Bhan, JL Strominger and MB Brenner, 1989. Human lymphocytes bearing T cell receptor γ/δ are phenotypically diverse and evenly distributed throughout the lymphoid system. **J. Exp. Med.**, 169:1277.

Guy-Grand D, N Cerf-Bensussan, B Malissen, M Malassis-Seris, C Briottet and P Vassalli, 1991. Two gut intraepithelial CD8+ lymphocyte populations with different T cell receptors: A role for the gut epithelium in T cell differentiation. **J. Exp. Med.**, 173:471.

Havran WL and JP Allison, 1988. Developmentally ordered appearance of thymocytes expressing different T-cell antigen receptors. **Nature**, 335:443.

Havran WL and JP Allison, 1990. Origin of Thy-1+ dendritic epidermal cells of adult mice from fetal thymic precursors. **Nature**, 344:68.

Havran WL, S Grell, G Duwe, J Kimura, A Wilson, AM Kruisbeek, RL O'Brien, W Born, RE Tigelaar and JP Allison, 1989. Limited diversity of T-cell receptor γ-chain expression of murine Thy-1+ dendritic epidermal cells revealed by Vγ3-specific monoclonal antibody. **Proc. Natl. Acad. Sci. USA**, 86:4185.

Havran WL, M Poenie, RE Tigelaar, RY Tsien and JP Allison, 1989. Phenotypic and functional analysis of gamma/δ T cell receptor-positive murine dendritic epidermal clones. **J. Immunol.**, 142:1422.

Haynes BF, KH Singer, SM Denning and ME Martin, 1988. Analysis of expression of CD2, CD3, and T cell antigen receptor molecules during early human fetal thymic development. **J. Immunol.**, 141:3776.

Ito K, M Bonneville, Y Takagaki, N Nakanishi, O Kanagawa, EG Krecko and S Tonegawa, 1989. Different $\gamma\delta$ T-cell receptors are expressed on thymocytes at different stages of development. **Proc. Natl. Acad. Sci. USA**, 86:631.

Itohara S, AG Farr, JJ Lafaille, M Bonneville, Y Takagaki, W Haas and S Tonegawa, 1990. Homing of a $\gamma\delta$ thymocyte subset with homogeneous T-cell receptors to mucosal epithelia. **Nature**, 343:754.

Janeway CA Jr, B Jones and A Hayday, 1988. Specificity and function of T cells bearing $\gamma\delta$ receptors. **Immunol. Today**, 9:73.

Kaufmann SHE, 1990. Heat shock proteins and the immune response. **Immunol. Today**, 11:129.

Kaufmann SHE, B Schoel, JDA Van Embden, T Koga, A Wand-Wurttenberger, ME Munk and U Steinhoff, 1991. Heat shock protein 60: Implications for pathogenesis of and protection against bacterial infections. **Immunol. Reviews**, 121:67.

Krangel MS, H Yssel, C Brocklehurst and H Spits, 1990. A distinct wave of human T cell receptor γδ lymphocytes in the early fetal thymus: Evidence for controlled gene rearrangement and cytokine production. **J. Exp. Med.**, 172:847.

Kuziel WA, J Lewis, J Nixon-Fulton, RE Tigelaar and PW Tucker, 1991. Murine epidermal γδ T cells express Fcγ Receptor II encoded by the FcγRα gene. **Eur. J. Immunol.**, 21: 1563.

Kuziel WA, A Takashima, M Bonyhadi, PR Bergstresser, JP Allison, RE Tigelaar and PW Tucker, 1987. Regulation of T-cell receptor γ-chain RNA expression in murine Thy-1 dendritic epidermal cells. **Nature**, 328:263.

Kyes S, E Carew, SR Carding, CA Janeway Jr and A Hayday, 1989. Diversity in T-cell receptor γ gene usage in intestinal epithelium. **Proc. Natl. Acad. Sci. USA,** 86:5527.

Lafaille JJ, A DeCloux, M Bonneville, Y Takagaki and S Tonegawa, 1989. Junctional sequences of T cell receptor γδ genes: Implications for γδ T cell lineages and for a novel intermediate of V-(D)-J joining. **Cell**, 59:859.

Lerner AB, T Shiohara, RE Boissy, KA Jacobson, ML Lamoreux and GE Moellmann, 1986. A mouse model for vitiligo. **J. Invest. Dermatol.**, 87:299.

Lewis JM and RE Tigelaar, 1989. Thymic dependence of Thy-1 dendritic epidermal cells (DEC). **J. Invest. Dermatol.**, 92:471A.

Lewis JM and RE Tigelaar, 1991. Recognition of an epidermal stress antigen by murine γ/δ dendritic epidermal T cells (DETC). **J. Invest. Dermatol.**, 96:538A.

Lindquist S and EA Craig, 1988. The heat-shock proteins. **Annu. Rev. Genet.**, 22:631.

McVay LD, SR Carding, K Bottomly and AC Hayday, 1991. Regulated expression and structure of T cell receptor gamma/δ transcripts in human thymic ontogeny. **EMBO J.**, 10: 83.

Miyauchi S and K Hashimoto, 1989. Thy-1 dendritic epidermal cells undergo mitosis in vivo. **J. Invest. Dermatol.**, 93:429.

Modlin RL, J Lewis, K Uyemura and RE Tigelaar, 1992. T-lymphocytes bearing γδ antigen receptors in skin. **Chem. Immunol.**, 53:61.

Mosmann TR and RL Coffman, 1989. Heterogeneity of cytokine secretion patterns and functions of helper T cells. **Adv. Immunol.**, 46:111.

Nixon-Fulton JL, PR Bergstresser and RE Tigelaar, 1986. Thy-1+ epidermal cells proliferate in response to concanavalin A and interleukin 2. **J. Immunol.**, 136:2776.

Nixon-Fulton JL, J Hackett, PR Bergstresser, V Kumar and Tigelaar, 1988. Phenotypic heterogeneity and cytotoxic activity of Con A and IL-2-stimulated cultures of mouse Thy-1+ epidermal cells. **J. Invest. Dermatol.**, 91:62.

Nixon-Fulton JL, WA Kuziel, B Santerse, PR Bergstresser, PW Tucker and RE Tigelaar, 1988. Thy-1+ epidermal cells in nude mice are distinct from their counterparts in thymus-bearing mice. A study of morphology, function, and T cell receptor expression. **J. Immunol.**, 141:1897.

Nixon-Fulton JL, PL Witte, RE Tigelaar, PR Bergstresser and V Kumar, 1987. Lack of dendritic Thy-1+ epidermal cells in mice with severe combined immunodeficiency disease. **J. Immunol.**, 138:2902.

O'Brien RL, MP Happ, A Dallas, E Palmer, R Kubo and WK Born, 1989. Stimulation of a major subset of lymphocytes expressing T cell receptor γδ by an antigen derived from *Mycobacterium tuberculosis*. **Cell**, 57:667.

Parker CM, V Groh, H Band, SA Porcelli, C Morita, M Fabbi, D Glass, JL Strominger and MB Brenner, 1990. Evidence for extrathymic changes in the T cell receptor γ/δ repertoire. **J. Exp. Med.**, 171:1597.

Payer E, A Elbe and G Stingl, 1991. Circulating CD3+/T cell receptor Vγ3+ fetal murine thymocytes home to the skin and give rise to proliferating dendritic epidermal T cells. **J. Immunol.**, 146:2536.

Porcelli S, MB Brenner, JL Greenstein, SP Balk, C Terhorst and PA Bleicher, 1989. Recognition of cluster of differentiation 1 antigens by human CD4-CD8- cytolytic T lymphocytes. **Nature**, 341:447.

Rheins LA, MR Palkowski and JJ Nordlund, 1986. Alterations in cutaneous immune reactivity to dinitrofluorobenzene in graying C57BL/vit/vit mice. **J. Invest. Dermatol.**, 86:539.

Rigdon RH and AA Packchanian, 1974. Histologic study of the skin of congenitally athymic "nude" mice. **Tex. Rep. Biol. Med.**, 32:711.

Rocha B, P Vassalli and D Guy-Grand, 1991. The Vβ repertoire of mouse gut homodimeric α CD8+ intraepithelial T cell receptor α/β+ lymphocytes reveals a major extrathymic pathway of T cell differentiation. **J. Exp. Med.**, 173:483.

Romani N, G Stingl, E Tschachler, MD Witmer, RM Steinman, EM Shevach and G Schuler, 1985. The Thy-1-bearing cell of murine epidermis. **J. Exp. Med.**, 161:1368.

Rocken M, KM Muller, J-H Saurat and C Hauser, 1991. Lectin-mediated induction of IL-4-producing CD4+ T cells. **J. Immunol.**, 146:577.

Shiohara T, N Moriya, C Gotoh, J Hayakawa, M Nagashima, K Saizawa and H Ishikawa, 1990a. Loss of epidermal integrity by T cell-mediated attack induces long-term local resistance to subsequent attack. I. Induction of resistance correlates with increases in Thy-1+ epidermal cell numbers. **J. Exp. Med.**, 171:1027.

Shiohara T, N Moriya, C Gotoh, J Hayakawa, H Ishikawa, K Saizawa and M Nagashima, 1990b. Loss of epidermal integrity by T cell-mediated attack induces long term local resistance to subsequent attack: II. Thymus dependency in the induction of the resistance. **J. Immunol.**, 145:2482.

Steiner G, F Koning, A Elbe, E Tschachler, WM Yokoyama, EM Shevach, G Stingl and JE Coligan, 1988. Characterization of T cell receptors on resident murine dendritic epidermal T cells. **Eur. J. Immunol.**, 18:1323.

Stingl G, KC Gunter, E Tschachler, H Yamada, RI Lechler, WM Yokoyama, G Steiner, RN Germain and EM Shevach, 1987. Thy-1+ dendritic epidermal cells belong to the T-cell lineage. **Proc. Natl. Acad. Sci. USA**, 84:2430.

Stingl G, F Koning, H Yamada, WM Yokoyama, E Tschachler, JA Bluestone, G Steiner, LE Samelson, AM Lew, JE Coligan and EM Shevach, 1987. Thy-1+ dendritic epidermal cells express T3 antigen and the T-cell receptor γ chain. **Proc. Natl. Acad. Sci. USA**, 84:4586.

Strominger JL, 1989. The $\gamma\delta$ T cell receptor and class Ib MHC-related proteins: Enigmatic molecules of immune recognition. **Cell**, 57:895.

Sullivan S, PR Bergstresser, RE Tigelaar and JW Streilein, 1986. Induction and regulation of contact hypersensitivity by resident, bone marrow-derived, dendritic epidermal cells: Langerhans cells and Thy-1 epidermal cells. **J. Immunol.**, 137:2460.

Takagaki Y, A DeCloux, M Bonneville and S Tonegawa, 1989. Diversity of $\gamma\delta$ T-cell receptors on murine intestinal intra-epithelial lymphocytes. **Nature**, 339:712.

Takashima A, JL Nixon-Fulton, PR Bergstresser and RE Tigelaar, 1988. Thy-1 dendritic epidermal cells in mice: Precursor frequency analysis and cloning of Concanavalin A-reactive cells. **J. Invest. Dermatol.**, 90:671.

Tigelaar RE, JM Lewis and PR Bergstresser, 1990. TCR gamma/δ+ dendritic epidermal T cells as constituents of skin-associated lymphoid tissue. **J. Invest. Dermatol.**, 94 Suppl.:58S.

Tschachler E, G Schuler, J Hutterer, H Leibl, K Wolff and G Stingl, 1983. Expression of Thy-1 antigen by murine epidermal cells. **J. Invest. Dermatol.**, 81:282.

Vidovic D, M Roglic, K McKune, S Guerder, C MacKay and Z Dembic, 1989. Qa-1 restricted recognition of foreign antigen by a $\gamma\delta$ T-cell hybridoma. **Nature**, 340:646.

Wu M, L Van Kaer, S Itohara and S Tonegawa, 1991. Highly restricted expression of the thymus leukemia antigens on intestinal epithelial cells. **J. Exp. Med.**, 174:213.

Young RA, 1990. Stress proteins and immunology. **Annu. Rev. Immunol.**, 8:401.

MORPHO-ANTIGENIC FEATURES OF DENDRITIC CELLS AS A CLUE TO THE INTERPRETATION OF SKIN IMMUNE SYSTEM-RELATED DISORDERS

Nicola Pimpinelli*
Paolo Romagnoli†
Marco Santucci‡
Benvenuto Giannotti*

*   Dermatology Clinic II
†   Department of Human Anatomy and Histology, Section "E. Allara"
‡   Institute of Morbid Anatomy and Histopathology
University of Florence
Florence, Italy

Correspondence to: Dr. N. Pimpinelli, Clin. Dermatol. II,
Univ. degli Studi, Via della Pergola 58,
I-50121 Florence, Italy

ABSTRACT

Investigation of the morpho-antigenic features and distribution of dendritic cells (DC) in different pathologic models may greatly contribute to a better understanding of their role in local immune systems, and of their differentiation pathways. Careful analysis of the differences in DC pattern found in normal versus pathologic skin and mucous membranes allows speculations on i) influence of the tissue microenvironment and iatrogenic insults on the number, distribution, morphology, differentiation, and expression of functionally relevant molecules by DC, and ii) possible role of DC alterations in the development and/or persistence of skin immune system-related disorders. Moreover, evaluation of the morpho-antigenic and topographic features of DC may have diagnostic and histogenic relevance in specific conditions.

Basic Mechanisms of Physiologic and Aberrant Lymphoproliferation in the Skin
Edited by W.C. Lambert *et al.*, Plenum Press, New York, 1994

DENDRITIC CELLS IN THE SKIN AND ORAL MUCOSA

Dendritic cells (DC), otherwise known as dendritic leukocytes or dendrocytes, represent a relatively homogeneous population within lymphoid organs, epithelia, connective tissue and lymph (Nussenzweig and Steinman, 1980; Nussenweig et al., 1981). They are defined by their typical shape, bone marrow origin (Staquet, 1988), constitutive expression of MHC class II antigens (van Voorhis et al., 1983), usually low phagocytic activity (van Voorhis et al., 1983), and high efficiency in stimulating ("antigen- presenting cells") and regulating T cell dependent immune responses (Inaba et al., 1983; 1984; 1985; Steinman and Inaba, 1989; Steinman, 1991). Ultrastructurally, DC share some basic features: a roundish to oval body and long, thin dendrites; an indented nucleus with pale chromatin (except for a thin peripheral rim); a cytoplasm containing cytoskeletal filaments (but no fibrils), mitochondria, few cisternae of rough endoplasmic reticulum, few dense bodies (primary lysosomes), many smooth vesicles and tubules; and a large Golgi apparatus (Nussenzweig et al., 1981). This group is comprised of inter-digitating reticulum cells (T cell areas) and dendritic reticulum cells (B cell areas) of secondary lymphoid organs, veiled cells in the afferent lymph, Langerhans cells of squamous stratified epithelia, dendritic leukocytes of epithelial surfaces other than squamous stratified epithelia, and interstitial dendritic leukocytes.

Langerhans cells

Langerhans cells (LC) are the best known and most extensively studied DC. Their morphologic, antigenic, environmental and functional features, their origin and life cycle, and their modifications by ageing and physical/chemical stimuli have been extensively reviewed elsewhere (Breathnach, 1988; Bos et al., 1988; Romagnoli et al., 1991; Schuler, 1991). Therefore, only a synthetic overview will be given here.

Morpho-antigenic and functional features of LC. Epidermal LC -- first described by Paul Langerhans in 1868 (Langerhans, 1868) -- are gold chloride and osmium iodide positive, are intensely reactive for ATPase, and express S-100 protein, features all shared by melanocytes. The cardinal features of LC are the presence of specific inclusions on electron microscopy (Birbeck et al., 1961), the so-called Birbeck granules, and the expression of CD1a antigen on the plasma membrane. Application of the above listed methods for the identification of LC has led to some confusion in terminology. Strictly speaking, only cells containing Birbeck granules should be considered LC; the identification of all epidermal (and dermal, when present) CD1a[+] cells as LC is an approximation, which is not generally accepted. CD1a[+] DC not containing Birbeck granules are currently interpreted as putative precursors of Langerhans cells, and correspond to so-called indeterminate cells. The findings of recent reports (Bartosik, 1992), however, suggest that the identification of Birbeck granules is very often made possible by the careful analysis of a large number of ultrathin sections. Consequently, use of the term indeterminate cells seems unnecessarily confusing and should be avoided.

Langerhans cells express many membrane molecules, relevant to their functional role in physiology and pathology (T cell activation, cytokine production, adhesion to the extracellular matrix, migration, etc.): the receptors for the Fc of IgG (Schmitt et al., 1990) and IgE (Torresani et al., 1991; Bieber et al., 1992; Wollenberg et al., 1993), the third component of the complement system (De Panfilis et al., 1990a), and interleukin-2; MHC class I and II antigens; leukocyte common antigen (CD45); CD4 antigen; at least some of the β_2-containing integrins (CD11/CD18) (De Panfilis et al., 1989); the β_1- containing integrins (VLA, Very Late Antigens) (Le Varlet et al., 1991); the leucocyte function-associated antigen-3 (LFA-3, CD58) (De Panfilis et al., 1991); and the inter-cellular adhesion molecule-1 (ICAM-1, CD54) (De Panfilis et al., 1990b). These antigenic and functional features justify the definition of these cells as the "sentinels" of the skin-associated lymphoid tissue (SALT) (Toews et al., 1980; Streilein, 1983) or skin immune system (SIS) (Bos and Kapsenberg, 1986).

Origin and life cycle of LC. Langerhans cells are thought to be derived from bone marrow HLA-DR⁻ precursor cells of monocyte/macrophage lineage (Bowers and Goodell, 1989; Hsiao et al., 1989). Thus, the finding of numerical and morphologic abnormalities of epidermal LC in diseases characterized by defective leukopoiesis is not surprising (Sepp et al., 1991). In some specific conditions, characterized by a dramatic decrease in number of epidermal LC, the number of CD1a⁺ cells in the peripheral blood clearly increases (Gothelf et al., 1988 and 1989; De Fraissinette et al., 1991); it is still unclear whether these circulating CD1a⁺ cells are true LC precursors, however, and what are their functional features. Epidermal LC may undergo mitosis, but this process seems to involve only a small fraction of these cells (Czernielewski et al., 1986; De Fraissinette et al., 1989; Hume and Moore, 1989; Miyauchi and Hashimoto, 1989).

Environmental features of LC. The influence of the epithelial microenvironment induces the maturation of precursor cells into morphologically and antigenically mature LC (Murphy et al., 1985 and 1986; Bani et al., 1988a and 1989; Haftek, 1988; Pimpinelli and Bani, 1989). This statement is in line with the findings that i) LC are regularly recognized in areas of epidermoid metaplasia (Wong and Buck, 1971); and ii) they are morphologically altered in skin disorders characterized by perturbed epidermal differentiation, either inherited (Ford et al., 1983; Kolde and Happle, 1985) or acquired (Chardonnet et al., 1986; Smolle et al., 1986; Sudo et al., 1987; Azizi et al., 1987; Drijkoningen et al., 1988; Alcalay et al., 1989). Although the possibility cannot be excluded that CD1a antigen may be acquired by LC before they enter the epithelium (Gothelf et al., 1988 and 1989; De Fraissinette et al., 1991), Birbeck granules appear only after this entry.

Modifications of LC induced by ageing and physical/chemical stimuli. There is a progressive increase in the density of LC in human epidermis during both fetal and postnatal life. Furthermore, LC have been demonstrated to undergo progressive maturation with time: expression of CD1a, HLA-DR and S-100 antigens begins during fetal life, whereas Birbeck granules appear only after birth. Ageing is associated with reduced ability of the skin not only to respond to recall antigens, but also to be sensitized to neoantigens (e.g., dinitrochlorobenzene). In mice, the number of Langerhans cells decreases with ageing, most probably because of a deficiency in the bone marrow precursors of these cells. In man, on the contrary, it has been proposed that only the functional activity of LC is reduced with ageing, since the number of these cells has not been demonstrated to be affected (Thivolet and Nicolas, 1990).

The effects of electromagnetic waves on LC have been the subject of extensive studies. Most of these studies indicate that LC are functionally impaired by ultraviolet (UV) and X-rays, at least for some time, and suggest that a functional alteration of LC plays some role in the damage induced by UV irradiation on the epidermis. In any case, the subtle interactions between UV irradiation and the SIS are not yet clearly understood: the established importance of UV light type and dose, of irradiation modalities, and of genetic features of the host (so called "UV-susceptibility" and "UV-resistance") makes the enormous amount of available data difficult to interpret from both the biologic and clinical point of view (Cruz & Bergstresser, 1991).

Concerning the effects of major and widely used immunosuppressive drugs on LC, the very numerous data of the literature may be synthesized as follows: i) corticosteroids and antimitotic agents negatively affect the number and structure of LC (Cruz & Bergstresser, 1991); and ii) a specific functional impairment of LC induced by cyclosporine-A has been claimed by some authors (Demidem et al., 1991; Dupuy et al., 1991), but contradicted by the results of others (Peguet-Navarro et al., 1991).

In mouse skin, another type of epidermal DC has been recognized. These DC are characterized by the expression of Thy-1 antigen (Tschachler et al., 1983; Bergstresser et al., 1983 and 1984; Romani et al., 1985), and have been recently identified as lymphoid DC, i.e., **dendritic epidermal T cells** (DETC) (Stingl et al., 1987). No epidermal Thy-1$^+$ DC is demonstrable in human skin (Cohen et al., 1986). A subset of T cells with functional analogies with murine DETC has been described in human skin, however; these cells bear the τ/δ T cell receptor (Foster & Stingl, 1990).

Dermal dendritic cells

The role of dermal dendritic cells (DC) in both murine and human SIS is convincingly supported by experimental evidence that they are capable of initiating delayed-type hypersensitivity responses (Cooper et al., 1987; Streilein, 1989; Sontheimer, 1989; Sontheimer et al., 1989; Tse and Cooper, 1990). There is substantial agreement concerning some common features of these dermal DC, variably termed **dermal dendrocytes** (Headington, 1986; Drijkoningen et al., 1987; Cerio et al., 1989; Arrese Estrada and Pierard, 1990), **perivascular veil cells** (Braverman et al., 1986), or **perivascular dendritic macrophages** (Sontheimer, 1989;

Sontheimer et al., 1989): expression of class II MHC antigens; mainly perivascular location (predominantly around the superficial vascular plexus); lacking expression of CD1a antigen and vascular markers (factor VIII-RA and Ulex Europaeus lectin); and ultrastructural features of dendritic macrophages. The antigenic phenotype of dermal DC, however, is actually an object of controversy; in fact, they have been defined as factor XIII$^+$ (Headington, 1986; Cerio et al., 1989; Arrese Estrada and Pierard, 1990; Headington and Cerio, 1990), CD11b$^+$/CD11c$^+$/CD36$^-$ (Sontheimer, 1989; Sontheimer et al., 1989), CD11b$^+$/CD11c$^+$/CD14$^+$/CD68$^+$/KiM8$^+$/CD36$^-$ (Weber-Matthiesen and Sterry, 1990), or CD11b$^-$/CD11c$^+$/CD14$^+$/CD36$^+$ (Headington, 1986; Cerio et al., 1989; Headington and Cerio, 1990; Tse and Cooper, 1990). Furthermore, it is presently not known whether the dermal CD36$^+$ DC identified in normal dermis correspond to those demonstrated in the skin upon UV irradiation, which show melanin phagocytosis and are reported to activate suppressor cell responses (Cooper et al., 1985 and 1986; Baadsgaard et al., 1988 and 1990), thus supporting the speculation that they are possibly interrelated with a CD36$^+$ subset of blood monocytes (Shen et al., 1983).

CD36$^+$/CD1a$^-$ DC have been found in normal epidermis (Smolle et al., 1985; Soyer et al., 1988), but this finding has not been confirmed regularly (Lisby et al., 1990a and 1990b). It remains to be established if and how these CD36$^+$ epidermal cells, if present, are related to those found in the dermis. Results of immunohistochemical investigations have in any case to be interpreted cautiously, since the expression of CD36 antigen does not seem to identify unequivocally monocyte-derived, possibly antigen-presenting DC. In fact, CD36$^+$ cells -- variably dendritic in shape but not expressing class II MHC antigens or CD45 antigen (the latter indicative of bone marrow origin) -- have been found by some authors at the dermo-epidermal junction (Weber-Matthiesen and Sterry, 1990).

On the basis of preliminary reports, dermal perivascular DC have been described as having a folded nucleus, a ruffled surface and a relatively dark cytoplasm, containing mitochondria and occasional lysosomes (Sontheimer et al., 1989). Cells corresponding in shape and location to CD36$^+$ DC have been recently identified in human oral mucosa and defined in their fine structure (Pimpinelli et al., 1991). These cells are characterized by the presence of many lysosomes (both primary and secondary, often containing melanin) outside the Golgi region; a variable, sometimes high number of cisternae of rough endoplasmic reticulum; and focal adhesion sites to the extracellular matrix.

MORPHO-ANTIGENIC FEATURES OF DC AS A CLUE TO THE INTERPRETATION OF SIS-RELATED DISORDERS

The aim of this chapter is to stress the possible value of the routine morphologic and antigenic typing of DC as a clue to the interpretation of skin -- and oral mucosa -- diseases characterized by aberrant lymphoid cell migration and proliferation, possibly related to a qualitative and/or quantitative alteration of the local immune system.

In this regard, we will mainly review the results obtained by our group in the last five years, schematically distinguishing and concerning three main groups or pathologic conditions: i) those in which DC alterations may have a relevant role in the pathogenesis and/or progression of the disease; ii) those in which the morpho-antigenic features of DC may have a diagnostic and/or histogenetic relevance; and iii) those in which it is uniquely possible to investigate the resistance of DC to iatrogenic insults, their homing, and their differentiation in the skin microenvironment, i.e., bone marrow transplantation and graft-versus-host disease.

Possible role of DC alterations in the pathogenesis and/or progression of the disease

In **mycosis fungoides** (MF), the prototype of cutaneous T-cell lymphoma, a clear-cut correlation between the number, distribution and ultrastructure of $CD1a^+$ DC and the stage-related histoimmunologic modifications has been documented. In the plaque stage, dermal $CD1a^+$ DC are numerous, form an extended cellular network, show morphologic signs of enhanced functional activity (abundant cytoplasm with large amounts of mitochondria, multiple Golgi stacks, and numerous cisternae of rough and smooth endoplasmic reticulum), and establish close contacts with $CD4^+$ neoplastic T cells often showing blastic/anaplastic morphology and activated/proliferating phenotype ($HLA-DR^+/CD25^+/CD71^+/Ki-67^+$). In the tumor stage, blastic/anaplastic T cells markedly increase in number and lose their mature $CD4^+$ phenotype, while $CD1a^+$ DC are sparse and less rich in organelles, and show only occasional contacts with T cells (Bani et al., 1988b). Notwithstanding the large numbers of epidermal $CD1a^+$ LC, close contacts between these cells and T cells are occasional, even in initial patches (Bani et al., 1990), thus raising doubts regarding the previously proposed hypothesis of a persistent stimulatory action of LC on T cells, eventually leading to the malignant transformation of the latter (van der Loo et al., 1979; Mackie, 1981). Therefore, it has been hypothesized that dermal $CD1a^+$ DC are possibly involved in the proliferation and neoplastic progression of T cells; on the other hand, $CD1a^+$ DC may differentiate and persist only under the influence of a mature T cell microenvironment. This latter point seems to be confirmed by the finding of very high numbers of $CD11c^+$ $CD1a^-$ monocytoid cells -- putative monocytic precursor of both epidermal LC and dermal $CD1a^+$ DC -- in the patch and plaque stage, but not in the tumor stage of MF (Bani and Giannotti, 1989). In this context, the large numbers of $CD1a^+$ LC in the epidermis of MF patches and plaques may be considered an epiphenomenon related to the migration of precursors of DC from the dermis into the epidermis, possibly attracted by specific cytokines such as interleukin-1 (Tron et al., 1988). In light of this, the recent finding of a positive correlation between higher numbers of epidermal $CD1a^+$ LC and a better prognosis in patients with MF is not surprising (Meissner et al., 1990). On the other hand, the report that only intraepidermal T cells are cycling in MF (Nickoloff & Griffiths, 1990) suggests that one should be very cautious about the exclusion of a possible role of epidermal LC in the pathophysiology of MF. In MF, neoplastic T-cells are more or less strictly interspersed with reactive T cells. Therefore, any speculation on the possible role of host immune response in the stage-related modifications of the cell/lymphocyte ratio is doubtful. Recent reports indicate possible clues for the recognition of functionally operating, antigen-presenting DC subsets in MF lesional epidermis (Hansen et al., 1990), and this approach may prove useful to address the issue of the role of host immune response against neoplastic T cells. Factor XIIIa$^+$ dermal dendrocytes are found in increased numbers in the papillary dermis of MF plaques, and possibly co-express Thy-1 (Fivenson et al., 1990) and CD1a antigens (Dréno et al., 1992). At the moment, no definite conclusion may be suggested concerning the possible role of these cells in the selective activation of suppressor pathways that allow malignant T cells to escape immune surveillance. The same holds true for the CD36$^+$/CD1a$^+$ dendritic cells found in MF lesional epidermis (Lisby et al., 1990a; 1990b).

In the well-developed lesions of **lichen planus** (LP), a classic model of immune-mediated benign dermatosis, DC form -- as in MF plaques -- an extended cellular network in the dermis and frequently establish close appositions with activated T cells. Unlike MF, nevertheless, no DC is found showing cytomorphological signs of activation, thus suggesting that in LP the mechanism of lymphocyte activation is similar to that operating in T cell areas of lymphoid organs under physiologic conditions, and does not lead to hyperfuction of DC. In the epidermis of LP lesions, LC were regularly found near or in close contact with infiltrating T cells; in some cases, an individual DC showed close contact with both a lymphocyte and a damaged keratinocyte. These findings suggest an active role of epidermal LC in the pathogenesis of LP (Pimpinelli and Bani, 1988).

Our findings in **chronic discoid** (CDLE) and **subacute cutaneous** (SCLE) **lupus erythematosus** (Mori et al., 1994) do not entirely confirm the notion that epidermal CD1a$^+$ LC are constantly reduced in number and perturbed in morphology in lesional skin (Sontheimer and Bergstresser, 1982). The number and dendriticity of epidermal CD1a$^+$ DC clearly appear inversely related to the degree of histologic epidermal atrophy, without any significant difference between CDLE and SCLE; only in the atrophic epidermal areas are CD11c$^+$/CD14$^+$ putative precursors to DC found in the basal layer. These results indicate that, in cutaneous LE, the differentiation of precursors into antigenically mature LC is clearly impaired in a morphologically -- and maybe functionally -- abnormal epidermal microenvironment and suggest that the previously claimed overall reduction in the numbers of epidermal LC (possibly due to the average figure resulting from both atrophic and non-atrophic areas) is not likely to have a relevant pathogenic significance. Independent of the number of CD1a$^+$ DC, however, their expression of HLA-DR antigens seems to be reduced on the basis of quantitative evaluation, thus suggesting a possible immunologic deficiency of epidermal LC. In the lesional dermis of cutaneous LE, both CD1a$^+$/HLA-DR$^+$ DC and CD36$^+$/Factor XIIIa$^+$/HLA-DR$^+$ DC (mainly in a perivascular location) were found, associated with CD4$^+$ and CD8$^+$ T cells, respectively. These findings indicate that in cutaneous LE the dermal infiltrate shows the immunohistologic profile of a typical delayed-type immune response, possibly modulated by a suppressor T cell response in which CD36$^+$/Factor XIIIa$^+$ DC may act as accessory cells.

In vulvar **lichen sclerosus et atrophicus** (LSA), the number of CD1a$^+$/HLA-DR$^+$ epidermal LC is constantly increased, independent of the evolutionary phase of the disease, amount of dermal infiltrate, presence and degree of sclerosis and fibrosis, and -- interestingly and uniquely -- degree of epidermal atrophy. Furthermore, a conspicuous number of CD11c$^+$ DC is constantly found in both the superficial dermis and basal layers of the epidermis; these cells may represent a precursor pool of cells which are destined to acquire the features of fully differentiated LC within the epidermis (Carli et al., 1991). These findings are consistent with a condition of persistent activation of the afferent limb of the skin immune system (SIS), which accordingly seems actively involved in the pathogenesis of LSA.

Involvement of LC during **HIV infection** deserves special consideration. Dendritic cells, including LC, are susceptible to HIV infection beginning in the very early phases of infection, via CD4 antigen as well as other mechanisms (Stingl et al., 1990; Langhoff & Haseltine, 1992). Langerhans cells have been described as diminished in number in the epidermis of subjects infected by HIV, although this report has not been univocally confirmed (Kanitakis et al., 1989; Manganoni and Groh, 1989).

In **hairy leukoplakia** (HL), a disease of tongue mucosa typically -- although not exclusively -- associated with HIV infection and often preceding the full blown acquired immune deficiency syndrome (AIDS), fully differentiated CD1a$^+$ LC are virtually absent in the lesional epithelium (Daniels et al., 1987) in which putative morphologic and antigenic precursors of LC (CD11c$^+$, CD14$^+$ cells with bluntly dendritic shape) are regularly found (Riccardi et al., 1990). Intracisternal particles, reminiscent of A particles typical of retroviral infections, have been found in occasional intraepithelial in HL lesional mucosa (Riccardi et al., 1990). In the lamina propria, on the contrary, CD1a$^+$ DC are regularly found associated with CD8$^+$ T cells. In the clinically healthy oral mucosa of HIV$^+$ subjects, with or without HL, the density of CD1a$^+$ LC in the epithelium and of CD36$^+$ perivascular DC in the lamina propria -- corresponding in shape and location to dendritic macrophages observed on electron microscopy -- is not significantly different from that of HIV$^-$ subjects, while the expression of class II antigens by these cells is clearly reduced (Pimpinelli et al., 1991). Altogether, these findings suggest a possible functional impairment of mucosal DC in HIV$^+$ subjects. Further insults, ineffective if isolated, could be crucial in determining a major alteration in the differentiation of these cells, and consequently in local cell-mediated immune responses. Hairy leukoplakia, in which Epstein-Barr virus produces an evident alteration of the epithelial microenvironment, may be a good example of a condition of greatly hampered differentiation of antigen-presenting cells in immune deficient subjects.

In HIV-related **Kaposi sarcoma** (KS), the reactive lymphohistiocytic infiltrate is always less pronounced than in classic KS lesions of comparable age. In particular, it is characterized by the virtual absence of CD4$^+$ T-cells and extreme paucity of CD1a$^+$ DC, even in patients with no detectable impairment of the systemic immunologic parameters (Santucci et al., 1988). These findings suggest a specific and early impairment of the SIS, with possible defective antigen presentation by epidermal LC, absence of CD4$^+$ T cell proliferation, and consequent further immune deficiency.

Morpho-antigenic features of DC: Possible diagnostic and/or histogenic relevance

Concerning **non-Hodgkin B-cell lymphomas**, previous studies suggest that skin infiltrating neoplastic B-cells are able to induce the development of a specialized microenvironment consisting of B-zone specific DC (dendritic reticulum cells, DRC; Smolle et al., 1985), although with a limited degree of morphologic differentiation (Pimpinelli et al., 1988).

Cutaneous B-cell lymphoma (CBCL) represents a clinically homogeneous group, characterized by non-aggressive course, good response to local treatment, rare extracutaneous spread, and excellent prognosis (Willemze et al., 1987a and 1987b; Berti et al., 1988; Pimpinelli et al., 1989). These features make reasonable the idea of CBCL as a unique type of low-grade lymphoma (Santucci et al., 1991), despite its histo-immunologic heterogeneity, mainly related to the evolutionary modifications of its skin lesions. Histologically, CBCL has features comparable to those typical of MALT (Mucosa-Associated Lymphoid Tissue) lymphomas, showing a wide spectrum of cytologic appearances (Pimpinelli et al., 1990; Santucci et al., 1991). Immunologically, neoplastic cells have a CD19$^+$/CD20$^+$/CD22$^+$/CD45RA$^+$/Leu-δ^+/CD5$^-$/CD10$^-$ phenotype; the immunoarchitecture of CBCL show different features according to the age and growth rate of skin lesions. In CBCL, both follicle-like nodules (clusters of monoclonal Leu-8$^+$/IgD$^+$ B cells and DRC) and true reactive, polyclonal follicles are found. In the former, DRC have a CD35$^+$/DRC-1$^+$/NGFr (Nerve Growth Factor receptor)$^+$/CD21$^{(+)-}$/CD14$^-$ phenotype, and often show an aberrant "centrifugal" pattern; in the latter, the phenotype of DRC is CD35$^+$/DRC-1$^+$/NGFr$^+$/CD21$^+$/CD14$^{(+)-}$. The immunophenotype and architectural fashion of DRC are interesting clues to the diagnostic (differentiation between neoplastic and true reactive follicle-like nodules) and histogenic interpretation of CBCL (B-cell lymphomas of the Skin-Associated Lymphoid Tissue?; Giannotti & Santucci, 1993).

The skin after bone marrow transplantation and in graft-versus-host disease

The sequential morphologic and immunologic analysis of the skin after allogeneic **bone marrow transplantation** (BMT) provides a very unique clue to the interpretation of bone marrow-derived cell homing and differentiation in the skin microenvironment. We performed a sequential immunohistologic and ultrastructural study of the skin in 29 patients treated with allogeneic BMT, with the aim of highlighting the treatment- and time-related modifications in the number, distribution, morphology, and immunophenotype of cutaneous DC after BMT, and the possible variations occurring during **acute graft-versus-host disease** (aGVHD), as a step to understand the role played by such cells in this disease. For this purpose, biopsies from clinically normal skin were taken before the conditioning treatment for BMT (-10 days), before

(-1 day) and after the bone marrow infusion (+14 days, +28 days and +60 days). If clinically evident aGVHD occurred, biopsies were taken from lesional skin and from clinically normal skin upon pharmacological resolution of the disease (at +60-70 days). In **clinically normal skin**, perivascular CD36$^+$ DC and Factor XIII$^+$ DC, corresponding in shape and location to dendritic

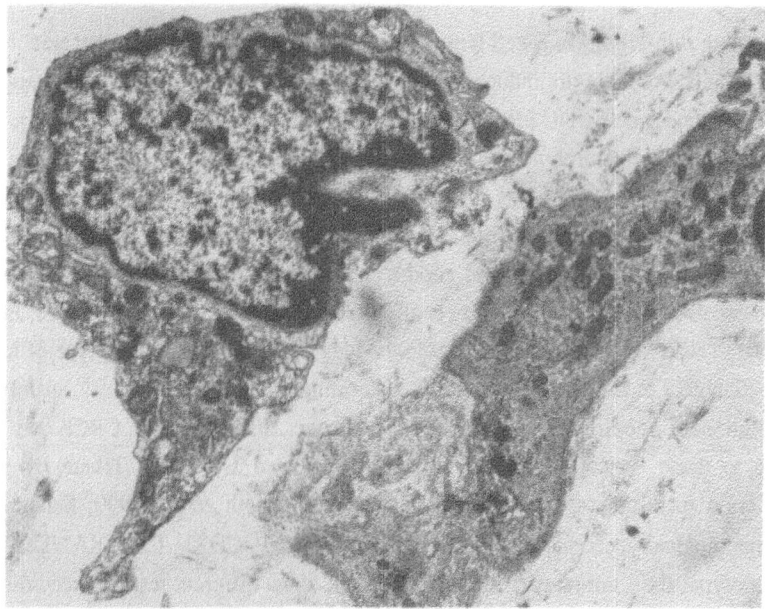

Figure 1. Perivascular dendritic macrophages in clinically normal skin after BMT (+14 days). Lysosomes containing melanin granules are clearly shown.

macrophages found on electron microscopy (Figure 1), were virtually the only bone marrow-derived cells found in the first month after BMT. Acute GVHD was characterized by the presence of numerous CD1a$^+$/HLA-DR$^+$/CD11a$^+$/CD18$^+$/CD54$^+$ DC in the basal epidermis and in the papillary dermis close to the dermo-epidermal junction, corresponding in shape and location to the LC-like cells observed on electron microscopy (Figure 2). The number of CD1a$^+$ DCs was lower than that found in biopsies taken before starting the conditioning treatment, but was clearly higher than that found in biopsies from patients without aGVHD at the same -- or comparable -- time point after BMT. Increased numbers of perivascular CD36$^+$ DC, some of them interspersed among collagen bundles, were also found. On electron microscopy, both dendritic macrophages and immature monocytoid cells were observed. Neither dividing cells nor transitional forms between putative LC and dendritic macrophages were found. Two months after BMT, the morpho-antigenic features of cutaneous DC were similar in all subjects, independent of the previous occurrence of aGVHD (Pimpinelli et al., 1993). Our results speak against a dramatic reduction of epidermal Langerhans cells during aGVHD, previously claimed (Lampert et al., 1982; Perreault et al., 1984; Sloane et al., 1984; Murphy et al., 1985) and only recently challenged (Vol-Platzer et al., 1988; Zambruno et al., 1991). Conversely, a definite reduction -- up to virtual absence -- of CD1a⁺ DC observed in the epidermis is presumably related to the iatrogenic insults of the conditioning treatment (Volc-Platzer et al., 1988; Zambruno et al., 1991). Different from LC, CD36⁺/Factor XIIIa⁺ dermal dendrocytes are resistant to this treatment (Pimpinelli et al., 1993).

Our results suggest that the CD1a⁺, LC-like DC may have a pivotal role in cutaneous aGVHD. In this situation, these cells are present in very large numbers (even higher than those of lymphocyes), show antigenic and morphologic signs of activation (expression of functionally relevant adhesion molecules, such as CD54 and CD11/CD18 antigens; well developed endoplasmic reticulum and Golgi apparatus), and appear polarized towards the epidermis (Figures 2 and 3). We do not know whether the many indeterminate cells observed in the skin

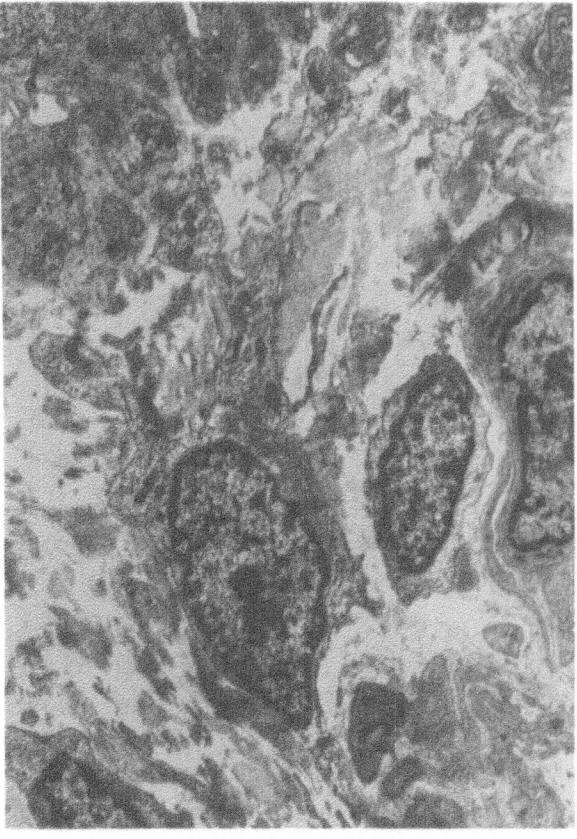

Figure 2. aGVHD. Dendritic cells with LC-like features, although devoid of typical Birbeck granules, close to the dermo-epidermal junction. The cells appear polarized, with most cytoplasm toward the epidermis.

during aGVHD were of recipient or donor origin. In the former case, they might have differentiated from perivascular DC which had survived after the conditioning treatment (Murphy et al., 1985 and 1986). Since neither dividing cells nor cells with clearcut intermediate features between perivascular dendritic macrophages and indeterminate cells were seen in the dermis during aGVHD, however, and in accordance with the finding of a large number of CD1a[+] cells in the peripheral blood after BMT (De Fraissinette et al., 1991), the hypothesis that the LC-like

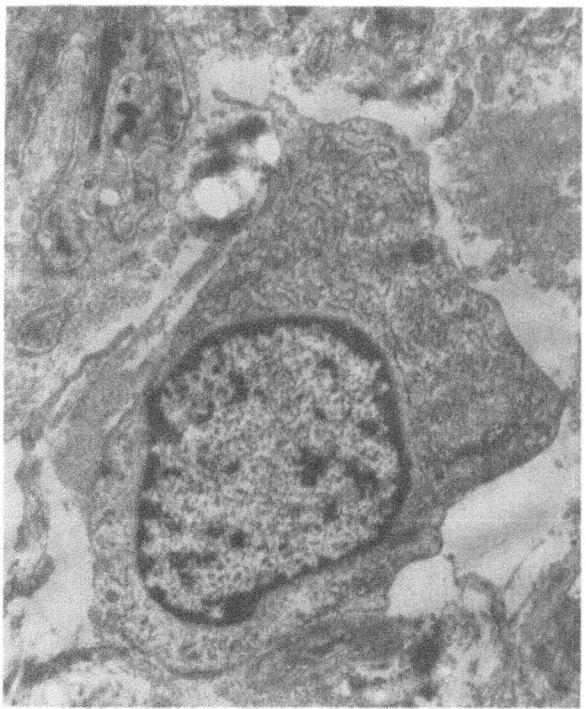

Figure 3. aGVHD. Dendritic cell with well developed smooth (besides rough) endoplasmic reticulum and Golgi apparatus and very few lysosomes, but devoid of typical Birbeck granules. The cell is clearly polarized towards the epidermis.

DC found in the skin during aGVHD are of donor origin should be kept under appropriate consideration. It can be speculated that the skin during aGVHD is "colonized" by CD1a[+] putative precursors of epidermal LC. This colonization seems transient, however, and followed by slow -- but long-lasting -- reconstitution of the LC population in the epidermis by cells of graft origin. In fact, our findings seem to indicate that the presence of putative LC in the skin during aGVHD has no correlation with the long-term repopulation of the epidermis by LC. The histoimmunologic and ultrastructural pattern of the skin 60-70 days after BMT is similar in patients who did not develop aGVHD and in those who had aGVHD and healed after treatment (Pimpinelli et al., 1993), in contrast to previous reports (Perreault et al., 1984; Murphy et al., 1985).

CONCLUSIONS

Review of results obtained by our and other groups indicates that investigation of the morpho-antigenic features and distribution of DC in different pathologic models may greatly contribute to a better understanding of their role in local immune systems, and of their differentiation pathways. These data have to be matched with the continuously increasing amount of data concerning the functional properties of DC under physiologic and pathologic conditions.

Analysis of the differences in DC pattern found between normal and pathologic skin and mucous membranes allows speculations on i) influence of the tissue microenvironment and iatrogenic insults on the number, distribution, morphology, differentiation, and expression of functionally relevant molecules by DC; ii) possible role of DC alterations in the pathogenesis of skin (and mucosal) immune system-related disorders; and iii) possible diagnostic and histogenic relevance of the morpho-antigenic and topographic features of DC.

ACKNOWLEDGEMENTS

This work was in part supported by grants from the Italian Ministries of Public Education, and of University and Scientific and Technologic Research

REFERENCES

Alcalay J, LH Goldberg, JE Wolff and ML Kripke, 1989. Variations in the number and morphology of Langerhans cells in the epidermal component of squamous cell carcinomas, **Arch. Dermatol.**, 125:917.

Arrese Estrada J and GE Pierard, 1990. Factor-XIIIa-positive dendrocytes and the dermal microvascular unit, **Dermatologica**, 180:51.

Azizi E, C Bucana, L Goldberg and ML Kripke, 1987. Perturbation of epidermal Langerhans cells in basal cell carcinomas, **Am. J. Dermatopathol.**, 9:465.

Baadsgaard O, DA Fox and KD Cooper, 1988. Human epidermal cells from ultraviolet light-exposed skin preferentially activate autoreactive CD4+2H4+ suppressor-inducer lymphocytes and CD8+ suppressor/cytotoxic lymphocytes, **J. Immunol.**, 140:1738.

Baadsgaard O, B Salvo, A Mannie, B Dass, DA Fox and KD Cooper, 1990. In vivo ultraviolet-exposed human epidermal cells activate T suppressor cell pathways that involve CD4$^+$CD45RA$^+$ suppressor-inducer T cells, **J. Immunol.**, 145:2854.

Bani D, S Moretti, N Pimpinelli and B Giannotti, 1988a. Differentiation of monocytes into Langerhans cells in human epidermis. An ultrastructural study, In: J. Thivolet, D. Schmitt, Eds., **The Langerhans cell**, Coll. INSERM 172, John Libbey Eurotext, London, Montrouge.

Bani D, S Moretti, N Pimpinelli and B Giannotti, 1988b. Interdigitating reticulum cells in the dermal infiltrate of mycosis fungoides. An ultrastructural and immunohistochemical study, **Virchows Arch. A: Pathol. Anat. Histopathol.**, 412:451.

Bani D and B Giannotti, 1989. Differentiation of interdigitating reticulum cells and Langerhans cells in the human skin with T-lymphoid infiltrate. An immunocytochemical and ultrastructural study, **Arch. Histol. Cytol.**, 52:361.

Bani D, N Pimpinelli, S Moretti and B Giannotti, 1990. Langerhans cells and mycosis fungoides: A critical overview of their role in the disease, **Clin. Exp. Dermatol.**, 15:7.

Bartosik, J, 1991. The non-keratinocytes in normal epidermis, **Eur. J. Dermatol.**, 1:131.

Bergstresser PR, T Tigelaar, JH Dees and JU Streilein, 1983, Thy-1 antigen-bearing dendritic cells populate murine epidermis, **J. Invest. Dermatol.**, 81:286.

Bergstresser PR, RE Tigelaar and JW Streilein, 1984. Thy-1 antigen-bearing dendritic cells in murine epidermis are derived from bone marrow precursors, **J. Invest. Dermatol.**, 83:83.

Berti E, E Alessi, R Caputo, R Gianotti, D Delia and P Vezzoni, 1988. Reticulohistiocytoma of the dorsum, **J. Am. Acad. Dermatol.**, 19:259.

Bieber T, C de la Salle and A Wollenberg et al, 1992. Human Langerhans cells express the high-affinity receptor for immunoglobulin E (Fc$\in$RI). **J. Exp. Med.**, 175:1285.

Birbeck MSC, AS Breathnach and JD Everall, 1984. An electron microscopic study of basal melanocytes and high level clear-cells (Langerhans cells) in vitiligo, **J. Invest. Dermatol.**, 37:51.

Bos JD and ML Kapsenberg, 1986. The skin immune system (SIS): Its cellular constituents and their interactions, **Immunol. Today**, 7:235.

Bos JD, MBM Teunissen and ML Kapsenberg, 1988. Dendritic cells of the skin immune system (SIS), In: J. Thivolet, Schmitt D., Eds., **The Langerhans Cell**, Coll. INSERM, vol. 172, John Libbey Eurotext, London, Montrouge.

Bowers WE and EM Goodell, 1989. Dendritic cell ontogeny, **Res. Immunol.**, 140:880.

Braverman IM, J Sibley and A Keh-Yen, 1986. A study of the veil cells around normal, diabetic, and aged cutaneous microvessels, **J. Invest. Dermatol.**, 86:57.

Breathnach SM, 1988. The Langerhans cell, **Br. J. Dermatol.**, 119:463.

Carli P, A Cattaneo, N Pimpinelli et al., 1991. Immunohistochemical evidence of skin immune system involvement in vulvar lichen sclerosus et atrophicus, **Dermatologica**, 182:18.

Cerio R, CEM Griffiths, XD Cooper et al., 1989. Characterization of factor XIIIa and dermal dendritic cells in normal and inflamed skin, **Br. J. Dermatol.**, 121:421.

Chardonnet Y, J Viac and J Thivolet, 1986. Langerhans cells in human warts, **Br. J. Dermatol.**, 109:309.

Cohen RL, JM Crawford and DA Chambers, 1986. Thy-1+ epidermal cells are not demonstrable in rat and human skin, **J. Invest. Dermatol.**, 87:30.

Cooper KD, P Fox, G Neises and SI Katz, 1985. Effects of ultraviolet radiation on human epidermal cell alloantigen presentation: Initial depression of Langerhans cell-dependent function is followed by appearance of T6Dr$^+$ cells that enhance epidermal alloantigen presentation, **J. Immunol.**, 34:129.

Cooper KD, G Neises and SI Katz, 1986. Antigen presenting OKM5[+] melanophages appear in human epidermis after ultraviolet radiation, **J. Invest. Dermatol.**, 86:363.

Cooper KD, N Duraiswamy, S Kang et al., 1987. Murine dermal cells in suspension contain T cell-activating presenting cells, **J. Invest. Dermatol.**, 88:482.

Cruz PJ, Jr. and PR Bergstresser, 1991. The influence of ultraviolet radiation and other physical and chemical agents on epidermal Langerhans cells, In: G. Schuler Ed., **Epidermal Langerhans Cells**, CRC Press, Boca Raton.

Czernielewski J, P Vaigot and M Prunieras, 1985. Epidermal Langerhans cells - a cycling population, **J. Invest. Dermatol.**, 84:424

Daniels TE, D Greenspan, JS Greenspan, E Lennette, E., M Schiodt, V Petersen and Y de Souza, 1987. Absence of Langerhans cells in oral hairy leukoplakia, an AIDS-associated lesion, **J. Invest. Dermatol.**, 89:178.

De Fraissinette A, MJ Staquet, C Dezutter-Dambuyant et al., 1988. Langerhans cells in S-phase in normal skin detected by simultaneous analysis of cell surface antigen and BrdU incorporation, **J. Invest. Dermatol.**, 91:603.

De Fraissinette A, C Dezutter-Dambuyant, D Guyotat and D Schmitt, 1991, High level of CD1a putative peripheral blood precursors of epidermal Langerhans cells after bone marrow transplantation, **Thymus**, 18:129.

Demidem A, JR Taylor, SF Grammer and JW Streilein, 1991, Comparison of effects of transforming growth factor-β and cyclosporin-A on antigen-presenting cells of blood and epidermis, **J. Invest. Dermatol.**, 96:401.

De Panfilis G, D Soligo, GC Manara et al., 1989. Adhesion molecules on the plasma membrane of epidermal cells, I. Human resting Langerhans cells express two members of the adherence promoting CD11/CD18 family, namely, H-Mac-1 (CD11b/CD18) and gp 150,95 (CD11c/CD18), **J. Invest. Dermatol.**, 93:60.

De Panfilis G, D Soligo, GC Manara et al., 1990a. Human normal resting epidermal Langerhans cells do express the type 3 complement receptor, **Br. J. Dermatol.**, 122:127.

De Panfilis G, GC Manara, C Ferrari and C Torresani, 1990b. Adhesion molecules on the plasma membrane of epidermal cells, II. The intercellular adhesion molecule-1 is constitutively present on the cell surface of human resting Langerhans cells, **J. Invest. Dermatol.**, 94:317.

De Panfilis G, GC Manara, C Ferrari and C Torresani, 1991. Adhesion molecules on the plasma membrane of epidermal cells. III. Keratinocytes and Langerhans cells express the lymphocyte function-associated antigen-3, **J. Invest. Dermatol.**, 96:512.

Dréno B, M Fleischmann, P Célérier and P Litoux, 1992. Dermal FXIIIa, CD1 positive cells in mycosis fungoides, **J. Invest. Dermatol.**, 99:113s (abs.).

Drijkoningen M, C de Wolf-Peeters, H de Greef and V Desmet, 1988. Epidermal Langerhans cells, dermal dendritic cells, and keratinocytes in viral lesions of skin and mucous membranes: An immunohistochemical study, **Arch. Dermatol. Res.**, 280:220.

Drijkoningen M, C De Wolf-Peeters, K Van der Steen, P Moerman and V Desmet, 1987. Epidermal Langerhans cells and dermal dendritic cells in human fetal and neonatal skin: An immunohistochemical study, **Pediatr. Dermatol.**, 4:11.

Dupuy P, M Bagot, M Michel, B Descourt and L Dubertret, 1991. Cyclosporin-A inhibits the antigen-presenting function of freshly isolated human Langerhans cells in vitro, **J. Invest. Dermatol.**, 96:408.

Fivenson DP, MC Douglass, BJ Nickoloff and EA Krull, 1990. Thy-1[+] dermal dendrocytes in mycosis fungoides, **Clin. Res.**, 38:835 (abs.).

Ford G P, PS Friedman and J Ross, 1983. Langerhans cells in autosomal dominant ichthyosis vulgaris, **Br. J. Dermatol.**, 109;309.

Foster CA and G Stingl, 1990. T cell receptor τ/δ bearing cells in the epidermis, In: W. A. van Vloten, R. Willemze, G. Lange Vejlsgaard and K. Thomsen, Eds., **Cutaneous Lymphoma, Current Problems in Dermatol.**, vol. 19., Karger, Basel.

Giannotti B and M Santucci, 1993. S.A.L.T.-related B cell lymphoma (primary cutaneous B cell lymphoma): A concept and a clinicopathologic entity, **Arch. Dermatol.**, in press.

Gothelf Y, D Hanau, H Tsur et al., 1988. T6 positive cells in the peripheral blood of burn patients: Are they Langerhans cells precursors? **J. Invest.Dermatol.**, 90:142.

Gothelf Y, CA Dinarello, M Yamin et al., 1989. IL-1 production by T6 (CD1a) positive cord blood mononuclear cells (Langerhans cell precursors), **Lymphokine Res.**, 8:373.

Haftek M, 1988. Langerhans cells in cutaneous pathology, In: J. Thivolet, D. Schmitt, Eds., **The Langerhans Cell**, Coll. INSERM 172, John Libbey Eurotext, London, Montrouge.

Hansen ER, O Baadsgaard, S Lisby et al., 1990. Cutaneous T cell lymphoma lesional epidermal cells activate autologous CD4[+] T lymphocytes: Involvement of both CD1[+]OKM5[+] and CD1[+]OKM5 antigen-presenting cells, **J. Invest. Dermatol.**, 94:485.

Headington JT, 1986. The dermal dendrocyte, In: J. P. Callen, M. V. Dahl, L. E. Golitz, et al., Eds., **Advances in Dermatol.**, Vol. 1, Chicago Year Book Medical Publishers, Chicago.

Headington JT and R Cerio, 1990. Dendritic cells and the dermis. **Am. J. Dermatopathol.**, 12:217.

Hsiao L, M Takeya, T Arao and K Takahashi, 1989. An immunohistochemical and immunoelectron microscopic study of the ontogeny of rat Langerhans cell lineage with antimacrophage and anti-Ia monoclonal antibodies, **J. Invest. Dermatol.**, 93:780.

Hume WJ and JK Moore, 1989. DNA synthesis in Langerhans cells of mouse ear epithelium revealed by tritiated thymidine autoradiography and histochemical staining for non-specific esterase and beta-glucuronidase activity, **Cell Tissue Kin.**, 22:311.

Kanitakis J, C Marchand, H Su et al, 1989. Immunohistochemical study of normal skin of HIV-infected patients shows no evidence of infection of epidermal Langerhans cells by HIV, **AIDS Res. Human Retrovir.**, 5:293.

Kolde G and R Happle, 1985. Langerhans cells degeneration in X-linked dominant ichthyosis: A quantitative and ultrastructural study, **Arch. Dermatol. Res.**, 277:245.

Inaba K, RM Steinman, WC Van Voorhis and S Muramatsu, 1983, Dendritic cells are critical accessory cells for thymus-dependent antibody responses in mouse and in man, **Proc. Natl. Acad. Sci. USA**, 80:6041.

Inaba K, MD Witmer and RM Steinman, 1984. Clustering of dendritic cells, helper T lymphocytes, and histocompatible B cells during primary antibody responses in vitro, **J. Exp. Med.**, 160:858

Inaba K and RM Steinman, 1985. Protein-specific helper T lymphocyte formation initiated by dendritic cells, **Science**, 229:475.

Lampert I A, G Janossy, AJ Suitters et al., 1982. Immunological analysis of the skin in graft-versus-host disease, **Clin. Exp. Immunol.**, 50:123.

Langerhans P, 1868. Uber die Nerven der menschlichen Haut, **Virchows Arch.**, 44:325.

Langhoff E and WA Haseltine, 1992. Infection of accessory dendritic cells by human immunodeficiency virus type 1, **J. Invest. Dermatol.**, 95:89s.

Le Varlet B, C Dezutter-Dambuyant, MJ Staquet, P Delorme and D Schmitt, 1991, Human epidermal Langerhans cells express integrins of the β_1 subfamily, **J. Invest. Dermatol.**, 96:518.

Lisby S, O Baadsgaard, KD Cooper et al., 1990a. Phenotype, ultrastructure, and function of CD1$^+$DR$^+$ epidermal cells that express CD36 (OKM5) in cutaneous T-cell lymphoma, **Scand. J. Immunol.**, 32:111.

Lisby S, E Ralfkiaer, ER Hansen and GL Vejlsgaard, 1990b. Keratinocyte and epidermal leukocyte expression of CD36 (OKM5) in benign and malignant skin diseases, **Acta Dermatovenerol.**, 70:18.

MacKie R, 1981. Initial event in mycosis fungoides of the skin is viral infection of epidermal Langerhans cells, **Lancet**, 11:283.

Manganoni AM and V Groh V, 1989. Langerhans cells in HIV-1 infection: Immunophenotypic characteristics of apparently healthy skin and their correlation with the stage of disease, **It. Gen. Rev. Dermatol.**, 26:169.

Meissner K, K Michaelis, W Rehpenning and T Loning, 1990. Epidermal Langerhans cell densities influence survival in mycosis fungoides and Sézary syndrome, **Cancer**, 65:2069.

Miyauchi S and K Hashimoto, 1989. Mitotic activities of normal epidermal Langerhans cells, **J. Invest. Dermatol.**, 92:120.

Mori M, N Pimpinelli, P Romagnoli, E Bernacchi, P Fabbri and B Giannotti, 1994. Dendritic cells in cutaneous lupus erythematosus: A hint to the pathogenesis of lesions. **Histopathology**, in press.

Murphy GF, Y Merot, AKF Tong et al., 1985. Depletion and repopulation of epidermal dendritic cells after allogeneic bone marrow transplantation in humans, **J. Invest. Dermatol.**, 84:210.

Murphy GF, D Messadi, E Fonferko and WW Hancock, 1986, Phenotypic transformation of macrophages to Langerhans cells in the skin, **Am. J. Pathol.**, 123:401.

Nickohoff BJ and CEM Griffiths, 1990. Intraepidermal but not dermal T lymphocytes are positive for a cell-cycle-associated antigen (Ki-67) in mycosis fungoides, **Am. J. Pathol.**, 136:261.

Nussenzweig MC and RM Steinman, 1980. Contribution of dendritic cells to stimulation of the murine syngenic mixed leukocyte reaction, **J. Exp. Med.**, 151:1196.

Nussenzweig MC, MD Witner, N Nogueira and ZA Cohn, 1981. A comparison of dendritic cells and macrophages, In: O. Forster, M. Landy Eds., **Heterogeneity of Mononuclear Phagocytes**, Academic Press, London.

Peguet-Navarro J, M Slaats and J Thivolet, 1991. Lack of demonstrable effect of cyclosporin-A on human epidermal Langerhans cell function, **Arch. Dermatol. Res.**, 283:198.

Perreault C, M Pelletier, D Landry et al., 1984. Study of Langerhans cells after allogeneic bone marrow transplantation, **Blood**, 63:807.

Pimpinelli N, P Romagnoli, S Moretti and B Giannotti, 1988. Nonlymphoid accessory cells in the cutaneous infiltrate of B cell lymphomas. An immunohistochemical and ultrastructural study, **Br. J. Dermatol.**, 118:353.

Pimpinelli N and Bani D, 1988. Non-lymphoid accessory cells in lichen planus and mycosis fungoides, **It. Gen. Rev. Dermatol.**, 25:82.

Pimpinelli N and D Bani, 1989. Langerhans cells and epidermal microenvironment, **Am. J. Dermatopathol.**, 11:188.

Pimpinelli N, M Santucci, A Bosi, S Moretti, C Vallecchi, A Messori and B Giannotti, 1989. Primary cutaneous follicular centre-cell lymphoma: A lymphoproliferative disease with favourable prognosis, **Clin. Exp. Dermatol.**, 14:12.

Pimpinelli N, M Santucci, A Bosi et al, 1990. Primary cutaneous follicular center-cell lymphoma: Clinical and histologic features, In:WA van Vloten, R Willemze, G Lange Vejlsgaard and K Thomsen, eds., **Cutaneous Lymphoma, Current Problems in Dermatol.**, vol. 19 (H. Honigsmann, ed.), Krager, Basel.

Pimpinelli N, L Borgognoni, R Riccardi, G Ficarra, M Mori, D Gaglioti and P Romagnoli, 1991. CD36(OKM5)[+] dendritic cells in the oral mucosa of HIV[-] and HIV[+] subjects, **J. Invest. Dermatol.**, 97:537.

Pimpinelli N, P Romagnoli, A Bosi et al., 1993. Dendritic cells in the skin after allogeneic bone marrow transplanation: Immunohistochemical and electron microscopic monitoring, **Eur. J. Dermatol.**, in press.

Riccardi R, N Pimpinelli, G Ficarra, L Borgognoni, D Gaglioti, D Milo and P Romagnoli, 1990. Morphology and membrane antigens of non-lymphoid accessory cells in oral hairy leukoplakia, **Human Pathol.**, 21:897.

Romagnoli P, N Pimpinelli and T Lotti, 1991. Dendritic cells in the skin and oral mucosa, **It. Gen. Rev. Dermatol.**, 28:49.

Romani N, G Stingl, E Tschachler, MD Witmer,MR Steinman, EM Shevach and G Schuler, 1985. The Thy-1 bearing cell of murine epidermis. A distinctive leukocyte perhaps related to natural killer cells, **J. Exp. Med.**, 161:1368.

Santucci M, N Pimpinelli, S Moretti and B Giannotti, 1988. Classic and immunodeficiency-associated Kaposi's sarcoma: Clinical, histologic, and immunologic correlations, **Arch. Pathol. Lab. Med.**, 112:1214.

Santucci M, N Pimpinelli and L Arganini, 1991. Primary cutaneous B cell lymphoma: A unique type of low-grade lymphoma, **Cancer**, 67:2311.

Schmitt DA, D Hanau, T Bieber et al., 1990. Human epidermal Langerhans cells express only the 40-kilodalton Fc receptor (Fc RCII), **J. Immunol.**, 144:4284.

Schuler G, ed., 1991. **Epidermal Langerhans Cells**, CRC Press, Boca Raton.

Sepp N, H Zwierzina, J Smolle, F Schmalzl, P Fritsch and G Schuler, 1991. Epidermal Langerhans cells in myelodysplastic syndromes are abnormal, **J. Invest. Dermatol.**, 96:932.

Shen H H, MA Talle, G Goldstein and L Chess, 1983. Functional subsets of human monocytes defined by monoclonal antibodies: A distinct subset of monocytes contains the cells capable of inducing the autologous mixed lymphocyte culture, **J. Immunol.**, 130:698.

Sloane JP, JA Thomas, SF Imrie et al., 1984. Morphological and immunological changes in the skin in allogeneic bone marrow recipients, **J. Clin. Pathol.**, 37:919.

Smolle J, R Ehall and H Kerl, 1985. Inflammatory cell types in normal human epidermis: An immunohistochemical and morphometric study, **Acta Dermatovenereol.**, 65:479.

Smolle J, P Kaudewitz, G Burg et al., 1985. Significance of non-lymphoid (accessory) cells in malignant lymphomas and pseudolymphomas of the skin, **Br. J. Dermatol.**, 113:677.

Smolle J, HP Soyer, R Ehall et al., 1986. Langerhans cell density in epithelial skin tumors correlates with epithelial differentiation but not with the peritumoral infiltrate, **J. Invest. Dermatol.**, 87:477.

Sontheimer RD and PR Bergstresser, 1982. Epidermal Langerhans cell involvement in cutaneous lupus erythematosus, **J. Invest. Dermatol.**, 79:237.

Sontheimer RD, T Matsubara and LL Seelig, 1989. A macrophage phenotype for a constitutive, class II antigen expressing, human dermal perivascular dendritic cell, **J. Invest. Dermatol.**, 95:154.

Sontheimer RD, 1989. Perivascular dendritic macrophages as immunobiological constituents of the human dermal microvascular unit, **J. Invest. Dermatol.**, 93:S96.

Soyer HP, J Smolle and H Kerl, 1988. Distribution patterns of the OKM5 antigen in normal and diseased human epidermis, **J. Cutan. Pathol.**, 16:60.

Staquet MJ, Origin and precursors of Langerhans cells, 1988, In: J. Thivolet, D. Schmitt, Eds., **The Langerhans Cell**, Coll. INSERM 172, John Libbey Eurotext, London, Montrouge.

Steinman R and K Inaba, 1989, Immunogenicity: Role of dendritic cells, **BioEssays**, 10:145.

Steinman RM, 1991. The dendritic cell system and its role in immunogenicity, **Ann. Rev. Immunol.**, 9:271.

Streilein JW, 1983. Skin-associated lymphoid tissue (SALT): Origins and functions, **J. Invest. Dermatol.**, 80:12.

Streilein JW, 1989. Antigen-presenting cells in the induction of contact hypersensitivity in mice: Evidence that Langerhans cells are sufficient but not required, **J. Invest. Dermatol.**, 93:443.

Stingl G, K Rapperberger, E Tschachler et al., 1990. Langerhans cells in HIV-1 infection, **J. Am. Acad. Dermatol.**, 22:1210.

Stingl G, F Koning, H Yamada, WM Yokoyama, E Tschachler, JA Bluestone, G Steiner, LE Samelson, AM Lew, JE Coligan and EM Shevach, 1987. Thy-1+ dendritic epidermal cells express T3 antigen and the T cell receptor δ chain, **Proc. Natl. Acad. Sci. USA**, 84:4586.

Sudo S, A Saito and M Morohashi, 1987. Immunohistochemical study of Langerhans cells in skin tumors, **Dermatologica**, 174:76.

Thivolet J and JF Nicolas, 1990. Skin ageing and immune competence, **Br. J. Dermatol.**, 122 (Suppl. 35):77.

Toews GB, PR Bergstresser and JW Streilein, 1980. Langerhans cells: Sentinels of the skin-associated lymphoid tissue, **J. Invest. Dermatol.**, 75:78.

Torresani C, GC Manara, C Ferrari and G De Panfilis, 1991. Immunoelectron microscopic characterization of a subpopulation of freshly isolated epidermal Langerhans cells that reacts with anti-CD23 monoclonal antibody, **Br. J. Dermatol.**, 124:533.

Tron VA, D Rosenthal and DN Sauder, 1988. Epidermal interleukin-1 is increased in cutaneous T cell lymphoma, **J. Invest. Dermatol.**, 90:378.

Tschachler E, G Schuler, J Hutterer et al., 1983. Expression of Thy-1 antigen by murine epidermal cells, **J. Invest. Dermatol.**, 81:282.

Tse Y and KD Cooper, 1990. Cutaneous dermal Ia+ cells are capable of initiating delayed type hypersensitivity responses, **J. Invest. Dermatol.**, 94:267.

van der Loo EM, GNP van Muijen, WA van Vloten et al., 1979. C-type virus-like particles specifically localized in Langerhans cells and related cells of skin and lymph nodes of patients with mycosis fungoides and Sézary syndrome, **Virchows Arch. B (Cell. Pathol.)**, 31: 193.

Volc-Platzer B, X Rappersberger, I Mosberger et al., 1988. Sequential immunohistologic analysis of the skin following allogeneic bone marrow transplantation, **J. Invest. Dermatol.**, 91:162.

Voorhis WC van, MD Witmer and RM Steinman, 1983. The phenotype of dendritic cells and macrophages, **Fed. Proc.**, 42:3114.

Weber-Matthiesen K and W Sterry, 1990. Organization of the monocyte/macrophage system of normal human skin, **J. Invest. Dermatol.**, 95:83.

Willemze R, CJLM Meijer, H Sentis et al., 1987a. Primary cutaneous large cell lymphomas of follicular center cell origin, **J. Am. Acad. Dermatol.**, 16:518.

Willemze R, CJLM Meijer, E Scheffer et al., 1987b. Diffuse large cell lymphomas of follicular center cell origin, **Am. J. Pathol.**, 126:325.

Wollenberg A, H de la Salle, D Hanau, E Kolodziejczyk, FT Liu and T Bieber, 1993. Surface expression and characterization of the endogenous ß-galactoside specific soluble lectin ∈ BP (IgE-binding protein) on human Langerhans cells, **Clin. Exp. Allergy**, in press.

Wong Y and RC Buck, 1971. Langerhans cells in epidermoid metaplasia, **J. Invest. Dermatol.**, 56:10.

CELL TRAFFICKING NETWORKS IN CUTANEOUS T CELL LYMPHOMA

David P. Fivenson, M.D.*
Brian J. Nickoloff, M.D., Ph.D.†

* Department of Dermatology
  Henry Ford Hospital
  Detroit, Michigan

† Department of Pathology
  University of Michigan
  Ann Arbor, Michigan

Correspondence to: Dr. B. J. Nickoloff, Department of Pathology,
University of Michigan School of Medicine, 1301 Catherine Road,
Ann Arbor, MI 48109, U.S.A.

ABSTRACT

An extensive network of Thy-1$^+$/Factor XIIIa$^+$ dermal dendrocytes (DD) (Table 1) exists within the papillary dermis in lesions of cutaneous T cell lymphoma (CTCL). To further characterize these cells and to study the role that activation signals and adhesion molecules play in the cellular dynamics of CTCL, immunohistochemical staining of formalin fixed, paraffin embedded tissue sections was used to study expression of high endothelial cell antigen-1 (HECA-452) and proliferating cell nuclear antigen (PCNA) in lesions of CTCL as compared to those of psoriasis, Rhus dermatitis and normal skin. In diseased skin, 10-60% of epidermotropic lymphocytes were PCNA$^+$, comparable to the numbers of Ki-67$^+$ and human mucosal leukocyte antigen (HML)-1$^+$ cells seen in previous studies. HECA-452 expression by dermal lymphocytes ranged from 1-42%. Only in lesions of CTCL were appreciable numbers of epidermal HECA-452$^+$ lymphocytes present (mean = 31%+). PCNA$^+$ lymphocytes were routinely seen only in CTCL and were limited to a subset of cells within the epidermis.

Basic Mechanisms of Physiologic and Aberrant Lymphoproliferation in the Skin
Edited by W.C. Lambert *et al.*, Plenum Press, New York, 1994

77

Dermal dendrocytes (DD) were HECA-452$^+$ in all cases. The expression of intercellular adhesion molecule (ICAM)-1, HECA-452 and vascular cell adhesion molecule (VCAM)-1 by Thy-1$^+$/FXIIIa$^+$ DD as well as Thy-1, endothelial leukocyte adhesion molecule (ELAM)-1 and VCAM-1 by the microvasculature, and LFA-1 by CD4$^+$ T cells, suggest a pivotal role for adhesion molecules in the pathogenesis of CTCL. These studies suggest that distinct cellular compartments exist within both the epidermis and dermis, which undergo differential activation and antigenic expression of dendritic and lymphoid components in all stages of CTCL. Enterance into the epidermis appears to allow a change to a proliferative phenotype (Ki-67$^+$, PCNA$^+$) and propagation of the CTCL lesion. The role of DD in the pathogenesis of CTCL is unknown, but selective adhesion molecule expression may be a mechanism by which LFA-1$^+$ malignant and reactive T cells are guided through the skin by these cells.

Table 1. Abbreviations used in this chapter. (See also "Terms and Abbreviations in Cutaneous Lymphoproliferative Phenomena" at the end of this book).

ACD	-	Allergic Contact Dermatitis
APC	-	Antigen Presenting Cell
CTCL	-	Cutaneous T Cell Lymphoma
DD	-	Dermal Dendrocyte
DETC	-	Dendrotic Epidermal T Cells, Thy-1$^+$ cells (present in mice)
EC	-	Endothelial Cell
ELAM-1	-	Endothelial Leukocyte Adhesion Molecule-1
FITC	-	Fluorescein Isothiocyanate
FXIIIa	-	Factor XIIIa
FXIIIs	-	Factor XIIIs
GMCAF	-	Granulocyte-Macrophage Cell Activating Factor
HECA-452	-	High Endothelial Cell Antigen-1
HML-1	-	Human Mucosal Leukocyte Antigen-1
HPF	-	High Power Field
ICAM-1	-	Intercellular Adhesion Molecule-1 (CD54)
KC	-	Keratinocyte
LC	-	Langerhans Cell
LFA-1	-	Leukocyte Function Antigen 1 (CD18)
MCAF	-	Mononuclear Cell Activating Factor
MF	-	Mycosis Fungoides
mAb	-	Monoclonal Antibody
Rhus ACD	-	Rhus/poison Ivy Allergic Contact Dermatitis
SLEX	-	Sialylated Lewis X Antigen
TCR	-	T Cell Receptor
VCAM-1	-	Vascular Cell Adhesion Molecule-1
VLA-4	-	Very Late Antigen-4

INTRODUCTION

Within the past few years, several new adhesion molecules have been described, along with their potential ligands. Among those of relevance to investigative skin biologists are (Table 1) endothelial leukocyte adhesion molecule-1 (ELAM-1), vascular cell adhesion molecule-1 (VCAM-1), intercellular adhesion molecule-1 (ICAM-1, CD54), leukocyte function antigen-1 (LFA-1, CD18), very late antigen-4 (VLA-4), sialylated lewis X (SLEX), and HECA-452 (Nickoloff, 1991a; Nickoloff and Griffiths, 1990a; 1990b; Table 1). Unique ligand-receptor relationships have been described for LFA-1/CD18 and ICAM-1, for VLA-4 and VCAM-1, and for SLEX and ELAM-1 (Stoolman, 1989). HECA-452 has been described as a "skin specific" homing receptor on T cells, similar to the peripheral lymph node homing receptor, Leu-8 (Picker et al., 1990). This antigen has been described as present on polymorphonuclear leukocytes, monocytes, a subpopulation of lymphocytes, and on high endothelial vessels (Duijvestin et al., 1988; Kruse et al., 1984; Kucherer et al., 1987). Homology with other glycoproteins involved in intercellular adhesion has been presented in support of adhesive functions for HECA-452 in skin-lymphocyte interactions (Duijvestin et al., 1988; Kruse et al., 1984; Kucherer et al., 1987).

Ongoing studies in our laboratories and in others have begun to elucidate the various cutaneous compartments and specific cell types which express these adhesion molecules. Previous reports have shown a characteristic temporal profile of adhesion molecule expression by T cells, dermal dendrocytes (DD), microvascular endothelial cells (EC), keratinocytes (KC) and Langerhans cells (LC) in psoriasis and in Rhus allergic contact dermatitis (ACD) (Griffiths et al., 1991; Nickoloff and Griffiths, 1990b). Observations of a rich network of Thy-1[+]/FXIIIa[+], ICAM-1[+] and VCAM-1[+] DD throughout the papillary dermis of CTCL along with the unique localization of proliferative (Ki-67[+]) T cells in the epidermis have lead us to speculate regarding the functional role these adhesion molecules play in the cellular dynamics of CTCL (Fivenson et al., 1991b; 1992). To further investigate the potential impact these molecules have on cellular trafficking in CTCL, we have now evaluated the expression of HECA-452 and PCNA in the same series of CTCL patients previously reported (Fivenson et al., 1991b; 1992), and have compared these to the expression profiles in normal skin, early rhus ACD and psoriasis.

MATERIALS AND METHODS

Patients: Punch biopsies from 29 patients, 11 with untreated MF (5 patch and 6 plaque-stage patients), 2 with premycotic parapsoriasis (pre-MF), 4 with plaque type psoriasis, 10 with early ACD (48 hours after antigen exposure, N = 4; 1 week after antigen exposure, N = 3; and 2 weeks after antigen exposure, N =3), and two with normal skin were obtained after informed consent. Pre-MF, as defined here, is represented by a particular histopathology characterized by a lichenoid and epidermotropic infiltrate of lymphocytes (some hyperchromatic and hyperconvoluted) but without Pautrier microabcesses and not warranting the diagnosis of MF (Griffiths et al., 1989b).

Immunohistochemistry: A highly sensitive avidin/biotin-linked immunoperoxidase staining technique was performed as reported previously using 4 micron paraffin sections of all skin biopsies (Griffiths et al., 1989b). An irrelevant, isotype-matched mAb was included with each set of patient slides as a control.

The mAb used and their sources included: HECA-452/CLA, provided by Louis Picker, MD, Stanford, CA, PCNA, obtained from Novocastra Laboratories, Newcastle upon Tyne, Great Britain, HM-1 and Ki67.

Preliminary experiments on reactive lymph node and patient specimens were performed to determine the optimal dilution for each antibody. All sections were examined by light microscopy, and the numbers of reactive cells for each monoclonal antibody recorded. Epidermotropic lymphocytes were quantified as the percentage of round lymphoid cells that were reactive with the mAb seen in 10 consecutive high power (40x) fields (HPF). Dermal lymphocytes were evaluated based on the percentage of round lymphoid cells that were reactive. At least 500 cells from at least five HPF were reviewed.

RESULTS and DISCUSSION

The results of this series of immunostaining studies are summarized in Figure 1 and Tables 2 and 3. HECA-452 was expressed by 1-85% of epidermotropic T cells as compared to 0-42% of dermal T cells in lesional CTCL. As shown in Figure 1 and Table 2, HECA-452 expression displayed a slight preference for the epidermal compartment in CTCL, but varied considerably among patients with different stages of disease. Figures 2 and 3 demonstrate HECA-452 staining of plaque stage MF, with both positive epidermal and dermal round cells seen. However, in Figure 4, also showing plaque stage MF, only a minority of dermal round cells were positive. Among the normal and benign inflammatory skin specimens studied, only two of the five psoriasis specimens had similar numbers of HECA-452+ dermal lymphoid cells, as compared to the MF specimens. Epidermal lymphoid expression of HECA-452 varied from 0-20% in psoriasis, 0-10% in Rhus ACD, and was negative in normal skin (summarized in Table 2). Of particular interest was the prominent staining seen with this antibody by both epidermal (i.e. LC) and dermal (i.e. DD) dendritic cells in most specimens. (Figure 5, from a case of pre-MF).

PCNA expression by lymphocytes in normal skin, psoriasis, and Rhus ACD was very rare. Basal keratinocytes routinely expressed this antigen in a nuclear distribution. As predicted by the classic studies of Van Scott and his associates (Van Scott and Ekel, 1963), the number of PCNA+ (i.e. proliferative fraction, in the S phase of the cell cycle) keratinocytes was greatly expanded in the psoriasis specimens compared to that of the other diseases and of normal skin (unquantified observation). CTCL expression of nuclear PCNA reactivity by lymphocytes is summarized in Table 3 alongside our previous data for ten of these same patients which

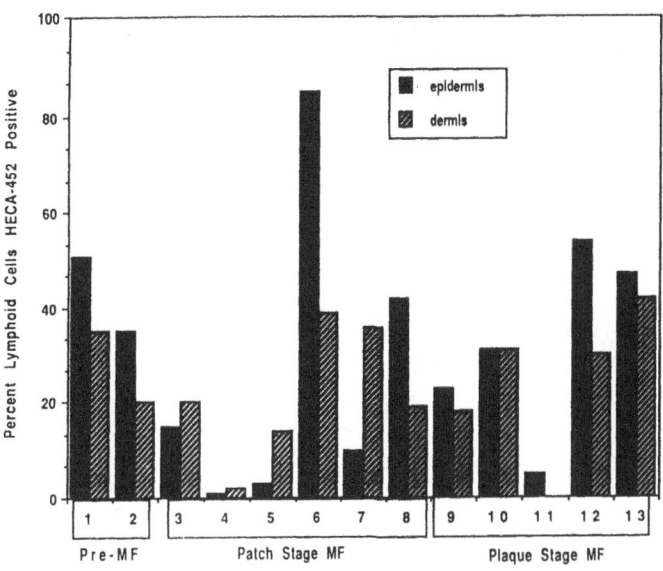

Figure 1. HECA-452 expression in mycosis fungoides and pre-MF. The percentage of positively stained, round lymphoid cells was calculated for epidermis and dermis separately in each case.

Table 2. Lymphocyte expression of HECA 452 in mycosis fungoides and benign dermatoses

Disease Entity	No. of Specimens	Epidermis*	Dermis**
Pre-MF	2	43%	28%
MF-patch Stage	5	28%	24%
MF-plaque Stage	6	30%	22%
Psorasis	5	8%	5%
Rhus ACD			
48 hours	4	3%	2%
1 week	3	4%	1%
2 weeks	3	4%	4%
Normal Skin	2	rare	rare

*Epidermal average is based on the percentage of round lymphoid appearing cells positively stained per 100 round cells in the epidermis per case.

**Dermal score is based on the percentage of round lymphoid appearing cells positively stained per 500 round cells in the dermis per case. One case of pre-MF had only 215 round cells in the dermis.

Table 3. Lymphocyte expression of activation antigens in mycosis fungoides

Disease Entity	No. of Specimens	PCNA		Ki-67†		HML-1†	
		Epidermis*	Dermis*	Epidermis	Dermis	Epidermis	Dermis
Pre-MF	2	7.5	0	32.0	0	34.0	53.0
MF-patch stage	5	6.4	0	56.0	0	7.0	30.0
MF-plaque stage	6	26.0	16.0**	49.0	2.0	69.0	138.0

†Ki-67 and HML-1 data represent a summary of previously published results (Fivenson et al., 1991a; 1992).

*Epidermal and dermal average are based on the number of round lymphoid cells positively stained per round cells present in 10 high power (40X) fields round cells per case.

**PCNA+ dermal cells were limited to the papillary dermis in these cases.

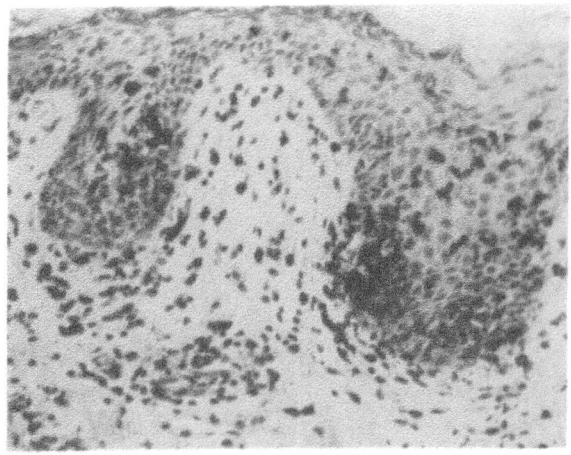

Figure 2. HECA-452 expression in plaque stage mycosis fungoides. Note the prominent reactivity of both epidermal and dermal lymphocytes. (Immunoperoxidase stain; magnification X 80)

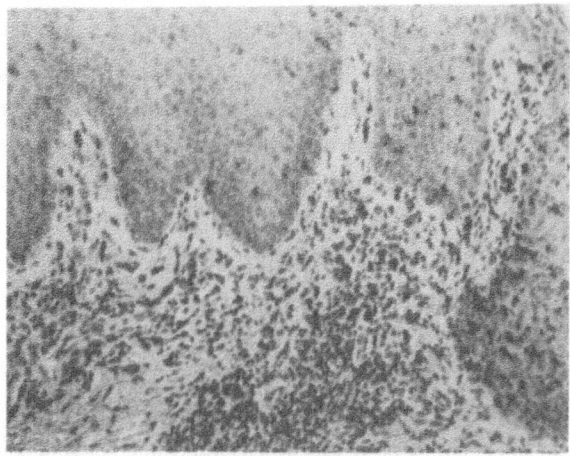

Figure 3. HECA-452 expression in plaque stage mycosis fungoides. Note the prominent reactivity of both epidermal and dermal lymphocyte. (Immunoperoxidase stain; magnification X 50)

examined the activation antigens, Ki-67 and HML-1. PCNA reactivity was limited to 10-50% of the Ki-67$^+$ lymphocytes in the epidermis, as was expected due to its restriction to S-phase expression. Dermal lymphocyte expression of PCNA was seen only in plaque stage CTCL in the dermal papillae, in close proximity to areas of epidermis where PCNA$^+$ cells were present.

Our previous reports have partially elucidated a network of adhesion molecules on Thy-

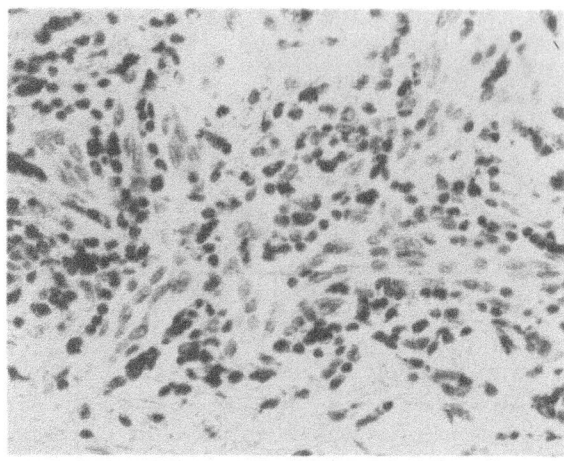

Figure 4. HECA-452 expression in plaque stage mycosis fungoides. Note that only a minority of round lymphoid cells are positive. (Immunoperoxidase stain; magnification X 150)

1$^+$/FXIIIa$^+$ DD in CTCL, in Rhus ACD and in psoriasis (Fivenson et al., 1991a; 1991b; 1992; Nickoloff, 1991a; Nickoloff and Griffiths, 1990a; 1990b). We have shown that Thy-1$^+$/FXIIIa$^+$ DD are seen in all cases of MF and pre-MF and that they form a complex dendritic network within the upper dermis. Thy-1 is also extensively expressed on endothelial cells (EC) of the superficial vascular plexus (Fivenson et al., 1991a; 1991b). We have further shown that these FXIIIa$^+$ DD co-express other bone marrow derived monocyte/macrophage/dendritic cell markers in cutaneous T cell lymphoma with an immunophenotype for these cells in CTCL as follows: Thy-1$^+$, FXIIIa$^+$, EBM-11$^+$, CD14$^+$, HLA-DR$^+$, HeL$^+$, ICAM-1$^+$, VCAM-1$^+$, CD4$^+$, CD18$^+$, CD36$^+$, CD1a$^-$, S100$^-$, FXIIIa$^-$, KP-1$^-$, MAC387$^-$ (Fivenson et al., 1991a; 1991b). Double immunofluorescence labelling has confirmed coexpression of Thy-1 and FXIIIa on identical cells (Fivenson et al., 1991a; 1992).

Ultrastructurally, DD are characterized by active phagocytosis, extensive rough endoplasmic reticulum and dendritic processes which closely interact with other dermal cell types including T cells and endothelial cells (Altman et al., 1992). DD phagocytic function in situ has been documented in cases of minocycline-induced hyperpigmentation and by hemosiderin phagocytosis in Kaposi sarcoma (Altman et al., 1992; Nickoloff and Griffiths, 1989). The expression of the monocyte/macrophage antigens, CD14 and EBM-11, but not KP-1 or MAC 387, by DD suggests they are part of the family of antigen presenting cells (APC), yet distinct from Langerhans cells (LC) and indeterminant cells (Cerio et al., 1989).

After making the initial observation that, within the dermis of MF, there is a significant number of dendritic Thy-1$^+$ cells (Fivenson, et al., 1991b), we subsequently stained a series of MF cases with a large panel of mAb to better characterize these cells (Fivenson et al., 1991b;

1992). In this study we demonstrated an extensive network of Thy-1$^+$, FXIIIa$^+$, CD4$^+$, CD14$^+$, CD1a$^-$ dermal dendrocytes that was consistently present within the papillary dermis of all stages of CTCL. CD34$^+$ dendritic cells were also present in the deep dermis of MF lesions as reported in normal skin (Nickoloff, 1991b). There was, however, a trend towards a decrease in CD34$^+$ cells in lesions rich in FXIIIa$^+$/Thy-1$^+$ DD.

Our earlier studies have suggested that at least two sources can be theorized to account for the expanded numbers of DD seen in CTCL. As these cells express HLe and HLA-DR along with monocyte markers, it is reasonable to assume at least some of them are derived from

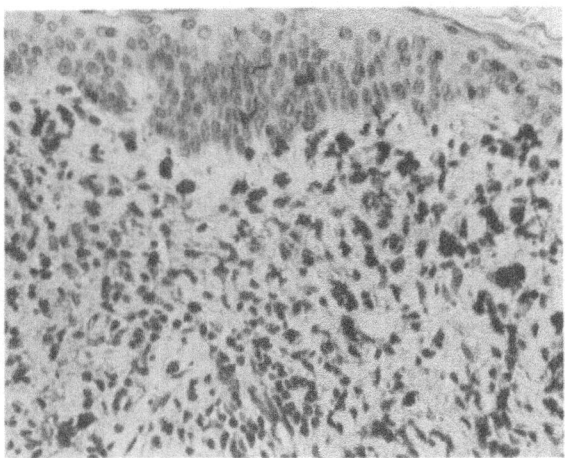

Figure 5. HECA-452 expression in pre-MF. Note positively stained dendritic epidermal (i.e., Langerhans cells) and dermal (i.e., dermal dendrocytes) cells. (Immunoperoxidase stain; magnification X 100)

circulating bone marrow-derived monocyte precursors (Cerio et al., 1989; 1990; Headington, 1986). A complimentary second site of origin is from the dendritic CD34$^+$ mesenchymal stem cell population that resides in the deep reticular dermis (Nickoloff, 1991b). CD34 antigen has been associated with less than 1% of bone marrow cells, and is reported to identify the pluripotent stem cell (Nickoloff, 1991b). Interestingly, Thy-1 antigen has been identified on bone marrow derived hematopoietic stem cells in mice (Basch and Berman, 1982). The extensive network of CD34$^+$ DD in the skin suggests that a reservoir of stem cells is present in the dermis. These cells could become activated and proliferate in the deep dermis in response to local inflammatory cytokines, and migrate into the upper dermis when they change their

Table 4. Expression of Adhesion Molecule Antigens by Dermal Dendrocytes and Endothelial Cells in Mycosis Fungoides†

Disease Entity	No. of Specimens	ELAM-1		VCAM-1		ICAM-1		Thy-1	
		DD*	Vessels**	DD*	Vessels**	DD*	Vessels**	DD*	Vessels**
PRE-MF	2	0	5.0	8.2	5.5	all	6.0	all	6.0
MF-patch stage	5	0	3.3	7.8	5.0	all	6.0	all	6.0
MF-plaque stage	6	0	4.8	12.4	5.0	all	6.0	all	6.0

†Adapted from previously reported data (Fivenson et al., 1991b; 1992).

*DD average is based on the average number of dendritic cells positively stained per at least 10 high power (40X) fields in the dermis

**Endothelial cell antigen expression was assessed semi-quantitatively by the following scoring system:

0 = negative or no vessel reactivity

2 = weak reactivity that was generally detectable on < 5 vessels/section

4 = moderate reactivity easily detectable on 6-10 vessels/section

6 = strong reactivity with easily detectable and diffuse staining of > 10 vessels/section.

phenotype by acquiring adhesion molecules and FXIIIa and EBM-11 antigens in addition to Thy-1. This concept supports the notion that much, if not all of the proliferative (i.e. Ki-67[+]/PCNA[+] see below) and immunomodulatory (i.e. Thy-1[+], FXIIIa[+], VCAM-1[+]) components that are active in cutaneous T cell lymphoma infiltrates are contained locally within the skin. This hypothesis is further corroborated by immunohistochemical studies which have shown increases in FXIIIa[+] cells which coincide with decreased CD34[+] cells during inflammatory dermatoses (Altman et al., 1992).

Adhesion molecule expression by APCs has been proposed as important in pathways of cell recognition, trafficking and communication, particularly duration the afferent/pro-inflammatory phases of cutaneous immune reactions (Griffiths et al., 1991; Nickoloff 1991a; Nickoloff and Griffiths, 1990b). We have shown that the DD present throughout lesional CTCL express the adhesion molecules CD54 (ICAM-1), CD18 (LFA-1), HECA-452 and VCAM-1 (Fivenson et al., 1991b; 1992; Table 2 and 4). These antigens are strongly expressed by DD in all stages of MF/CTCL. ELAM-1 is also expressed strongly and persistently by the papillary dermal EC in all stages of MF (Fivenson et al., 1991b; 1992; Nickoloff et al., 1991). KC also express ICAM-1 and HLA-DR in lesional CTCL skin (Griffiths et al., 1989b).

These observations have led us to conclude that DD are important cells in the etiopathophysiology of CTCL. The rich adhesion molecule network formed by inter-digitating dendrites would be viewed as a form of "dermal scaffolding" over which circulating malignant T cells could climb from the VCAM-1[+], ELAM-1[+], Thy-1[+] endothelium on their way to the epidermis expressing ICAM-1 and HLA-DR. The juxtaposition of Thy-1[+], VCAM-1[+], HECA-452[+] DD between the vasculature of the papillary dermis and the surrounding extracellular matrix, combined with T cells expressing their own compliment of ligands for these adhesion molecules, place the DD in a unique location to coordinate migration of cells to and from the epidermis, wherein the proliferative T cell compartment apparently exists (see below).

Braun-Falco et al., reported HML-1 to be an activation antigen specific for epidermotropic cells in CTCL (Sperling et al., 1989). Nickoloff and Griffiths reported Ki-67[+] to be specific for proliferating epidermal lymphocytes in CTCL. Our earlier findings that Ki-67[+] lymphocytes are limited to the epidermis, while HML-1 is expressed by both epidermal and dermal cells, supported the specificity of Ki-67 over HML-1 for the proliferative population in MF. In the current study, anti-PCNA mAb was applied to sections from the same biopsy specimens and similar confirmation of an epidermal T cell proliferative compartment was found (see Table 3). This mAb is interesting in that it recognizes DNA polymerase delta, which is only transcribed during the S-phase of the cell cycle (Waseem and Lane, 1990). Thus, it is predicted that a smaller fraction of epidermotropic T cells would be PCNA[+] than would be Ki-67[+] since the latter is expressed by any cell not in G_o (i.e. S, G_1, M, or G_2) (Bergstresser et al., 1985). As noted above, this mAb also nicely recognizes the expanded growth fraction of keratinocytes in psoriasis, which serves as a good internal positive control for the immunostaining technique.

In this report, Thy-1 antigen expression by DD and endothelial cells has been discussed in the context of this antigen possibly functioning as an adhesion molecule. While this is not proven in humans, adhesion properties have been proposed for Thy-1 antigen in the mouse (Nakashima et al., 1991). Thy-1 is a member of the Ig supergene family and is closely linked to N-CAM (Nguyen et al, 1986). Ongoing studies in our laboratory are currently focusing on showing whether Thy-1 functions as a typical adhesion molecule. As we have reported, Thy-1 is not expressed in the epidermis; thus we expect to find that its adhesive properties parallel other dermal and/or matrix adhesion molecules, such as fibronectin (Stoolman, 1989).

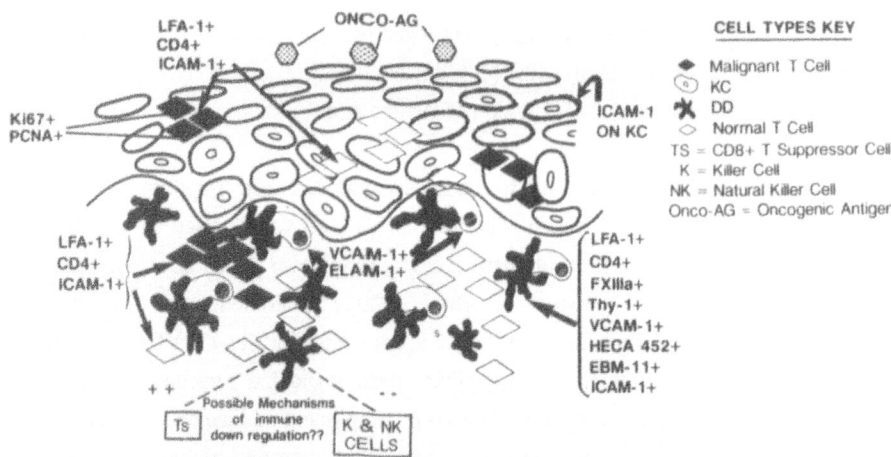

Figure 6. Cell trafficking networks in the development of CTCL.

Our findings of HECA-452 expression in CTCL are somewhat at odds with those of Picker et al. (1990). They refer to this antigen as a skin specific homing marker, and they found, on average, 85% of cutaneous T cells in CTCL to be HECA-452$^+$. In our series of 11 cases of CTCL, cutaneous T cells varied between 1 and 85% HECA-452$^+$ in the epidermis (mean = 31%) and 0-42% in the dermis (mean = 24%). We agree that this antigen appears to be preferentially expressed in the skin (only rare peripheral blood mononuclear cells (PBMC) were HECA-452$^+$). We could not, however, support the hypothesis that it serves as a skin specific homing marker, because the majority of lymphocytes in the case of CTCL, psoriasis, Rhus ACD, and normal skin studies were HECA-452 negative.

These studies suggest that a complex network of cutaneous compartments exists within lesions of inflammatory skin disease. The sheer numbers of Thy-1[+] DDs within the papillary dermis in lesions of CTCL would suggest a possible pathophysiological role for these cells in MF. To attempt to construct a unifying hypothesis from these various studies in CTCL and benign inflammatory dermatoses, we have developed the following model (Figure 6): In response to antigenic stimulation modulated by APCs (LC, DD, CD36[+] cells, macrophages??), T cells are recruited to the skin. EC adhesion molecules (VCAM-1, ELAM-1, Thy-1) are up-regulated during the pro-inflammatory and pro-elicitation phases of early ACD, psoriasis or "pre-MF", possibly mediated via KC derived cytokines (IL-1, GMCSF, MCAF, TGF-β, etc.). Coincident with this is upregulation of their adhesion molecule profile (HECA-452, ICAM-1, LFA-1, CD4, VCAM-1, Thy-1), again probably under local cytokine control. Proliferation/differentiation of DD within the dermis from the CD34[+] reservoir, as well as recruitment from circulating monocyte precursors, occurs concurrently. We have observed occasional PCNA[+], Ki-67[+] dendritic cells within the dermis, which support the concept of this local proliferation (results not shown).

Developing cutaneous T cell infiltrates and the subsequent histologic patterns would then be dictated by a combination of the inciting antigen(s) and the relative contribution of cutaneous APCs. Using the Rhus contact dermatitis model, Griffiths, Nickoloff and colleagues have shown that DD have a rich supply of TNF-α (the principle pro-inflammatory cytokine in cutaneous inflammatory reactions) (Griffiths et al, 1991; Nickoloff, 1991a; Nickoloff and Griffiths 1990a). TNF-α release from DD could induce keratinocyte ICAM-1 and IL-8 production, with subsequent increases in T cell aggregation and IFN-γ release (Barker et al., 1990; Griffiths et al, 1989a; Nickoloff, 1991a: Nickoloff and Griffiths, 1990a). Keratinocytes also make TGF-β, as well as mononuclear cell activating factor (MCAF) and granulocyte/macrophage cell activating factor (GMCSF), both of which are chemoattractants for monocytes (i.e., for DD precursors) (Barker et al., 1990; 1991; Nickoloff, 1991a). Thus, KC and DD appear to work synergistically via local and systemic cytokine pathways to augment the developing cutaneous inflammatory reaction.

Thy-1[+] DD may function as a selective activator of suppressor pathways. Thy-1[+] cells in mice and the T6[-], DR[+], CD36[+] macrophage in humans have been associated with suppressor cell activation (Bergstresser et al., 1985; Libsy et al., 1989). We have suggested that the role of the Thy-1[+] DD in MF would involve not only the important, albeit nonspecific, positional function outlined above, but also a specific suppressor-inducer function (like the murine Thy-1[+] dendritic epidermal T cells (Thy-1[+] DETC). An important role in cutaneous physiology and pathophysiology then emerges for this cell type. DD may function as the immune cell which counter-regulates inflammatory reactions in the skin. Just as LC activate the afferent limb of cutaneous immune responses, the DD could shut it off. A balance between these two types of cutaneous APCs can thus be envisioned. Initial LC activity would result in dermatitis with cutaneous inflammation. When DD activity "catches up", or the antigen is cleared, homeostasis is again achieved. While it is naive to assume that such a simple yin/yang relationship controls all cutaneous inflammatory processes, this model helps us to visualize the basic concepts of intercellular interactions in inflammatory dermatoses. It would probably be more realistic to consider the interplay of multiple cell types and cytokines in this balance.

Cutaneous T cell lymphoma could result from excess DD activity in response to a persistent oncogenic antigen, alone or in association with other factors (e.g. viruses, immunogenetic predisposition, oncogenes, etc.). As T cell lymphoma progresses from "pre-MF" to a well defined plaque, there is a continuous influx of Thy-1$^+$/FXIIIa$^+$ DD, paralleling the increasing T cell infiltrate. This chronic antigenic stimulation theory of CTCL pathogenesis is controversial, but a considerable amount of circumstantial evidence has been reported in support of it (Knobler and Edelson, 1986; Tan et al, 1984). Observations of large numbers of APCs within lesional skin, made by both us and others (Fivenson et al, 1991b; 1992; Hansen et al, 1990) would favor this theory. LC have also been reported to play an important role in this hypothesis, having been shown to be intimately associated with atypical, epidermotropic T cells within Pautrier microabcesses (Rowden et al., 1979). DD also may, via APC function, present tumor antigens in a way which either selectively activates a suppressor/inducer (CD8) signal or nonspecifically inhibits cytotoxic (K) and/or natural killer (NK) cell function. The result of either mechanism would be to down-regulate immune responses to the malignant T cells of CTCL, allowing indolent progression. Additional circumstantial evidence for a common etiologic factor in CTCL comes from the report by Jack et al. (1990), in which 10 of 16 cases of CTCL had malignant clones restricted to the TCR Vβ8 family. This report suggests that a common etiological factor exists in these unrelated patients. If the Thy-1$^+$/FXIIIa$^+$ DD population is involved in both the pathogenesis and propagation of CTCL, then therapeutic targeting of DD would be an important approach to the treatment of CTCL.

Our model shows how developing T cell infiltrates could be facilitated by a "scaffolding" of DD dendritic processes bearing adhesion molecules to guide lymphocytes from the vascular space through the dermis and into the epidermis. Persistent expression of these adhesion molecules by DD and EC may serve to augment migration of CD4$^+$, ICAM-1$^+$, LFA-1$^+$ T-cells as well as dendritic cell precursors into the dermis and/or epidermis of the MF lesion, much the same as in lesions of psoriasis and ACD (Griffiths et al., 1991; Nickoloff, 1991a; Nickoloff and Griffiths, 1990a; 1990b). As described above, it is in the epidermal compartment that, at least in CTCL, T cell proliferation (i.e., presence of PCNA$^+$, Ki-67$^+$) occurs in the developing lesion.

In conclusion, within the lesional biopsies of CTCL patients, the upper dermis contains an extensive network of DD bearing numerous adhesion molecules. Activation and adhesion marker studies suggest that DD may participate in the propagation of lesions of CTCL by facilitating cytokine mediated efflux of T cells beween various compartments of the skin.

Additional studies are underway to assess the APC function of the Thy-1$^+$ DD in CTCL, as well the effects of therapeutic targeting of DD and/or adhesion molecules.

ACKNOWLEDGEMENTS

The authors thank Dr. CEM Griffiths for his assistance in obtaining some of the biopsies used in this study. Supported in part by NIH grants AR31857, AR40065, AR01823, and AR40488 (BJN). This work was presented in part at the combined Society of Investigative Dermatology and American Federation of Clinical Research Meetings, Seattle, Washington, May 1991.

REFERENCES

Altman, DA, DP Fivenson and MW Lee, 1992. Minocycline hyperpigmentation as a model for in-situ phagocytic activity of factor XIIIa positive dermal dendrocytes. **J. Cutan. Pathol.**, 19; 345-350.

Barker, JNWN, V Sarma, V Dixit, RS Mitra and BJ Nickoloff, 1990a. Marked synergism between tumor necrosis factor-alpha and interferon gamma in regulation of keratinocyte derived chemotactic factors and adhesion molecules. **J. Clin. Invest.**, 85:605-608.

Barker, JNWN, RS Mitra, CEM Griffiths, VM Dixit and BJ Nickoloff, 1990b. Keratinocytes as initiators of inflammation. **Lancet**, 337:211-214.

Basch, RS and JW Berman, 1982. Thy-1 determinants are present on many murine hematopoietic cells other than T cells. **Eur. J. Immunol.**, 12:359-364.

Bergstresser, PR, S Sullivan, JW Streilein and RE Tigelaar, 1985. Origin and function of Thy-1$^+$ dendritic epidermal cells in mice. **J. Invest. Dermatol.**, 85:85s-9Os.

Cerio, R, CEM Griffiths, KD Cooper, BJ Nickoloff and JT Headington, 1989. Characterization of Factor XIIIa positive dermal dendritic cells in normal and inflamed skin. **Brit. J. Dermatol.**, 121:421-432.

Cerio, R, J Spaull, GF Oliver and E Wilson Jones, 1990. A study of factor XIIIa and Mac 387 immunolabelling in normal and pathological skin. **Am. J. Dermatopathol.**, 12:221-233.

Duijvestin, AM, E Horst, ST Pals, BN Rouse, AC Steere, LJ Picker, CJLM Meijer and EC Butcher, 1988. High endothelial differentiation in human lymphoid and inflammatory tissues defined by monoclonal antibody HECA-452. **Am. J. Pathol.**, 130:147-155.

Fivenson, DP, LA Rheins, JJ Nordlund and EA Krull, 1991a. Thy-1 expression and T cell receptor type in mycosis fungoides and benign dermatoses. **J. Natl. Canc. Inst.**, 83:1088-1092.

Fivenson, DP, RW Dunstan, MC Douglass, BJ Nickoloff and PF Moore, 1991b. Thy-1$^+$ dermal dendrocytes in mycosis fungoides. **J. Invest. Dermatol.**, 96:599A.

Fivenson, DP, MC Douglass and BJ Nickoloff, 1992. Cutaneous expression of Thy-1 in mycosis fungoides. **Am. J. Pathol.**, 141:1373-1380.

Griffiths, CEM, JJ Voorhees and BJ Nickoloff, 1989a. Gamma interferon induced different keratinocyte cellular patterns of expression of HLA-DR and DQ and intercellular adhesion molecule-1 (ICAM-1). **Br. J. Dermatol.**, 120:1-8.

Griffiths, CEM, J Voorhees and BJ Nickoloff, 1989b. Characterization of intercellular adhesion molecule-1 and HLA-DR in normal and inflamed skin: Modulation by recombinant interferon gamma and tumor necrosis factor. **J. Am. Acad. Dermatol.**, 20:617-629.

Griffiths, CEM, JNWN Barker, S Kunkel and BJ Nickoloff, 1991. Induction, distribution and dimunition of leukocyte adhesion molecules, T cell chemotaxin and a modulatory cytokine during the evolution of allergic contact dermatitis. **Br. J. Dermatol.**, 124:519-526.

Hansen, ER, O Baadsgaard, S Lisby, KD Cooper, K Thomsen and GL Vejlsgaard, 1990. Cutaneous T cell lymphoma lesional epidermal cells activate autologous $CD8^+$ T lymphocytes: Involvement of both $CD1^+$, $OKM5^+$ and $CD1^+$, $OKM5^-$ antigen-presenting cells. **J. Invest. Dermatol.**, 94:485-491.

Headington, JT, 1986. The dermal dendrocyte. In Callen JP, Dahl MV, Golitz LE et al. Eds: **Advances in Dermatology**, Vol. 1, Chicago: Year Book Medical Publishers Inc., 159-71.

Jack, AS, AW Boylston, S Carrell and I Grigor, 1990. Cutaneous T cell lymphoma cells employ a restricted range of T cell antigen receptor variable region genes. **Am. J. Pathol.**, 136(1):17-21.

Kruse, J, R Maihammer, H Wernecke, A Faissner, I Sommer, C Goridis and M Schachner, 1984. Neural cell adhesion molecules and myelin-associated glycoprotein share a common carbohydrate moiety recognized by monoclonal antibodies L2 and HNK-1. **Nature**, 311:153-155.

Knobler, RM and RL Edelson, 1986. Cutaneous T cell lymphoma. **Med. Clin. North. Am.**, 70:109-13.

Kucherer, A, A Faissner and M Schachne, 1987. The novel carbohydrate epitope L3 is shared by some neural cell adhesion molecules. **J. Cell Biol.**, 104:1597-1602.

Libsy, S, O Baadsgaard, KD Cooper and GL Vejlsgaard, 1989. Decreased number and function of antigen-presenting cells in the skin after application of irritating agents: Relevance for skin cancer? **J. Invest. Dermatol.**, 92:842-847.

Nakashima, I, Y Zhang, SMJ Rahman, T Yoshida, K Isobe, L Ding, T Iwamoto, M Hamaguchi, H Ikezawa and R Taguchi, 1991. Evidence of synergy between Thy-1 and CD3/TCR complex in signal delivery to murine thymocytes for cell death. **J. Immunol.**, 147:1153-1162.

Nguyen, C, M-G Mattei, J-F Mattei, MJ Santoni, C Goridis and BR Jordan, 1986. Localization of human N-CAM gene band to q23 of chromosome 11: The third gene coding for a cell interaction molecule mapped to the distal portion of the long arm of chromosome 11. **J. Cell Biol.**, 102: 711-715.

Nickoloff, BJ and CEM Griffiths, 1989. Factor XIIIa expressing dermal dendrocytes are increased in AIDS associated Kaposi's sarcoma. **Science**, 243:1736-1737.

Nickoloff, BJ, 1991a. The cytokine network in psoriasis. **Arch. Dermatol.**, 127:871-884.

Nickoloff, BJ, 1991b. CD34 expression in normal skin and Kaposi's sarcoma. **Arch. Dermatol.**, 127:523-529.

Nickoloff, BJ, DP Fivenson, CEM Griffiths and R Modlin, 1991. Preferential but not unique cutaneous endothelial cell (EC) expression of ELAM-1. **Clin. Res.**, 39:153A.

Nickoloff, BJ and CEM Griffiths, 1990a. Abnormal cutaneous topobiology: The molecular basis for dermatopathological mononuclear cell patterns in inflammatory skin disease. **J. Invest. Dermatol.**, 95:128s-131s.

Nickoloff, BJ and CEM Griffiths, 1990b. Lymphocyte trafficking in psoriasis: A new perspective emphasizing the dermal dendrocyte with active dermal recruitment medicated via endothelial cells followed by intra-epidermal T cell activation. **J. Invest. Dermatol.**, 95:355-375.

Nickoloff, BJ and CEM Griffiths, 1990c. Intraepidermal but not dermal T lymphocytes are positive for a cell-cycle associated antigen (Ki-67) in mycosis fungoides. **Am. J. Pathol.**, 136:261-266.

Picker, LJ, SA Michie, LS Rott and EC Butcher, 1990. A unique phenotype of skin-associated lymphocytes in humans: Preferential expression of the HECA-452 epitope by benign and malignant T cells at cutaneous sites. **Am. J. Pathol.**, 136:1053-1068.

Rowden, G, T Phillips, M Lewis et al., 1979. Target role of Langerhans cells in mycosis fungoides: Transmission and immunoelectron microscopic studies. **J. Cutan. Pathol.**, 6:364-382.

Sperling, M, P Kaudewitz, O Braun-Falco and H Stein, 1989. Reactivity of T cells in mycosis fungoides exhibiting marked epidermotropism with the monoclonal antibody HML-1 that defines a membrane molecule on human mucosal lymphocytes. **Am. J. Pathol.**, 134:955-960.

Stoolman, LM, 1989. Adhesion molecules controlling lymphocyte migration. **Cell**, 56:907-910.

Tan, R, C Butterworth, H McLaughlin et al., 1974. Mycosis fungoides: A disease of antigen persistence. **Br. J. Dermatol.**, 91:607-616.

VanScott, EJ and TM Ekel, 1963. Kinetics of hyperplasia in psoriasis. **Arch. Dermatol.**, 88:373-381.

Waseem, NH and DP Lane, 1990. Monoclonal antibody analysis of the proliferating cell nuclear antigen (PCNA): Structural conservation and the detection of a nucleolar form. **J. Cell Sci.**, 96:121-129.

CYTOKINE NEUROPEPTIDE INTERACTIONS IN THE SKIN

T. A. Luger*

A. Köck*

E. Schauer†

A. Schwarz*

F. Trautinger†

T. Schwarz*

* Department of Dermatology, Ludwig Boltzmann Institute of Cell Biology
and Immunology of the Skin
University of Munster
Munster, Germany

† Department of Dermatology II
University of Vienna
Vienna, Austria

Correspondence to: Prof. Dr. T. A. Luger, Department of Dermatology,
University of Ulm, von Esmarch Strasse 56,
D-4400 Munster, Germany

ABSTRACT

There is clear evidence that there is a close relationship between immunoregulatory cytokines which have recently been demonstrated to be synthesized and released by epidermal cells and pituitary-derived neuropeptides such as adrenocorticotropin (ACTH) and melanocyte stimulating hormone (αMSH). Therefore, it was investigated whether keratinocytes are capable of producing neuropeptides. Supernatant fluids derived from normal human keratinocytes and from epidermoid carcinoma cell lines (A431, KB) contained significant levels of both αMSH and ACTH. Northern blot analysis using a cDNA probe for the αMSH/ACTH precursor,

Basic Mechanisms of Physiologic and Aberrant Lymphoproliferation in the Skin
Edited by W.C. Lambert *et al.*, Plenum Press, New York, 1994

95

proopiomelanocortin (POMC), revealed the expression of POMC specific mRNA in normal keratinocytes as well as in epidermoid carcinoma cell lines. The production of αMSH as well as ACTH was significantly upregulated, at both the protein and mRNA level, after stimulation with the tumor promoters, phorbol myristate acetate (PMA) or ultraviolet (UV) light, or with interleukin-1 (IL-1). Since it has recently been shown that αMSH exhibits immunomodulatory capacities, the effect of αMSH on MHC class I and class II as well as on ICAM-1 expression was investigated. αMSH (10^{-9}M) antigen significantly blocked MHC class I expession on peripheral blood mononuclear cells, cells from a monomyelocytic cell line (U937) and A431 cells, but MHC class II antigen and ICAM-1 expression were not affected. These data indicate that keratinocytes, in addition to cytokines, produce neuropeptides which also appear to function as regulatory elements of the skin immune system.

INTRODUCTION

The role of the epidermis as a fully developed immune organ is well established. Accordingly, the epidermis harbors all cellular constituents necessary for the initiation of an immune response, including dendritic cells with antigen presenting capacities and cells belonging to the T cell lineage (Bos et al., 1989; Stingl et al., 1989; Streilein et al., 1991). In addition, cytokines which mediate immune and inflammatory reactions have been shown to be released by several types of epidermal cell such as keratinocytes, melanocytes and Langerhans cells (Köck et al., 1991; Kupper, 1990; Luger and Schwarz, 1991). Cytokines produced by epidermal cells include interleukins, colony stimulating factors, tumor necrosis factor and growth factors. There is also evidence for a complex network of interacting cytokines and a close relationship between the cytokine cascade and other mediators such as eicosanoids and hormones.

An increasing amount of data has accumulated linking the immune and neuroendocrine systems (Bateman et al., 1989). Accordingly, immunosupression turned out to be a characteristic feature of the stress syndrome, which appears to be exerted via two peripheral effectors, the glucocorticosteroids and catecholamines (Khansari et al., 1990). In addition, corticotropin releasing hormone (CRH), initially isolated from the hypothalamus and named for its property of stimulating adrenocorticotropin (ACTH) and glucocorticoid secretion, has been found to directly stimulate the production of proopiomelanocortin (POMC) related peptides (Brown and Blalock, 1990). POMC is a large prohormone which, via the action of specific proteases, is cleaved into several peptide hormones such as ACTH, melanocyte stimulating hormone (MSH), endorphins and lipotrophins (Brown and Blalock 1990). There is also stong evidence that CRH and POMC derived peptides have direct effects on the immune and inflammatory systems (Bateman et al., 1989). On the other hand, mediators of immunity and inflammation, such as cytokines including interleukin (IL)-1, IL-6 and tumor necrosis factor α (TNFα), appear to stimulate CRH and POMC production and functions (Bateman et al., 1989; Brown and Blalock, 1990). Therefore, cytokines may be regarded as additional important mediators of the immune-hypothalamic-pituitary-adrenal-axis (immune-HPA).

96

KERATINOCYTE PRODUCTION OF PROOPIOMELANOCORTIN-DERIVED HORMONES

A number of extrapituitary sources of POMC have been identified, including brain, gastrointestinal tract, placenta, gonads and leukocytes (Bateman et al., 1990). Moreover, the POMC product, αMSH, has recently been isolated from the skin (Thody et al., 1983). Therefore, and because of the immunosecretory capacity of epidermal cells, it seemed likely that keratinocytes may also serve as a source for POMC.

The human epidermoid carcinoma cell lines, A431 and KB, as well as long term cultured human normal foreskin keratinocytes (HNK) were investigated for their capacity to produce the POMC derived hormones, αMSH and ACTH. Cells were plated at a density of 1×10^6/ml and supernatant fluids were harvested at different time points (24, 48 and 72 hours). To stimulate hormone production, cells were treated with phorbol myristate acetetate (PMA), recombinant human IL-1β and UVB-light. For the detection of αMSH, a radioimmunoassay (Milab Corp., Malmo, Sweden) was used and ACTH was measured using an IRMA (Allegro-HS-ACTH, Nichols Institute, San Juan, CA). Both human epidermoid carcinoma cells and normal human keratinocytes spontaneously produced detectable levels of αMSH and ACTH (Köck et al., 1990). Moreover, partially purified epidermal cell derived αMSH was found to be biologically active using the tyrosinase assay (data not shown). Treatment of the cells with PMA resulted in a significant induction of keratinocyte hormone production, with highest yields achieved after cultivation for 72 hours (Table 1). Among a variety of other cytokines tested for their capacity to enhance αMSH production by epidermal cells so far, only IL-1β proved to be effective (data not shown) (Köck, et al., 1990). Moreover, upon treatment with UV-B light, a significant enhancement of A431 cell αMSH production was observed (Table 1).

In order to investigate whether the prohormone, POMC, is expressed in human epidermal cells, Northern blot analysis was performed. Using a 0.9 kb cDNA probe (provided by Dr. K. Boehm, Cleveland, Ohio, USA) specific transcripts with a size of 1.3 kb were detected in A431 cells after 4 hours. Only small amounts of POMC were found to be transcribed spontaneously; this was significantly upregulated upon treatment with PMA (10 ng/ml) or IL-1 (100 U/ml) (Figure 1). Moreover, whereas POMC specific mRNA was not detectable in untreated normal human keratinocytes, treatment with IL-1 or PMA resulted in stimulation of POMC mRNA after 4 hours (data not shown).

These findings demonstrate for the first time that normal and malignant human keratinocytes produce neuropeptides such as the POMC products, αMSH and ACTH. In addition to its function as a melanotropic hormone, αMSH is now well known to be a mediator of immune and inflammatory reactions. Accordingly, αMSH has been demonstrated to block several functions of IL-1, i.e., thymocyte proliferation and prostaglandin release as well as induction of fever and acute phase proteins (Bateman et al., 1989; Cannon et al., 1986). αMSH has also been found to reverse the inhibitory effects of IL-1 or TNF-α on the effector phase of contact hypersensitivity in animals (Bateman et al., 1989). Recently, it was found that epicutaneous application of αMSH suppressed both the sensitization and elicitation limb of the cutaneous immune response to potent contact sensitizers (Rheins et al., 1989). Since UV light is well known to block the induction of contact hypersensitivity (CHS), it is possible that keratinocytes may participate, through the UV-induced production of αMSH, in the regulation of contact hypersentivity (Kripke and Morison, 1986). This

Table 1. Production of αMSH and ACTH by human epidermal cells.

cells	stimulius	αMSH (pg/ml)	ACTH (pg/ml)
HK[*]	-	32	n.t.
	PMA	78	n.t.
A431[*]	-	45	96
	PMA	120	204
	UVB	67	n.t.

*HNK or A431 cells were left untreated or stimulated with PMA (10 ng/ml) or UVB (120 J/m²). Supernatant fluids were harvested after 72 hours incubation and tested for αMSH or ACTH using specific immunoassays. Results are expressed as mean value of 3 different experiments. SD were within the 10% range. n.t., not tested.

is further supported by a previous finding that keratinocytes, upon UV irradiation, are able to produce an inhibitor of CHS which is distinct from αMSH and other inhibitory cytokines such as transforming growth factor β (TGFβ) or an IL-1 receptor antagonist (IL-1ra) (Schwarz and Luger, 1989).

EFFECT OF PROOPIOMELANOCORTIN DERIVED HORMONES ON MHC ANTIGEN AND ICAM-1 EXPRESSION

Keratinocytes are well known to release a variety of distinct mediators affecting immune functions. Accordingly, several cytokines and growth factors have been detected in epidermal cells on a transcriptional as well as a translational level (Kupper, 1990; Luger and Schwarz, 1991). However, keratinocyte supernatant fluids also may contain other mediators which, to date, have been only partially characterized. One of these previously described secretory products of keratinocytes is a factor of approximately 1 kD which is capable of reducing major histocompatibility (MHC) class I antigen expression in several cell lines (Schwarz et al., 1988). Since the biochemical characteristics of this inhibitor appeared to be similar to those of MSH, it was tested whether αMSH may influence the expression of MHC class I antigen and β_2 microglobulin. In addition, MHC class II antigen and intercellular adhesion molecule 1 (ICAM-1) expression were investigated. Human peripheral blood mononuclear adherent cells (PBMC), a monomyelocytic cell line (U937) and A431 (epidermal) cells were evaluated by FACS analysis using monoclonal antibodies.

Incubation of U937 cells with αMSH resulted in a significant reduction of spontaneous MHC class I antigen and β_2 microglobulin expression in a dose dependent manner. αMSH in a concentration of 10^{-9} M was most effective (Figure 2). Since interferon-γ (IFN-γ) is known to be a potent inducer of class I antigen expression, it was investigated whether αMSH could overcome the stimulating effect of IFN-γ. αMSH completely blocked the U937 cell class I antigen and β_2 microglobulin inducing capacity of IFN-γ (Figure 2). In addition, αMSH was able to inhibit spontaneous as well as IFN-γ induced MHC class I antigen expression by PBMC

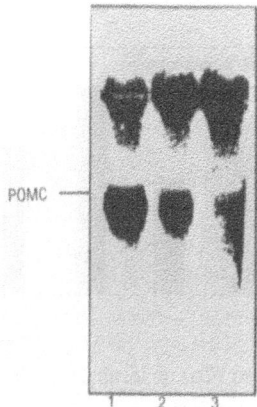

Figure 1. POMC mRNA expression in A431 cells. Confluent A431 cells were treated with PMA, 10 ng/ml (lane 1), IL-1β, 100 U/ml (lane 2), or left untreated (lane 3), and incubated for 4 hours. Total cellular RNA was extracted and hybridized with a ^{32}P labelled POMC cDNA probe.

and A431 cells (data not shown). In order to obtain further insight into the mechanisms by which αMSH affects MHC class I antigen expression, it was tested whether αMSH is effective at the transcriptional level. Upon Northern blot analysis using a cDNA probe of the constant region of class I antigen (Seeman et al., 1986) αMSH was found to block the IFN-γ mediated transcription of MHC class I antigen (data not shown). By contrast, αMSH did not affect MHC class II or ICAM-1 expression on PBMC, U937 or A431 cells (data not shown).

The HLA class I/β_{2m} complex, consisting of 3 highly variable heavy chains noncovalently associated with an invariant light chain (β_{2m}), is involved in the presentation of antigen to cytotoxic T-lymphocytes (Lopez De Castro et al., 1985). The expression of class I antigens plays an important role in host defense against microorganisms and in rejection of allografts and tumors (Lopez De Castro et al., 1985; Miller et al., 1989). In certain tumors, a down-regulation of polymorphic HLA class I antigens has been reported, which may account for the impaired recognition by the host immunosurveillance (Bernards et al., 1983; Hui et al., 1984). Therefore, the regulation of class I expression appears to be an important mechanism of host defense against transformed cells (Halloran and Madrenas, 1990). Interferons have been reported to upregulate class I molecules on various target cells. Although all 3 types of IFN's can induce an increase in class I expression, IFNγ is the most potent (David-Watine et al., 1990). In addition, TNFα, which is also produced by epidermal cells, appears to be involved in the regulation of class I expression (David-Watine et al., 1990). Down-regulation of class I antigens is known to be mediated by several viruses via reduction in class I gene transcription and mRNA accumulation (Halloran and Madrenas, 1990). A novel mechanism for reducing class I antigen expression appears to be exerted through the POMC gene product, αMSH. The

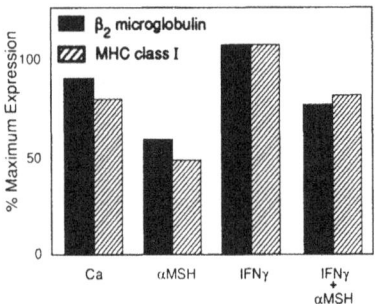

Figure 2. U937 cells were left untreated (Co) or incubated with MSHα (10^{-9} M) and/or IFN-γ (1000 U/ml) and evaluated for MHC class I antigen or β_2 microglobulin expression using specific monoclonal antibodies and FACS analysis. Results are expressed as % of maximum expression of 3 different experiments. SD values were within the 10% range. Maximum expression is defined as degree of MHC class I or β_2 microglobulin expression which was achieved upon IFN-γ treatment.

production of αMSH in keratinocytes is upregulated by tumor promoters such as PMA and UVB light. Moreover, malignant keratinocyte cell lines were found to produce significantly increased amounts of αMSH in comparison to normal human keratinocytes. Therefore, αMSH production by malignant cells may reflect one of the mechanisms needed to escape immune detection by class I restricted cytotoxic lymphocytes.

In summary, the present data demonstrate that human keratinocytes, in addition to their capacity to produce cytokines and growth factors, are also able to release POMC derived neuropeptides such as αMSH and ACTH. Awareness of the production of these hormones, which have been recognized as potent mediators of immunity and inflammation, may further add to our understanding of the complex interactions within the skin immune system. Moreover, these findings further support the concept of the close relationship between the neuroendocrine and immune systems.

ACKNOWLEDGEMENTS

We wish to thank Mrs. M.L. Hülsmann for her expert secretarial assistance. This work was supported by the Deutsche Forschungsgemeinschaft Projekt Nr. Lu 443/1-1.

REFERENCES

Bateman A, A Singh, T Kral and S Solomon, 1989. The immune-hypothalamic-pituitary-adrenal axis, **Endocrine Rev.**, 10:92.

Bernards R, PI Schrier, A Houweling, JL Bos, AJ van der Eb, M Zijlstra and CJM Melief, 1983. Tumorigenicity of cells transformed by adenovirus type by evasion of T cell immunity, **Nature**, 305:776.

Bos JD, PR Das and ML Kapsenberg, 1989. The Skin Immune System (SIS), In: J.D. Bos, Ed., **The Skin Immune System (SIS)**, CRC Press, Boca Raton, Florida pp. 3-9 .

Brown SL and JE Blalock, 1990. Neuroendocrine immune interactions, In: J.J. Oppenheim, E. Shevach, Eds., **Immunophysiology**, Oxford University Press, Oxford and New York p. 306-320.

Cannon JG, JB Tatro, S Reichlin and CA Dinarello, 1986. α Melanocyte stimulating hormone inhibits immunostimulatory and inflammatory actions of interleukin 1, **J. Immunol.**, 137:2232.

David-Watine B, A Israel and P Kourilsky, 1009. The regulation and expression of MHC class I genes, **Immunol. Today**, 11:286.

Halloran PF and J Madrenas, 1990. Regulation of MHC transcription, **Transplantation**, 50:725.

Hui K, F Grosveld and H Festenstein, 1984. Rejection of transplantable AKR leukaemia cells following MHC DNA-mediated cell transformation, **Nature**, 311:750.

Khansari DN, AJ Murgo and RE Faith, 1990. Effects of stress on the immune system, **Immunol. Today**, 11:170.

Köck A, E Schauer, T Schwarz and TA Luger, 1990. αMSH and ACTH production by human keratinocytes: A link between the neuronal and the immune system, **J. Invest. Dermatol.**, 94:543.

Köck A, T Schwarz, M Micksche and TA Luger, 1991. Cytokines and human malignant melanoma immuno- and growth-regulatory peptides in melanoma biology, In: L. Nathanson, Ed., **Melanoma Research: Genetics, Growth Factors, Metastases, and Antigens**, Kluwer Academic Publishers, Boston p. 41-65.

Kripke ML and WL Morison, 1986. Studies on the mechanism of systemic suppression of contact hypersensitivity by ultraviolet B radiation, **Photodermatology**, 3:4.

Kupper TS, 1990. Role of epidermal cytokines, In: J.J. Oppenheim, E. Shevach, Eds., **Immunophysiology**, Oxford University Press, Oxford and New York pp. 285-306.

Lopez De Castro JA, JA Barbosa, MS Krangel, PA Biro and JL Strominger, 1985. Structural analysis of the functional sites of class I HLA antigens, **Immunol. Rev.**, 85:149.

Luger TA and T Schwarz, 1991. Epidermal cell-derived secretory regulins, In: G. Schuler, Ed., **Epidermal Langerhans Cells**, CRC Press, Boca Raton, Florida p. 217- 253.

Miller JFAP, G Morahan, J Allison, PS Bhathal and KO Cox, 1989. T cell tolerance in transgenic mice expressing major histocompatibility class I molecules in defined tissues, **Immunol. Rev.**, 107:109.

Rheins LA, AL Cotleur, RS Kleier, WB Hoppenjans, DN Sauder and JJ Nordlund, 1989. Alpha-melanocyte stimulating hormone modulates contact hypersensitivity responsiveness in C57/BL6 mice, **J. Invest. Dermatol.**, 95:511.

Schwarz T, M Danner, E Schauer, R Kirnbauer, A Urbanski and TA Luger, 1988. Regulation of MHC class I and class II antigen expression by different epidermal cytokines, **J. Invest. Dermatol.**, 90:607.

Schwarz T and TA Luger, 1989. Effect of UV irradiation on epidermal cell cytokine production, **J. Photochem. Photobiol.**, B 4:1.

Seemann GHA, RS Rein, CS Brown and HL Ploegh, 1986. Gene conversion-like mechanisms may generate polymorphism in human class I genes, **EMBO J.**, 5:547.

Stingl G, C Hauser, E Tschachler, V Groh and K Wolff, 1989. Immune Functions of Epidermal Cells, In: D.A. Norris, Ed., **Immune Mechanisms in Cutaneous Disease**, Marcel Dekker, New York and Basel, pp.3-73.

Streilein JW, 1989. Skin-associated lymphoid tissue, In: D.A. Norris, Ed., **Immune Mechanisms in Cutaneous Disease**, Marcel Dekker, New York and Basel pp. 73-97.

Thody AJ, K Ridley, RJ Penny, R Chalmers, C Fisher and S Shuster, 1983. MSH peptides are present in mammalian skin, **Peptides**, 4:813.

EFFECT OF UV LIGHT ON CYTOKINE PRODUCTION BY EPIDERMAL CELLS

Thomas Schwarz*†
Agatha Urbanski‡
Franz Trautinger†
Peter Neuner‡
Thomas A.Luger†

* Department of Dermatology
  Hospital Lainz
  Vienna, Austria

† LBI-DVS
  Laboratory of Cell Biology
  Department of Dermatology
  University of Munster
  Munster, Germany

‡ Department of Dermatology II
  University of Vienna
  Vienna, Austria

Correspondence to: Prof. Dr. Th. Schwarz, Department of Dermatology,
University Hospitak, von Esmarch Strasse 56,
D-4400 Munster, Germany

ABSTRACT

The epidermis has been recently recognized as a potent source for cytokines, including interleukins (IL), colony stimulating factors (CSF), tumor necrosis factor (TNF) and growth factors. In addition, ultraviolet B (UVB) light (290-320nm) has turned out to be a strong

Basic Mechanisms of Physiologic and Aberrant Lymphoproliferation in the Skin
Edited by W.C. Lambert *et al.*, Plenum Press, New York, 1994

stimulus for cytokine production by keratinocytes. UVB-irradiation induces the release of IL-1, IL-6, granulocyte macrophage colony stimulating factor (GM-CSF), IL-3 and TNFα, which can be demonstrated at both the protein and the mRNA level. The release of these mediators may be important in the pathogenesis of inflammatory skin reactions following ultraviolet light exposure. In addition, TNFα seems to be involved in the generation of sunburn cells, since intralesional injection of a TNFα antiserum following UV-exposure results in a significant reduction of sunburn cell formation. Since UV-light generally induces the release of proinflammatory cytokines, the effect of psoralen (8-methoxypsoralen; 8MOP) plus long wavelength (320-400 nm) ultraviolet light (PUVA) on the release of IL-1, IL-6 and TNFα by peripheral blood mononuclear cells (PBMC) was tested. Treatment of PBMC with 8-MOP and UVA resulted in significant down-regulation of the secretion of these mediators by PBMC demonstrated at both the protein and the mRNA level. This effect may contribute to the antinflammatory activity of PUVA.

INTRODUCTION

Within the last decade, it has been demonstrated that epidermal cells are a potent source of cytokines (Luger and Schwarz, 1991), indicating that the epidermis is a site where immune responses and inflammatory reactions can originate independently. Although keratinocytes appeared to be the major source of these soluble mediators, there is evidence that dendritic epidermal cells and melanocytes can also produce such factors (Kock et al., 1991; Schreiber et al., 1991). Today it is definitely known that murine keratinocytes produce interleukin (IL) 1α, IL-1β, IL-3, IL-7, granulocyte/macrophage colony stimlating factor (GM-CSF), tumor necrosis factor α (TNFα), and transforming growth factor β (TGFβ); human keratinocytes release IL-1α, IL-1β, IL-6, IL-8, granulocyte colony stimulating factor (G-CSF), macrophage colony stimulating factor (M-CSF), basic fibroblast growth factor (bFGF), platelet derived growth factor (PDGF) and transforming growth factor α (TGFα) (Luger and Schwarz, 1991). Melanocytes and melanoma cells have been reported to secrete IL-1α, IL-1β, IL-3, IL-6, IL-8, TNFα, GM-CSF, PDGF and bFGF (Kock et al., 1991). Langerhans cells exhibit the capacity to release IL-1 and IL-6 (Sauder et al., 1984; Schreiber et al., 1991). Through the production of these mediators, epidermal cells may be able to significantly influence immunologic and inflammatory reactions within the skin.

The constitutive production of these mediators by epidermal cells, both in vivo and in vitro is rather low, but is found to be increased under pathologic conditions and can be dramatically enhanced by various stimuli. These include bacterial and viral products, tumor promotors and cytokines themselves. Since keratinocytes are uniquely exposed to ultraviolet (UV)-light by virtue of their anatomic location, and since UVB light influences inflammatory and immune reactions, the effect of UV-light on the release of cytokines by keratinocytes appeared to be of interest and has been addressed by a variety of studies.

INTERLEUKIN 1

The first cytokine demonstrated to be secreted by keratinocytes was IL-1, originally described according to its property to co-stimulate the proliferative response of thymocytes to mitogens (Luger et al., 1991). Soon thereafter it was shown that exposure of keratinocyte cell lines to relatively high doses of UVB-light results in a significant up-regulation of IL-1 activity in the supernatant fluid (Ansel et al., 1983). Similar findings were reported with murine macrophages and macrophage cell lines (P388 D1) (Ansel et al., 1984). In addition to these biodata, increase of mRNA expression in murine and human keratinocytes in response to UV-light was detected by Northern blot analysis (Ansel et al., 1988) and the S1 nuclease protection assay (Kupper et al., 1987), demonstrating that UV-light regulates IL-1 production in keratinocytes at the transcriptional level. From these findings it was concluded that IL-1 release following UV-irradiation may be of importance in the mediation of UV-induced inflammation (Ansel et al., 1987). In addition, it has recently been reported that increased IL-1 levels are found in the circulation in psoriatics undergoing phototherapy (Konnikov et al., 1989). In this study, IL-1 activity was measured with the thymocyte costimulator assay and, interestingly, IL-1 activity in plasma samples could not be completely blocked by IL-1 antibodies. According to more recent studies, it appears to be very likely that the activity not neutralized by IL-1 antibodies is due to IL-6, which also exhibits some thymocyte costimulator activity and is found to be enhanced after UV-irradiation as well (Kirnbauer et al., 1991; see below).

In addition, in supernatant fluids of UV-exposed epidermal cells, an activity was found which inhibited particular biologic functions of IL-1 (Schwarz et al., 1987). Although attempts so far have failed to isolate and clone this inhibitor, named Contra-IL-1, this observation supports the concept of a balanced network of interacting cytokines, called the cytokine cascade. Recently, an IL-1 inhibitor which acts via IL-1 receptor blockade was isolated and cloned from macrophages (Eisenberg et al., 1990) and this IL-1 receptor antagonist was also found to be expressed in keratinocytes (Bigler et al, 1991, our unpublished observation). Whether its release is induced by UV-light remains to be determined.

INTERLEUKIN 6

It has been shown that human epidermal carcinoma cell lines, freshly isolated epidermal cells and long term cultured human keratinocytes exhibit the capacity to release IL-6 (Kirnbauer et al., 1991), a multifunctional mediator of immunity and inflammation (Wong and Clark, 1989). Exposure of epidermal cells to UVB-light results in a significantly enhanced release of IL-6, as detected by the B9-hybridoma bioassay and Western blot analysis (Kirnbauer et al., 1991). In addition, IL-6 mRNA expression in keratinocytes was found to be increased after UVB exposure in a dose dependent manner. Irradiation of keratinocytes with UVA-light up to 1500 kJ/m^2 did not affect IL-6 production. In contrast, exposure of fibroblasts to UVA-light (up to 350 kJ/m^2) has recently been found to result in enhanced IL-6 release, which might activate collagenase

(Scharfetter et al., 1991). Since UVA is able penetrate through the epidermis into the dermis, IL-6 may play a role in solar actinic damage of the dermis. Moreover, it has been reported that addition of corticosteroids down-regulates UVB induced IL-6 release by keratinocytes. This effect of corticosteroids is dose dependent and affects IL-6 production at the protein and mRNA level (Kirnbauer et al., 1991). IL-6, similarly to IL-1, is pyrogenic and mediates the acute phase response, reaction to both of which are observed during a severe sunburn reaction. Therefore, whether these effects could be mediated via circulating IL-6 was investigated. In fact, it was demonstrated that total body UVB-exposure of human volunteers with four minimal erythema doses results in a significant increase in plasma IL-6 levels which correlate with fever and CRP levels (Urbanski et al., 1990). Whether UVB-light in vivo induces the release of IL-6 directly or via other cytokines, like IL-1, which is a potent stimulus for IL-6 production, remains to be determined. Because of its B-cell stimulatory capacity, increased IL-6 production following UV-exposure may be responsible for UV-induced exacerbation, of inflammatory disorders. It is noteworthy in this regard that enhanced serum IL-6 levels have recently been detected in patients with systemic lupus erythematosus (Linker-Israeli et al., 1991).

COLONY STIMULATING FACTORS

There is evidence that epidermal cells produce all known types of CSFs, i.e., IL-3, GM-CSF, G-CSF, and M-CSF (Luger et al., 1991). The production of these mediators appears of relevance since GM-CSF plays an important role in the maturation of Langerhans cells (Heufler et al., 1988). It also has been demonstrated that CSF, and, in particular, GM-CSF activity present in normal skin, is enhanced by UVB-light, suggesting that UVB-irradiation induces the cutaneous release of CSF in amounts sufficient to reverse acute myelosuppression (Birchall et al., 1988). Thus the UV-induced release of epidermal cell derived cytokines may play a role in recovery from bone marrow suppression. Recently, it has been reported that augmentation of GM-CSF expression in the murine keratinocyte cell line, Pam 212, by UVB-light is mediated via IL-1 (Nozaki et al., 1991). In addition to GM-CSF, IL-3 is found to be released in enhanced amounts by Pam 212 cells following UV-exposure (Gallo et al., 1991).

TUMOR NECROSIS FACTOR ALPHA

TNFα has become relevant in cutaneous biology for a variety of reasons. TNFα seems to affect Langerhans cell maturation (Kock et al., 1990), to be involved in the elicitation phase of contact hypersensitivity reactions (Piguet et al., 1991) and to play a role in the occurrence of cutaneous lesions during graft-versus-host disease (Piguet et al., 1987). In addition, there is evidence that TNFα plays a role in the pathogenesis of UV-induced immunosuppression, since injection of a TNFα antibody prevents UV-induced inhibition of contact hypersensitivity induction (Yoshikawa and Streilein, 1990). Therefore, it was investigated whether UV-irradiation induces the release of TNFα by keratinocytes. UVB exposure stimulates both normal human keratinocytes and human epidermal carcinoma cell lines to release TNFα (Kock et al., 1990). This has been demonstrated by the use of ELISA, bioassay and Western blot analysis. In addition, UVB irradiation results in a dose dependent upregulation of TNFα-specific mRNA in keratinocytes. Accordingly, enhanced expression of TNFα in situ by keratinocytes was detected in epidermis after UV-exposure by immunohistochemical methods (Oxholm et al., 1988). It has been recently reported that keratinocytes express the 55 kD type I receptor for TNFα (TNFRI) and that TNFα appears to play an important role in the UV-induced regulation of the adhesion molecule, ICAM-1 (Trefzer et al., 1991).

TNFα AND SUNBURN CELL FORMATION

Within 24 hours of moderate exposure to sunlight, a cell of unusual and distinct morphology may be observed in the epidermis. The sunburn cell (SC), as it has come to be known, has been described as having a "shrunken, homogenized, densely staining, glassy cytoplasm and a hyperchromatic, condensed, pyknotic nucleus" (Young, 1987). Although the existence of the SC has been known for a long time, the origin of these cells is quite unclear. Recently, it has been suggested that SC be regarded as examples of apoptosis, controlled individual cell death (Young, 1987). Hypotheses of SC formation include decreased DNA repair capacity and cell cycle dependence. It has been shown that SC generation is dependent on oxygen supply (Youn et al., 1988), and can be prevented by administration of antioxidants (Hanadam et al., 1991). In addition, it has been demonstrated that pretreatment with infrared light reduces the formation of SC (Danno et al., 1991). Nevertheless, the particular mechanisms involved are quite unclear.

TNFα was originally described as a factor responsible for hemorrhagic necrosis of tumors following infection of animals and humans. Since (i) TNFα is produced by keratinocytes (Kock et al., 1990), (ii) its release is induced by UV-light (Kock et al., 1990) and, (iii) keratinocytes bear type I receptors for TNFα (Trefzer et al., 1991), the question of whether TNFα is involved in the formation of SC was investigated. C3H/HeN mice were exposed to UVB-light (FS20 bulbs, 2000-3000 kJ/m^2) on their shaved abdomen and biopsies were performed 24 hours later. This treatment resulted in a significant formation of SC, which were quantitatively evaluated by counting shrunken epidermal cells with eosinophilic cytoplasms and pyknotic nuclei.

Table 1. Effect of anti-TNFα on sunburn cell formation.

	UV[a]	UV + antiTNF[b]	UV + control serum[c]
sunburn cells/mm	8.1±0.9	4.6±0.7	8.2±0.6

[a]) C3H/HeN mice were exposed to UVB-light (2000kJ/m^2)
and SC counted after 24 hours.

[b]) Immediately after UV-treatment, TNFα antiserum
was injected into the irradiated skin area.

[c]) Immediately after UV-treatment, rabbit control serum
was injected into the irradiated skin area.

Immediately after UV-exposure, a rabbit TNFα antiserum was injected subcutaneously and, 24 hours later, biopsies obtained. Injection of the TNFα antiserum resulted in a significant reduction of SC, while the injection of PBS or a nonspecific rabbit control antiserum had no effect on SC formation (Table 1).

The reducing effect of the TNFα antiserum was dose dependent. Maximal reduction was observed when the antiserum was injected immediately or one hour after UV-exposure. When the antiserum was administered 6 hours after UV-exposure or later, the reducing effect was no longer observed. The SC-suppressing antiserum appeared to be specific, since pre-incubation of the antiserum with recombinant murine TNFα resulted in the loss of the reducing capacity. In further experiments, we have investigated whether injection of TNFα results in the formation of SC-like cells. So far, however, we have not been able to induce this effect. Therefore, based on the present data, one can speculate that TNFα appears to be necessary, but not sufficient, for SC formation. On the other hand, it may be necessary to up-regulate TNFα receptors on keratinocytes before injecting TNFα. Whether this modification in the experimental design succeeds in the induction of SC remains to be determined. In summary, these findings contribute to a better understanding of the pathogenesis of SC and, furthermore, indicate that TNFα is an important mediator involved in the mediation of UV-induced changes within the skin.

EFFECT OF 8-MOP PLUS UVA ON THE RELEASE OF CYTOKINES

Studies dealing with the effect of UV-light on cytokine release have shown that UVB generally induces the release of these mediators (Schwarz et al., 1989), while UVA, so far, has not been found to affect cytokine production. Under no circumstances has suppression of cytokine secretion by UV-light been observed, although UV-light can cause immunosuppression and reduce certain inflammatory skin diseases. Since the combination of 8-methoxpsoralen (8-MOP) plus UVA has been shown to affect the immune system (Kripke et al., 1983) and is successful in the treatment of a variety of inflammatory skin disorders, the effect of PUVA on the release of cytokines in vitro was tested. Peripheral blood mononuclear cells (PBMC) were isolated by separation via Lymphoprep, resuspended in phosphate buffered saline (PBS) (1×10^6/ml) and 8-MOP (dissolved in ethanol) was added at different concentrations (100-1000 ng/ml). One hour later cells were irradiated with UVA-light (20 kJ/m^2) and supernatant fluids harvested after 24 hours. Supernatant fluids were then evaluated for IL-1, IL-6 and TNFα content. IL-1 was determined by the use of an IRMA and a bioassay (D10 cells), IL-6 by the use of the B9-hybridoma assay and TNFα by an ELISA and the L929 bioassay. As shown in Table 2, treatment of cells with 8-MOP plus UVA resulted in a significant reduction of IL-1, IL-6 and TNFα released by PBMC compared to supernatant fluids derived from untreated PBMC. UVA-treatment alone did not affect cytokine release; and the same was true for the effect of 8-MOP on the production of IL-1 and TNFα. Recently, we have reported that 8-MOP alone can affect IL-6 release by PBMC and epidermal cells (Neuner et al., 1991); this issue, however, is still controversial and the effects observed may be due to differences in the drug formulations or the solvent. In addition, the effect of 8-MOP plus UVA on the release of IL-1 by murine keratinocytes has recently been investigated. Similar to our findings, IL-1 release was significantly reduced after in vitro PUVA-treatment (Tokura et al., 1991).

Table 2. Effect of 8-MOP plus UVA on the release of IL-1β, IL-6 and TNFα by PBMC.

Treatment	IL-1β[a]	IL-6[b]	TNFα[c]
None (control)	33.8	15.5	15.0
8-MOP+UVA	13.6	1.3	8.7
8-MOP	58.4	11.3	14.8
UVA	46.4	13.3	15.3

[a] IL-1β was evaluated by the use of an IL-1β specific IRMA. Data are expressed as cpm x 1000.
[b] IL-6 was evaluated by the use of the B9 hybridoma bioassay. Data are expressed as cpm x 1000.
[c] TNFa was evaluated by the use of a TNFα specific IRMA. Data are expressed as cpm x 1000.

In addition, RNA was extracted from PBMC four hours after in vitro treatment with PUVA, 8-MOP, UVA or sham treatment. Northern blot analysis was performed and showed significant reduction of mRNA encoding for IL-1, IL-6 and TNFα in PUVA treated cells when compared to untreated controls, while UVA and 8-MOP alone had no remarkable effects (data not shown). These results demonstrate that 8-MOP plus UVA is able to suppress the release of pro-inflammatory cytokines like IL-1, IL-6 and TNFα; this effect may contribute to the anti-inflammatory activity of PUVA therapy. Whether these in vitro data also reflect the in vivo situation remains to be determined by appropiate methods such as in situ hybridization.

ACKNOWLEDGEMENTS

The authors thank Mrs. M. Bednar for excellent secretarial assistance. This work was supported by "Deutsche Forschungsgemeinschaft" grant LU443/1-1 (TAL) and "Jubilaumsfonds der Osterreichischen Nationalbank" grant 3987 (PN).

REFERENCES

Ansel JC, TA Luger and I Green, 1983. The effect of in vitro and in vivo UV irradiation on the production of ETAF activity by human and murine keratinocytes. **J. Invest. Dermatol.**, 81:519.

Ansel JC, TA Luger, A Kock, A Hochstein and I Green, 1984. The effect of in vitro UV irradiation on the production of IL-1 by murine macrophages and P388D1 cells. **J. Immunol.**, 133:1350.

Ansel JC, TA Luger and I Green, 1987. Fever and increased serum IL-1 activity as a systemic manifestation of acute phototoxicity in New Zealand white rabbits. **J. Invest. Dermatol.**, 89:32.

Ansel JC, TA Luger, D Lowry, P Perry, DR Roop and JD Mountz, 1988. The expression and modulation of IL-1α in murine keratinocytes. **J. Immunol.**, 140:227.

Bigler CF, DA Norris, WL Weston, and WP Arend, 1991. Interleukin-1 receptor antagonist production by human keratinocytes. **Clin. Res.**, 98:38.

Birchall N, C Gamba and T Kupper, 1988. Cutaneous UVB irradiation enhances recovery from bone marrow suppression. **Clin. Res.**, 36:801A (Abstract).

Danno K, T Horio and S Imamura, 1991. Infrared radiation suppresses ultraviolet B-induced sunburn cell formation. **J. Invest. Dermatol.**, 96:1007.

Eisenberg SP, RJ Evans, WP Arend, E Verderber, MT Brewer, CH Hannum and RC Thompson, 1990. Primary structure and functional expression from complementary DNA of a human interleukin-1 receptor antagonist. **Nature**, 343:341.

Gallo RL, R Staszewski, DN Sauder, TL Knisely and RD Granstein, 1991. Regulation of GM-CSF and IL-3 production from the murine keratinocyte cell line Pam 212 following exposure to ultraviolet radiation. **J. Invest. Dermatol.**, 97:203.

Hanadam KH, RW Gange and MJ Comor, 1991. Effect of glutathione depletion on sunburn cell formation in the hairless mouse. **J. Invest. Dermatol.**, 96:838.

Heufler C, F Koch and G Schuler, 1988. Granulocyte/macrophage colony-stimulating factor and interleukin 1 mediate the maturation of murine epidermal Langerhans cells into potent immunostimulator dendritic cells. **J. Exp. Med.**, 167:700.

Kirnbauer R, A Kock, T Schwarz, A Urbanski, J Krutmann, W Borth, JC Ansel and TA Luger, 1989. B-cell differentiation factor-2, hybridoma growth factor (interleukin-6) is expressed and released by human epidermal cells and epidermoid carcinoma cell lines. **J. Immunol.**, 142:1922.

Kirnbauer R, A Kock, P Neuner E Forster, J Krutmann, A Urbanski, E Schauer, JC Ansel, T Schwarz and TA Luger, 1991. Regulation of epidermal cell interleukin-6 production by UV light and corticosteroids. **J. Invest. Dermatol.**, 96:484.

Koch F, C Heufler, D Schneeweiss, E Kaempgen and G Schuler, 1990. Tumor necrosis factor alpha maintains viability of murine epidermal Langerhans cell in culture, but in contrast to GM-CSF without inducing functional maturation. **J. Exp. Med.**, 171:159.

Kock A, T Schwarz, R Kirnbauer, A Urbanski, P Perry, JC Ansel and TA Luger, 1990. Human keratinocytes are a source for tumor necrosis factor: Evidence for synthesis and release upon stimulation with endotoxin or ultraviolet light. **J. Exp. Med.**, 172:1609.

Kock A, T Schwarz, M Micksche and TA Luger, 1991. Cytokines and human malignant melanoma. Immuno- and growth-regulatory peptides in melanoma biology. In: L. Nathanson, Ed: **Melanoma Research: Genetics, Growth Factors, Metastases**, Kluwer Academic Publishers, Boston, p. 41.

Konnikov N, SH Pincus and CA Dinarello, 1989. Elevated plasma interleukin-1 levels in humans following ultraviolet light therapy for psoriasis. **J. Invest. Dermatol.**, 92:235.

Kripke ML, WL Morrison and JA Parrish, 1983. Systemic suppression of contact hypersensitivity in mice by psoralen plus UVA radiation (PUVA). **J. Invest. Dermatol.**, 81:87.

Kupper TS, AO Chua, P Flood, J McGuire and U Gubler, 1987. Interleukin-1 gene expression in cultured human keratinocytes is augmented by ultraviolet irradiation. **J. Clin. Invest.** 80: 430.

Linker-Israeli M, RJ Deans, DJ Wallace, J Prehn, T Ozeri-Chen and JR Klinenberg, 1991. Elevated levels of endogenous IL-6 in systemic lupus erythematosus. A putative role in pathogenesis. **J. Immunol.**, 147:117.

Luger TA, BM Stadler, SI Katz and JJ Oppenheim, 1981. Epidermal cell (keratinocyte) derived thymocyte activating factor (ETAF). **J. Immunol.**, 127:1493.

Luger TA and T Schwarz, 1991. Epidermal cell derived secretory regulins, In: G Schuler, Ed: **Epidermal Langerhans Cells**, CRC Press, Boca Raton, FL, p. 217.

Neuner P, A Moller, R Kirnbauer, Ch. Grunwald, A Urbanski, R Knobler, TA Luger and T Schwarz, 1991. Effect of 8-methoxypsoralen (8-MOP) plus UVA on the release of IL-6 by PBMC and epidermal cells. **Arch. Derm. Res.**, 283:24.

Nozaki S, JS Abrams, MK Pearce and DN Sauder, 1991. Augmentation of granulocyte/macrophage colony stimulating factor expression by ultraviolet irradiation is mediated by interleukin-1 in Pam 212 keratinocytes. **J. Invest. Dermatol.**, 97:10.

Oxholm A, P Oxholm, B Staberg and K Bendtzen, 1988. Immunohistological detection of interleukin-1 like molecules and tumour necrosis factor in human epidermis before and after UVB-irradiation in vivo. **Brit. J. Dermatol.**, 118:369.

Piguet PF, GE Grau, B Allet and P Vasalli, 1987. Tumor necrosis factor/cachectin is an effector of skin and gut lesions of the acute phase of graft-vs.-host disease. **J. Exp. Med.**, 166:1280.

Piguet PF, GE Grau, C Hauser and P Vassalli, 1991. Tumor necrosis factor is a crititcal mediator in hapten-induced irritant and contact hypersensitivity reactions. **J. Exp. Med.**, 173:673.

Sauder DN, CA Dinarello and VB Morhenn, 1984. Langerhans cell production of interleukin-1. **J. Invest. Dermatol.**, 82:605.

Sharffetter K, F Wilmroth, M Wlaschek, K Bolsen, P Lehmann, T Krieg, G Goerz, G Plewig and PC Heinrich, 1991. UV-induced autocrine stimulation of fibroblast derived collagenase by IL-6: A possible mechanism in dermal photodamage? **Arch. Derm. Res.**, 283:58.

Schreiber S, O Kilgus, E Payuer, R Kutil, A Elbe C Müller and G Stingl, 1992. Cytokine pattern of Langerhans cells isolated from murine epidermal cell cultures. **J. Immunol.**, 149:3525

Schwarz T, A Urbanska, F Gschnait and TA Luger, 1987. UV-irradiated epidermal cells produce a specific inhibitor of interleukin 1 activity. **J. Immunol.**, 138:1457

Schwarz T and TA Luger, 1989. Effect of UV irradiation on epidermal cell cytokine production. **J. Photochem Photobiol.**, 84:1.

Tokura Y, J Yagi, RL Edelson and FP Gasparro, 1991. Inhibitory effect of 8-MOP plus UVA on IL1 production by murine epidermal keratinocytes. **Photochem. Photobiol.**, 53:517.

Trefzer U, M Brockhaus, H Loetscher, F Parlow, A Kapp, E Schöpf and J Krutmann, 1991. 55-kd tumor necrosis factor receptor is expressed by human keratinocytes and plays a pivotal role in regulation of human keratinocyte ICAM-1 expression. **J. Invest. Dermatol.**, 96:543A (Abstract).

Urbanski A, T Schwarz, P Neuner, J Krutmann, R Kirnbauer, A Kock and TA Luger, 1990. Ultraviolet light induces increased circulating interleukin-6 in humans. **J. Invest. Dermatol.**, 94:808.

Wong GG and SC Clark, 1989. Multiple actions of interleukin 6 within a cytokine network. **Immunol. Today**, 9:137.

Yoshikawa T and JW Streilein, 1990. TNF-alpha released by UVB-treated keratinocytes impairs induction of contact hypersensitivity. **J. Invest. Dermatol.**, 94:593.

Youn JI, RW Gange, D Maytum and JA Parrish, 1988. Effect of hypoxia on sunburn cell formation and inflammation induced by ultraviolet radiation. **Photodermatology**, 5:252.

Young AR, 1987. The sunburn cell. **Photodermatology** 4:127.

ADHESION MOLECULES INVOLVED IN THE EXTRAVASATION OF LYMPHOCYTES IN LYMPHOID ORGANS AND CHRONICALLY INFLAMED TISSUES

A.C.H.M. van Dinther-Janssen*
G. Kraal†
R.J. Scheper*
R. Willemze‡
C.J.L.M. Meijer‡

* Department of Pathology
  Free University Hospital

† Department of Histology
  Faculty of Medicine
  Free University

‡ Department of Dermatology
  Free University Hospital
  Amsterdam, The Netherlands

Correspondence to: Dr. C. J. L. M. Meijer, Department of Pathology,
University Hospital, de Boelelaan 1117,
1081 HV Amsterdam, The Netherlands

INTRODUCTION

Cell adhesion molecules play an important role in many cellular processes, such as sperm-egg binding, organogenesis (Hoffmann et al., 1982) and lymphocyte migration (Springer, 1990; Albelda, 1991). Furthermore, in the immune system, they are crucial in T lymphocyte-

Basic Mechanisms of Physiologic and Aberrant Lymphoproliferation in the Skin
Edited by W.C. Lambert *et al.*, Plenum Press, New York, 1994

113

accessory cell and T lymphocyte-target cell interactions which are required, respectively, for the induction of immune responses or for effector cell function (Dustin et al., 1987; Springer et al., 1987; Martz, 1987). They also mediate a variety of other, non-antigen-specific, cell-cell and cell-substrate interactions in the immune system, including lymphocyte adhesion to endothelium during lymphocyte recirculation through lymphoid organs and lymphocyte extravasation in chronic inflammation (Stoolman, 1989; Chin et al., 1990; Jalkanen et al., 1990). Here we will highlight the role of cell adhesion molecules in lymphocyte - endothelium interactions in lymphocyte extravasation in lymph nodes and in chronically inflamed tissues.

ORGAN SPECIFIC RECIRCULATION OF LYMPHOCYTES

Lymphocyte recirculation between the blood and the lymphoid organs is essential for dissemination of the immune response. It is a dynamic, non-random process which does not require the presence of antigen (Butcher, 1986). One of the purposes of this recirculation is to facilitate the interaction between antigen specific lymphocytes and antigen-presenting cells required for the induction and regulation of antigen-specific immune responses in the secondary lymphoid organs. In addition, lymphocyte recirculation may also be important in the segregation of lymphocytes with particular functions in different lymphoid tissues.

The majority of lymphocytes enter the lymph node directly from the blood via specialized post-capillary high endothelial venules (HEV) in the paracortical areas (Gowans et al., 1964; Marchesi et al., 1964). This migration, or "homing", of lymphocytes is directed by specific receptors on lymphocytes (homing receptors) which recognize complementary ligands (addressins) on HEV (Butcher et al., 1980; Chin et al., 1984; Jalkanen et al., 1986; Pals et al., 1989). Lymphocyte-HEV interactions have been extensively studied, both in short-term in vivo homing experiments, and in an in vitro adhesion assay developed by Stamper and Woodruff (1976), in which lymphocytes overlaid on frozen tissue sections of lymphoid organs specifically adhere to HEV (Stamper et al., 1976; Streeter et al., 1988a; Streeter et al., 1988b; Butcher, 1990).

One of the most exciting observations made in these studies, both in vivo and in vitro, is that lymphocytes can discriminate between HEV in different lymphoid tissues. For example, in vivo recirculation studies in sheep have demonstrated that lymphocytes from gut-associated lymphoid tissue (GALT) preferentially recirculate back to the gut, whereas lymphocytes from peripheral lymph nodes (PLN) return to the peripheral lymph nodes. (Scollay et al., 1970; Hall et al., 1977; Cahill et al., 1977; Reynolds et al., 1982). The greatest difference in organ-related homing was found, however, by comparing lymphocyte subsets: B cells in comparison to T cells showed a relative preference for GALT over PLN, independent of the organ source of the lymphocytes (Stevens et al., 1982; Fossum et al., 1983). A similar observation was made for CD4$^+$ T cells (helper/inducer phenotype) as compared with CD8$^+$ T cells (cytotoxic/suppressor phenotype) (Kraal et al., 1983). Of different cell populations, memory and blast cells especially show strong tissue origin-related homing preferences (Smith et al., 1980). By contrast, lymphocyte (sub)class is thought to be the major determinant of the migratory properties of the mature "virgin" lymphocyte. These in vivo homing characteristics correspond with their in vitro adherence patterns to HEV of different lymphoid organs. Thus, certain murine and human lymphoma cell lines were shown to bind selectively to PLN or GALT-HEV (Butcher et al., 1980; Jalkanen et al., 1986; Jalkanen et al., 1987). The existence of organ-selective homing of lymphocytes has been confirmed by the generation of monoclonal antibodies (mAb) that selectively inhibit lymphocyte-HEV interaction (Sheeter et al., 1988a; Streeter et al., 1988b; Butcher et al., 1990).

In sites of chronic inflammation, extravasation of lymphocytes is often associated with a change in the appearance of small venules, which come to resemble HEV. It has therefore been suggested that lymphocyte-endothelial cell interaction in chronic inflammation also bears an element of organ-specificity. Indeed, evidence for the existence of distinct homing specificities to inflamed skin (Chin et al., 1990; Jalkanen et al., 1990), and rheumatoid synovium (Jalkanen et al., 1986) has been described.

ADHESION MOLECULES INVOLVED IN LYMPHOCYTE RECIRCULATION

The existence of specific homing receptors mediating lymphocyte-HEV interaction has been supported by the development of monoclonal antibodies that inhibit lymphocyte binding to endothelium in man (Camerini et al., 1990; Kishimoto et al., 1990; Picker et al., 1990; Tedder et al., 1990a; 1990b) and rodents (Gallatin et al., 1983).

Lymphocyte adhesion molecules

Molecules on lymphocytes known to be involved in lymphocyte-HEV interactions are: L-Selectin (LECAM-1), a member of the Selectin (LECCAM) family; antigens clustered in the CD44 group, and two members of the integrin family of adhesion molecules: LFA-1 and VLA-4.

The selectin, or LECCAM, family

The selectin family consists of three similar single chain integral membrane glycoproteins, each of which consists of a Ca^{++} dependent amino-terminal lectin domain, a proximal epidermal growth factor-like motif and a backbone composed of repeated units homologous to the complement regulatory protein repeat units (Lasky et al., 1989; Bowen et al., 1990; Siegelman et al., 1989). Three of the most important members of this family are presently known as: L-selectin (LECAM-1; the peripheral lymph node homing receptor (LHR); murine homologue MEL14) and E-selectin (ELAM-1) on endothelium, and P-selectin (GMP-140) on endothelium and platelets (Bowen et al., 1990; Bevilacqua et al., 1989, 1991; Johnson et al., 1989). The fact that these molecules contain a lectin domain and that carbohydrates can block the interactions of lymphocytes with HEV (Stoolman et al., 1983; Stoolman et al., 1987) has led to the idea that carbohydrates are ligands for these molecules. Indeed, each of the molecules involved has been found to bind carbohydrates, with E-selectin and P-selectin binding sialyl Lewis X (Springer et al., 1990; Larsen et al., 1990, Lowe et al., 1990, Philips et al., 1990; Goelz et al., 1990) while L-selectin can bind mannose-6-phosphate and fructose-1-phosphate (Imai et al., 1990; Stoolmann et al., 1984). Studies of the genomic organization of the selectins have shown that all three molecules in this family are coded for within a 300 kilobase stretch of human and mouse chromosome 1 (Watson et al., 1990; Tedder et al., 1989). In this section, L-selectin will be described. E-selectin will be discussed in the section describing endothelial adhesion molecules.

L-Selectin (LECAM-1, LAM-1, Leu 8, TQ1, Dreg 56, MEL-14)

L-selectin (first named MEL14 or gp90^{mel}) was initially described as a mouse lymphocyte surface glycoprotein involved in homing of lymphocytes to HEV in PLN, but not to HEV in Peyer's Patches (Gallatin et al., 1983; Jalkanen et al., 1986; Pals et al., 1988). In man, an equivalent of the mouse MEL-14 mAb, called Dreg56, has been described (Kishimoto et al., 1990). This mAb defines a 80-85 kD molecule involved in human lymphocyte recognition of peripheral lymph node HEV. In addition, Dreg56 recognizes the gp80 antigen on lymphoid cell lines that specifically interacts with peripheral lymph node HEV (Kishimoto et al., 1990).

L-Selectin is constitutively expressed on all recirculating lymphocytes. Low levels of L-selectin are expressed on bone marrow pre-B cells and thymocytes (Gallatin et al., 1983; Lewinsohn et al., 1987), whereas sessile activated B cells of germinal centers do not express L-selectin (Reichert et al., 1983). Upon activation, as well as after initial adhesive interaction in vitro, the antigen is shed from the cell surface (Kishimoto et al., 1989; Dinther-Janssen et al., 1991; Stoolman et al., 1990; Picker et al., 1990). Soluble L-selectin has been shown to inhibit the migration of neutrophils into acute inflamatory sites (Lewinsohn et al., 1987; Yednock et al., 1989; Julita et al., 1989).

The CD44 family of adhesion molecules

Also involved in lymphocyte-HEV interaction is the CD44/Hermes group of membrane antigens, which are structurally unrelated to the MEL-14 group (Berg et al., 1989). The CD44 antigen consists of an extracellular domain which bears homology to cartilage link proteins and proteoglycan core proteins, a transmembrane domain, and a cytoplasmic domain (Idzerda et al., 1989; Goldstein et al., 1989). The 85-95 kD forms of these proteins have been shown to be identical to the murine Phagocytic Protein-1 (PgP-1) (Trowbridge et al., 1982; Picker et al., 1989), Extracellular Matrix Protein III (ECMIII) (Carter et al., 1988; Wayner et al., 1987), In(Lu) related p80 (Picker et al., 1989), Hutch-1 (Gallatin et al., 1987) and B cell p80

(Letarte et al., 1985). The CD44 molecule is encoded on the short arm of chromosome 11 (Forsberg et al., 1989).

On epithelium, a structurally related form of 160 kD has been described (Stamenkovic et al., 1991). The CD44 family of membrane antigens is widely distributed on hematopoietic and non-hematopoietic cells. Expression on hematopoietic cells appeares to correlate with the state of maturation and migration, e.g., mature and non-activated lymphocytes express high levels of CD44, whereas immature and activated lymphocytes express low levels of this antigen.

Functionally, CD44 has been shown not only to be involved in normal leukocyte circulation but also in leukocyte traffic to sites of inflammation (Jalkanen et al., 1986; Jalkanen et al., 1987; Lewinsohn et al., 1987). Apart from serving as a mediator of leukocyte-endothelial cell binding, CD44 also plays a role in other lymphocyte adhesion events, such as induction of T cell adhesion to red blood cells, homotypic T and B cell aggregation and T cell activation and proliferation (Haynes et al., 1989; Koopman et al., 1990; Denning et al., 1990; Shimizu et al., 1989; Huet et al., 1989). Moreover, CD44 also binds to hyaluronate (Aruffo et al., 1990; Stamenkovic et al., 1991).

The CD44 molecule can, therefore, mediate various interactions involving a large number of different cell types.

The integrin family of adhesion molecules

The integrins form a large family of heterodimeric glycoproteins involved in a variety of cell adhesion functions (Hynes et al., 1987; Hemler et al., 1987a). All integrins are formed by two non-covalently linked subunits: the larger termed α chain and the smaller β chain. Both subunits are integral membrane proteins with a small C-terminal cytoplasmic domain, a large N-terminal extracellular domain and a transmembrane segment.

The integrins concerned can be classified into three subfamilies: the β_1 or VLA (very late antigen) family, the β_2 or leu-cam family (leukocyte adhesion molecules), and the β_3 or cytoadhesins (Hemler et al., 1987a). Additional β chains have recently been described (Kajiji et al., 1989; Hemler et al., 1989; Cheresh et al., 1989; Holzman et al., 1989; Freed et al., 1989), however. Most members of the integrins form receptors for extracellular matrix and plasma proteins, e.g., collagen, laminin, and fibronectin (Wayner et al., 1988; Pytela et al., 1985), by recognizing a sequence of only three amino acids (Arg-Gly-Asp; RGD) (Ruoslahti et al., 1986).

Only two members of the integrin family, LFA-1 and VLA-4, are involved in lymphocyte adhesion to endothelium.

Lymphocyte function-associated antigen-1 (LFA-1)

LFA-1 belongs to the β_2 integrin subfamily of adhesion molecules. This leu-cam family consists of three CD11/CD18 complexes which have been shown to be of great importance in mediating both neutrophil, monocyte, natural killer and lymphocyte cell-cell interactions (Harlan et al., 1987; Arnaout, 1990; Sanchez-Madrid et al., 1983). The LFA-1 molecule is a heterodimer consisting of a 180 kD α chain, encoded on chromosome 16, and a 95 kD ß chain encoded on chromosome 21 (Springer et al., 1987; Arnaout, 1990). MAb against the α chain are referred to as CD11a and mAb against the β chain as CD18.

LFA-1 is expressed on leukocytes and predominates on lymphocytes (Springer et al., 1987). Initially, LFA-1 was defined on lymphocytes by mAb mediating inhibition of killing by cytolytic T cells (CTL) and natural killer cells (Krensky et al., 1983). Later LFA-1 has also been shown to block T cell adhesion to both epidermal keratinocytes and endothelial cells in culture (Dustin et al., 1988; Dustin et al., 1988). Here LFA-1 acts as a receptor for ICAM-1 and ICAM-2 (Marlin et al., 1987; Staunton et al., 1989; Nortamo et al., 1991) or more probably ICAM-3 (De Fougerolles et al., 1991; 1992). In lymphocyte migration, the role of LFA-1 is thought to be accessory, since mAb to LFA-1 only partially inhibited lymphocyte binding to HEV in frozen sections of both PLN and MALT (Pals et al., 1988; Hamann et al., 1988).

Very late antigen-4 (VLA-4)

VLA-4 was first described as an $\alpha_4\beta_1$ heterodimer appearing as the predominant VLA protein complex on T lymphoblastoid cell lines (Hemler et al., 1987a). Monoclonal Ab against VLA-4 were initially found to block cytolytic T cell function (Clayberger et al., 1987; Takada et al., 1989a) as well as homotypic T cell aggregation (Bednarcyk et al., 1990). On B cells, the molecule was reported to play a role in the interaction with follicular dendritic cells (Koopman et al., 1991).

VLA-4 is present in substantial quantities on normal peripheral blood T and B cells, thymocytes, monocytes, natural killer cells, activated T cells and eosinophils (Clayberger et al., 1987; Hemler et al., 1987; Bochner et al., 1991). In the mouse, homologues of the human VLA-4 (LPAM-1 and LPAM-2) have been found to mediate homing of lymphocytes to Peyer's Patches (Holzmann et al., 1989; Holzmann et al., 1989; Takada et al., 1989). VLA-4 is the only member of the β_1 integrins which mediates both cell-cell and cell-matrix interactions (Hemler et al., 1987a; Tadaka et al., 1989; Hemler et al., 1990; Gismondi et al., 1991; Holzmann et al., 1989; Wayner et al., 1989). In adhesion to the extracellular matrix, VLA-4 acts as a receptor of fibronectin (FN) via a cell attachment domain (called CS1) in an alternatively spliced region of FN (Wayner et al., 1989; Ager et al., 1990). This domain does not contain the well-known Arg-Gly-Asp (RGD) sequence. Cell adhesion to the latter sequence of FN is mediated by VLA-5 (Ruoslathi et al., 1987). Recently, VLA-4 has also been implicated in binding to VCAM-1 (Osborn et al., 1989; Elices et al., 1990), a member of the immunoglobulin (Ig) gene super family (see below).

High endothelial adhesion molecules

The vascular endothelium contains a counter-repertoire of adhesion molecules involved in binding of lymphocytes to HEV. Most of these molecules belong to three families of adhesion molecules, notably the Ig gene superfamily, the selectin family, and the vascular addressins. Molecules involved are ICAM-1, ICAM-2, ICAM-3 and VCAM-1, all four being members of the Ig gene superfamily, E-selectin (ELAM-1), belonging to the Selectin, or LECCAM, family of adhesion molecules, and MECA-79 and MECA-367, the peripheral lymph node addressin (PNad) and mucosal addressin (Mad), respectively. The addressins have, to date, only been identified in the mouse (Streeter et al., 1989a; 1989b).

The immunoglobulin supergene family

Members of the Ig superfamily share common structural features. A typical Ig-like domain consists of about 100 amino acids arranged in two sheets of antiparallel β-strands, stabilized by a disulfide bond (Williams et al., 1988; Alzari et al., 1988). Loops of amino acids connecting the β-strands usually define the specificity of the molecule for its cognate ligand. Examples include the adhesion molecules CD2, CD3/TCR, CD4, CD8, LFA3, ICAM-1 and ICAM-2, ICAM-3, ICAM-2, VCAM-1, PECAM, MHC classes I and II, NCAM and CEA. Four of these molecules (i.e., ICAM-1, -2, -3, and VCAM-1) play a role in leucocyte-endothelial cell interaction. In particular, the up-regulated, or inducible, expression of these molecules at sites of inflammation seems to contribute substantially to the course of the inflammatory process. The counter-structures on lymphocytes for the adhesion of members of the immunoglobulin family are each members of the integrin family of adhesion molecules, c.q., LFA-1 for ICAM-1, ICAM-2 and ICAM-3 (Staunton et al., 1989; De Fougerolles et al., 1992) and VLA-4 for VCAM-1 (Osborn et al., 1989; Elices et al., 1990).

ICAM-1

ICAM-1 is a cell adhesion molecule with a central role in mediating cell-cell adhesion. It is a heavily glycosylated cell surface protein, with a molecular weight of about 90 kD, containing five tandem extra-cellular Ig-like domains (Williams et al., 1988; Alzari et al., 1988). Only the first two domains are required for function. On endothelium, ICAM-1 is constitutively expressed at a low level, but expression is strongly increased after stimulation of the endothelial cells with cytokines such as IL-1 and TNFα (Dustin et al., 1986; Pober et al., 1986). ICAM-1 was first defined using mAb which blocked lymphocyte functions dependent on LFA-1 (Rothlein et al., 1986; Rothlein et al., 1986; Marlin et al., 1987). In addition, using purified ICAM-1, it was demonstrated that ICAM-1 interacts directly with LFA-1 molecules (Narlin et al., 1987). Whereas LFA-1 mAb could block lymphocyte interaction with high endothelial cells, however, mAb to ICAM-1 frequently did not, although ICAM-1 is highly expressed on high endothelium.

Thus, LFA-1 dependent/ICAM-1 independent, as well as LFA-1/ICAM-1 dependent, interaction systems in several cell-cell adhesion processes have been described (Dustin et al., 1988; Berg et al., 1991; Tamatani et al., 1991). In addition to expression on endothelium, ICAM-1 is also expressed on a variety of other cell types, including thymic epithelial cells, fibroblasts, macrophages, FDC, peripheral blood lymphocytes, and stimulated T cells (Rothlein et al., 1986, Dustin et al., 1986). Here, also, expression of ICAM-1 can be up-regulated upon activation (Dustin et al., 1986; Wawrijk et al., 1989; Pober et al., 1986), for example, on dermal and synovial fibroblasts and epidermal keratinocytes, by TNF and interferon-γ and on fibroblasts also by IL-1 (Dustin et al., 1988; Rothlein et al., 1988; Dustin et al., 1986).

ICAM-2 and ICAM-3

Functional studies have revealed that, apart from the ICAM-1 molecule, at least two other ligands mediate LFA-1 dependent adhesion of lymphocytes to cultured endothelial cells (Rothlein et al., 1986; Makgoba et al., 1988; Dustin et al., 1988). Indeed, recently a homologue of ICAM-1, named ICAM-2, has been described (Staunton et al., 1989; Nortamo et al., 1991; De Fougerolles et al., 1991). ICAM-2 has two Ig like domains (ICAM-1 has five), which are 35% identical to the two N-terminal domains of ICAM-1. ICAM-2 is expressed on lymphoblastoid B cells, resting lymphocytes, monocytes and on hematopoietic cell lines. In contrast to ICAM-1, ICAM-2 is highly expressed on non-activated endothelium and cannot be up-regulated by inflammatory mediators (Nortamo et al., 1991). Recently, it was found that the LFA-1 dependent aggregation of a T cell lymphoma cell line could be blocked by neither anti-ICAM-1 nor anti-ICAM-2. This finding showed the existence of a third ligand for LFA-1, and this ligand has recently been defined and termed ICAM-3 (De Fougerolles et al., 1991; 1992).

VCAM-1

VCAM-1 was defined by cloning of cytokine-induced endothelial cell cDNAs (Rice et al., 1989; 1990). It is a glycosylated cell-surface molecule with a molecular weight of about 110 kD, containing six or seven extracellular Ig domains generated by alternative splicing (Osborn et al., 1989; Cybulski, et al., 1991). Both forms are fully functional, and, as is the case for the ICAM-1 molecule, only the first two domains of VCAM-1 are required for its adhesive function. VCAM-1 is normally not detectable on endothelial cells, but, like ICAM-1, its expression is induced upon activation with LPS, IL-1, IL-4 or TNFα, requires de novo synthesis, and follows the same induction curve as ICAM-1 (Rice et al., 1990; Thornhill et al., 1990; Masinovsky et al., 1990; Graber et al., 1990). The leukocyte receptor for VCAM-1 is VLA-4 (CD49d/CD29), a member of the β_1 integrin family, present on all leucocytes except granulocytes (Elices, et al., 1990; Shimizy et al., 1990).

Evidence for VLA-4/VCAM-1 interaction was obtained in dual transfection experiments in which VLA-4-transfected K-562 cells bound to VCAM transfected COS cells. Furthermore, a

VLA-4 positive cell line specifically bound to VCAM-1 on COS cells and anti-VLA-4 mAb completely inhibited VLA-4 dependent binding to VCAM-1 (Elices et al., 1990).

Recently, it has been shown that the interaction site of VCAM-1 with VLA-4 is distinct from the CS1/VLA-4 binding site. This finding implies that within the VLA-4 molecule different binding sites for the two ligands exist (Elices et al., 1990; Dinther-Janssen et al., submitted).

E-Selectin (ELAM-1)

E-selectin is a member of the Selectin family of adhesion molecules, with a characteristic aminoterminal carbohydrate binding (lectin) domain (Pober et al., 1986; Doukas et al., 1990; Leeuwenberg et al., 1989). E-selectin was first identified by mAb studies as an endothelial cell molecule involved in neutrophil adhesion to endothelium activated with IL-1, TNFα or LPS (Bevilaqua et al., 1987). The induction is rapid (peak at 4 hours) and transient (gone by 20 hours; Doukas et al., 1990; Leeuwenberg et al., 1989) despite the continuous presence of these cytokines (Cotran et al., 1986; Leeuwenberg et al., 1990). Therefore, E-selectin is likely to mediate acute cellular infiltration. The molecule binds specifically to the carbohydrate group, sialyl Lewis X, a terminal structure found on cell surface glycoproteins of neutrophils, monocytes and tumor cells (Philips et al., 1990; Walz et al., 1990). In addition, memory CD4$^+$ T cells have also recently been found to interact via a sialyl Lewis X with E Selectin on cytokine-activated endothelium (Graber, et al., 1990; Shimizu, et al., 1991). The leukocyte receptor for E-selectin has not yet been exactly defined, but it may also be a selectin, for example, L-selectin (Kishimoto et al., 1991). Likewise, Picker et al. (1991) demonstrated that L-Selectin bears oligosaccharide sequences recognized by E-selectin and P-selectin (Picker et al., 1991). Berg, et al. have shown, in E-selectin transfected mice, that the counter-structure of E-selectin is the cutaneous lymphocyte antigen defined by HECA-452 (Berg et al., 1991).

Recirculation through PLN

Lymphocyte recirculation via HEV in secondary lymphoid organs is controlled by the expression of several adhesion molecules (LHR) on the surface of both lymphocytes and high endothelial cells (Jalkanen et al., 1986; Hamann et al., 1988; Butcher et al., 1990; Butcher 1990, Michl et al., 1991; see Table 1). As described above, distinct adhesion molecules have been described that mediate lymphocyte extravasation into lymphoid tissue. The first LHR described was the 80-95 kD glycoprotein on murine lymphocytes recognized by the MEL-14 mAb, L-selectin. L-selectin is expressed on all recirculating lymphocytes and, in contrast to mAb to CD44, mAb to L-selectin could selectively block lymphocyte binding to PLN-HEV, whereas the binding to mucosal-HEV was not affected. During a recent study, we could confirm these findings. Lymphocyte binding to PLN-HEV was found to be strongly dependent on CD44

Table 1. Molecules involved in lymphocyte-endothelial cell interaction.

Family	Molecule on endothelium	Molecule on lymphocyte	MW(kD)	Expression	Receptor	Reference
?	Mad	-	58-66	mucosal HEV	Hermes 3?	Streeter et al 1988a,b; Berg et al 1989; Picker et al 1989.
?	pNad	-	90,100	PLN-HEV	L-selectin	Streeter et al 19881,b; Berg et al 1989.
Selectin	E-selectin		100,120	activated endothelium	sialyl Lewis X HECA-452	Pober et al 1986; Doukas et al 1990; Leeuwenberg et al 1990; Lowe et al 1990; Picker et al 1990, 1991.
		L-selectin	80-100	leukocytes	PLN-HEV	Streeter et al 1988a,b; Berg et al 1991.
Ig supergene	ICAM-1		90-114	endothelium leukocytes	$\alpha_1\beta_2$ integrin (LFA-1)	Rothlein et al 1986; Dustin et al 1986, 1988.
	ICAM-2		55-65	endothelium leukocytes	$\alpha_4\beta_1$ integrin (LFA-4)	Staunton et al 1989.
	VCAM-1		110	activated endothelium	$\alpha_4\beta_1$ integrin (VLA-4)	Osborn et al 1989; Graber et al 1990.
Integrins $\alpha_1\beta_2$		LFA-1	95-180	leukocytes	ICAM-1/2/3	Wawrijk et al 1989; Dustin et al 1988; Fougerolles et al 1992.
$\alpha_4\beta_1$		VLA-4 (LPAM-2)	150/130	leukocytes	VCAM-1 CS1/FN	Elices et al 1990; Shimizu et al 1990; Freedman et al 1990.
$\alpha_4\beta_p$		LPAM-1	160/130	lymphocytes	MALT-HEV	Holzmann et al 1989.

Family	Molecule on endothelium	Molecule on lymphocyte	MW(kD)	Expression	Receptor	Reference
CD 44		Hermes 3	97/150	broad tissue distribution	CD44	Streeter et al 1988a,b; Berg et al 1989; Picker et al 1989.
		CD 44	90,150/200	broad tissue distribution	HA	Stamenkovic et al 1991; Aruffo et al 1990
?	HA		?	PLN-HEV	CD44	Stamenkovic et al 1991; Aruffo et al 1990.
site on FN CS1	?	PLN-HEV			$\alpha_4\beta_1$ integrin (VLA-4)	Hemler et al 1990; Wagner et al 1989; Ager et al, 1990
					synovial HEV	Van Dinther et al, submitted.

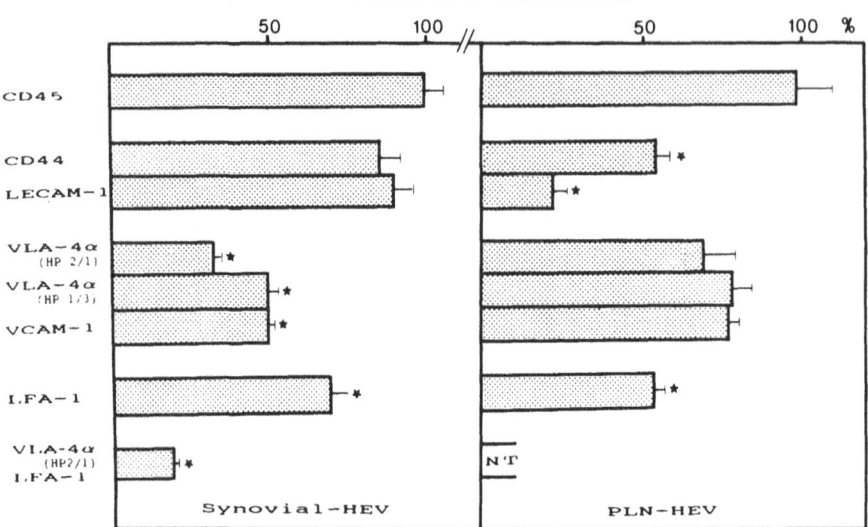

Figure 1. Inhibition of adhesion of normal human PB-T [normal (non-activated) peripheral blood-T cells] to synovial (A) and PLN HEV (B) by mAb against various adhesion molecules. Adherence is expressed as percentage of control (no mAb added). Each value represents the mean ± SE of at least three experiments. The antiVCAM-1 mAb 2G7 and 4B9 gave identical results. Absolute binding of PB-T: SM HEV, 5.75±0.52/mm HEV; PLN HEV, 18.59±2.94/mm HEV; *, significantly different from control by two-tailed Student t-test. (SM, synovial membrane).

and L-selectin (Pals et al., 1989; Dinther-Janssen et al., 1991). L-selectin has been described as the receptor for PLN vascular addressin (PNAd), since L-selectin mediates lymphocyte binding to carbohydrate determinants on PNAd (Berg et al., 1991). Importantly, E-selectin has also been found to mediate leukocyte adhesion by recognition of a carbohydrate ligand, i.e., sialyl Lewis X (Philips et al., 1990) and via the cutaneous lymphocyte antigen (CLA, HECA-452) expressed on memory T cells in the skin (Berg et al.,1991).

Another important molecule involved in lymphocyte-HEV interaction in man is the 90 kD form of CD44, as recognized by the HERMES antibodies (Jalkanen et al., 1986; 1987).

MAb Hermes-1 did not interfere with lymphocyte-HEV binding, whereas Hermes-3 inhibited lymphocyte binding to mucosal HEV only. The Hermes-3 defined epitope appeared to be a lymphocyte receptor for the mucosal addressin, Meca-367 (Berg et al., 1989). We showed that another anti-CD44 mAb (Pals et al., 1989) blocked lymphocyte binding to PLN-HEV up to 40%, whereas this mAb did not interfere with lymphocyte-synovial HEV interaction (Dinther-Janssen et al., 1991). On the other hand, synovial binding could be inhibited by a polyclonal anti CD44 (Jalkanen et al., 1986). It has been shown that the hematopoietic, but not the epithelial, forms of CD44 could bind to cultured rat PLN high endothelium and that this adhesion could be blocked by hyaluronidase treatment of both cultured high endothelial cells and

PLN sections (Stamenkovic et al., 1991). This strongly suggests that CD44 is a cell surface receptor for hyaluronate (Pals et al., 1989; Aruffo et al., 1990). Coming to an explanation of the conflicting data described above, it was furthermore shown that the Hermes-3 mAb recognizes an epitope on CD44 that is distinct from the hyaluronate binding domain (Goldstein et al., 1989; Jalkanen et al., 1987). This suggests that the selective recirculation of lymphocytes throughout the body is regulated within distinct regions of the CD44 molecules. Whereas LFA-1 mAb partially inhibit adhesion of lymphocytes to PLN-HEV in frozen section assays (Pals et al., 1988), mAb to ICAM-1 did not block this adhesion (unpublished results), although ICAM-1 is strongly expressed on HEV. The inability of ICAM-1 mAb to inhibit this interaction suggests that ICAM-1 is not the sole ligand for LFA-1 but rather a member of a family of related LFA-1 ligands, only one of which is recognized by the ICAM-1 mAb (Springer et al., 1987). Indeed, in several cell-cell adhesion studies, LFA-1/ICAM-1 dependent as well as LFA-1/ICAM-1 independent pathways have been described (Lewinsohn et al., 1987; Dustin et al., 1988; Tamatani et al., 1991). Furthermore, evidence for a third counter-receptor for LFA-1 has been provided (De Fougerolles et al., 1991; De Fougerolles et al., 1992).

The VLA-4/VCAM-1 pathway did not seem to contribute to lymphocyte interaction with PLN-HEV as both anti-VLA-4 and anti-VCAM-1 mAb were only marginally inhibitory (Dinther-Janssen et al., 1991) (Figure 1). This is in accordance with the fact that HEV in PLN show no or only weak expression of VCAM-1. Recently, the CS1 motif on the type IIICS of fibronectin has been discovered as a second receptor of VLA-4 (Wayner et al., 1989). This motif supports the adhesion of rat lymphocytes to PLN cultured high endothelial cells (Ager et al., 1990). The CS1 peptide also supports lymphocyte binding to HEV in frozen sections of PLN (Dinther-Janssen et al., submitted). The clear inhibition of lymphocyte binding by the CS1 peptide, as compared with the marginal blocking with the VLA-4 mAb, suggests that another, as yet unidentified, molecule on lymphocytes can bind to the CS1 motif of FN.

Upon activation, the ability of lymphocytes to adhere to PLN-HEV was greatly abolished (Dinther-Janssen et al., 1991). For example, in vivo activated T cells, isolated from either rheumatoid synovium or peritoneal fluid from continuous ambulatory peritoneal dialysis patients, as well as in vitro stimulated T cells, showed poor binding to PLN-HEV, as compared to non-activated T cells (Figure 2). Interestingly, FACS-analysis of these T cells clearly showed a down-regulation of L-selectin, whereas CD44 and LFA-1 expression levels were increased, as has also been found by others (Smith, 1991; Kishimoto et al., 1990).

Taken together, the above findings indicate that L-selectin and CD44 largely determine the adhesion of peripheral blood lymphocytes to PLN-HEV, with the VLA-4/VCAM-1 pathway of minor importance in this interaction. LFA-1 and the CS1 adhesion motif of FN probably serve as accessory molecules, stabilizing the tissue specific interaction of CD44 and L-selectin.

ADHESION MOLECULES INVOLVED IN HOMING TO TISSUES WITH CHRONIC INFLAMMATION

Under physiological conditions, recirculation of lymphocytes through extra-lymphoid tissues is marginal (Parrot et al., 1981). In the course of an inflammatory reaction, however, lymphocyte traffic through inflamed tissue is increased. Adhesion of lymphocytes to the microvascular endothelium is essential for lymphocyte retention and mediation of endothelial cell damage that characterizes many inflammatory sites. In Figure 3 a scheme is shown for the adhesion molecules involved in lymphocyte interaction with endothelial cells in both lymphoid organs and in areas of inflammation. The initiation of these adhesions is apparently through the

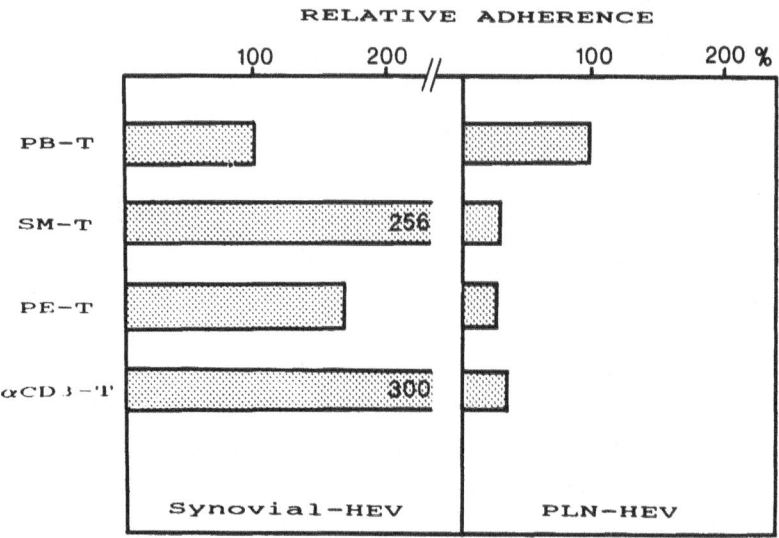

Figure 2. Binding of activated T lymphocytes to synovial (A), and PLN HEV (B). PB-T, normal (non activated) peripheral blood T cells; SM-T, T cells from rheumatoid synovium; PE-T, peritoneal T cells; anti-CD3-T, anti-CD3 stimulated T cells. Adherence is expressed as percentage of the binding of PB-T. Each value represents the mean of at least three experiments. Absolute binding of different T cell populations to synovial and PLN HEV is shown in Table 1.

upregulated and/or induced expression of adhesion molecules on endothelium such as E-selectin, VCAM-1 and ICAM-1. The expression of adhesion molecules on lymphocytes (CD44, VLA-4) can also be increased (Dinther-Janssen et al., 1991; Kishimoto et al., 1990). Interestingly, the simultaneously decreased expression of L-selectin on activated lymphocytes reduces their entry into lymph nodes (Dinther-Janssen et al., 1991). In addition, for LFA-1 it has been shown that an up-regulation and conformational change leads to a high affinity cellular contact (Julita et al., 1989; Kooyk, 1989; Spertini et al., 1991), which is mediated through the β subunit (Hibbs et al., 1991). Since L-selectin can also exist in two affinity states (Spertini et al., 1991), it is likely that this is a general phenomenon for cell adhesion molecules.

E-selectin is normally not detectable on endothelial cells, but has been found to be predominanly expressed on endothelium in acute inflammatory reactions (Cotran et al., 1986). In skin, E selectin can be induced by intracutaneous injection with TNFα and IL-1 in baboons (Bevilacqua et al., 1987), and is present on microvascular endothelium of human skin in allergic and delayed hypersensitivity reactions (Munro et al., 1989; Kyan-Aung et al., 1991) and in cutaneous discoid lupus erythematosus (CDLE) (unpublished results).

Recently, Picker et al. suggested that E-selectin might be a major vascular addressin for the skin homing receptor (Picker et al., 1991). This view is based on the preferential expression of E-selectin on inflamed cutaneous vessels, as compared to inflamed non-cutaneous vessels, and the selective extravasation of skin homing memory T cells (Shimizu et al., 1991; Picker et al., 1990). They also suggested that E-selectin might be the ligand for HECA-452, on the basis of i) the preferential expression of the HECA-452 epitope on cutaneous T cells, ii) the exclusive binding of HECA-452 memory T cells to E-selectin positive skin venules, and iii) the binding of E-selectin transfected mouse cells to HECA-452 memory T cells. Consequently, the name, cutaneous lymphocyte associated antigen (CLA), was proposed for the antigen detected by HECA-452 on T cells. Several findings are in conflict with this suggestion, however, since i) E-selectin is not only expressed on venules in inflamed skin but also on venules in inflamed synovium (Koch et al., 1991) and inflamed lung, where memory T cells do not express the HECA-452 antigen (Dinther-Janssen et al., 1993), and ii) E-selectin transfected COS cells do not bind to a HECA 452 positive cell line (J.M. Harlan, personal communication). In an early study we reported that the HECA-452 defined antigen is exclusively expressed on cutaneous T non Hodgkin lymphomas (T-NHL), while it is absent from most nodal T-NHL (Meijer et al., 1989). More recently, HEV in cutaneous T-NHL were generally found to be HECA-452 negative, while HEV were positive in lymph node based T-NHL (Noorduyn et al., 1992), suggesting that localization of T cells within nodal and extranodal lymphomas is probably mediated via different mechanisms. The data reported by Picker, et al. (1990) and Berg, et al. (1991) suggest that HECA-452 is indeed involved in homing to the skin, leaving the role of E Selectin in lymphocyte extravasation in other non-lymphoid, non-cutaneous tissues unresolved.

VCAM-1 is a cell adhesion protein which is normally not expressed on endothelial cells, but is induced by cytokine stimulation of cultured HUVEC (Rice et al., 1990; Graber et al., 1990). VCAM-1 is found on endothelial cells in both acute and chronic inflammation in synovium and lung (Koch et al., 1991; Dinther-Janssen et al., 1993). VCAM-1 expression was also strongly expressed on endothelium in skin lesions of CDLE (unpublished results). Functionally, VCAM-1 was found to support the adhesion of lymphocytes to inflamed synovium (Dinther-Janssen et al., 1991). Whether this molecule also mediates lymphocyte migration to the skin remains to be established. ICAM-1 is constitutively present on vascular endothelium (Dustin et al., 1986) and its surface expression is enhanced during cytokine stimulation of endothelial cells in vivo and in vitro (Pober et al., 1986). At sites of cutaneous inflammatory responses, ICAM-1 expression is found on endothelial cells, fibroblasts, some leucocytes and keratinocytes (Singer et al., 1989). Here, ICAM-1 was found to mediate the binding of activated T cells to epidermal keratinocytes

(Dustin et al., 1988). ICAM-1 expression on keratinocytes was also found to strongly correlate with various inflammatory skin lesions and malignant cutaneous lymphomas (Lisby et al., 1989; Nickoloff et al., 1990). For example, all benign cutaneous disorders characterized by more chronic dermal inflammation showed strong ICAM-1 expression on the keratinocytes. These results suggest that keratinocytes may also actively participate in lymphocyte trafficking to the skin. The expression of vascular cell adhesion molecules appears to be "non-organ specific", since, in other sites of inflammation (e.g., rheumatoid arthritis (RA) synovium, sarcoidosis of the lung and PLN and Usual Interstitial Pneumonitis), E selectin, VCAM-1 and ICAM-1 could also be detected (Dinther-Janssen et al., 1993). The expression of these adhesion molecules in

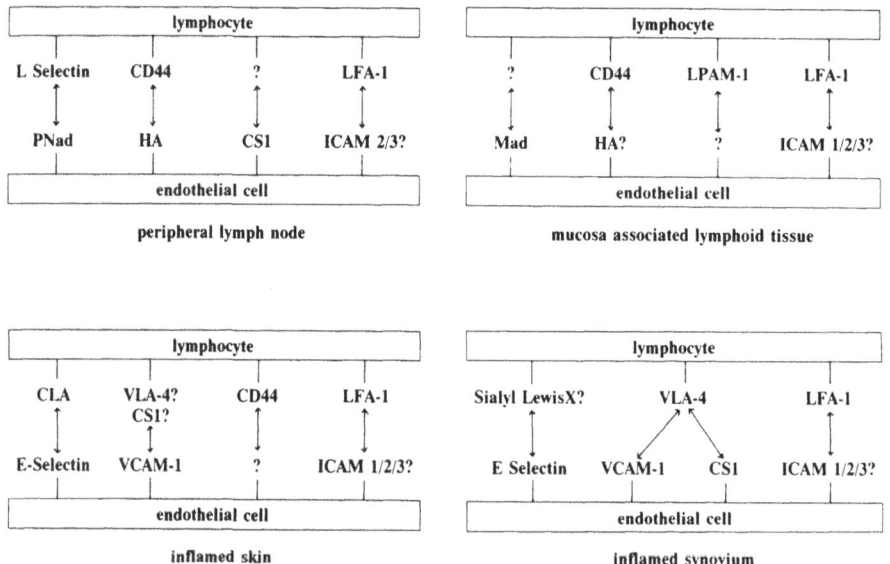

Figure 3. Molecules involved in the interaction between lymphocytes and high endothelial cells in different tissues. HA = hyaluronate.

the inflamed tissues studied differs from those on vessels in PLN. Here neither VCAM-1 nor E-selectin expression was found. E-selectin expression was exclusively found on vessels surrounded by a cellular infiltrate, i.e., either granulocytes in acute, or lymphocytes in chronic, inflammation. These results support the view that E-selectin not only mediates the extravasation of granulocytes but also that of lymphocytes (Shimizu et al., 1991; Picker et al., 1991). In addition, E-selectin was also found to mediate lymphocyte adhesion to synovial-HEV (van Dinther, manuscript in preparation). ICAM-1 and VCAM-1 could be detected on endothelium in the acute and chronic phases of both diseases. With respect to the inflammatory infiltrate, lymphocytes in inflamed skin, synovium and lung were LFA-1 and VLA-4 positive, suggesting a role for the LFA-1/ICAM-1 and VLA-4/VCAM-1 pathways in lymphocyte extravasation in these lesions.

Indeed, in a recent report, we showed that two adhesion pathways are of particular importance in lymphocyte recruitement in inflamed synovium, i.e., LFA-1/ICAM-1 and the VLA-4/VCAM-1 pathways (Dinther-Janssen et al., 1991). We observed that LFA-1 mAb partially blocked lymphocyte binding to synovial HEV, whereas VLA-4 and VCAM-1 mAb strongly inhibited this interaction, as can be explained by the expression of VCAM-1 on synovial endothelial cells. Whether the VLA-4/VCAM-1 pathway also mediates lymphocyte-endothelial cell interaction in inflamed skin remains to be established. Besides supporting the adhesion of lymphocytes to PLN-HEV, the CS1 motif of FN was also capable of supporting lymphocyte adhesion to synovial HEV. This suggests that CS1 mediates both physiological and pathological lymphocyte recirculation. Notably, FN staining was observed on endothelium in both PLN and synovial membrane. An attractive hypothesis to explain these observations is that CS1, like LFA-1, acts as an accessory molecule in lymphocyte homing. The fact that the VLA-4 mAb and CS1, together, did not completely inhibit lymphocyte binding to synovial HEV, however, confirms the notion that lymphocytes use a complex receptor system of multiple adhesion molecules to recognize and adhere to HEV. Activated (memory) T cells were, in contrast to naïve T cells, extremely prone to adhere to synovial HEV, as could be explained by their increased expression of VLA-4, CD44 and LFA-1 and their decrease in L-selectin expression. This binding could also be strongly inhibited by anti-VLA-4 and anti-VCAM-1 antibodies (Dinther-Janssen et al., 1991). Thus, the similar expression of homing receptors on leukocytes (LFA-1 and VLA-4) and endothelium (E selectin, VCAM-1 and ICAM-1) in inflammatory tissues suggests that both the LFA1/ICAM-1 and the VLA-4/VCAM-1 pathways are important in lymphocyte homing to these sites. The role of the HECA-452 antigen in this process is still unclear and needs further investigation.

CONCLUSIONS

Adhesion molecules play an important role in lymphocyte recirculation and extravasation in sites of inflammation. A large variety of these molecules have now been identified, both on endothelial cells and on leukocytes (Figure 3). High endothelial cells in organized secondary lymphoid organs seem to express several adhesion molecules constitutively, whereas at sites of inflammation their expression is up-regulated after activation. Many receptor-ligand systems have now been described, and it is becoming clear that adhesion molecules can interact with more than one ligand. In addition, it has been shown, for various molecules, that conformational changes of the molecule can occur, leading to enhanced interaction. From these data it can be understood that cell-cell interactions, as seen in lymphocyte recirculation, are extremely complex. They are not just based on the mere expression of the right receptors but are also dependent on the activation status of the cell. This may lead to a delicate fine-tuning of such interactions and, therefore, of the immune/inflammatory responses.

ACKNOWLEDGEMENTS

The authors wish to thank Miss Y. Duiker and Mrs. C. van Rijn for secretarial assistance.

REFERENCES

Ager A and MJ Humphries, 1990. Use of synthetic peptides to probe lymphocyte-high endothelial cell interactions. Lymphocytes recognize a ligand on the endothelial surface which contains the CS-1 adhesive motive. **Intern. Immunol.**, 2(10):921.

Albelda SM, 1991. Endothelial and epithelial cell adhesion molecules. **Am. J. Respir. Cell Mol. Biol.**, 4:195-203.

Alzari PM, MB Lascombe and RJ Poljak, 1988. Three-dimensional structure of antibodies. **Ann. Rev. Immunol.**, 6:555.

Arnaout MA, 1990. Structure and function of the leucocyte adhesion molecules CD11/CD18. **Blood**, 75(5):1037.

Aruffo A, I Stamenkovic, M Melnick, CB Underhill and B Seed, 1990. CD44 is the principal cell surface receptor for hyaluronate. **Cell**, 61:1303.

Bednarczyk JL and BW McIntyre, 1990. A monoclonal antibody to VLA-4α chain (CDW4ad) induces homotypic lymphocyte aggregation. **J. Immunol.**, 144:777.

Berg EL, MA Goldstein, M Julita, LJ Nakache, PR Picker, NW Streeter, D Wu, DFH Zhou and EC Butcher, 1989. Homing receptors and vascular addressins: Cell adhesion molecules that direct lymphocyte traffic. **Immunol. Rev.**, 108:1.

Berg EL, MK Robinson, RA Warnock and EC Butcher, 1991. The human peripheral lymph node vascular addressin is a ligand for LECAM-1, the peripheral lymph node homing receptor. **J. Cell Biol.**, 114 (2):343.

Berg EL, T Yoshino, LS Rott, MK Robinson, RA Warnock, TK Kishimoto, LJ Picker and EC Butcher, 1991. The cutaneous lymphocyte antigen is a skin lymphocyte homing receptor for the vascular lectin endothelial cell-leukocyte adhesion molecule 1. **J. Exp. Med.**, 174:1461.

Bevilacqua MP, JS Pober, DL Mendrick, RS Cotran and MA Gimbrone Jr., 1987. Identification of an inducible endothelial-leucocyte adhesion molecule. **Proc. Natl. Acad. Sci. USA**, 84: 9238.

Bevilacqua MP, S Stengelin, MA Gimbrone Jr and B Seed, 1989. Endothelial leucocyte adhesion molecule-1: An inducible receptor for neutrophils related to regulatory proteins and lectins. **Science**, 243:1160.

Bevilacqua M, E Butcher, B Furie, M Gallatin, M Gimbrone, J Harlan, K Kishimoto, L Lasky, R McEver, J Paulson, S Rosen, B Seed, M Siegelman, T Springer, L Stoolman, T Ledder, A Varki, D Wagner, I Weissman and G Zimmerman, 1991. Selectins: a family of adhesion receptors. **Cell**, 67:233.

Bochner BS, FW Luscinskas, MA Gimbrone, W Newman, SA Sterbinsky, CP Derse Anthony, D Klunck and RP Schleimer, 1991. Adhesion of human basophils, eosinophils and neutrophils to interleukin-1 activated human vascular endothelial cells: Contribution of endothelial cell adhesion molecules. **J. Exp. Med.**, 173:1553.

Bowen B, C Fennie and LA Lasky, 1990. The MEL-14 antibody binds to the lectin domain of the murine peripheral lymph node homing receptor. **J. Cell Biol.**, 110:147.

Butcher EC, 1986. The regulation of lymphocyte traffic. **Current Topic Microbiol. and Immunol.**, 128:85.

Butcher EC, 1990. Cellular and molecular mechanisms that direct leucocyte traffic. **Am. J. Pathol.**, 136:3.

Butcher EC, RG Scollay and IL Weissman, 1979. Lymphocyte adherence to high endothelial venules: Characterization of a modified in vitro assay and examination of the binding of syngeneic and allogeneic lymphocyte populations. **J. Immunol.**, 123:1996.

Butcher EC, RG Scollay and JL Weissman, 1980. Organ specificity of lymphocyte migration: Mediation by highly selective lymphocyte interaction with organ-specific determinants on high endothelial venules. **Eur. J. Immunol.**, 10:556.

Cahill RNP, DC Poskitt, H Frost and Z Trnka, 1977. Two distinct pools of recirculation T lymphocytes: Migration characteristics of nodal and intestinal T lymphocytes. **J. Exp. Med.**, 145:420.

Camerini D, SP James, I Samenkovic and B Seed, 1990. Leu-8/TQ1 is the human equivalent of the MEL14 lymph node homing receptor. **Nature**, 342:78.

Carter WG and EA Wayner, 1988. Characterization of a collagen-binding phosphorylated transmembrane glycoprotein expressed in nucleated human cells. **J. Biol. Chem.**, 263:4193.

Cheresh DA, JW Smith, HM Cooper and V Quaranta, 1989. A novel vitronectin receptor intergin (alpha V beta X) is responsible for distinct adhesive properties of carcinoma cells. **Cell**, 57: 59.

Chin Y-H, JP Cai and K Johnson, 1990. Lymphocyte adhesion to cultured Peyer's patch high endothelial venule cells is mediated by organ-specific homing receptors and can be regulated by cytokines. **J. Immunol.**, 145:3669.

Chin YH, RA Rasmussen, AG Cahiroglu and JL Woodruff, 1984. Lymphocyte recognition of lymph node high endothelium. VI. Evidence of distinct structures mediating binding to high endothelial cells of lymph nodes and Peyer's patches. **J. Immunol.**, 133:2961.

Clayberger C, AM Krensky, BW McIntyre, TD Koller, R Parham, F Brodsky, DJ Linn and AL Evans, 1987. Identification and characterization of two novel lymphocyte-function-associated antigens, L24 and L25. **J. Immunol.**, 138:1510.

Cotran RS, MA Gimbrone Jr, MP Bevilacqua, DL Mendrick and JS Pober, 1986. Induction and detection of a human endothelial activation antigen in vivo. **J. Exp. Med.**, 164:661.

Cybulski MI, JWH Fries, AJ Williams, P Sultan, VM Davis, MA Gimbrone Jr and T Collins, 1991. Alternative splicing of human VCAM-1 in vascular endothelium. **Am. J. Pathol.**, 138(4):815.

Denning SM, PT Le, KH Singer and BF Haynes, 1990. Antibodies against the CD44 p80, lymphocyte homing receptor molecule augment human peripheral blood T cell activation. **J. Immunol.**, 144:7.

Diamond MS, DE Staunton, AR de Fougerolles, SA Stacker, J Garcia-Aguilar, ML Hibbs and TA Springer, 1990. ICAM-1 (CD54): a counter receptor for Mac-1 (CD11b/CD18). **J. Cell Biol.**, 111:3129.

Dinther-Janssen ACHM van, E Horst, G Koopman, W Newman, RJ Scheper, CJLM Meijer and ST Pals, 1991. The VLA-4/VCAM-1 pathway is involved in lymphocyte adhesion to endothelium in rheumatoid synovium. **J. Immunol.**, 147:4207.

Dinther-Janssen ACHM van, ST Pals and RJ Scheper, CJLM Meijer. The CS1 motif of fibronectin is involved in binding to both synovial and peripheral lymph node endothelium. Submitted.

Dinther-Janssen ACHM van, TCMTh van Maarsseveen, H Eckert, W Newman and CJLM Meijer. Identical expression of ELAM-1, VCAM-1 and ICAM-1 in sarcoidosis and usual interstitial pneumonitis. **J. Pathol.** (in press)

Doukas J and JS Pober, 1990. INF-gamma enhances endothelial activation induced by tumor necrosis factor but not by IL-1. **J. Immunol.**, 145:1727.

Dustin ML, R Rothlein, AK Bhan, CA Dinarello and TA Springer, 1986. Induction by IL-1 and IFN-gamma: Tissue distribution, biochemistry and function of a natural adhesion molecule (ICAM-1). **J. Immunol.**, 137:245.

Dustin ML, KH Singer, DT Tuck and TA Springer, 1988. Adhesion of T lymphoblasts to epidermal keratinocytes is regulated by interferon-gamma and is mediated by intercellular adhesion molecule-1 (ICAM-1). **J. Exp. Med.**, 167:1323.

Dustin M, P Selvara, RJ Mattaliano and TA Springer, 1987. Anchoring mechanisms for LFA-3 cell adhesion glycoprotein at membrane surface. **Nature**, 329: 846.

Dustin ML and TA Springer, 1988. Lymphocyte-function-associated antigen (LFA-1) interaction with intercellular adhesion molecule (ICAM-1) is one of at least three mechanisms for lymphocytes to adhere to cultured endothelial cells. **J. Cell Biol.**, 107:321.

Elices MJ, L Osborn, Y Takada, C Crouse, S Luhowskyj, ME Hemler and RR Lobb, 1990. VCAM-1 on activated endothelium interacts with the leukocyte Integrin VLA-4 at a site distinct from the VLA-4/Fibronectin binding site. **Cell**, 60:577.

Forsberg UH, ST Jalkanen and J Schroder, 1989. Assignment of the human lymphocyte homing receptor gene to the short arm of chromosome 11. **Immunogenetics**, 29:405.

Fossum S, ME Smit and WL Ford, 1983. The recirculation of lymphocytes in the rat. **Proc. R. Soc. Lond. (Biol).**, 159:257.

Fougerolles AR de, SA Stacker, R Swarting and TA Springer, 1991. Characterization of ICAM-2 and evidence for a third counter receptor for LFA-1. **J. Exp. Med.**, 174: 253.

Fougerolles AR de and TA Springer, 1992. Intercellular adhesion molecule 3, a third adhesion counter-receptor for lymphocyte function-associated molecule 1 on resting lymphocytes. **J. Exp. Med.**, 175:185.

Freed A, J Gailit, P van der Geer, E Ruoslahti and T Hunter, 1989. A novel integrin β subunit is associated with the vitronectin receptor α subunit in a human osteosarcoma cell line and is a substrate for protein kinase C. **EMBO J.**, 8:2955.

Gallatin M, TP St John, M Siegelman, R Reichert, EC Butcher and IL Weissman, 1987. Lymphocyte homing receptors. **Cell**, 44: 673.

Gallatin WM, IL Weissman and EC Butcher, 1983. A cell surface molecule involved in organ-specific homing of lymphocytes. **Nature**, 303: 30.

Gismondi A, S Morrone, MJ Humphries, M Piccolo, L Frati and A Santoni, 1991. Human natural killer cells express the VLA-4 and VLA-5, which mediate their interaction with fibronectin. **J. Immunol.**, 146:384.

Goelz SE, C Hession, D Goff, B Griffiths, R Tizard, B Newman, G Chi-Rosso and R Lobb, 1990. ELFT: a gene that directs the expression of an ELAM-1 ligand. **Cell**, 63:1349.

Goldstein LA, DFH Zhou, LJ Picker, CN Minty, RF Bargatze, JF Ding and EC Butcher, 1989. A human lymph node homing receptor, the Hermes antigen, is related to cartilage proteoglycan core and link proteins. **Cell**, 56:1063.

Gowans JL and EJ Knight, 1964. The route of recirculation of lymphocytes in the rat. **Proc. R. Soc. Lond. Biol. Sci.**, 159:257.

Graber N, TV Gopal, D Wilson, LD Beall, R Polte and W Newman, 1990. T-cells bind to cytokine activated endothelial cells via a novel inducible sialoglycoprotein and endothelial adhesion molecule-1. **J. Immunol.**, 145:819.

Hall JG, J Hopkins aand E Orlans, 1977. Studies on the lymphocyte of sheep. III Destination of lymph borne immunoblasts in relation to their tissue of origin. **Eur. J. Immunol.**, 7:30.

Hamann AD, D Jablonski-Westrich, KU Scholz, A Duijvestijn, EC Butcher and HG Thiele, 1988. Regulation of lymphocyte homing 1. Alternations in homing receptor and organ-specific high endothelial venule binding of lymphocytes upon activation. **J. Immunol.**, 140:737.

Hamann A, D Jablonski-Westrich, AM Duijvestijn, EC Butcher, J Baisch, R Harder and HG Thiele, 1988. Evidence for an accessory role of LFA-1 in lymphocyte-high endothelium interaction during homing. **J. Immunol.**, 140:693.

Harlan JM, BR Schwartz, WJ Wallis and TH Pohlman, 1987. The role of neutrophil membrane proteins in neutrophil emigration. In: ZH Movat, Ed. **Leucocyte emigration and its sequelae.** Karger Press, Basel, p.94.

Haynes BT, MJ Telen, LP Hale and SM Denning, 1989. CD44-A molecule involved in leucocyte adherence and T-cell activation. **Immunol. Today**, 10 (12):423.

Hemler ME, C Huang and L Schwarz, 1987. The VLA protein family: Characterization of five distinct cell surface heterodimers each with a common 130,000 molecular weight β subunit. **J. Biol. Chem.**, 262:3300.

Hemler ME, C Huang, Y Takada, L Schwarz, LJ Strominger and ML Clabby, 1987. Characterization of the cell surface heterodimer VLA-4 and related peptides. **J. Biol. Chem.**, 263:1478.

Hemler ME, C Crouse and A Sonnenberg, 1989. Association of the VLA alpha 6 subunit with a novel protein. A possible alternative to the common VLA beta 1 subunit on certain cell lines. **J. Biol. Chem.**, 264:6529.

Hemler ME, MJ Elices, C Parker and Y Takada, 1990. Structure of the integrin VLA-4 and its cell-cell and cell-matrix adhesion functions. **Immunol. Rev.**, 114:45.

Hibbs ML, H Xu and Stacker, 1991. Regulation of adhesion of ICAM-1 by the cytoplasmic domain of LFA-1 integrin beta subunit. **Science**, 251:1611.

Hoffman JF and GH Giebisch, Eds. **Membranes in growth and development.** Alan R. Liss, New York, 1982.

Holzmann B, BK McIntyre and IL Weissman, 1989. Identification of a murine Peyer's patch-specific lymphocyte homing receptor as an integrin with an α chain homologous to human VLA-4α. **Cell**, 56:37.

Holzmann B and IL Weissman, 1989. Peyer's Patch specific homing receptor consists of a VLA-4 like α chain associated with either of two integrin chains, one of which is novel. **EMBO J.**, 8:1735.

Holzmann B and IL Weissman, 1989. Integrin molecules involved in lymphocyte homing to Peyer's patches. **Immunol. Rev.**, 108:45.

Huet S, H Groux, B Caillou, A Valentin, A Prieur and A Bernard, 1989. CD44 contributes to T cell activation. **J. Immunol.**, 143: 798.

Hynes RO, 1987. Integrins: a family of cell surface receptors. **Cell**, 48:549.

Idzerda RL, WG Carter, C Nottenburg, EA Wayner, WM Gallatin, J St John, 1989. Isolation and DNA sequence of a cDNA clone encoding a lymphocyte adhesion receptor for high endothelium. **Proc. Natl. Acad. Sci. USA**, 86:4659.

Imai Y, DD True, MS Singer and SD Rosen, 1990. Direct demonstration of the lectin activity of gp90[MEL], a lymphocyte homing receptor. **J. Cell Biol.**, 111:1225.

Jalkanen S, AC Steere, RI Fox and EC Butcher, 1986. A distinct endothelial recognition system that controls lymphocyte traffic to inflamed synovium. **Science**, 233:556.

Jalkanen S, RA Reichert, WM Gallatin, RPF Bargatze, IL Weissman and EC Butcher, 1986. Homing receptors and the control of lymphocyte migration. **Immunol. Rev.**, 91:39.

Jalkanen S, R Bargatze, L Herron and EC Butcher, 1986. A lymphoid cell surface glycoprotein involved in endothelial recognition and lymphocyte homing in man. **Eur. J. Immunol.**, 16:1195.

Jalkanen S, RF Bargatze, J de los Toyos and EC Butcher, 1987. Lymphocyte recognition of high endothelium: Antibodies to distinct epitopes of an 8595 kD glycoprotein antigen differentially inhibit lymphocyte binding to lymph node, mucosal or synovial endothelial cells. **J. Cell Biol.**, 105:983.

Jalkanen S, N Wu, RF Bargatze and EC Butcher, 1987. Human lymphocyte and lymphoma homing receptors. **Ann. Rev. Med.**, 38:467.

Jalkanen S, M Jalkanen, R Bargatze, M Tammi and EC Butcher, 1988. Biochemical properties of glycoproteins involved in lymphocyte recognition of high endothelial venules in man. **J. Immunol.**, 141:1615.

Jalkanen S, S Saari, H. Kalimo, K Lamminitausta, E Vainio, R Leino, AM Duyvestein, and K Kalimo, 1990. Lymphocyte migration to skin: The role of lymphocyte homing receptor (CD44) and endothelial cell antigen (HECA-452). **J. Invest. Dermatol.**, 94:789.

Johnson GI, RG Cock and RP McEver, 1989. Cloning of GMP-140, a granule membrane protein of platelets and endothelium: Sequence similarity to proteins involved in cell adhesion and inflammation. **Cell**, 56: 1033.

Jutila M, L Rott, EL Berg and EC Butcher, 1989. Function and regulation of the neutrophil MEL-14 antigen in vivo: comparison with LFA-1 and Mac-1. **J. Immunol.**, 143: 3318.

Kajiji S, RN Tamura and V Quaranta, 1989. A novel integrin (alpha E beta 4) from human epithelial cells suggest a fourth family of integrin adhesion receptors. **EMBO J.**, 8:673.

Kishimoto TK, ME Jutila, EL Berg and EC Butcher, 1989. Neutrophil Mac-1 and MEL-14 adhesion proteins inversely regulated by chemotactic factors. **Science**, 245:1238.

Kishimoto TK, MA Jutila and EC Butcher, 1990. Identification of a human peripheral lymph node homing receptor: A rapidly down-regulated adhesion molecule. **Proc. Natl. Acad. Sci. USA**, 87:2244.

Kishimoto TK, RA Warnock, MA Jutila, EC Butcher, C Lane, DC Anderson and CW Smith, 1991. Antibodies against human neutrophil LECAM-1 (LAM-1/Leu8/Dreg56 antigen) and endothelial cell ELAM-1 inhibit a common CD18-independent adhesion pathway in vitro. **Blood**, 78:805.

Koch AE, JC Burrows, KG Haines, TM Carlos, JM Harlan, S Joseph and S Leibovich, 1991. Immunolocalization of endothelial and leucocyte adhesion molecules in human rheumatoid and osteoarthritic synovial tissues. **Lab. Invest.**, 64:313.

Koopman G, HK Parmentier, HJ Schuurman, W Newman, CJLM Meijer and ST Pals. 1991. Adhesion of human B cells to follicular dendritic cell involves both the LFA-1/ICAM-1 and the Very Late Antigen 4/VCAM-1 pathways. **J. Exp. Med.**, 173:1297.

Koopman G, Y van Kooyk, M de Graaff, CJLM Neijer, CG Figdor and ST Pals, 1990. Triggering of the C44 antigen on T lymphocytes promoted the T cell adhesion through the LFA-1 pathway. **J. Immunol.**, 145:3589.

Kooyk Y van, P van de Wiel, P van Kemenade Weder, TW Kuypers and CG Figdor, 1989. Enhancement of LFA-1 mediated cell adhesion by triggering through CD2 or CD3 on T lymphocytes. **Nature**, 342:811.

Kraal G, IL Weissman and EC Butcher, 1983. Differences in in vivo distribution and homing of T cell subsets to mucosal versus nonmucosal lymphoid organs. **J. Immunol.**, 130:1097.

Krensky AM, F Sanchez-Madrid, E Robbins, JA Nagy, TA Springer and SJ Burskoff, 1983. The functional significance, distribution and structure of LFA-1, LFA-2 and LFA-3: Cell surface antigens associated with CTL target interaction. **J. Immunol.**, 131:611.

Kyan-Aung U, DO Haskard, RN Poston, MH Thornhill and TH Lee, 1991. Endothelial leucocyte adhesion molecule-1 and intercellular adhesion molecule-1 mediate the adhesion of eosinophils to endothelial cells in vitro and are expressed by endothelium in allergic cutaneous inflammation in vivo. **J. Immunol.**, 145:521.

Larsen E, T Palabrica, S Sajer, GE Gilbert, DD Wagner, BC Furie and B Furie, 1990. PADGEM-dependent adhesion of platelets to monocytes and neutrophils is mediated by a lineage-specific carbohydrate LNF 111 (CD15). **Cell**, 63:467.

Lasky LA, MS Singer, TA Yednock, D Dowbenko, C Fenny, H Rodrigues, T Nguyen, S Stachel and SD Rosen, 1989. Cloning of a lymphocyte homing receptor reveales a lectin domain. **Cell**, 56:1045.

Leeuwenberg JFM, EJU von Asmuth, TMAA Jeunhomme and WA Buurman, 1990. IFN-gamma regulates the expression of the adhesion molecule ELAM-1 and the IL-6 production by human endothelial cells in vitro. **J. Immunol.**, 145:2110.

Leeuwenberg JFM, TMAA Jeunhomme and WA Buurman, 1989. Induction of an activation antigen on human endothelial cells in vitro. **Eur. J. Immunol.**, 19:715.

Letarte M, S Iturbe and J Quackenbush, 1985. A glycoprotein of molecular weight 85,000 on human cells of the B-cell lineage: Detection with a family of monoclonal antibodies. **Mol. Immunol.**, 22:113.

Lewinsohn DM, RF Bargatze and EC Butcher, 1987. Leucocyte-endothelial cell recognition: Evidence of a common molecular mechanism shared by neutrophils, lymphocytes and other leucocytes. **J. Immunol.**, 138:4313.

Lisby S, E Ralflkiaer, R Rothlein and G Lange Vejlsgaard, 1989. Intercellular adhesion molecule-1 (ICAM-1) expression correlated to inflammation. **Br. J. Dermatol.**, 120:479.

Lowe JB, LM Stoolman, RP Nair, RD Larsen, TL Berhend and RM Marks, 1990. ELAM-1 dependent cell adhesion to vascular endothelium determined by a transfected human fucosyltransferase cDNA. **Cell**, 63:475.

Makgoba MW, ME Sanders, LGA Ginther, EA Gugel, ML Dustin, TA Springer and S Shaw, 1988. Functional evidence that intercellular adhesion molecule-1 (ICAM-1) is a ligand for LFA-1 dependent adhesion in T-cell mediated cytotoxicity. **Eur. J. Immunol.**, 18:637.

Marchesi VT and JL Gowans, 1964. The migration of lymphocytes through the endothelium of venules in lymph nodes. **Proc. R Soc. Lond. B. Biol. Sci.**, 159:283.

Marlin SD and TA Springer, 1987. Purified intercellular adhesion molecule 1 (ICAM-1) is a ligand for lymphocyte-function-associated antigen-1 (LFA-1). **Cell**, 51:813.

Martz E, 1987. LFA-1 and other accessory molecules functioning in adhesion of T and B lymphocytes. **Hum. Immunol.**, 18:3.

Masinovsky B, D Urdal and WM Gallatin. 1990. IL-4 acts synergistically with IL-1β to promote lymphocyte adhesion to microvascular endothelium by induction of vascular cell adhesion molecule-1. **J. Immunol.**, 145:2886.

Meijer CJLM, R Beljaards, E Horst, R Willemze, P van der Valk and ST Pals, 1989. Differences in antigen expression between primary cutaneous and node based T cell lymphomas. **J. Invest. Dermatol.**, 92:479.

Michl J, QY Qui and HM Kuere, 1991. Homing receptors and addressins. **Current Opinion in Immunology**, 3:373.

Munro JM, JS Pober and RS Cotran, 1989. Tumor necrosis factor and interferon-gamma induce distinct patterns of endothelial activation and associated leucocyte accumulation in skin of Papio anubis. **Am. J. Pathol.**, 135:121.

Nickoloff BJ, CEM Griffiths and JNWN Barker, 1990. The role of adhesion molecules, chemotactic factors and cytokines in inflammatory and neoplastic skin disease. **J. Invest. Dermatol.**, 94:1515.

Noorduyn LA, RC Beljaards, ST Pals, P van Heerde, T Radaszkiewicz, R Willemze and CJLM Meijer, 1992. Differential expression of the HECA-452 antigen (cutaneous lymphocyte associated antigen, CLA) in cutaneous and non cutaneous T-cell lymphomas. **Histopathology**, 21:59.

Nortamo P, R Salcedo, T Timonen, M Patarroyo and CG Gahmberg, 1991. A monoclonal antibody to the human leucocyte adhesion molecule intercellular adhesion molecule-2. Cellular distribution and molecular characterization of the antigen. **J. Immunol.**, 146:2530.

Osborn L, C Hession, R Tizard, C Vassalo, S Lukowskyj, G Chi Rosso and R Lobb, 1989. Direct expression cloning of vascular cell adhesion molecule-1, a cytokine-induced endothelial protein that binds to lymphocytes. **Cell**, 59:1203.

Pals ST, A den Otter, F Niedema, P Kabel, GD Keizer, RJ Scheper and CJLM Meijer,1988. Evidence that leucocyte-function-associated antigen-1 is involved in recirculation and homing of human lymphocytes via high endothelial venules. **J. Immunol.**, 140:1851.

Pals ST, F Hogervorst, GD Keizer, T Thepen, E Horst and CG Figdor, 1989. Identification of a widely distributed 90 kDa glycoprotein that is homologous to the Hermes-1 human lymphocyte homing receptor. **J. Immunol.**, 143:851.

Pals ST, E Horst, RJ Scheper and CJLM Meijer, 1989. Mechanisms of human lymphocyte migration and their role in the pathogenesis of disease. **Imm. Rev.**, 108:111.

Parrot DMV, 1981. Lymphocyte circulation outside the lymphoid system. In: de Sousa, M., Ed. **Lymphocyte circulation: Experimental and clinical aspects**, Wiley Interscience Publications, New York.

Phillips ML, E Nudelman, FCA Gaeta, M Perez, AK Singhal, SI Hakomor and JC Paulson, 1990. ELAM-1 mediates cell adhesion by recognition of a carbohydrate ligand Sialyl-Le^x. **Science**, 250:1130.

Picker LJ, MW Terstappen, LS Rott, R Streeter, H Stein and EC Butcher, 1990. Differential expression of homing associated adhesion molecules by T cell subsets in man. **J. Immunol.**, 45:3247.

Picker LJ, J de los Toyos, MJ Telen, BF Haynes and EC Butcher, 1989. Monoclonal antibodies against the CD44 [In(lu)-related p80] and the Pgp-1 antigens in man recognize the Hermes class of lymphocyte homing receptors. **J. Immunol.**, 142:2046.

Picker LJ, TK Kishimoto, CW Smith, RA Warnock and EC Butcher, 1991. ELAM-1 is an adhesion molecule for skin homing T cells. **Nature**, 349:796.

Picker LJ, RA Warnock, AR Burns, CM Doershuk, EL Berg and EC Butcher, 1991. The neutrophil selectin LECAM-1 presents carbohydrate ligands to the vascular selectins ELAM-1 and GMP140. **Cell**, 66:921.

Picker LJ, LWMM Terstappen, LS Rott, PR Streeter, H Stein and EC Butcher, 1990. Differential expression of homing-associated adhesion molecules by T cell subsets in man. **J. Immunol.**, 145:3247.

Picker LJ, SA Michie, LS Rott and EC Butcher, 1990. A unique phenotype of skin-homing associated lymphocytes in humans. Preferential expression of the HECA-452 epitope by benign and malignant T cells at cutaneous sites. **Am. J. Pathol.**, 136(5):1053.

Pober JS, MP Bevilacqua, DL Mendrick, LA Lapierre, W Fiers and MA Gimbrone Jr, 1986. Two distinct monokines, IL-1 and tumor necrosis factor each independently induce biosynthesis and transient expression of the same antigen on the surface of cultured human vascular endothelial cells. **J. Immunol.**, 136:1680.

Pober JS, MA Gimbrone Jr, LA Lapierre, DL Mendrick, W Fiers, R Rothlein and TA Springer, 1986. Overlapping patterns of activation of human encothelial cells by interleukin-1, tumor necrosis factor, and immune interferon. **J. Immunol.**, 137:1893.

Pytela R, MD Piersbacher and E Ruoslathi, 1985. A 125/115 kDa cell surface receptor specific for vitronectin interacts with the arginine-glycine-aspartic acid adhesion sequence derived from fibronectin. **Proc. Natl. Acad. Sci. USA,** 82:5766.

Reichert RA, IL Weissman and EC Butcher, 1983. Germinal center cells lack homing receptor expression necessary for normal lymphocyte migration. **J. Exp. Med.,** 157:813.

Reynolds J, I Heron, L Dudler and Z Trnka, 1982. T-cell recirculation in the sheep: Migratory properties of cells from lymph nodes. **Immunol.,** 47:415.

Rice GE and MP Bevilacqua, 1989. An inducible endothelial cell surface glycoprotein mediates melanoma adhesion. **Science,** 246:1303.

Rice GE, M Munro and MP Bevilacqua, 1990. Inducible cell adhesion molecule 110 (INCAM-llO) is an endothelial receptor for lymphocytes. A CD11/CD18 independent adhesion mechanism. **J. Exp. Med.,** 171:1369.

Rothlein R, ML Dustin, SD Marlin and TA Springer, 1986. A human intercellular adhesion molecule (ICAM-1) distinct from LFA-1. **J. Immunol.,** 137:1270.

Rothlein R and TA Springer, 1986. The requirement for lymphocyte function associated antigen-1 in homotypic leucocyte adhesion stimulated by phorbol ester. **J. Exp. Med.,** 163:1132.

Ruoslahti E and MD Pierschbacher, 1986. Arg-Gly-Asp: a versatile cell recognition signal. **Cell,** 44:517.

Ruoslahti E and MD Pierschbacher, 1987. New perspectives in cell adhesion: RGD and integrins. **Science,** 238:491.

Sanchez-Madrid F, P Simons, S Thompson and TA Springer, 1983. Mapping of antigenic and functional epitopes on the α and the β-subunits of two related mouse glycoproteins involved in cell interactions LFA-1 and Mac-1. **J. Exp. Med.,** 158:586.

Scollay R, J Hopkins and J Hall, 1970. Possible role of surface Ig in non-random recirculation of lymphocytes. **Nature,** 260:528.

Shimizu Y, GA van Seventer, R Siraganian, L Wahl and S Shaw, 1989. Dual role of the CD44 molecule in T cell adhesion and activation. **J. Immunol.,** 143:2457.

Shimizu Y, S Shaw, N Graber, TV Gopal, KJ Horgan, SA van Seventer and W Newman, 1991. Activation independent binding of human memory T cells to adhesion molecule ELAM-1. **Nature,** 349:799.

Shimizy Y, G van Seventer, KJ Horgan and S Shaw, 1990. Regulated expression and binding of three VLA-β-1 integrin receptors on T cells. **Nature,** 345:250.

Siegelman MH, M van Rijn and IL Weissman, 1989. Mouse lymph node homing receptor cDNA clones encodes a glycoprotein revealing tandem interaction domains. **Science,** 243:1165.

Singer KH, DT Tuck, HA Sampson and RP Hall, 1989. Epidermal keratinocytes express the adhesion molecule intercellular adhesion molecule-1 in inflammatory dermatoses. **J. Invest. Dermatol.,** 92:746.

Smith CW, TK Kishimotot, O Abbas, B Hughes, R Rotlein, LV McIntire and EC Butcher, DC Anderson, 1991. Chemotactic factors regulate lectin adhesion molecule-1 (LECAM-1)-dependent neutrophil adhesion to cytokine-stimulated endothelial cells in vitro. **J. Clin. Invest.,** 87:609

Smith CW, TK Kishimoto, O Abbas, B Hughes, R Rothlein, LV McIntire, EC Butcher and DC Anderson, 1991. Chemotactic factors regulate Lectin Adhesion Molecule-1 (LECAM-1)-dependent neutrophil adhesion to cytokine-stimulated endothelial cells in vitro. **J. Clin. Invest.**, 87:609.

Smith ME, AF Martin and WL Ford, 1980. Migration of lymphoblasts in the rat: Preferential localization of DNA-synthesizing lymphocytes in particular lymph nodes and other sites. **Monogr. Allergy**, 16:203.

Spertini O, GS Kansas, JM Munro, JD Griffin and TF Tedder, 1991. Regulation of leucocyte migration by activation of the leucocyte adhesion molecule-1 (LAM-1) selectin. **Nature**, 349:691.

Springer TA, ML Dustin, TK Kishimoto and SD Marlin, 1987. The lymphocyte-function-associated antigens LFA-1, CD2, and LFA-3 molecules: Cell adhesion receptors of the immune system. **Annu. Rev. Immunol.**, 5:223.

Springer TA, 1990. Adhesion receptors of the immune system. **Nature**, 346:425.

Stamenkovic I, A Aruffo, M Amiot and B Seed. 1991. The hematopoietic and epithelial forms of CD44 are distinct polypeptides with different potentials for hyaluronate- bearing cells. **EMBO J.**, 10:343.

Stamper HB Jr and JJ Woodruff, 1976. Lymphocyte homing into lymph nodes: In vitro demonstration of the selective affinity of recirculating lymphocytes for high endothelial venules. **J. Exp. Med.**, 144:828.

Staunton DE, ML Dustin and TA Springer, 1989. Functional cloning of ICAM-2, a cell adhesion ligand for LFA-1 homologous to ICAM-1. **Nature**, 339:61.

Stevens SK, IL Weissman and EC Butcher, 1982. Differences in the migration of B and T lymphocytes: Organ localization in vivo and the role of lymphocyte-endothelial recognition. **J. Immunol.**, 128:844.

Stoolman LM, TS Tenforde and SD Rosen, 1984. Phosphomannosyl receptors may participate in the adhesive interaction between lymphocytes and high endothelial venules. **J. Cell Biol.**, 99:1535.

Stoolman LM and SD Rosen, 1983. Possible role for cell-surface carbohydrate-binding molecules in lymphocyte recirculation. **J. Cell Biol.**, 96:722.

Stoolman LM, TA Yednock and SD Rosen, 1987. Homing receptors on human and rodent lymphocytes. Evidence for a conserved carbohydrate-binding specificity. **Blood**, 70:1842.

Stoolman LM, 1989. Adhesion molecules controlling lymphocyte migration. **Cell**, 56:907.

Streeter PR, EL Berg, BTM Rouse, RR Bargatze and EC Butcher, 1988a. A tissue-specific endothelial cell molecule involved in lymphocyte homing. **Nature**, 331:41.

Streeter PR, BTN Rouse and EC Butcher, 1988b. Immunohistologic and functional characterization of a vascular addressin involved in lymphocyte homing into peripheral lymph nodes. **J. Cell Biol.**, 107:1853.

Takada Y, MJ Elices, C Crouse and ME Nealer, 1989. The primary structure of the $\alpha4$ subunit of VLA-4: Homology to other integrins and possible cell-cell adhesion function. **EMBO J.**, 8:1361.

Tamatani T, M Kotani, T Tanaka and M Miyasaka, 1991. Molecular mechanisms underlying lymphocyte recirculation, II: Differential regulation of LFA-1 in the interaction between lymphocytes and high endothelial cells. **Eur. J. Immunol.**, 21:855.

Tedder TF, AC Penta, HB Levine and AS Freedman, 1990a. Expression of the human adhesion molecule LAM-1: Identity with the TQ1 and Leu-8 differentiation antigens. **J. Immunol.**, 144:532.

Tedder TF, T Matsuyama, D Rothstein, SF Schlossman and C Morimoto, 1990b. Human antigen-specific memory T cells express the homing receptor (LAN-1) necessary for lymphocyte recirculation. **Eur. J. Immunol.**, 20:1351.

Tedder TF, CM Isaacs, TJ Ernst, GD Demetri, DA Adler and CD Disteche. 1989. Isolation and chromosomal localisation of cDNAs encoding a novel human lymphocyte cell surface molecule, LAM-1. Homology with the mouse lymphocyte homing receptor and other human adhesion proteins. **J. Exp. Med.**, 170:123.

Thornhill NH and D Haskard, 1990. IL-4 regulates cell activation by IL-1, tumor necrosis factor or IFN-gamma. **J. Immunol.**, 145:865.

Trowbridge IS, J Lesley, R Schulte, R Hyman and J Trotter, 1982. Biochemical characterization and cellular distribution of polymorphic murine cell-surface glycoprotein expressed on lymphoid tissues. **Immunogenetics**, 15:299.

Walz G, A Aruffo, W Kolanus, M Bevilaqua and B Seed, 1990. Recognition by ELAM-1 of the Sialyl-Le^x determinant on meyeloid and tumor cells. **Science**, 250:1132.

Wassarman, PN, 1983. In: Yamada, KN, Ed. **Fertilization in cell interaction and development: Molecular mechanisms**, John Wiley and Sons, New York.

Watson NL, SF Kingsmore, GI Johnson, MH Siegelman, MM Le Beau, RS Lemons, NS Bora, TA Howard, IL Weissman, RP NcEver and MF Seldin, 1990. Genomic organization of the selectin family of leucocyte adhesion molecules on human and mouse chromosome 1. **J. Exp. Med.**, 172:263.

Wawrijk SO, JR Novotny, IP Wicks, D Wilkinson, D Naher, E Salvaris, R Welch and J Fecondo, Boyd, 1989. The role of LFA-l/ICAM-1 interaction in human leucocyte homing and adhesion. **Immunol. Rev.**, 108:135.

Wayner EA and WG Carter, 1987. Identification of multiple cell adhesion receptors for collagen and fibronectin in human fibrosarcoma cells possessing unique α and β chains. **J. Cell Biol.**, 105:1873.

Wayner EA, A Garcia-Pardo, NJ Humphries, JA McDonald and WG Cartger, 1989. Identification and characterization of the lymphocyte receptor for an alternative cell attachment domain in plasma fibronectin. **J. Cell Biol.**, 109:1321.

Wayner EA, WG Carter, R Piotrowicz and TJ Kunicki, 1988. The function of multiple extracellular matrix receptors (ECMRs) in mediating cell adhesion to ECM: Preparation of monoclonal antibodies to the fibronectin receptor that specifically inhibit cell adhesion to fibronectin and react with platelet glycoproteins CD11/CD18. **J. Cell Biol.**, 107:1881.

Williams AF and AN Barclay, 1988. The immunoglobulin superfamily domains for cell surface recognition. **Ann. Rev. Immun.**, 6:381.

Yednock T and SD Rosen, 1989. Lymphocyte homing. **Adv. Immuunol.**, 44:313.

ADHESION RECEPTORS IN NORMAL SKIN AND CUTANEOUS MALIGNANT LYMPHOMAS: PATHOPHYSIOLOGICAL AND CLINICAL CORRELATIONS

Wolfram Sterry*
Volker Mielke*
Ulrich Kontert†
Imke Kellner*
Wolf-Henning Boehncke*

* Department of Dermatology
University of Ulm
Ulm, Germany

† Department of Maxillary Surgery
University of Cologne
Cologne, Germany

Correspondence to: Dr. W. Sterry, Department of Dermatology
University of Ulm, Oberer Eselsberg 40
W-7900 Ulm, Germany

ABSTRACT

The molecular mechanisms underlying the phenomenon of epidermotropism are still poorly understood. To determine the importance of adhesion molecules and their ligands in the process of T-cell migration into the epidermis, we analyzed, by immunohistochemistry, the expression pattern of adhesion molecules belonging to the integrin and immunoglobulin superfamilies in inflammatory skin disorders and malignant T-cell lymphomas. Cases with diffuse, focal, or no epidermotropism were distinguished in the lymphomas investigated. LFA-1 and LFA-3 were present on infiltrating cells in all cases of epidermotropic and nonepidermotropic cutaneous T-cell lymphoma (CTCL) as well as in reactive processes. β1-integrins showed differential

Basic Mechanisms of Physiologic and Aberrant Lymphoproliferation in the Skin
Edited by W.C. Lambert *et al.*, Plenum Press, New York, 1994

141

expression, most prominent in the case of VLA-1 and VLA-6: These molecules were expressed on infiltrating cells in the majority of cases, with epidermotropic MF comparable to inflammatory conditions, and were absent in most other CTCLs. Thus, differential expression and regulation of avidity seem to contribute to the phenomenon of epidermotropism, with VLA-1 being the most influential $\beta 1$ integrin.

INTRODUCTION

Involvement of adhesion molecules in the pathophysiology of cutaneous T-cell lymphomas

Adhesion molecules and their ligands, with a multitude of interactions and various regulatory mechanisms, provide an ideal means of organizing complex processes like differentiation of multicellular organisms or coordination of activities of the immune system (Springer 1990). They are also known to be involved in cutaneous inflammation and malignancies (Nickoloff et al., 1990; Kellner et al., 1990).

Based on their molecular structure, three families of cell adhesion receptors have been defined: The integrin family (Hynes, 1987) is characterized by a heterodimeric structure with a subfamily-specific unique β-chain and an individual α-chain. So far, five subfamilies have been distinguished by their β-subunits, with the $\beta 1$-, $\beta 2$- and $\beta 3$-integrins being the most important. Among the $\beta 1$-integrins (Hemler, 1987) are cell receptors that bind to the extracellular matrix components, fibronectin, collagen, and laminin. VLA-4 serves as both matrix and cell receptor (Hemler, 1990). LFA-1, a member of the $\beta 2$-integrins (Kishimoto et al., 1987), interacts with ICAM-1 (Dustin et al., 1986; Marlin et al., 1987) and ICAM-2 (Staunton et al., 1989), both belonging to the immunoglobulins. Two other members of the immunoglobulin family form the receptor-ligand pair, LFA-3/CD2 (Springer et al., 1987; Wallner et al., 1987).

Cutaneous T-cell lymphomas (CTCLs) are caused by malignant transformation and proliferation of T-cells, mainly of the CD4$^+$ subset (Slater et al., 1991). T-cell epidermotropism is a prominent feature in the histopathology of CTCLs. In early mycosis fungoides (MF), this migration is accompanied by the aggregation of T-cells within the epidermis, thus leading to the formation of Pautrier's abscesses. Progression of the disease into tumor stage is often accompanied by a loss of epidermotropism and subsequent systemic dissemination of tumor cells (Sterry, 1985).

The key to understanding both the initial epidermotropism as well as the subsequent dissemination of T-cells in CTCLs might be provided by changes in the expression pattern of adhesion molecules, namely of ICAM-1: Expression of this molecule can be found on a variety of cells, including keratinocytes. Its inducibility by inflammatory mediators is an important mechanism for the regulation of its interaction with LFA-1, resulting in a mononuclear cell infiltrate at the site of inflammation (Nickoloff et al., 1990). As in inflammatory sites, early stages of CTCL also exhibit the presence of ICAM-1 positive keratinocytes and T-cells within the epidermis (Nickoloff, 1988). In contrast to these findings in early CTCL, Nickoloff and coworkers described a case of Sézary's syndrome lacking epidermotropism. Here, ICAM-1 expression of keratinocytes could not be detected (Nickoloff et al., 1989). Those authors concluded that, due to this lack of ICAM-1 expression, malignant T-cells were released from the epidermal compartment, and thus caused systemic disease.

MATERIALS AND METHODS

Immunohistochemical approach to determine the role of adhesion molecules in T-cell epidermotropism

To further determine the role of adhesion molecules in the phenomenon of epidermotropism, we analyzed and compared, in relation to inflammatory skin diseases, the expression pattern of nine adhesion molecules on keratinocytes and the mononuclear infiltrate in cases of epidermotropic and non-epidermotropic CTCLs. For this purpose, we investigated biopsy material from patients with CTCLs and inflammatory dermatoses comprising MF (n=15), pleomorphic T-cell lymphoma (n=10), high-grade T-cell lymphoma (n=7), psoriasis (n=15), pityriasis lichenoides (n=11), parapsoriasis en plaques (n=11), contact dermatitis (n=7) and lichen planus (n=5). Specimens were excised under local anesthesia prior to systemic or topical treatment. Informed consent was obtained. Biopsies were snap-frozen in 0.9% NaCl solution with liquid nitrogen and stored at -80°C in a freezer. Serial six micrometer frozen sections were cut from each block on a cryostat, air dried for 24 hours and stored at -20°C until used.

A set of monoclonal antibodies (mAb) was employed for routine three step immunoperoxidase staining: The anti-ICAM-1 mAb, RR1/1 (Rothlein, 1986), anti-LFA-3 mAb, TS2/9 (Sanchez-Madrid, 1982) and anti-VLA-1 mAb, TS2/7 (Hemler, 1985) were kind gifts from Dr. T.A. Springer (Boston). Anti-VLA-β1 mAb, A-1A5 (Hemler, 1983) and anti-VLA-4 mAb, B-5G10 (Hemler, 1987) were given to us by Dr. M.E. Hemler (Boston). R. Kantor (New York) provided us with the anti-VLA-3 mAb, J143 (Kaufmann, 1989). 1OG11 (Hemler, 1988), detecting VLA-2, and GoH3 (Sonnenberg, 1989), directed against VLA-6, were kind gifts from Dr. von dem Borne (Amsterdam) and Dr. Sonnenberg (Amsterdam), respectively. Dr. Damsky (San Fancisco) provided us with the anti-VLA-5 mAb, BIIG2 (Werb, 1989). Horseradish peroxidase conjugated rabbit anti-mouse antibodies and goat anti-rabbit antibodies were purchased from Dakopatts (Denmark) and Medac (Germany) (Table 1).

RESULTS

Expression patterns of adhesion molecules on keratinocytes are comparable in different entities of CTCLs and inflammatory dermatoses

Keratinocytes in different entities of CTCLs show a very similar pattern of adhesion molecule expression (Table 2). LFA-1, VLA-1, VLA-4 and VLA-5 were not detectable on keratinocytes (Table 1). LFA-3 was found to be expressed by keratinocytes basally and in the stratum spinosum, whereas VLA-2 was restricted to basal keratinocytes. Thus, these two markers showed the same distribution in these dermatoses as in normal skin. Compared to normal skin, keratinocytes in CTCLs exhibit focal neoexpression of ICAM-1. This neo-expression was restricted to cases of CTCL with epidermotropism. VLA-3 expression was found both on basal keratinocytes as well as in suprabasal layers. VLA-6 was the only adhesion molecule included in this study revealing differential expression: As in normal skin, basal keratinocytes in pleomorphic and high grade T-cell lymphoma stained positive for this marker,

Table 1. Adhesion molecules of the integrin and immunoglobulin superfamilies, cluster of differentiation, ligand and antibody name. (from Boehnke W.H. et al., 1991b)

Superfamily Molecule	Adhesion	CD	Ligand	Antibody
Integrin				
β1-integrins	VLA-1	-	col, lam	TS2/7
	VLA-2	CD49b	col, lam	10G11
	VLA-3	-	col, fib, lam	J 143
	VLA-4	CD49d	fib, VCAM-1	B-5G10
	VLA-5	-	fibronectin	BIIG2
	VLA-6	CD49f	laminin	GoH3
β2-integrin	LFA-1	CD11a	ICAM-1	IOT16
Immunoglobulin	LFA-3	CD58	CD2	T52/9
	ICAM-1	CD54	LFA-1	RR1/1

col = collagen
fib = fibronectin
lam = laminin

whereas in MF, VLA-6 expression was also detectable suprabasally. In MF, keratinocytes expressing ICAM-1, VLA-3 or VLA-6 were localized close to Pautrier's microabscesses.

As is the case in normal skin and in the CTCLs studied by us, keratinocytes in all inflammatory dermatoses included in this study exhibited a phenotype negative for LFA-1, VLA-1 and VLA-4. The focal neoexpression of ICAM-1 described in the cases with CTCL was a feature shared by the inflammatory dermatoses under investigation. Moreover, VLA-3 and VLA-6 expression, also on keratinocytes located suprabasally, paralleled our findings in CTCLs (Table 2). By contrast, VLA-5 was differentially upregulated: It was present focally in the basal layer of keratinocytes in psoriasis, lichen planus and pityriasis lichenoides. Keratinocytes in the other dermatoses lacked VLA-5 expression. Lichen planus represents an exception with regard to LFA-3 expression in as much as in this dermatosis LFA-3 was restricted to the basal and suprabasal layers.

Differential expression of some β1-integrins corresponds to the intradermal localization of infiltrating mononuclear cells

Cases with CTCL were grouped, according to their distribution of infiltrating cells, as strongly epidermotropic, focally epidermotropic or non-epidermotropic (Tables 3, 4 and 5). MF turned out to be the CTCL most frequently exhibiting the phenomenon of epidermotropism: eight cases were classified as epidermotropic; one case was considered focally epidermotropic and three cases not epidermotropic. By contrast, only two of ten cases of pleomorphic T-cell

Table 2. Expression of adhesion molecules on keratinocytes in mycosis fungoides, pleomorphic and high-grade T cell lymphoma. (from: Sterry et al., 1991)

	MF	**Pleo. TCL**	**High-grade TCL**	**Normal skin**
LFA-1	neg	neg	neg	neg
LFA-3	basal/spin	basal/spin	basal/spin	basal/spin
ICAM-1	focal	focal	focal	neg
VLA-1	neg	neg	neg	neg
VLA-2	basal	basal	basal	basal
VLA-3	basal/sb.	basal/sb.	basal/sb.	basal
VLA-4	neg	neg	neg	neg
VLA-5	neg	neg	neg	neg
VLA-6	basal/sb.	basal	basal	basal

basal = basal layer
sb. = suprabasal layers
spin = stratum spinosum

lymphoma and two of seven cases of high-grade lymphoma showed pronounced epidermotropism (Tables 3,4,5). Infiltrating cells located epidermally in cases with epidermotropic MF regularly expressed LFA-1 (Table 3). This molecule was also demonstrable on the majority of cells infiltrating the dermis in both epidermotropic and non-epidermotropic cases. Parallel findings were obtained for LFA-3 and ICAM-1 expression, respectively. VLA-1$^+$ cells could be demonstrated in the dermal and epidermal infiltrate of epidermotropic MF, but its expression was less frequent compared to LFA-1, LFA-3 and ICAM-1. VLA-1 expression was rare on dermally located cells in non-epidermotropic MF. This holds true also for VLA-4 and VLA-5. Some cases of epidermotropic MF lacked expression of these markers on cells infiltrating the

Table 3. Expression of adhesion molecules on infiltrating cells in cases of mycosis fungoides. Groups of cases with diffuse, focal and no epidermotropism can be distinguished according to the distribution pattern of infiltrating cells. (from: Sterry et al., 1991)

Case		LFA-1	LFA-3	ICAM-1	VLA-1	VLA-2	VLA-3	VLA-4	VLA-5	VLA-6
Diffuse epidermotropism:										
1	E:	++++	++	++	+	—	—	++	+	—
	S:	++++	+++	+++	++	—	+	+++	++	+
2	E:	++++	+	—	+++	—	—	+++	+	—
	S:	++++	+++	+++	++	—	+	+++	+++	++
3	E:	+++	+++++	++	+++	—	—	+	++	+
	S:	++++	++++	+++++	++	—	—	+++	+++	++
4	E:	++++	++++	++++	—	—	++	—	++	—
	S:	++++	++++	++++	+++	—	+++	+++	++++	++
5	E:	+++++	+++++	++++	++	—	—	++++	++	—
	S:	++++	+++++	++++	++	—	+	++++	+++	++
6	E:	++++	++	++	+	—	+	++	+	—
	S:	++++	++++	++++	+	—	—	++	+++	—
7	E:	+++	++++	++	++	—	—	+	—	—
	S:	++++	++++	++++	+	—	+	+++	+++	—
8	E:	+++	++++	+	+++	—	—	+	—	—
	S:	+++	+++	++++	++	—	+	+++	+++	++

146

Case		LFA-1	LFA-3	ICAM-1	VLA-1	VLA-2	VLA-3	VLA-4	VLA-5	VLA-6
Focal epidermotropism:										
9	E:	+ + + +	+ + + +	+ + +	–	–	–	+	–	–
	S:	+ + + +	+ + + +	+ + + +	–	–	–	+ +	+ +	–
No epidermotropism:										
10	E:	0	0	0	0	0	0	0	0	0
	S:	+ + + +	+ + + +	+ + +	+	–	+	+ +	+ + +	+
11	E:	0	0	0	0	0	0	0	0	0
	S:	+ + + +	+ + + +	+ + + +	–	–	–	+ +	+ +	–
12	E:	0	0	0	0	0	0	0	0	0
	S:	+ + + +	+ + + +	+ + +	+	–	+	+ +	+ +	–

E = epidermal

S = subepidermal

O = no infiltrate

– = no cells express marker

+ = 1- 25% express marker

+ + = 25- 50% express marker

+ + + = 50- 75% express marker

+ + + + = 75-100% express marker

147

epidermis, however. VLA-2 expression was not detectable in any case, expression of VLA-3 and VLA-6 was usually restricted to the dermal infiltrate of only a few cases.

The expression patterns described for MF were paralleled by our results in cases with pleomorphic T-cell lymphomas and high-grade T-cell lymphomas (Tables 4,5) with regard to LFA-1, LFA-3 and ICAM-1. Moreover, infiltrating cells lacked VLA-2 expression, and, in five of 17 cases, VLA-3$^+$ cells were detected on cells infiltrating the dermis. The other members of the β1-integrin subfamily, however, showed differences when compared to MF.

VLA-1$^+$ cells were found in only 4 cases of pleomorphic T- cell lymphoma where they accounted for less than 50% of the dermal infiltrate. Expression of this marker was absent in high-grade T-cell lymphoma. Although staining for VLA-4 and VLA-5 yielded patterns comparable to MF on cells infiltrating the epidermis in epidermotropic CTCLs, expression of these markers was also increased in the dermal infiltrate of non-epidermotropic high-grade T-cell lymphomas. In the case of VLA-4, this is also true for pleomorphic T-cell lymphomas. Finally, VLA-6$^+$ cells were not detectable, with the exception of one case of epidermotropic high-grade T-cell lymphoma where some VLA-6$^+$ cells were found in the dermal infiltrate.

When compared to CTCLs, infiltrating cells in the inflammatory dermatoses investigated exhibited a similar phenotype with regard to markers other than β1-integrins: Here, too, the vast majority of cells stained positive for LFA-1, LFA-3 and ICAM-1 (Table 6). Again, as described for CTCLs, differential expression was documented for members of the β1-integrin family: VLA-1 was positive on intraepidermal lymphocytes in psoriasis and pityriasis lichenoides, whereas the subepidermal infiltrate lacked this marker. VLA-2 was never observed in our biopsy material. Cells in epidermal localization were characterized by a VLA-3 negative phenotype. Expression of VLA-4 and VLA-5 was detectable on the majority of infiltrating cells. Expression of VLA-1, VLA-3 and VLA-6 was absent or moderate on the subepidermal infiltrate in most inflammatory dermatoses investigated. In contrast, lichen planus exhibited a high percentage of cells staining positive for these molecules.

DISCUSSION

Differential expression of several adhesion molecules is likely to contribute to the phenomenon of epidermotropism

The discovery of cell surface receptors which play a central role in adhesive interactions of T cells with other cells, as well as with the extracellular matrix (Springer, 1990), has yielded new perspectives in understanding the tumor cell biology of cutaneous T cell lymphomas (CTCLs). These adhesion molecules are involved in the regulation of immune functions like

Table 4. Expression of adhesion molecules on infiltrating cells in cases with pleomorphic T cell lymphoma. (from: Sterry et al., 1991)

Case no		LFA-1	LFA-3	ICAM-1	VLA-1	VLA-2	VLA-3	VLA-4	VLA-5	VLA-6
Diffuse epidermotropism:										
1	E:	+++	++	++	—	—	—	+++	+++	—
	S:	+++	++++	++++	—	—	—	++	+++	—
2	E:	+++	+++	++	—	—	—	++	++	—
	S:	+++	++++	++++	—	—	—	++	++	—
Focal epidermotropism:										
3	E:	++	++	++	—	—	—	++	++	—
	S:	+++	+++	++++	—	—	—	+++	++	—
4	E:	+++	++++	+++	—	—	—	+	+++	—
	S:	+++	++++	++++	+	—	+	++	+++	—
5	E:	+++	+++	++	—	—	—	+	++	—
	S:	+++	++++	++++	++	—	++	+++	++	—
6	E:	+++	+++	+++	—	—	—	+	+	—
	S:	+++	+++	++++	++	—	+	++	++	—
7	E:	++	++	++	—	—	—	—	+	—
	S:	+++	+++	++++	—	—	—	++	++	—
No epidermotropism:										
8	E:	O	O	O	O	O	O	O	O	O
	S:	++++	++++	++++	+	—	—	++	+	—
9	E:	O	O	O	O	O	O	O	O	O
	S:	+++	++++	++++	—	—	—	+++	-	—
10	E:	O	O	O	O	O	O	O	O	O
	S:	+++	+++	++++	—	—	—	++	+	—

E	= epidermal	+	= 1- 25 % express marker
S	= subepidermal	++	= 25- 50 % express marker
O	= no infiltrate	+++	= 50- 75 % express marker
—	= no cells express marker	++++	= 75-100 % express marker

adherence to vascular endothelial cells (Picker et al., 1991; Kyan-Aung et al., 1991), migration of lymphocytes into extravascular tissue (Springer, 1990), T-cell interactions with antigens and accessory cells (Shimizu et al., 1990) as well as non-random recirculation (Mackay, 1991).

Table 5. Expression of adhesion molecules on infiltrating cells in cases with high-grade T cell lymphoma. (from: Sterry et al., 1991)

Case		LFA-1	LFA-3	ICAM-1	VLA-1	VLA-2	VLA-3	VLA-4	VLA-5	VLA-6
Diffuse epidermotropism:										
1	E:	++++	++++	++++	—	—	—	—	+	—
	S:	++++	++++	++++	—	—	—	++	++	—
2	E:	++++	++++	++++	—	—	—	+++	+	—
	S:	++++	++++	++++	—	—	++	+++	+++	+
Focal epidermotropism:										
3	E:	+++	+++	++	—	—	—	+	+	—
	S:	++++	++++	++++	—	—	—	+++	++	+
4	E:	++++	++++	++	—	—	—	+	+	—
	S:	++++	++++	+++	—	—	+	++	+++	—
No epidermotropism:										
5	E:	O	O	O	O	O	O	O	O	O
	S:	++++	++++	++++	—	—	—	+++	+++	—
6	E:	O	O	O	O	O	O	O	O	O
	S:	++++	++++	++++	—	—	—	++++	++++	—
7	E:	O	O	O	O	O	O	O	O	O
	S:	++++	+++	+++	—	—	—	+++	++	—

E	= epidermal	+	= 1- 25% express marker
S	= subepidermal	++	= 25- 50% express marker
O	= no infiltrate	+++	= 50- 75% express marker
—	= no cells express marker	++++	= 75-100% express marker

CTCLs are caused by the malignant transformation and subsequent autonomous proliferation of CD4[+] T-cells of the memory subset (Sanders et al., 1988; Sterry and Mielke, 1989). These cells are characterized by increased expression levels of LFA-1, LFA-3, VLA-4, VLA-5, and VLA-6 (Shimizu et al., 1990). Expression of these molecules is accompanied by increased binding capacity and, therefore, results in facilitated binding of this cell type to endothelium and emigration into the skin (Picker et al., 1991, Sterry et al., 1990). These findings are reflected by our observation that LFA-1, LFA-3, VLA-4, and VLA-5 were readily detectable on infiltrating cells in all cases of CTCLs and inflammatory dermatoses investigated.

If migration of T-cells into the epidermis is indeed influenced by adhesion molecules, one would expect either increased expression or increased avidity of these markers on cells infiltrating the epidermis. This should be paralleled by a down-regulated expression, or lower avidity, on dermally located cells, and in cases without epidermotropism. Reviewing our data, we could not identify any adhesion molecule included in this study that was expressed exclusively in epidermotropic CTCLs or on intraepidermal cells in inflammatory processes, and not in others. Thus, we conclude that the phenomenon of epidermotropism in CTCLs or epidermal infiltration under inflammatory conditions cannot be explained by the differential expression of a single adhesion molecule.

Besides changes in the number of molecules expressed, regulation of cellular adhesion might also be explainable by regulatory events influencing the avidity of a given type of molecule. Two examples for this mode of regulation are the interaction of LFA-1 with its counter-receptor ICAM-1, and the LFA-3/CD2 receptor-ligand pair (Springer, 1990). Thus, the unchanged expression pattern of a given adhesion molecule does not necessarily exclude this marker as possible cause for epidermotropism. Therefore, we cannot rule out a possible contribution of LFA-1 and LFA-3 to the phenomenon of epidermotropism, despite their expression on the cellular infiltrate in both epidermotropic and non-epidermotropic CTCLs.

Although we cannot exclude adhesion molecules with unchanged expression patterns in epidermotropic versus nonepidermotropic CTCLs from the list of candidates of those that may have epidermotropic effects, we can do so for those markers which are absent in the infiltrate of epidermotropic CTCLs. We observed infiltrating cells lacking expression of ICAM-1 and all $\beta 1$ integrins in cases of epidermotropic CTCL. Therefore, we feel that these molecules are dispensable as candidaes for epidermotropism. One should, however, keep in mind that there are differences between MF, pleomorphic T cell lymphoma and high-grade T cell lymphoma with regard to the percentage of epidermotropic cases staining negative for a given marker. This is particularly true for VLA-1, which was present in seven of nine cases with epidermotropic MF. In particular, one case of MF, characterized by the presence of a $V\beta 8^+$ epidermotropic T-cell clone (Boehncke 1991a), revealed a strong preference for VLA-1 expression on T-cells located in the epidermis. By contrast, only three of seven epidermotropic pleomorphic T-cell lymphomas and no high grade lymphoma were VLA-1^+. Interestingly, this preference for VLA-1 positive cells to migrate into the epidermis was also demonstrable in psoriasis and pityriasis lichenoides, whereas the other inflammatory dermatoses lacked epidermal VLA-1 positive infiltrating cells. Therefore, it is possible that epidermotropism in CTCLs and infiltration of cells into the epidermis in inflammatory skin diseases are differentially regulated in different entities.

Table 6. Expression of adhesion molecules of the integrin and immunoglobulin superfamilies on cells of the epidermal and dermal infiltrate in several cutaneous inflammations. (from Boehnke et al., 1992b).

	Psoriasis vulgaris	Pityriasis lichenoides	Parapsoriasis en plaques	Contact dermat.	Lichen planus
Epidermal infiltrate					
LFA-1	+ + + +	+ + + +	+ + + +	+ + + +	+ + + +
ICAM-1	+ + +	+ + +	+ +	+ + +	+ + + +
LFA-3	+ + + +	+ + + +	+ + + +	+ + + +	+ + + +
VLA-1	+ +	neg/+ +*	neg	neg	neg
VLA-2	neg	neg	neg	neg	neg
VLA-3	neg	neg	neg	neg	neg
VLA-4	+ + +	+ +	neg/+ +*	+ + +	+ + +
VLA-5	+ +	+ +	neg	+ + +	+ +
VLA-6	neg	neg	neg	neg	neg
Subepidermal infiltrate					
LFA-1	+ + + +	+ + + +	+ + + +	+ + + +	+ + + +
ICAM-1	+ + +	+ + +	+ + + +	+ + + +	+ + + +
LFA-3	+ + + +	+ + + +	+ + + +	+ + + +	+ + + +
VLA-1	neg/+*	neg	neg/+*	neg	+ +
VLA-2	neg	neg	neg	neg	neg
VLA-3	neg	neg/+ +*	neg/+*	neg/+ +*	+ +
VLA-4	+ + +	+ + +	+ + +	+ + +	+ + +
VLA-5	+ + +	+ + +	+ + +	+ + +	+ +
VLA-6	neg	neg/+ +*	neg/+ +*	neg/+ +*	+ + +

+	= 1-25% of cells expressing a particular marker
+ +	= 25-50% of cells expressing a particular marker
+ + +	= 50 - 75% of cells expressing a particular marker
+ + + +	= 75 - 100% of cells expressing a particular marker
*	= individual cases show expression of a particular marker

The postulated function of adhesion molecules in epidermotropism is a means of explaining dissemination of a disease initially affecting only the skin. Investigating low-grade lymphomas, Medeiros and coworkers (1989) found that 90% of LFA-1 positive cases turned LFA-1 negative during the course of disease. Thus, epidermally located malignant cells could be released from this compartment due to a loss of expression of adhesion molecules. Those authors were unable to correlate LFA-1 expression and clinical course, however. This release of malignant cells could be caused not by a loss of adhesion molecule expression on infiltrating cells, but rather by a failure of resident cells to further express their ligands, as observed by Nickoloff and colleages (1989): They described a patient with erythrodermic CTCL in whom epidermotropism was absent, and suggested that this could be most likely due to a failure of keratinocytes to express ICAM-1. Our data fit into this hypothesis, in as much as we observed up-regulation of ICAM-1 on keratinocytes in epidermotropic CTCLs at sites neighboring infiltrating T cells.

One explanation for a loss of keratinocytic ICAM-1 expression might be the emergence of T -cells that do not produce inducers of ICAM-1, such as interferon gamma (Nickoloff et al., 1989). Moreover, lack of certain cytokines would most likely not result in isolated ICAM-1 down-regulation, but instead might also affect expression of other adhesion molecules, e.g. LFA-1. In this case, both components of the receptor-ligand pair LFA-1/ICAM-1 would contribute to a dissemination of the disease due to a loss of epidermotropism by the malignant T cells.

We conclude that the tendency of infiltrating cells to migrate into the epidermis, and, in particular, the phenomenon of epidermotropism in CTCLs cannot be explained by differential expression of a single adhesion molecule. We favor the view that several adhesion molecules, namely LFA-1, LFA-3, and, in some instances, VLA-1, contribute to this phenomenon. Moreover, different entities of CTCL or inflammatory dermatoses might utilize different sets of adhesion molecules. Finally, since several adhesion molecules were not expressed on epidermotropic T cells in individual cases, they can be ruled out as major contributors to the phenomenon of epidermotropism. This is true for all β1-integrins except VLA-1.

REFERENCES

Boehncke W-H, S Krettek, MR Parwaresch and W Sterry, 1992a. Demonstration of clonal disease in early mycosis fungoides. **Am. J. Dermatopathol.**, 14:95-99.

Boehncke W-H, I Kellner, U Konter and W Sterry, 1992b. Differential expression of adhesion molecules on infiltrating cells in inflammatory dermatoses. **J. Am. Acad. Dermatol.**, 26:907-913.

Berger CL, D Warburton, J Raafat, P Logerfo and RL Edelson, 1979. Cutaneous T cell lymphoma: Neoplasm of T cells with helper activity. **Blood**, 53:642.

Dustin ML, R Rothlein, AR Bahn and CA Dinarello, 1986. Induction by IL-1 and interferon beta: Tissue distribution, biochemistry and function of a natural adherence molecule (ICAM--1). **J. Immunol.**, 137:245.

Hemler ME, C Huang and L Schwarz, 1987. The VLA protein family. Characterization of five distinct cell surface heterodimers, each with a common 130,000 molecular weight β subunit. **J. Biol. Chem.**, 262:3300.

Hemler ME, 1990. VLA proteins in the integrin family: structures, functions, and their role on leukocytes. **Ann. Rev. Immunol.**, 8:365.

Hemler ME, JG Jacobson and JL Strominger, 1985. Biochemical characterization of VLA-1 and VLA-2: Cell surface heterodimers on activated T cells. **J. Biol. Chem.**, 260:15246.

Hemler ME, CF Ware and JL Strominger, 1983. Characterization of a novel differentiation antigen complex recognized by a monoclonal antibody (A-lA5): Unique activation-specific molecular forms on stimulated T cells. **J. Immunol.**, 131:334.

Hemler ME, C Huang, Y Takada, L Schwarz, JL Strominger and ML Clabby, 1987. Characterization of the cell surface heterodimer VLA-4 and related peptides. **J. Biol. Chem.**, 262:11478.

Hemler ME, C Crouse, Y Takada and A Sonnenberg, 1988. Multiple very late antigen (VLA) heterodimers on platelets. Evidence for distinct VLA-2, VLA-5 (fibronectin receptor) and VLA-6 structures. **J. Biol. Chem.**, 263:7660.

Hynes R.O., 1987. Integrins: a family of cell surface receptors. **Cell**, 48:549.

Kaufmann R, D Frosch, C Westphal, L Weber and CE Klein, 1989. Integrin VLA-3: Ultrastructural localization at cell-cell contact sites of human cell cultures. **J. Cell Biol.**, 109:1807.

Kellner I, U Konter and W Sterry, 1990. Up-regulation of adhesion molecules in inflammatory skin diseases. **Arch. Dermatol. Res.**, 281:550.

Kishimoto TK, K O'Connor, A Lee, TM Roberts and TA Springer, 1987. Cloning of the β subunit of the leucocyte adhesion proteins: Homology to an extracellular matrix receptor defines a novel supergene family. **Cell**, 48:681.

Kyan-Aung U, DO Haskard, RN Poston, NH Thornhill and Lee, 1991. Endothelial leukocyte adhesion molecule-1 and intercellular adhesion molecule-1 mediate the adhesion of eosinophils to endothelial cells in vitro and are expressed by endothelium in allergic cutaneous inflammation in vivo. **J. Immunol.**, 146:521.

MacKay C.R., 1991. Skin-seeking memory T cells. **Nature**, 349:737.

Marlin SD and TA Springer, 1987. Purified intercellular adhesion molecule-1 (ICAM-1) is a ligand for lymphocyte function associated antigen-1 (LFA-1). **Cell**, 51:813.

Nedeiros LJ, LN Weiss, LJ Picker, C Clayberger, SJ Horning, AN Krensky and RA Warnke, 1989. Expression of LFA-1 in Non- Hodgkin's Lymphoma. **Cancer**, 63:255.

Nickoloff BJ, CEN Griffith and JNWN Barker, 1990. The role of adhesion molecules, chemotactic factors, and cytokines in inflammatory and neoplastic skin disease, 1990 update. **J. Invest. Dermatol.**, 94(S):151.

Nickoloff BJ, 1988. The role of IFN gamma in cutaneous trafficking of lymphocytes with emphasis on molecular and cellular events. **Arch. Dermatol.**, 124:1835.

Nickoloff BJ, CEN Griffith, O Baadsgaard et al., 1989. Markedly diminished epidermal keratinocyte expression of ICAM-1 in Sézary syndrome. **JAMA**, 261:2217.

Picker LJ, TK Kishimoto, CW Smith, RA Warnock and EC Butcher, 1991. ELAM-1 is an adhesion molecule for skin homing T cells. **Nature**, 349:796.

Rothlein R, ML Dustin, SD Marlin and TA Springer, 1986. A human intercellular adhesion molecule (ICAM-1) distinct from LFA-1. **J. Immunol.**, 137:1270.

Ruoslahti E and ND Pierschbacher, 1987. New perspectives in cell adhesion: RGD and integrins. **Science**, 238:491.

Sanchez-Nadrid F, AN Krenzky, CF Ware, E Robbins, JL Strominger, SJ Burakoff and TA Springer, 1982. Three distinct antigens associated with human T-lymphocyte-mediated killing: LFA-1, LFA-2, LFA-3. **Proc. Natl. Acad. Sci. USA**, 79:7489 .

Sanders NE, MW Nakgoba and S Shaw, 1988. Human naive and memory T cells: Reinterpretation of helper-inducer and suppressor inducer subsets. **Immunol. Today**, 9:195.

Shimizu Y, GA van Seventer, KJ Horgan and S Shaw, 1990. Roles of adhesion molecules in T-cell recognition: Fundamental similarities between four integrins on resting human T cells (LFA-1, VLA-4, VLA-5, VLA-6) in expression, binding, and co-stimulation. **Immunol. Rev.**, 114:1.

Slater DN, 1991. Cutaneous lymphoproliferative disorders: An assessment of recent investigative techniques. **Br. J. Dermatol.**, 124:309.

Sonnenberg A, PW Modderman and F Hogervorst, 1989. Laminin receptor on platelets is the integrin VLA-6. **Nature**, 336:487.

Springer TA, 1990. Adhesion receptors of the immune system. **Nature**, 346:425.

Springer TA, 1990. The sensation and regulation of interactions with the extracellular environment: The cell biology of lymphocyte adhesion receptors. **Annu. Rev. Cell Biol.**, 6:359.

Springer TA, NL Dustin, TK Klshimoto and SDA Marlin, 1987. The lymphocyte function-associated LFA-1, CD2 and LFA-3 molecules: Cell adhesion receptors of the immune system. **Ann. Rev. Immunol.**, 5:223.

Staunton DE, ML Dustin and TA Springer, 1989. Functional cloning of ICAM-2, a cell adhesion ligand for LFA-1 homologous to ICAM-l. **Nature**, 339:61.

Sterry W, 1985. Mycosis fungoides. In: Berry CL, ed., **Current topics in Pathology**. Berlin, Springer, 74:167.

Sterry W, S Bruhn, N Kunne, B Lichtenberg, K Weber-Matthiesen, J Brasch and V Nielke, 1990. Dominance of memory over naive T cells in contact dermatitis is due to differential tissue immigration. **Br. J. Dermatol.**, 123:59.

Sterry W and V Mielke, 1989. CD4$^+$ cutaneous T cell lymphomas show the phenotype of helper/inducer T cells (CD45R$^-$, CDw29$^+$). **J. Invest. Dermatol.**, 93:413.

Wallner BP, AZ Frey, R Tizard, R Nattaliano, C Hession, ME Sanders, ML Dustin and TA Springer, 1987. Primary structure of lymphocyte function-associated antigen-3 (LFA-3). The ligand of the lymphocyte CD2 glycoprotein. **J. Exp. Med.**, 166:923.

Werb Z, PM Tremble, O Behrendtsen, E Crowley and CH Damsky, 1989. Signal transduction through the fibronectin receptor induces collagenase and stromelysin gene expression. **J. Cell Biol.**, 109:877.

INTEGRINS AND HOMING RECEPTORS IN CUTANEOUS LYMPHOMAS

Emilio Berti*
Paola Randi*
Elena Roscetti*
Domenico Delia†

*   First Department of Dermatology
      University of Milan and IRCCS, Ospedale Maggiore
      Milan, Italy

†   Istituto Nazionale dei Tumori
      Milan, Italy

      Correspondence to: Prof. Dr. E. Berti, Department of Dermatology I
      University of Milan, Via Pace 9
      I-20122 Milan, Italy

ABSTRACT

The aim of this study was to evaluate the expression on neoplastic cell membranes of some receptors involved in intercellular and cell-matrix adhesion. We used monoclonal antibodies (mAbs) directed against VLA-3, VLA-4, LFA-1, ICAM-1, Leu-8 and CD44 antigens, with an alkaline phosphatase-anti-alkaline phosphatase (APAAP) immunohistochemical method, in 40 cases of cutaneous B-cell lymphomas (CBCL) and 60 cases of cutaneous T-cell lymphomas (CTCL), which had been previously characterized employing a large panel of mAbs. Our results showed, in CBCL, consistent expression of CD44, CD11a, ICAM-1 and VLA-4 molecules. LEU-8 and VLA-3 receptors were detected, respectively, in 50% and in 25% of the cases examined. No significant difference was noted between the pattern of adhesion molecules of our CBCL and of 70 cases of nodal follicular lymphomas. In CTCL, CD44 reactivity was demonstrated in all cases; VLA-4, CD11a and ICAM-1 were negative in a case of γδ T-cell

Basic Mechanisms of Physiologic and Aberrant Lymphoproliferation in the Skin
Edited by W.C. Lambert *et al.*, Plenum Press, New York, 1994

157

lymphoma and in a case of highly malignant CD8[+] lymphoma. Furthermore, anti-VLA-4 mAb did not label a case with an NK-like phenotype, nor a case of Ki-1[+] lymphoma. Interestingly anti-VLA-3 mAb, normally weakly expressed on T-cell membranes, was strongly positive on blastic cells with an activated phenotype, particularly in Ki-1[+] lymphomas, including lymphomatoid papulosis. Reed-Sternberg cells in 5 cases of Hodgkin disease examined were VLA-2 negative. VLA-3 receptor seems to be involved not only in cell-matrix and cell-cell adhesion, but also in lymphocyte activation.

INTRODUCTION

Adhesion molecules play a central role in regulating cell-cell and cell-matrix interactions. Some of these molecules (e.g., LFA1-ICAM1) are mainly involved in the "recognition-facilitation" process of antigen specific dependent events, whereas other adhesion molecules (e.g., CD44 (Hermes Antigen)) determine the antigen-independent preferential migration of "homing" leukocytes to a site (Butcher, 1990; Haynes et al., 1989; Jalkanen et al., 1991; Makgoba et al., 1989; Picker et al., 1988; Rossien et al., 1989; Sun et al., 1991). The integrins consist of cell surface receptors binding to the extracellular matrix through the recognition of argenine-glycine-asparamine (RGD) as well as receptors involved in various aspects of cell-cell adhesion (Albelda and Buck, 1990; Elices et al., 1991; Hynes, 1987; Takada et al., 1988; Wayuner et al., 1988).

Integrin molecules consist of an alpha chain non-covalently associated with a beta subunit. At least 7 beta subunits and 15 α subunits have been identified. Integrins have been divided into 7 subfamilies, each member of which is composed of a unique alpha subunit associated with a beta subunit shared by every member of the subfamily. Integrin beta-1 is the common subunit of the VLA family; 6 different VLA molecules have been identified, and functional analysis has shown that they function as receptors for extracellular matrix, except for VLA-4, the human analogue to the murine LPAM-1 molecule involved in the "homing" of lymphocytes to Peyer's Patches (Holzmann et al., 1989).

The possibility that alpha chains (i.e., VLA-4) could be associated with more than one beta subunit has recently been proposed. In this study we have evaluated 60 cases of primary cutaneous T-cell lymphomas (CTCLs) and 40 cases of primary cutaneous B-cell lymphomas (CBCLs) for their reactivity with several monoclonal antibodies (mAbs) specific for some integrin molecules of the beta-1 (VLA-1, VLA-2, VLA-3, VLA-4, VLA-6) and beta-2 (LFA-1) subfamilies, for ICAM-1 molecules (the ligand for LFA-1), for the CD44-Hermes and for Leu8-Mel-14 (Camerini et al., 1989; Pals et al., 1991) "homing" receptors, by using an immunohisto-chemical alkaline phosphatase anti-alkaline phosphatase (APAAP) method on cryostat serial sections of pathological skin.

Seventy cases of extracutaneous B-cell lymphomas were also evaluated to compare the patterns of adhesion molecules in CBCLs and in extracutaneous B-cell lymphomas.

MATERIALS

Serial cryostat sections of 60 specimens of cutaneous T-cell lymphomas and of 40 specimens of cutaneous B-cell lymphomas, obtained from the First Department of Dermatology of the University of Milan, were dried for 12-24 hours at room temperature, fixed 10 minutes in acetone, dried for 30-60 minutes and kept at -20°C until used. CTCLs analyzed included 7 cases of "early" mycosis fungoides (MF), 26 cases of classical MF, 5 cases of erythrodermic MF, 5 cases of tumoral stage MF, 2 cases of pagetoid reticulosis, 8 cases of Ki-1[+] lymphoma, 4 cases of CD8[+] suppressor/cytotoxic T-cell lymphoma and 2 cases of other CTCLs. Finally, we included 2 elderly patients that simultaneously developed a very aggressive cutaneous and systemic peripheral T-cell lymphoma and one case of TCLL.

Cutaneous B-cell lymphomas were classified according to Kiel's classification: CB/CCD (19 cases), CB/CC F (2 cases), CB-CC F/D (8 cases), CB (3 cases), CC (1 case), CB multi-lobulated (M) (1 case), large cell (LC) (2 cases), lymphoplasmocytoid lymphoma (2 cases) and plasmocytic lymphoma (2 cases). The phenotype of all these cases was extensively studied by using a large panel of mAbs on serial cryostat sections.

The extracutaneous B-cell lymphomas analyzed included nine CLL, 15 CB/CC F, two CB/CC F/D, eight CB/CC D, 11 CB multilobulated, 11 CB, and five IMB. 45 cases were nodal, three involved the spleen, three the lung, three the stomach, two the colon, one the ovary and two the skin (secondarily).

METHODS

5 μ dried cryostat sections were hydrated in TBS for 15 minutes and then incubated for 15 minutes with normal rabbit serum, 10%, plus normal human AB serum, 10%, in TBS-BSA 1% - NaAz 0,1%, 0,05M, pH76 (TBS-BSA) and for 60 minutes with different mAbs, diluted 1:400 in TBS-BSA from ascites. After rinsing in TBS, the slides were incubated with rabbit anti mouse Igs (DAKOPATT GLOSTRUP-DENMARK, human serum adsorbed) for 1 hour, washed in TBS, and finally incubated for one hour with APAAP COMPLEX (SERA-LAB, ENGLAND 1:50 diluted). The last two steps were repeated using a shorter time (15-30 minutes), to amplify the reaction. Reactions were detected using New Fucsin and naphtol AS-Bi phosphate sodium salt in the presence of one mM levamisole for 20 minutes at room temperature.

Reagents. Specific mAbs used were: anti CD22 (T015), anti CD21 (1F8,DAKO), anti DRC-1 (DAKO), anti IgD (DAKO), anti Leu-8 (Becton Dickinson (BD)), anti CD1c (L161*), anti CD54 (RR-1), anti CD69 (FN61*), anti CD70 (HNC142*), anti CD44 (F-1044-2*), anti VLA-3 (J143*), anti VLA-4 (HP2/1*), anti VLA-1 (T-CELL SCIENCE), anti VLA-2 (CLB THROMB-4*), anti VLA-6 (GoH3*), anti CD11a (MHM2μ), anti CD3 (Leu4-BD), Ki-67 proliferating cells (DAKO), anti CD30 (Ber-h2*), anti CD25 (IL-2 R-BD.), anti CD4 (Leu-3a-BD), anti CD8 (Leu2a-BD), anti CD56 (Leu19-BD), anti CD16 (Leu11-BD), anti CD2 (Leu7), anti CD5 (Leu1), anti CD7 (G3-7*), anti CD29 (4B4*), anti CD45RA (F8.11.13*), anti CD45RO (A-6*), anti CD58, CD68(XP1) and anti CD32 (KB-61) Ag.

All asterisked(*) MABs were obtained from the 6th International Workshop on Leukocyte Differentiation Antigens, Vienna, 1989.

RESULTS
Cutaneous T-Cell Lymphomas

A study of 10 cases of CTCL demonstrated that mAbs anti VLA-1, anti VLA-2 and VLA-6 did not significantly react with the cell infiltrate, but only stained vessels and/or basal kera-tinocytes.

EARLY MYCOSIS FUNGOIDES (7 CASES)

Phenotypes (Table 1): the superficial dermis was occupied by a polymorphous infiltrate, formed by neoplastic cells (CD3$^+$, CD4$^+$), but also by a very high number of CD1a$^+$ dendritic cells located in perivascular areas and of monocyte-macrophagic elements (CD14$^+$) usually scattered on the superficial dermis but particularly frequent in the areas surrounding the periphery of the lymphoid infiltrate.

Furthermore, a variable number of CD8$^+$ cells (10 to 30% of the lymphoid infiltrate) were observed, and the lymphoid infiltrate often expressed variable "naive" (CD45RA$^+$), instead of the classical "memory" T-cell phenotype (CD45RO$^+$) of the MF cells. In some cases a percentage variable between one and five percent of the cells in the superficial dermis expressed TCR-delta-1$^+$ phenotype typical of the gamma-delta T-lymphocytes.

Only scattered lymphocytes or a few Pautrier micro-abscesses usually composed of mixed lympho-monocytic cells were seen in the epithelium. The intraepithelial large T-lymphocytes were more often CD3$^+$, CD45RA$^+$; some TCR-delta-1$^+$ cells were also detected. The lympho-monocytic cells forming the infiltrate strongly expressed class II (HLA-DR) molecules.

Adhesion molecules (Table 2): VLA-3 molecules were weakly expressed in all cases, except one, on the membrane of most lymphocytes in the superficial dermis. The basal and suprabasal keratinocytes, as well as vessels of the superficial dermis, were stained, whereas the infiltrating scattered lymphocytes or the lympho-monocytic cells forming the intraepithelial theques and Langerhans' cells were negative. VLA-4 molecules were clearly expressed in all cases by cells forming the infiltrate in the superficial dermis and in the epidermis. Some Langerhans' cells in the epidermis were labelled.

CD11a-LFA-1 strong reactivity was detected in all the lympho-monocytic cells forming the infiltrate. The CD54-ICAM-1 molecule (the ligand for LFA-1) was strongly expressed by all the infiltrating cells, many vessels of the superficial dermis and groups of keratinocytes.

Table 1. Phenotypes of cases studied.

mAb	Early MF (7 cases)		Classical MF (26 cases)		Erythrod. MF (5 cases)		Tumoral stage MF (5 cases)	Pagetoid reticulosis (2 cases)	
	der.	epider.	der.	epider.	der.	epider.	der.	case 1	case 2
CD3	++	++	++	++	++	++	++	++	+
CD4	++	++	++	++	++	++	++	++	+
CD8	+	+	+	+	+	+	−	−	−
CD1A	+	+	+	+	+	+	+	+	+
CD45RO	++	+	++	++	++	++	++	−	−
CD45RA	+	+	+/−	+	+	+	1/5	+	
HLA-DR	++	++	++	++	++	++	++	−	−
CD7	+	+/−	+	−	+	−	−	−	−
CD5	++	++	++	++	++	++	3/5	−	+/−
CD25	+	+	+	+	+	+	+	−	−
CD30	−	−	+/−	+/−	+	+	+	−	−
BETA-F-1	++	++	++	++	++	++	+	+	−
TCR1	−	−	−	−	−	−	−	−	+
DELTA-1	−	−	−	−					
BERACT-8	−	−	−	−	−	−	1/5	−	−

+, 30-70% of cells positive; ++, 70-100% of cells positive; −/+,
1-10% of cells positive; +/−, 10-30% of cells positive; −, negative or <10% of cells positive.

The CD44-Hermes antigen was expressed by all lympho-monocytic cells, epithelial cells, fibroblasts and vessels.

Leu-8-LECAM-1 molecules were variably expressed (30-50% with a weak positivity) by the infiltrating lymphocytes; only in areas of dense infiltrate surrounding some vessels of the superficial dermis was a strong positivity usually observed.

CLASSICAL MYCOSIS FUNGOIDES (26 CASES)

Phenotypes (Table 1): The number of CD3[+], CD4[+] T-lymphocytes was increased both in the superficial dermis and in the epidermis. Most infiltrating cells in the superficial dermis were characterized by the expression of the CD45RO antigen ("primed" T-cells); moreover the CD7 and the CD5 pan T-cell antigens were undetected, respectively, in 69% and in 12% of cases.

The infiltrate, and particularly the intraepithelial lymphocytes, expressed some activation anti-gens such as the CD25 or the CD30 (positive in a percentage variable from 1% to 40% of the infiltrating cells). Unexpectedly, the large roundish lymphoid CD3$^+$ "Mycosis Fungoides" cells in the epithelial layers, particularly in the basal layer, expressed the CD45RA "naive" T-cell phenotype instead of the CD45RO antigen.

Table 2. Adhesion molecules of cases studied.

mAb	Early Mycosis Fungoides (7 cases)	Classical Mycosis Fungoides (26 cases)	Erythroder-mic Mycosis Fungoides (5 cases)	Tumoral Stage Mycosis Fungoides (5 cases)
VLA-3	6/7 W	11/26 W	1/5 W	2/5 W
			1/5 S	1/5 S
VLA-4	7/7 M	26/26 M	5/5 M	5/5 M
CD11a-LFA-1	7/7 S	26/26 S	5/5 S	5/5 S
CD54-ICAM-1	7/7 S	26/26 M-S	5/5 S	5/5 S
CD44	7/7 S	26/26 S	5/5 S	5/5 S
Leu-8	7/7 W	12/26 W	4/5 W	1/5 W
				2/5 M

S = strong intensity   M = medium intensity   W = weak intensity

Adhesion molecules (Table 2): VLA-3 expression was not significantly different in comparison with the "early stage". Lymphoid cells forming the infiltrate in the superficial dermis weakly expressed VLA-3 molecules in 11 of 26 cases studied. Intraepithelial lymphocytes were usually negative. VLA-4 molecules were expressed on most infiltrating cells in all cases. Only in some cases was an irregular staining intensity observed, and usually small cells were strongly labelled.

Anti CD11a-LFA-1 reactivity was homogeneous and strong. All the lymphomonocytic cells, both in the superficial dermis and in the epidermis, were stained in all of the cases ana-lyzed.

CD54-ICAM-1: A labelling pattern similar to the one observed with anti LFA mAb was noted. The intensity of the reaction was variable; the vessels of the superficial dermis and groups of keratinocytes were also stained. CD44 Hermes antigen was strongly expressed on all cells of the infiltrate, epithelial cells, fibroblasts and vessels in all cases.

Leu-8 molecules, also identifying the suppressor-inducer subset of the CD4 T-helper lymphocytes, were irregularly expressed with a stronger staining of the dense perivascular infiltrate. The number of Leu-8 positive cells was clearly diminished in 12 of the 26 cases studied (46%).

ERYTHRODERMIC MYCOSIS FUNGOIDES (5 CASES)

Phenotypes (Table 1): No difference was observed in the phenotype in comparison with "classical" mycosis fungoides, except for one case, characterized by a lymphoid infiltrate occupying the whole dermis and showing the $CD3^+$, $CD4^+$, $CD25^+$, $CD30^+$ (with BerH-2 mAb, but negative with Ki-1 mAb), $CD16^+$, $CD45RO^+$ phenotype. The CD56-NK marker was also expressed in one case on 30% of the proliferating cells. All of the cases were beta Fl (TCR-beta chain) positive.

Adhesion molecules (Table 2): VLA-3 molecules were absent in neoplastic cells in two cases, weakly expressed in one case and strongly expressed in the case with the $CD25^+$, $CD30^+$ phenotype cited above. In the latter case an irregular intensity of positivity was seen.

Anti VLA-4 mAb stained the infiltrating cells in all cases examined. CD11a-LFA-1 was the same as for VLA-4.

CD54-ICAM1: was the same as for VLA4. Vessels and groups of keratinocytes were labelled in addition.

CD44-Hermes antigen: was the same as for VLA-4. Moreover, vessels, keratinocytes, and fibroblasts were stained.

Leu-8 antigen was also expressed in four of the five cases. In the last case, $CD3^+$, $CD4^+$, $CD25^+$, $CD30^+$ and VLA-3^+, Leu-8 molecules were not expressed.

TUMORAL STAGE MYCOSIS FUNGOIDES (5 CASES)

Phenotypes (Table 1): The infiltrate in two cases was strongly epidermotropic, whereas in the other three cases it lost the epidermotropism characteristic of CTCL. The infiltrate was dense, occupying the whole dermis, with a variable number of blasts. The phenotype of the cells was, in all cases, $CD2^+$, $CD3^+$, $CD4^+$, $CD7^-$; CD5 was negative in two of five cases. Coexpression of CD45RA and CD45RO markers was observed in one case. In the other cases we observed the CD45RO phenotype. The beta-Fl (TCR-beta) marker was expressed in four of five cases, whereas TCR-delta 1 was always negative. In one case a strong reaction with anti CD70 mAb was noted. Anti CD25 and anti CD30 mAbs reacted with 10-20% of the proliferating cells in two of five cases. The anti CD16 and CD56 NK-markers were negative. One of these cases showed reactivity with BER-ACT-8 analogous to HML-1 mAb, recognizing the intraepithelial $CD8^+$ activated T-lymphocytes of the gut.

Adhesion molecules (Table 3): No VLA-3 reactivity was detected in neoplastic cells in two of the five cases, whereas a weak positivity was observed in two other cases. In the last case, however, large blastic cells reactive with anti CD25 and CD30 activation antigens (10% of the infiltrate) were strongly stained with anti VLA-3 mAb.

Anti VLA-4 mAb labelled most of the infiltrating cells in all of the cases examined.

Anti CD11a-LFA-1 mAb strongly labelled all the infiltrating cells in all of the cases examined.

CD54 (ICAM-1): The same results as for anti LFA-1 were obtained.

CD44-Hermes antigen: The same results as for LFA-1 were obtained.

Leu 8-Mel-14 was completely absent in one case (CD70[+]), reduced in the case BER-ACT-8[+], weakly expressed in one case and normally expressed in the last two cases.

PAGETOID RETICULOSIS (2 CASES)

One case was a localized variant (Woringer-Kolopp), whereas the second was a disseminated type (Berti et al., 1991).

Phenotypes (Table 1): The phenotype of the first case was CD3[+]/ CD4[+]/ CD5[-]/ CD7[-]/ beta-F1[+]/ CD45RA[+]. The phenotype of the second was CD3[+]/ CD4[-]/ CD8[-]/ CD5[+] (weak)/ CD7[+]/ CD45RA[+]/ beta-F1[-]/ TCR-delta-1[+]. Our second case was a very rare cutaneous T-cell lymphoma originating from gamma-delta lymphocytes.

Adhesion molecules (Table 3): Anti VLA-3 was negative in both cases.

Anti-VLA-4 was positive (weak reactivity) on the neoplastic intraepithelial cells in the first case; no reactivity was detected in the second case. Anti-CD11a-LFA-1 was strongly positive in the proliferating cells in the first case; no reactivity was observed in the second. Anti-CD54 (ICAM-1) mAb was strongly positive on the proliferating cells, keratinocytes and vessels in the first case. Only very weak staining, probably of the lymphoid intraepithelial cells, was observed in the second case.

CD44-Hermes antigen: Positive reactivity was clearly evident in both cases. Leu-8 molecules were not expressed in either case.

SUPPRESSOR-CYTOTOXIC CD8$^+$ T-CELL LYMPHOMAS (4 cases)

Phenotypes (Table 4): Three cases presented a very aggressive clinical course and were characterized by deep nodules, plaques and tumors. One case showed localized plaques with a very slow progression. All of the cases were CD3$^+$/ CD8$^+$; one case was CD25$^+$. CD5$^+$ and CD7$^+$ pan T-cell markers were lost in three of the four cases. The CD45RA antigen, identifying the suppressor subset of CD8$^+$ lymphocytes, was positive in only one case. In one case neither CD45, CD45RA nor CD45RO antigens were detected. Beta-F1 (TCR-beta), was demonstrated in all cases. In one case both CD4 and CD8 were expressed and CD16 NK marker and BER-ACT-8 (CD8 activation antigen) were detected.

Table 3. Adhesion molecules of cases studied.

mAb	Pagetoid reticulosis	Suppressor/ cytoxic CD8$^+$T-Cell lymphoma	Ki-1$^+$ lymphoma	Unclassifi- able lymphoma	Chronic T-cell leukemia (TCLL)
	(2 cases)	(4 cases)	(8 cases)	(4 cases)	(1 case)
VLA-3	0/2	2/4 W 2/4 S	6/8 M-S	0/4	0/1
VLA-4	1/2 M	3/4 M	7/8 M	2/4	1/l M
CD11a (LFA-1)	1/2 S	3/4 S	8/8 S	4/4 S	1/1 S
CD54 (ICAM-1)	1/2 S	3/4 S	7/8 S	3/4 S	1/1 S 1/4 W
CD44	2/2 S	4/4 S	8/8 S	4/4 S	1/1 S
Leu-8	0/2	2/4 M 1/4 W	2/8 M	2/4 S	0/1

S strong intensity   M medium intensity   W weak intensity

Adhesion molecules (Table 3): VLA-3 molecules were weakly expressed on neoplastic cellular membranes in two of the four cases. In the remaining two cases (one aggressive and one localized) all the infiltrating cells strongly expressed the VLA-3 molecules. They were strongly positive with anti HLA-DR; one was the case expressing the CD16 and BER-ACT-8 activation markers.

Anti VLA-4 mAb stained 3 of the 4 cases. The unstained case expressed the CD8$^+$/ CD45RA$^+$ phenotype of the suppressor subset.

Table 4. Phenotypes of suppressor/cytotoxic CD8⁺ T-cell lymphoma cases studied.

Case	1	2	3	4
mAb				
CD3	+ +	+ +	+ +	+ +
CD8	+ +	+	+	+
CD4	+	—	—	—
CD25	—	—	—	—
CD7	—	+	—	—
CD5	+ +	—	—	—
CD45RA	—	—	—	+
CD45RO	+	+	—	—
CD45	+ +	+ +	—	+ +
BETA-F-1	+	+	+	+
CD16-56	+	—	—	—
BER-ACT-8	+	—	—	—
CD2	+	+	+	ND
CD30	—	—	—	—
HLA-DR	+ +	+	+ +	+

—, negative;   + +, 70-100% of cells positive;
+, 30-70% of cells positive; ND = not done.

CD11a-LFA-1 molecules showed the same results as for VLA-4. CD54-ICAM-1 showed the same staining pattern as for VLA-4. Vessels and groups of keratinocytes were also labelled.

CD44-Hermes antigen: A strong labelling of all the cases was observed. Epithelial cells, vessels and fibroblasts were also reactive.

Leu-8: This was negative in one case (aggressive form VLA-3⁺), reduced (20-30% of all cells) in another case (localized form VLA-3⁺) and normally expressed in the remaining two cases.

Ki-l⁺ LYMPHOMA (8 cases)

This group was quite heterogeneous.

Phenotypes (Table 5): Case 1 clinically resembled MF; histologically it showed a pleomorphic infiltrate composed of medium and large lymphocytes which were CD30⁺/ EMA⁺/ CD15⁺. Cases 2 and 3 showed a large cell anaplastic lymphoma (ALC) concurrent with lymphomatoid papulosis. Case 4 was a typical large cell anaplastic Ki-1[+] lymphoma. Case 5 was an atypical regressing lymphoma characterized by a very deep pleomorphic, medium-large lymphoid infiltrate. Cases 7 and 8 showed papulo-nodular (lymphomatoid papulosis-like) lesions associated with stage Ib MF.

The phenotype was characterized by a strong expression of the CD30(Ber-h2), CD25(IL-2 receptor) (except case 6, a typical pleomorphic lymphoma) and HLA-DR markers in about 70% of the infiltrating cells. The large cells in two cases were CD3[-].

Table 5. Phenotypes of Ki-1[+] lymphomas cases studied.

CASE	1	2	3	4	5	6	7	8
mAb								
CD30	++	++	++	++	+	++	+	+
CD15	++	+/—	+/—	+/—	+	+	+	+
EMA	++	+	+	+	+	+	+	+
CD25	++	++	++	++	++	—	++	+
CD3	++	—	+	++	+	—	++	++
CD4	+	+	+	—	+	+	++	++
CD5	+	—	—	—	—	—	++	+
CD7	—	—	—	—	—	—	+	—
CD45RO	+	+	+	+	+	+	++	+
CD45RA	—	—	—	—	—	—	—	—
CD16	+	+	—	—	—	—	—	—
CD56	+	+	—	—	—	—	—	—
CD57	—	+	—	—	—	—	—	—
BETA-Fl	+	+	+	—	—	+	+	+
HLA-DR	++	+++	++	++	++	++	++	++

—, negative; +/—, 19-30% of cells positive; +, 30-70% of cells positive; ++, 70-100% of cells positive.

The CD4 helper T-cell antigen was lost in the typical large cell anaplastic lymphoma and in the intraepithelial cells in the pleomorphic MF. CD7 pan-T cell antigen was lost in all of the cases, except one; CD5 was expressed only in four of seven cases. All cases were CD45RO[+]; beta-F1 (beta chain T-cell marker) was detected in six of eight cases. In two cases a minor percentage of cells (20-30%) expressed the NK markers CD16, CD56 and CD57.

Adhesion molecules (Table 3): VLA-3 molecules, in six of the eight cases analyzed, were strongly expressed on the cell membrane of most infiltrating cells, particularly in the blastic large or giant Reed-Sternberg-like or multinucleated cells. The atypical regressing lympho-matoid-papulosis-like pleomorphic lymphoma and one case of ALC were negative.

The VLA-4 molecule was irregularly expressed on a minor percentage of infiltrating cells in one case and normally expressed in the other seven cases. Anti CD11a-LFA-1 mAb strongly stained the infiltrating cells in all the cases examined.

The CD54 (ICAM-1) molecule was detected in seven of the eight cases studied. The negative one was a case of large cell anaplastic lymphoma. The keratinocytes in close contact with the neoplastic infiltrate were labeled depending on the epidermotropism of the infiltrate. Vessels of the superficial dermis were also stained.

CD44-Hermes antigen: As for CD11a-LFA-1, a strong reactivity of all infiltrating cells was observed.

Leu-8 molecules in six of the eight cases were not expressed. The only positive ones were the two cases which were VLA3⁻.

OTHER CTCLs (2 cases)

These two cases showed isolated multiple nodules on the trunk characterized by a dense infiltrate over the entire dermis, composed in the former of small round lymphocytes and in the latter of medium-large clear cells with irregular and elongated nuclei.

Phenotypes: The phenotype of the first case was characteristic of T helper proliferation (CD3⁺/ CD4⁺/ CD5⁺), but expressed the CD45RA, marker of the "naive" T-cells. The phenotype of the second case was highly defective (CD2⁺/ CD3⁻/ CD4⁺/⁻/ CD5⁻/ beta-F1⁻/ TCR-delta-1⁻/ CD7⁺/ CD45RA⁺ CD56⁺/ CD16⁻).

Adhesion molecules (Table 3): In both cases anti-VLA-3 mAb reactivity was absent.

VLA-4 molecules were normally expressed in the first case, but were completely negative in the second. Anti CD11a-LFA-1 mAb labelled all of the neoplastic cells in both cases.

CD54 (ICAM-1) molecules were strongly expressed in the first case, but weakly expressed in the second.

Anti CD44(Hermes antigen) mAb strongly stained the lymphoid cells in both cases.

Leu-8 molecules were strongly expressed in both the first (suppressor-inducer) and the second case.

SIMULTANEOUS CUTANEOUS AND SYSTEMIC PERIPHERAL T-CELL LYMPHOMAS (2 CASES) AND CHRONIC T-CELL LEUKEMIA (1 CASE)

Cases 1 and 2 presented multiple deep skin nodules. The infiltrate involved the whole dermis and was formed by pleomorphic medium and large cells.

Phenotypes: Case 1 was: CD4$^+$/ CD45RA$^+$/ CD3$^-$/ CD2$^+$/ CD5$^-$/ CD7$^-$/ beta-F1$^-$/ TCR-delta-1$^-$. Case 2 was: CD4$^+$/ CD2$^-$/ CD3$^-$/ CD5$^-$/ CD7$^-$/ CD16$^-$/ CD56$^-$/ beta-F1$^-$/ TCR-delta-1$^-$/ CD45RO$^-$/ CD45RA$^-$. Case 3 (TCLL) expressed the CD3$^+$/ CD2$^+$/ CD4$^+$/ CD5$^+$ (30% of cells)/ CD45RA$^+$/ beta-F1$^-$ phenotype.

Adhesion molecules (Table 3): VLA-3 was negative in all cases, VLA-4 was positive in cases 1 and 3. CD11a(LFA-1) was positive on proliferating cells in all of the cases. CD54 (ICAM-1) was positive on proliferating cells in all cases. CD44$^-$ (Hermes antigen) was positive on proliferating cells in all cases. Leu-8 was negative in all cases.

Primary Cutaneous B-cell Lymphomas

These cases were CB/CC D, CB/CC F, CB/CC F/D,CB ,CB/M ,CC, LC (36 cases)

Skin lesions in all of the cases consisted of localized plaques and/or papulo-nodular elements (Berti et al., 1991; Willemze et al., 1987; Berti et al., 1989).

Phenotypes: The mAb anti CD22 labelled most of the cells in all of the cases analyzed. The mAb anti-CD21 stained 52% of cases. Dendritic reticulum cells of the follicle (DRC-1$^+$) were demonstrated in 65% of cases. The mAbs anti CD1c, KB-61 and anti IgD, recognizing the mantle-zone B subset, were positive in 34%, 32% and 38%, respectively, of cases.

Adhesion molecules (Table 6): Anti-VLA-3 mab detected a positive infiltrate only in seven cases, whereas in all the other cases only vessels of the superficial dermis and basal keratinocytes were stained. Six of the seven positive cases were negative for Leu-8 antigen. Anti-VLA-4 mab stained a large percentage of proliferating cells in all cases, except three characterized by a proliferation of multilobated or large cells lymphocytes. Anti-CD11a-LFA-1 mAb labelled most of the infiltrate in all of the cases, except for one case of multilobated lymphoma in which very weak staining was observed. CD54 (ICAM-1) molecules were detected on infiltrating cells in all the cases examined. Anti CD44 mAb strongly stained most infiltrating cells in all cases cited above. Anti Leu-8 mAb stained infiltrating cells in 50% of cases only.

LYMPHO-PLASMOCYTOID (LPC)(2 CASES) AND PLASMOCYTIC LYMPHOMAS (2 CASES)

These lymphomas were observed in 10% of the cutaneous B-cell lymphomas. Skin lesions were multiple nodules or localized plaques.

Phenotypes: all cases expressed the CD38 antigen and cyto-plasmic monotypic Kappa or Lambda light chains. The mature plasmocytes usually lost the CD22 and CD20 antigens. The CD45RA marker was positive.

Adhesion molecules (Table 6): Anti VLA-3 mAb was strongly positive in one case of plasmocytic lymphoma, characterized by a very pleomorphic infiltrate, and weakly positive in a case of LPC.

Anti VLA-4 mAb labelled most of the lympho-plasmocytic elements in all cases.

Table 6. Adhesion molecules of primary B-cell lymphomas studied

mAbs	Primary cutaneous CB/CC F,CB/CC /F/D, CB/CC D,CB,LC,CC, CB/M (36 cases)	Extracutaneous CB/CC F,CB/CC F/D, CB/CC D,CB,CB/M, CC,CB/P,CLL,IB (59 cases)	Lympho-plasmo-cytoid (2 cases)	Plasmo-cytic (2 cases)
VLA-3	7/36 W	24/59 W	1/2 W	1/2 S
VLA-4	33/36 M	51/59 M	2/2 M	2/2 M
CD11a-LFA-1	35/36 S 1/36 W	50/59 S	2/2 W	0/2
CD54-ICAM-1	36/36 S	47/59 S	2/2 S	1/2 S
CD44	36/36 S	54/59 S	2/2 S	1/2 S
Leu-8	18/36 M	26/59 M	1/2 M	0/2

S, strong intensity; M, medium intensity; W, weak intensity

Anti CD11a-LFA-1 mAb failed to stain the most differentiated plasmocytic elements in LPC and was negative in the plasmocytic lymphomas.

CD54 (ICAM-1) molecules were expressed in the two LPC cases and one plasmocytic lymphoma.

CD44 reactivity was not detected in the case of plasmocytic lymphoma strongly VLA-3[+].

Anti Leu-8 moAb reacted only with one of the two LPC cases.

Extracutaneous B-cell Lymphomas

Phenotype: All cases expressed the CD22 pan-B cell markers and showed a restricted expression of kappa or lambda light chains (on cell suspension analysis).

CB/CC F (15 CASES), CB/CC F/D (2 CASES), CB/CC D (8 CASES)

Adhesion molecules (Table 6): VLA-3 molecules were expressed in eight of the 25 cases with weak intensity (32%). Anti VLA-4 mAb stained most cells in all specimens except two cases. Anti CD11a-LFA-1 mAb stained most cells in all specimens, except in two cases. Anti CD54-ICAM-1 mAb stained most cells in all specimens, except in two cases. CD44-Hermes antigen was expressed in 22 of the 25 cases analyzed. Leu-8 antigen was expressed in 10 of the 25 cases studied (34%).

CB, CB/M, CB/P, CC (20 CASES)

Adhesion molecules (Table 6): VLA-3 mAb reacted with seven of the 20 cases with weak intensity, except in two cases. VLA-4 molecules were expressed in 17 of the 20 cases examined. CD11a-LFA-1 mAb stained most of the cells in 17 of the 20 cases analyzed. CD44-Hermes antigen reactivity was observed in 19 of the 20 cases studied. CD54 (ICAM-1) molecules were expressed on neoplastic cells of 18 cases. Anti Leu-8 mAb stained only 7 cases most with weak intensity)

CLL (9 CASES)

The phenotype of CLL is characterized by reactivity with the CD22(CD19) B-cell markers and the CD5 marker.

Adhesion molecules (Table 6): The VLA-3 molecule was expressed in most cases (7 of 9). VLA-4: The same positivity (7 of 9) was noted. The CD11a-LFA-1 marker was not detected in four of the nine cases examined. CD54 (ICAM-1) reactivity was observed only in three of the nine cases. Anti CD44 mAb strongly stained the proliferating cells in all cases. Leu-8 molecules were strongly expressed in eight of the nine cases.

IMMUNOBLASTIC B-CELL LYMPHOMA (5 CASES)

Adhesion molecules (Table 6): VLA-3 was positive with weak intensity in two of the five cases.

VLA-4 was positive in four of the five cases.

CD11a (LFA-1) was positive in four of the five cases.

CD54 (ICAM-1) was positive in three of the five cases.

CD44 (Hermes antigen) was positive in four of the five cases.

Leu8 was positive only in one of the five cases.

DISCUSSION

Adhesion molecules (CD44, ICAM-1, VLA-3, VLA-4, etc.) are not exclusively present on hemopoietic cells, but rather are present also in skin tissues such as vessels, epithelial cells, melanocytes, fibroblasts and nerves. Moreover, the expression of some of these molecules can be induced in many cell types by lymphokines released by infiltrating mononuclear cells. In our studies, we examined the VLA-3, VLA-4, LFA-1, CD44, ICAM-1 and Leu-8 molecules in cutaneous B or T-cell lymphomas to determine whether any of these proliferations presented a specific pattern of expression of cell-matrix, cell-cell or "homing" receptors. In normal lymphoid tissue (lymph nodes or tonsils) anti VLA-3 mAb weakly stains some germinal center cells of the follicles and T-lymphocytes in the T-cell areas. VLA-4 molecules show a peculiar distribution on T-lymphocytes in the T-cell areas and on mantle zone B-lymphocytes, whereas rapidly proliferating germinal center B-lymphocytes and intrafollicular T-lymphocytes are negative. The anti LFA-1 mAb stains all lympho-monocytic cells in lymphoid tissues similar to a pan leukocyte reagent. ICAM-1 molecules are strongly expressed by germinal center B-lymphocytes and dendritic reticulum cells of the follicle. Anti CD44 mAb displays a pan reactivity since it stains most cell types. Leu-8 marker, identifying the suppressor-inducer subset of $CD4^+$ T-helper lymphocytes, shows a distribution similar to that of VLA-4: it is negative on germinal center cells (both T and B lymphocytes) but reacts with T-cells in the T-areas of the lymph nodes and with the mantle zone B-cells. Surely the LFA-1 molecules are mainly involved in specific antigen-antibody mediated cell-cell interaction, whereas the CD44 antigen is a typical "homing" receptor determining the preferential migration of cells to a site. Structural homologies between VLA-4 and the murine LPAM-1 "homing" receptor and between Leu8 and the murine Mel-14 "homing" receptor have been demonstrated, and their similarity in distribution in normal lymphoid tissues thus is not surprising. The significance of VLA-3 receptors (a multi-ligand receptor for collagen, laminin, and fibronectin) in cell-matrix interactions has been extensively studied, but the role of expression of these molecules in cell-cell interactions is not known. The results of our studies on T-cell lymphomas show that the pattern of adhesion molecule expression in MF (early stages and classical form) is not significantly different from that of T-cells of normal lymphoid tissues or of inflammatory reactive skin diseases. No correlation was seen between "abnormal" phenotype expression (i.e. $CD7^-$, $CD5^-$) and the pattern of adhesion molecules analyzed. The only significant observation that we could obtain was the consistant expression of VLA-4 and the frequently reduced reactivity of Leu-8, which suggests that VLA-4 and Leu8 molecules may be differentially involved in "homing" to skin tissue and lymph nodes, respectively. In analyzing erythrodermic MF we observed no overall phenotypic differences, except for an interesting case showing the CD16[+], CD25[+] and CD30[+] phenotype. In this case VLA-4 was once more strongly positive and Leu 8 completely negative; however, VLA-3 molecules were also strongly expressed. In tumoral stage MF no correlation was seen between the atypical phenotypes, such as absence of CD5 and CD7 markers, absence of expression of beta-F1 (alpha-beta T-cell marker), expression of the CD70 activation antigen and particularly of the BER-ACT8 marker (analogous to HML-1 and specific for the intraepithelial CD8[+] activated lymphocytes of the gut) and some adhesion molecule patterns. Interestingly, in one case the large multinucleated and Reed-Sternberg like CD30[+] cells strongly expressed the VLA-3 molecule. The peculiar expression of the VLA-3 molecule on large blastic T-cells was confirmed from the results obtained in Ki-1[+] lymphomas, showing strong reactivity with anti VLA-3 in 6 of the 8 cases studied. Moreover, Leu-8 molecules were not detected in 6 of the 8 cases of Ki-1[+] lymphomas, confirming a down regulation of this molecule in rapidly proliferating cells. The expression of CD44, LFA-1, VLA-4 and ICAM-1 adhesion molecules seemed not to be significantly modified, independent of the highly defective phenotypes of these lymphomas, frequently showing NK marker expression as well. Moreover, VLA-3 receptors were strongly expressed in 2 of 5 cases of CD8[+] CTCLs analyzed (both strongly DR[+] and one case expressing both CD16 NK marker and BER-ACT-8 activation marker). In the same cases Leu-8 reactivity was not detected. Interestingly, in the case of gamma/delta pagetoid reticulosis (CD4[-]/ CD8[-]) no expression of VLA-3, VLA-4, ICAM-1, LFA-1, or Leu-8 molecules was detected and only expression of the CD44 antigen was observed. Leu 8 molecules were also absent in the second case of pagetoid reticulosis (localized form) and in the last 5 cases of T-lymphomas studied including the 2 cases with the simultaneous cutaneous and systemic involvement and the case of TCLL. Finally, VLA-4 molecules were not expressed in the 2 atypical cases showing an NK-like phenotype (CD2[+]/ CD3[-]/ CD56[+] and CD4[+]/ CD56[+]/ CD3[-]/ CD2[-]). No difference in expression of adhesion molecules was observed in correlation with the expression of CD45RO ("primed" T-lymphocytes) or of the CD45RA ("naive" T-cells) phenotype. In summary, the results of T-cell lymphomas analyzed indicate that CD11a-LFA-1, ICAM-1 and CD44 adhesion molecules are expressed in most cases; VLA-4 and not Leu-8 may be relevant for the "homing" of alpha-beta T-cells in CTCLs. Leu-8 seems down-regulated in highly proliferating tumors, whereas VLA-3 molecules are preferentially expressed on activated and proliferating cells positive for CD30 or, less frequently, for other activation markers. Our preliminary study of a few cases of Hodgkin disease, however, showed that typical Reed-Sternberg and Hodgkin cells do not react with anti VLA-3 mAb.

The results obtained from analysis of Primary Cutaneous B-cell Lymphomas showed that VLA-3 molecules are rarely expressed and usually with a weak intensity, whereas VLA-4 reactivity was detected in all cases analyzed. The same positive reactivity was noted by using anti ICAM-1 reagents; CD44 and LFA-1 were negative only in one of the 36 cases examined. Leu-8, identifying a subset of mantle zone B-lymphocytes, was expressed in 50% of the cases studied. In one plasmocytic lymphoma we noted a strong VLA-3 reactivity. The differences in the adhesion molecule pattern expression in the case of plasmocytic lymphomas was evident (negativity of LFA-1, ICAM-1 and Leu-8). Extracutaneous B-cell lymphomas (mainly nodal lymphomas) showed a similar pattern of adhesion molecules, even if the expression was more irregular. VLA-4 was negative or weak in 7, LFA-1 in 3, ICAM-1 in 6, and CD44 in 6 of the cases examined. Leu-8 molecules were expressed only in 34% of the cases and VLA-3 in 32%. In several cases expressing a strong VLA-3 reactivity, complementary Leu-8 negativity was observed as in T-cell lymphomas. In immunoblastic B-cell lymphomas reactivity with anti VLA-4, CD11a-LFA-1 and CD44 was confirmed in four of five cases, whereas VLA-3 molecules were observed in two (weak intensity) and Leu8 antigen expression only in one case.

More interesting, and peculiar, are the data about lymphocytic lymphomas with a phenotype and morphology similar to that of the B-cell lymphocytic leukemia (CD22+, CD5+). In fact, in all but one case, VLA-3 molecules were clearly expressed; the same reactivity was noted by using Leu-8, VLA-4 and CD44 mAbs, whereas LFA-1 and ICAM-1 molecules were absent, respectively, in 4 and 6 of the 9 cases analyzed. These results suggest some conclusions also for B-cell lymphomas. The adhesion molecule pattern expressed by cutaneous versus nodal B-cell follicular lymphomas were similar. In both, a weak expression of VLA-3 could be observed, whereas a strong expression of VLA-4, CD11a-LFA-1, ICAM-1 and CD44 was detected in most cases. Leu-8 molecules were positive in 50% of cases, usually with a weak intensity. There were no correlations between particular phenotypes (expression of mantle zone B-cell or of activation antigens) and the expression of the adhesion molecules studied. However, VLA-3 expression seemed to be more frequent in activated cells of large cell lymphomas or in cells expressing the CD22+ and CD5+ phenotype (CLL and CC lymphomas).

REFERENCES

Albelda SM and Buck CA: Integrins and other cell adhesion molecules. **FASEB J**, 4:2868-2880, (1990).

Berti A, A Cerri, S Cavicchini, D Delia, D Soligo, E Alessi and R Caputo, 1991. Primary cutaneous gamma-delta T-cell lymphoma presenting as disseminated pagetoid retiulosis. **J. Invest. Dermatol.**, 96(5):718-723.

Berti E, E Alessi and R Caputo, 1991. Reticulohistiocytoma of the dorsum (Crosti's disease) and other B-cell lymphomas. **Seminar in diagnostic pathology**, 8(2):82-90.

Berti E, R Gianotti, E Alesis and R Caputo, 1989. Primary cutaneous follicular center cell lymphoma: Immunophenotypical and immunogenotypical aspects. **Curr. Probl. Dermatol.**, 19:196-202.

Butcher EC, 1990. Cellular and molecular mechanism that direct leukocyte traffic. **Am. J. Pathol.**, 136(1).

Camerini D, SP James, I Stamenkovic and B Seed, 1989. Leu8/TQ1 is the human equivalent of the MEL-14 lymph node homing receptor. **Nature**, 342:78-82.

Elices MJ, LA Urry and ME Hemler ME, 1991. Receptor functions for the Integrin VLA3: Fibronectin, Collagen, and Laminin binding are differentially influenced by ARG-GLY-ASP peptide and by divalent cations. **J. Cell Biol.**, 112(1): 169-181.

Haynes BF, M Telen, L Hale and S Denning, 1989. CD44: A molecule involved in leukocyte adherence and T-cell activation. **Immunology** Today, 10(12):423-428.

Hynes RO, 1987. Integrins: A family of cell surface receptors. **Cell**, 48:549-554.

Hynes RO, 1992. Integrins: Versatility, modulation, and signalling in cell adhesion. **Cell**, 69:11-25.

Jalkanen S, H Joensuu, KO Soderstrom and P Klemi, 1991. Lymphocyte homing and clinical behavior of Non-Hodgkin's lymphoma. **J. Clin. Invest.**, 87:1835-1840.

Makgoba MW, ME Sanders and S Shaw, 1989. The CD2-LFA3 and LFA-l-ICAM pathways: Relevance to T-cell recognition. **Immunology Today**, 10 (12):417-422.

Pals ST, CJ Meijer and T Radaszkiewicz, 1991. Expression of the human peripheral lymph node homing receptor (LECAM-1) in nodal and gastrointestinal non-Hodgkin's lymphomas. **Leukemia**, 5(7):628-631.

Picker L, J Medeiros, L Weiss, R Warnke and EC Butcher, 1988. Expression of lymphocyte homing receptor antigen in Non-Hodgkin's Lymphoma. **Am. J. Pathol.**, 130(3):496-504.

Roossien FF, D de Rijk, A Bikker and E Roos, 1989. Involvement of LFA-1 in lymphoma invasion and metastasis demonstrated with LFA-l-deficient mutants. **J. Cell Biol.**, 108:1979-198.

Schwartz MA, 1992. Transmembrane signalling by integrins. **Trends Cell Biol.**, 2:304-308.

Sun Sy M, YJ Guo and I Stamenkovic, 1991. Distinct effects of two CD44 isoforms on tumor growth in vivo. **J. Exp. Med.**, 174: 859-866.

Takada Y, EA Wayner, WG Carter and ME Hemler, 1988. Extracutaneous matrix receptors, ECMRII and ECM RI, for collagen and fibronectin, correspond to VLA-2 and VLA-3 in the VLA family of heterodimers. **J. Cell Biochem.**, 37:385-393.

Wayuner EA, WG Carter, RS Piotrowica and TJ Kunicki, 1988. The function of exracellular matrix receptors in mediating cell adhesion to extracellular matrix: Preparation of monoclonal antibodies to the fibronectin receptor that specifically inhibit cell adhesion to fibronectin and react with platelet glycoproteins Ic-IIa. **J. Cell Biol.**, 107:1881-1891.

Willemze R, CJLM Meijer, HJ Sentis, E Scheffer, WA van Vloten, J Toonstra and C Van Der Putte, 1981. Primary cutaneous large cell lymphomas of follicular center cell origin. **J. Am. Acad. Dermatol.**, 16:518-526.

A NEW RETROVIRUS FROM CUTANEOUS T-CELL LYMPHOMA

Vittorio Manzari*
Loredana Albonici†
Marco Ciotti*
Maria Pia Lombardi‡
Ida Silvestri‡

* Department of Experimental Medicine and Biochemical Science
University of Rome "Tor Vergata"
Rome, Italy

† Institute of Biomedical Technology, CNR
Rome, Italy

‡ Department of Experimental Medicine
University of Rome "la Sapienza"
Rome, Italy

Correspondence to: Dr. V. Manzari, Inst. Pathologia Gen.,
University of Rome "Tor Vergata", Via Orazio Raimondo,
I-00173 Roma, Italy

ABSTRACT

Several years ago, our laboratory reported isolation of a virus, HTLV-5, from a Tac-negative T-cell lymphoma/leukemia. To date, however, no cell line has been obtained which consistently produces amounts of virus sufficient to permit detection of reverse transcriptase (RT) or to form the basis for a serologic test. In the process of attempting to develop such a cell line, we found that the lymphocyte cell line, GB, derived from a patient with cutaneous lymphoma/leukemia, produces an inhibitor of RT. Production of this inhibitory factor is

Basic Mechanisms of Physiologic and Aberrant Lymphoproliferation in the Skin
Edited by W.C. Lambert *et al.*, Plenum Press, New York, 1994

transmitted, both by infection and by transfection, to cell lines which do not produce it spontaneously.

INTRODUCTION

Known Human T-lymphotropic retroviruses belong to two families: i) the HTLV family, which includes HTLV-1 and HTLV-2, which are transforming viruses, and likely a new virus which has been provisionally named HTLV-5, and ii) the HIV family, which includes HIV I and HIV II, which are cytolytic viruses.

Fifteen out of one hundred fifty T-cell lymphomas, examined by hybridization with a HTLV-1 probe, showed low stringency reactivity; sera from these patients reacted with both HTLV-1 and HIV I antigens, mostly p24.

Definite proof of presence of a retrovirus was obtained in a lymphocyte culture derived from the blood of a patient affected by cutaneous lymphoma/leukemia. When these cells (GB) were cultured in RPMI 1640 medium, supplemented with 20% fetal calf serum (FCS), an immortalized cell line appeared after 90 days; unexpectedly, it was a B-cell line. One hypothesis to account for these results is that the virus may be cytolytic in vitro for T-cells but immortalizing for B-cells.

After a few months, the cell line began to produce a retrovirus identified by the presence of Mg^{+2} dependent reverse transcriptase activity associated with particles with a density of 1.16-1.19 gr/ml sucrose gradient. Electron microscopy showed typical viral budding, but, to date, we have not been able to obtain persistent production of reverse transcriptase activity in the supernatant fluids of these cells (Manzari et al., 1987).

DNAs from both cell culture and from fresh peripheral lymphocytes showed the same hybridization pattern: some regions which hybridized to HTLV-1 showed exogenous genomic sequences with low homology to HTLV-1 (i.e., they hybridized in low stringency but not in high stringency).

The main problem, to date, has been to obtain a cell line continuously producing adequate amounts of virus and to obtain an immunofluorescence-positive non-B cell line for a first serological screening. For this purpose we performed transfection and infection experiments using different cell lines (Manzari et al., 1990).

MATERIALS AND METHODS

The cell lines were cultured at variable cell densities, $2x10^5$-$1x10^6$, in RPMI 1640 medium supplemented with L-glutamine, penicillin, streptomycin, and 10-20% FCS, at 37° C in 5% CO_2.

We have two genomic libraries cloned in EMBL-3 phage, derived from two patients affected by mycosis fungoides. The first one was obtained from fresh peripheral lymphocytes and the second from a long-term lymphocyte culture. Some subclones derived from such libraries hybridized in low stringency with HTLV-1 DNA and in high stringency with DNAs extracted from neoplastic cells.

Transfection was carried out by a protoplast fusion technique. HL60, CEM, and U937 cell lines were transfected by protoplast fusion (PEG 1000 method) driving a recombinant plasmid pBlue Script M13(-) subclone carrying the HTLV-5 viral sequences. After transfection, the supernatant fluids from different experiments were collected and analyzed for presence of reverse transcriptase (RT; Table 1).

Table 1. Reverse transcriptase activity of transfected cells.

	R T activity after 4 days cpm	after 12 days cpm	after 1 month cpm
HL60/8	4876	650	390
U937/8	3828	960	482
CEN/	1180	900	472
MT2	3470		

Infection experiments were performed on many leukemic cell lines by co-culture with GB cells (Manzari et al., 1990). Briefly, 2×10^6 GB cells were irradiated with 1.2×10^4 rads or treated with $50 \mu g/ml$ mitomycin C for 20 minutes at 37° C, washed and added at a ratio 1:5 to the cell line which was in exponential growth in RPMI 1640 medium, supplemented with 20% fetal calf serum (FCS).

The level of reverse transcriptase was tested according to the method of Poiesz et al. (Pouesz et al., 1980). In our experiments 10 ml clarified supernatant fluid was centrifuged in a SW41 rotor at 30,000 rpm for 1 hour and resuspended 10x concentrated. Before the assay the virus was disrupted with 0.1% Triton X-100 and incubated one hour at 37° C with 50 mM Tris-HCl, pH 7.8; 10 mM $MgCl^2$; 10 mM DTT; poly A:oligo(dT)(12:18) and [^{3}H] dTTP. To test the interference of GB supernatant on the RT of other retroviruses, we added 10 μl or 20 μl of 10x concentrated GB supernatant before adding the RT cocktail.

At the end of incubation, each sample was treated with 100 μg of yeast tRNA and precipitated with chilled 20% trichloroacetic acid (TCA) containing phosphate buffer. The precipitate was collected on a Millipore filter, washed and dried, and its radioactivity determined with a LKB scintillation spectrometer.

Every experiment was carried out in duplicate with a blank of 250 cpm subtracted.

RESULTS

Infection experiments have shown that, upon co-culture of GB with HL60, syncythia and giant cells appeared in the culture and infected cells became readily distinguishable from untreated cells. Virus production, however, was low, as indicated by RT levels constantly near background over many months, even if a few budding viral particles could be evidenced by electron microscopy.

Transfection experiments, on the other hand, have shown erratic short term production of RT lasting a few days (Manzari et al, 1990).

On the basis of these data, the hypothesis of production of a RT inhibitor was tested: Table 2 shows interference of the reverse transcriptase activity of a 10x concentrated MT2 supernatant fluid or HIV I by GB supernatant fluid (10x) added to the reaction mixture. GB supernatant fluid strongly inhibited the RT level of both HTLV-1 and HIV I.

Table 2. Inhibitory effect of GB supernatant fluid on MT2 and HIV I reverse transcriptase levels.

	RT activity cpm
MT2	1346
MT2 + 10μl GB	550
MT2 + 20μl GB	450
HIV I	1572
HIV I + 10μl GB	570
HIV I + 20μl GB	480

A significant inhibition was also observed on commercial Molony murine leukemia virus (MoMuLV) RT cloned in E. coli (Table 3).

Moreover, we tried supernatant fluids from transfected cells in order to test whether the inhibitory effect was transmissable. Table 4 shows the inhibitory effect on MT2 RT of supernatant fluids from both untreated and transfected cells. Concentrated supernatant fluids from both U937/8 and CEM/8 cells (transfected cells) but not those from U937 and CEM cells (non-transfected cells), decreased the MT2 RT level.

Table 3. Inhibitory effect of GB supernatant fluid on MoMuLV reverse transcriptase activity.

	R T activity cpm	
MoMuLV	41,000	
MoMuLV + 10μl GB	27,300	

Table 4. Effects of supernatant fluids from untreated and transfected cells on MT2 reverse transcriptase activity.

	R T activity cpm	
MT2	1394	
MT2 + 20μl U937	1260	
MT2 + 10μl U937/8	976	
MT2 + 20μl U937/8	598	
MT2	2363	
MT2 + 20μl CEM	2149	
MT2 + 10μl CEM/8	755	
MT2 + 20μl CEM/8	325	

U 937 and CEM, untreated cells; U937/8 and CEM/8, transfected cells.

We questioned whether the inhibitor is a DNase or RNase. Table 5 shows that levels of RT of MT2 supernatant fluid treated with GB supernatant fluid are not affected by adding RNase inhibitor and that adding GB supernatant fluid after the MT2 RT reaction does not affect the outcome of the reaction (Table 6).

DISCUSSION

The main problem regarding HTLV-5, a virus isolated a few years ago (Manzari et al, 1987), is that, to date, no cell line has been obtained which consistently produces amounts of virus sufficient to permit RT detection or to form the basis for a serological test.

Table 5. Interference of GB supernatant on with MT2 reverse transcriptase activity in the presence of an RNase inhibitor.

	R T activity cpm
MT2	1990
MT2+10ul GB	930
MT2+RNasein	1975
MT2+10ul GB+RNasein	853

Table 6. Effect of adding DNase to MT2 reverse transcriptase after the reaction to test for presence of DNase in GB.

	R T activity cpm
MT2	2426
MT2+20μl GB	2363

In the last few years, therefore, we have focused our attention on induction of stable virus production either in GB cells or in other cell lines. This attempt has been unsuccessful; RT production has been erratic and non-reproducible, even if, as in the case of HL 60 cells, the cells appeared to have been infected. We thus tested the hypothesis that an inhibitor of RT is produced by GB cells, and this has been shown to be the case. The most interesting finding has been, however, that production of the factor was transmitted, both by infection and by transfection, to cell lines which do not produce inhibitory factor spontaneously.

The fact that RT inhibition is transmitted through infection implies that either the effect is produced directly by a viral product or that the virus activates a cellular mechanism at high efficency.

We are now trying to characterize the factor and to understand the close association between its production and infection, both in order to obtain unhinibited (i.e., virus-productive) cell lines and to understand the meaning of the factor in the viral infection cycle, i.e., whether it is a regulatory mechanism of the virus, itself, or a defense mechanism provided by the cell;

whether it is important in the pathogenesis of the disease; and whether it interferes with other retroviral infections.

REFERENCES

Manzari V, E Collalti, I Silvestri, A Santoni, A Modesti and L Frati, 1990. Human T lymphotropic virus V: HTLV-V. In: WA Blattner, Ed: **Human retrovirology: HTLV** Raven Press (New York), pp. 143-146.

Manzari V, A Gismondi, G Barillari, S Morrone, A Modesti, L Albonici, VM Fazio, A Gradilone, L Frati and A Santoni, 1987. HTLV-V: A new human retrovirus isolated in a Tac-negative T-cell lymphoma/leukemia. **Science**, 238:1581-1584.

Poiesz BJ, FW Ruscetti, AF Gazdar, PA Bunn, JD Minna and RC Gallo, 1980. Detection and isolation of type C retrovirus particles from fresh and cultured lymphocytes of a patient with cutaneous T-cell lymphoma. **Proc. Natl. Acad. Sci. U.S.A.**, 77:7415-7419.

SURVEY OF CUTANEOUS T CELL LYMPHOMAS FOR HUMAN T-LYMPHOTROPIC VIRUS INFECTION

Michel D'Incan*†
Pierre Souteyrand*
Yves-Jean Bignon‡
Claude Desgranges†

*   Dermatology Department
    Hotel-Dieu
    Clermont-Ferrand, France

†   Laboratory of Viral Hepatitis, AIDS and Human Retroviruses
    INSERM,
    Lyon, France

‡   Molecular Oncology Department
    Centre Jean Perrin,
    Clermont-Ferrand,   France

Correspondence to: Prof. Dr. Pierre Souteyrand, Department of Dermatology,
Hotel-Dieu, P. O. Box 69, F-63003 Clermont Ferrand Cedex, France

ABSTRACT

The etiology of cutaneous T cell lymphomas (CTCL) is still unknown, but the similarities it shares with the human T-lymphotropic virus type-1 (HTLV-associated adult T cell lymphoma led to the speculation that a retrovirus may be involved as a causative agent. Many studies using electron microscopy and serological tests have supported this hypothesis. The recently available powerful techniques of molecular biology (D'Incan et al., 1992a) have shown that some cases of cutaneous T cell lymphomas outside HTLV-1 endemic areas are associated with the genomic integration of a related or, more probably, a defective HTLV-1 provirus. To date, no viral isolate was established from a case of CTCL. Moreover, the incidence of a retroviral infection in CTCL seems to be low although highly underestimated.

Basic Mechanisms of Physiologic and Aberrant Lymphoproliferation in the Skin
Edited by W.C. Lambert *et al.*, Plenum Press, New York, 1994

INTRODUCTION

The generic term cutaneous T cell lymphoma (CTCL) encompasses a spectrum of diseases characterized by a malignant proliferation of T-lymphocytes with a major clinical expression in the skin. It includes mycosis fungoides and its leukemic form the Sézary syndrome, pagetoid lymphoma (WoringerKolopp disease), T cell chronic lymphocytic leukemia and the rare non epidermotropic T cell lymphomas (Abel, 1985; Edelson, 1987; Zackheim, 1981). Their etiology remains still unknown. Although some cases of drug induced epidermotropic T cell lymphomas have been reported (D'Incan et al, 1992b; Souteyrand, et al., 1990), the role of exposures to a toxic agent as a consistent causative factor has been ruled out by epidemiologic studies (Whittemore et al., 1989). The discovery at the beginning of the eighties of HTLV-1 (Human T Lymphotropic Virus Type I) and of its implication in the pathophysiology of the adult T cell lymphoma (ATL), a malignant proliferation of mature T lymphocytes in humans (Poiesz et al., 1980; 1981), encouraged many groups to look for a possible retroviral etiology in cutaneous T cell lymphomas. We now present an overview of the current status concerning this very stimulating field of research.

THE BIRTH OF AN HYPOTHESIS

The hypothesis of a retrovirus as a causative factor in cutaneous T cell lymphomas was first suggested by the discovery in 1979, of type-C retroviral-like particles in cutaneous and lymph node antigen-presenting cells from seven cases of mycosis fungoides and 2 cases of Sézary syndromes and the detection of a reverse transcriptase activity in one of the mycosis fungoides (Van der Loo et al., 1979). This fact led to the hypothesis that the initiating event in mycosis fungoides may be an infection of Langerhans cells by a type-C retrovirus (MacKie, 1981).

At the same time, HTLV-1 retrovirus was identified in T cell lines established from an American and a Carribean patients with an aggressive variant of mycosis fungoides and Sézary syndrome respectively (Poiesz et al., 1980; 1981). Another type C retrovirus isolated in Japan (Adult Tcell Leukemia Virus, ATLV) was shown to be identical to the US isolate (Watanabe et al., 1984). At this time, HTLV-1 is clearly associated with two distinct human diseases in Japan, the Carribean region and Africa: i) a degenerative neurologic disorder: the Tropical Spastic Paraparesis (TSP) or HTLV-1 Associated Myelopathy (HAM) (Gessain et al. 1985), and ii) the Adult T Cell lymphoma (Uchiyama et al., 1977).

Three clinical forms of ATL have been described (reviewed in Blattner et al., 1983; Takatsuki et al., 1989). The acute and aggressive form represents 50% of cases of ATL. It is a leukemia with extensive lymphadenopathy, visceral involvement, specific cutaneous lesions in 50 to 60% of the cases, and sometimes opportunistic infections. Biologically, it is characterized by an hypercalcemia and a leukocytosis with 5 to 99% atypical lymphocytes with a clover leaf-like nucleus and the immunophenotype of helper/inducer mature T cells. Smoldering ATL is characterized by skin erythema, papules or nodules as premonitory symptoms, but other clinical and laboratory data including white blood cells count, normal. Chronic ATL is defined as intermediate forms between the acute and the smoldering forms, with a less aggressive course and varied clinical abnormalities.

Striking similarities exist between typical CTCL and the chronic and smoldering forms of ATL (Kawano et al., 1985; Yamaguchi et al., 1983). In particular, the morphology and the immunophenotype of the neoplastic cells in ATL are closely similar to those in typical CTCL i.e. lymphocytes with a highly convoluted nucleus, and with the immunophenotype CD3$^+$, CD4$^+$, CD8$^-$. However, cells in ATL express the receptor for Interleukine-2 (CD25) and show a suppressive activity, whereas cells in CTCL do not (Waldmann et al., 1984; Yamada, 1983). Therefore, especially in some cases of smoldering ATL, the histological features of the cutaneous involvement may lead to diagnostic confusion with epidermotropic CTCL such as Sézary syndrome or mycosis fungoides (Chan et al., 1985; Detmar et al., 1991; Ikai et al., 1987; Lessana-Leibowitch et al., 1984; Maeda et al., 1987; Takahashi et al., 1988). In these conditions, the constant presence of antibodies reactive against HTLV-1 and the establishment of the proviral genomic integration are the major criterions for ATL (Takigawa et al., 1988; Dosaka et al., 1991). So, the two cases from which HTLV-1 was first isolated (Poiesz, et al.. 1980; 1981) are now considered as true ATL instead of mycosis fungoides or Sézary syndrome in spite of close histological analogies.

Together with previous ultrastructural data, however, these similarities between ATL and CTCL have been sufficient to generate speculation that a retrovirus may be involved in the pathogenesis of some cases of CTCL, leading to numerous studies whose results will be considered now.

ULTRASTRUCTURAL DATA

Following the aforementioned works of Van der Loo et al., Slater et al. reported two cases of Sézary syndrome with type C retroviral particles in reactive lymph nodes restricted to Langerhans cells (Slater et al., 1983; 1985). In 1988, Kaltoft et al. established the Se-Ax T cell line from peripheral blood of a 66 year-old woman with a Sézary syndrome. Under special culture conditions, type-C retroviral-like particles appeared in the extracellular medium, but no budding of particles was seen, nor was there reactivity using adult T cell leukemia serum with activity against envelope and core proteins of HTLV-1, nor was reverse transcriptase activity detected. Moreover, HTLV-1 provirus was not detected in southern blot assay with a specific viral probe (Kaltoft et al., 1987; 1988).

IMMUNOREACTIVITY AGAINST HTLV EPITOPES IN CTCL

Many publications report the finding of antibodies against HTLV-1 in patients with true CTCL. However, it is necessary to specify two important points concerning interpretation of the

HTLV-1 serology tests. First, many false positive results are due to the fact that reagents in commercially available tests utilize virus grown in human cell lines (Bolton et al., 1989) and it has been shown that cross-reactivities can occur between HTLV-1 antigenic epitopes, such as the protein p19, and mammalian cells one (Haynes et al., 1983). Second, a serological cross-reactivity is possible between human retroviruses, as has been demonstrated with HIV and HTLV-1 in HIV-infected individuals (Wong-Staal et al., 1985). These facts have two consequences. First, it is important to demonstrate reactivity to products of two or more viral genes to verify the presence of HTLV-1 antibodies (Fang et al., 1988). Second, the immunoreactivity against proteins encoded by just one HTLV-1 gene may be interpreted only as identifying an unknown human retrovirus, although one with close antigenic similarities with HTLV-1 (Ranki et al., 1988).

In northern Europe, a non endemic area for HTLV-1 infection, antibodies crossreacting with HTLV-1 core proteins have been found at a low titer in more than 10% of individuals with a CTCL (mycosis fungoides, Sézary syndromes and lymphomatoid papulosis) (Lange-Wantzin et al., 1984; 1986; Saxinger et al., 1985). A sole cross-reactivity against the HTLV-1 p24 gag-encoded protein and against the HIV-1 p24 gag-encoded product was detected in, respectively, 12 and 6 of 22 Finnish patients with a mycosis fungoides (Ranki et al., 1987; 1988). More recently (Sahai Srivastava et al., 1990), 6 of 27 mycosis fungoides patients tested gave a weak reaction on HTLV-1 ELISA and 3 of them gave multiple bands on western blot that was interpreted as an indeterminate reaction. Two isolated reports note, in one, the presence of HTLV-1 p19 antigen in skin and lymph node of a patient with mycosis fungoides (Turbitt et al., 1985) and the other, a weak reactivity against HTLV-1 p24 protein in a patient with a mycosis fungoides and a B cell chronic lymphocytic leukemia (Peterman et al., 1986).

DEMONSTRATION OF HTLV-1 RELATED SEQUENCES IN CTCL

The rapid expansion of the molecular biology technology in the past decade led to a better knowledge of viral diseases in detecting infectious agents with a greater sensitivity than with anyother techniques and in allowing an approach of the understanding of their pathophysiology. Using nucleic acid hybridization procedures, it has been possible to detect, in some cases of CTCL, the presence of HTLV-1-related proviral sequences, although, to date, establishment of a virus productive cell line has not been achieved.

In 1987, isolation of a HTLV-1-related retrovirus from EBV-transformed B cells of a CD25 negative mycosis fungoides patient in Italy was reported. Southern blot analysis of this virus, nammed HTLV-5, showed that although similar to HTLV-1, it was unique and may be involved in the etiology of CTCL. However, no isolate of this viral genome is available at present (Manzari et al., 1987). By the combined use of Southern blot analysis and the polymerase chain reaction, HTLV-1 genomic sequences have been detected in 6 of 6 CD30-positive large cell cutaneous T cell lymphomas in Germany, a non endemic area for HTLV-1 (Anagnostopoulos et al., 1990). Interestingly, in only one case, which was also the only case with antibodies against HTLV-1, did Southern blot analysis indicate integration of a complete HTLV-1 provirus, whereas in the 4 other cases tested the blot pattern showed smaller bands than expected, indicating the presence of a defective HTLV-1 genome. Additional similar results have also been reported, emphasizing the possible role of defective HTLV-1 viruses or of a HTLV-1-related one in the etiology of CTCL. Indeed (Hall et al., 1991), a HTLV-1-provirus, largely deleted in gag and env genes and completely deleted in pol gene, was shown to be monoclonally integrated in a B cell line established from peripheral lymphocytes and in uncultured circulating lymphocytes of a HTLV-1-seronegative patient with leukemic mycosis fungoides. Moreover, polymerase chain amplification with primers specific for the different genes of HTLV-1 was performed on DNAs extracted from cutaneous lesions of 5 HTLV-1-seronegative Swedish patients with a mycosis fungoides and showed, in each case, HTLV-1-related sequences but with variable deletions. HTLV-1 provirus monoclonally integrated in cultured circulating lymphocytes of a seronegative patient with Sézary syndrome has been also reported. A particular restriction enzyme pattern together with a weak molecular hybridization signal with polymerase chain products derived from the gag gene, suggested either a defective or variant HTLV-1 (Bazarbachi et al., 1991). Finally, using the polymerase chain reaction procedure (submitted for publication), we showed the presence of HTLV-1-related sequences with deletions in the pol gene in successive blood samples from one French CTCL among 51 tested.

DISCUSSION

Considering the aforementioned data, it appears that the hypothesis of a retrovirus as a causative factor for some CTCL is more and more consistent, but many questions remain still unanswerable. Definitive proof of this hypothesis will not be obtained as long as no viral isolate can be established from 51 tested cases of CTCL.

Nevertheless, the fact that HTLV-1 itself is not the causal agent seems to be established. Indeed, the conclusions issuing from molecular biology and serological data lead one to think that a close-related HTLV-1 virus or, more probably, a defective HTLV-1 is involved. A large deletion in viral genome may subsequently limit or prevent active replication and thus, no antibody response or perhaps only a limited antibody response can occur (Hall et al., 1991). This may explain: i) the weak reactivity of HTLV-1 serological tests in CTCL and, ii) the relative indolence of CTCL in comparison to ATL which is associated with the integration of a complete HTLV-1 genome. Indeed, it has been demonstrated (Ranki et al, 1990), CTCL associated with antibodies reactive with some HTLV-1 antigenic epitopes have a more fulminant course than seronegative CTCL.

A second question which has to be raised is the mechanism of leukemogenesis in virus-associated CTCL. The paradigm of the pathophysiology of HTLV-1-induced ATL, which involves, in the preliminary steps, the transactivation by HTLV-1 Tax protein of the genes encoding Interleukin-2 and its membranous receptor cannot be applied to CTCL since CTCL leukemic cells generally do not express the receptor for Interleukin-2 (CD25 antigen). Moreover, the role of cells other than lymphocytes, such as antigen presenting cells, is still unknown. Ultrastructural data seem to show that they may play an active role in virus-associated CTCL (Van der Loo et al., 1979; Slater et al., 1983) as they do in other retrovirus-associated human diseases (Zambruno et al., 1991).

The incidence of retroviral-infected CTCL is also a matter of speculation. At this time, only a few number of retrovirus-associated CTCL have been reported, but we can assume that this number is underestimated since searching HTLV infection in CTCL with sensitive technics is far from systematic. In our experience, only one CTCL among 51 is associated with the presence of HTLV-1 genomic sequences (submitted for publication) and in a recent series of 24 French and Portuguese mycosis fungoides and Sézary syndromes, no case was associated with a HTLV infection (Capesius et al., 1991).

In conclusion, establishing a causal relation between retroviruses and cutaneous T cell lymphomas remains a stimulating challenge for which the very powerful molecular biology technology will play a determinant role. This will contribute to a better understanding of the spectrum of human retroviral diseases, unknown just ten years ago, and of their mechanisms. This may encourage the development of new therapeutic modalities, especially concerning CTCL.

REFERENCES

Abel, EA, 1985. Clinical features of cutaneous T cell lymphoma. **Dermatol. Clinics,** 3:647.

Anagnostopoulos I, M Hummel, P Kaudewitz, H Herbst, O Braun-Falco and H Stein, 1990. Detection of HTLV-1 proviral sequences in CD30-positive large cell cutaneous T cell lymphomas. **Am. J. Pathol.,** 137:1317.

Anderson DW, JS Epstein, T-H Lee, MD Lairmore, C Saxinger, VS Kalyanaram, D Slamon, W Parkes, BJ Poiesz, LT Pierik, H Lee, R Montagna, PA Roche, A Williams and W Blattner, 1989. Serological confirmation of human T-lymphotropic virus type I infection in healthy blood and plasma donors. **Blood,** 74: 2585.

Bazarbachi A, F Saal, J Lasneret, L Laroche, F Galibert, J Peries and M-T Daniel, 1991. HTLV-1 like virus infection markers in a patient with Sézary syndrome. In: **"Current issues in human retrovirology: HTLV",** 4th Conference, Jamaica, February 10-13.

Blattner WA, K Takatsuki and RC Gallo, 1983. Human T cell leukemia-lymphoma virus and adult T cell leukemia. **JAMA,** 250: 1074.

Bolton WV, BR Wylie, KG Kenrick, GT Archer, CA Hyland, SL Parker, IF Young, RK Maloney, VA Armstrong, AJ Keller, PW Robertson, 1989. HTLV-I and blood donors. **Lancet,** ii: 1324.

Capesius C, F Saal, E Maero, A Bazarbachi, J Lasneret, L Laroche, A Gessain, F Hojman and J Peries, 1991. No evidence for HTLV-1 infection in 24 cases of French and

Portuguese mycosis fungoides and Sézary syndrome (as seen in France). **Leukemia,** 5:416.

Chan H-L, I-J Su, T-T Kuo, Y-Z Kuan, M-J Chen, L-Y Shih, T Eimoto, Y Maeda, M Kikuchi and M Takeshita, 1985. Cutaneous manifestations of adult T cell leukemia/lymphoma. Report of three different forms. **J. Am. Acad Dermatol.,** 13:213.

Detmar M, G Pauli, I Anagnostopoulos, U Wunderlich, H Herbst, C Garbe, H Stein and CE Orfanos, 1991. A case of classical mycosis fungoides associated with human T cell lymphotropic virus type I. **Brit. J. Dermatol.,** 124:198.

D'Incan M, Y Chardonnet and P Souteyrand, 1992a. Apport des techniques de biologie moléculaire au diagnostic et à l'étude des dermatoses virales. **Ann. Dermatol. Venereol. (Paris),** 119-335.

D'Incan M, P. Souteyrand, YJ Bignon, Y Fonckand H Roger, 1992b. Hydantoin-induced cutaneous pseudolymphoma with clinical, pathologic and immunologic aspects of Sézary syndrome. **Arch Dermatol.,** 128:1371.

Dosaka N, T Tanaka, Y Miyachi, S Imamura and A Kakizuka, 1991. Examination of HTLV-1 integration in the skin lesions of various types of adult T cell leukemia (ATL): independence of cutaneoustype ATL confirmed by southern blot analysis. **J. Invest. Dermatol.,** 96:196.

Edelson RL, 1987. Cutaneous T cell lymphoma. **J. Dermatol.,** 14:397.

Fang CT, AE Williams, SG Sandler, DJ Slamon and BJ Poiesz, 1988. Detection of antibodies to human T-lymphotropic virus type I (HTLV-1). **Transfusion,** 28:179.

Gessain A, F Barrin, JC Vernant, O Gout, L Maurs, A Calender and G De The, 1985. Antibodies to human T-lymphotropic virus type-1 in patients with tropical spastic paraparesis. **Lancet,** ii:40.

Hall WW, CR Liu, O Schneewind, H Takahashi, MH Kaplan, G Roupe and A Vahlne, 1991. Deleted HTLV-1 provirus in blood and cutaneous lesions of patients with mycosis fungoides. **Science,** 253:317.

Haynes BF, M Robert-Guroff, RS Metzgar, G Franchini, VS Kalyanaram, TJ Palker and RC Gallo, 1983. Monoclonal antibody against human T cell leukemia virus p19 defines a human thymic epithelial antigen acquired during ontogeny. **J. Exp. Med.,** 157:907.

Ikai K, T Uchiyama, M Maeda and M Takigawa, 1987. Sézary-like syndrome in a 10-year-old girl with serologic evidence of human Tcell lymphotropic virus type I infection. **Arch. Dermatol.,** 123:1351.

Kaltoft K, S Bisballe, HF Rasmussen, K Thestrup-Pedersen, K Thomsen and W Sterry, 1987. A continuous T cell line from a patient with Sézary syndrome. **Arch. Dermatol., Res.,** 279:293.

Kaltoft K, S Bisballe, HF Rasmussen, K Thestrup-Pedersen, W-H Boehncke, H Volker and W Sterry, 1988. C-type particles are inducible in Se-Ax, a continuous T cell line from a patient with Sézary syndrome. **Arch. Dermatol. Res.,** 280:264.

Kawano F, K Yamaguchi, H Nishimura, H Tsuda and K Takatsuki, 1985. Variation in the clinical courses of adult T cell leukemia. **Cancer,** 55:851.

Lange-Wantzin G, WC Saxinger, A Woods, JK Larsen, K Thomsen and RC Gallo, 1984. Human T cell leukemia virus in cutaneous T cell lymphoma in Denmark. A possible association of HTLV and aneuploidy. **Acta Derm. Venereol. (Stockh.)**, 64:395.

Lange-Wantzin G, K Thomsen, NI Nissen, C Saxinger and RC Gallo, 1986. Occurrence of human T cell lymphotropic virus (type I) antibodies in cutaneous T cell lymphoma. **J. Am. Acad. Dermatol.**, 15:598.

Lessana-Leibowitch M, J Leibowitch, C Frances, B Autran, I Gorin and JP Escande, 1985. Lymphome T pseudo-mycosis fungoides chez un africain associe a un retrovirus HTLV. **Ann. Dermatol. Venereol. (Paris)**, 111:725.

Mac Kie R, 1981. Initial event in mycosis fungoides of the skin is viral infection of epidermal Langerhans cells. **Lancet**, ii:283.

Maeda K, K Yamana, H Takahashi and K Jimbow, 1987. Dual surface markers and HTLV-1 proviral DNA in a cutaneous tumor nodule in a case of adult T cell leukemia/lymphoma. **Brit. J. Dermatol.**, 117:S61.

Manzari V, A Gismondi, G Barillari, S Morrone, A Modesti, L Albonici, L De Marchis, V Fazio, A Gradilone, M Zani, L Frati, and A Santoni, 1987. HTLV-5: a new human retrovirus related in Tac-negative T cell lymphoma /leukemia. **Science**, 238:1581.

Peterman A, M Jerdan, S Staal, B Bender, H Striecher, J Schupbach and L Resnick, 1986. Evidence for HTLV-1 associated with mycosis fungoides and B cell chronic lymphocytic leukemia. **Arch. Dermatol.**, 122:568.

Poiesz BJ, FW Ruscetti, AF Gazdar, PA Bunn, JD Minna and RC Gallo, 1980. Detection and isolation of type C retrovirus particles from fresh and cultured lymphocytes of a patient with cutaneous T cell lymphoma. **Proc. Natl. Acad. Sci. (USA).**, 77:7415.

Poiesz BJ, FW Ruscetti, MS Reitz, VS Kalyanaram and RC Gallo, 1981. Isolation of a new type C retrovirus (HTLV) in primary uncultured cells of a patient with Sézary T cell leukaemia. **Nature**, 294:268.

Ranki A and K Krohn, 1987. Cross-reacting antibodies to gag proteins of HTLV-1 and HTLV-3 in patients with mycosis fungoides or its prodrome, large-plaque parapsoriasis. In:"Viruses and human cancer", R.C. Gallo, W. Haseltine, G. Nein and H. Zur Hausen, Eds: Alan R. Liss; New York, p. 43. Ranki A, E Johansson and K Krohn, 1988. Interpretation of antibodies reacting solely with human retroviral core proteins. **N. Enql. J. Med.**, 318: 448.

Ranki A, K-M Niemi, P Niemi and K Krohn, 1990. Antibodies against retroviral core proteins in relation to disease outcome in patients with mycosis fungoides. **Arch. Dermatol. Res.**, 282:532.

Sahai Srivastava BI, C Gonzales, R Loftus, JE Fitzpatrick and CW Saxinger, 1990. Examination of HTLV-1 ELISA-positive leukemia/lymphoma patients by western blotting gave mostly negative or indeterminate reaction, In: **AIDS Research and Human Retroviruses, volume 6:** MA Liebert, Inc., p. 617.

Saxinger WC, G Lange-Wantzin, K Thomsen, M Hoh and RC Gallo, 1985. Occurrence of HTLV-1 antibodies in Danish patients with cutaneous T cell lymphoma. **Scand. J. Haematol.**, 34:455.

Slater D, S Bleehen, N Rooney and A Hamed, 1983. Type C retrovirus particles in mycosis fungoides. **Brit. J. Dermatol.**, 109:120.

Slater D, N Rooney, S Bleehen and A Hamed, 1985. The lymph node in mycosis fungoides: A light and electron microscopic and immunohistological study supporting the Langerhans' cell retrovirus infection hypothesis. **Histopathology**, 9:687.

Souteyrand P and M D'Incan, 1990. Drug-induced mycosis fungoides-like lesions. In: **"Current problems in dermatology, volume XIX: Cutaneous lymphomas"**. WA Van Vloten, R Willemze R, G Lange Vejlsgaard, K Thomsen, Eds.: Karger, p. 176.

Takahashi K, T Tanaka, M Fujita, Y Horiguchi, Y Miyachi and S Imamura, 1988. Cutaneous-type adult T cell leukemia/lymphoma. A unique clinical feature with monoclonal T cell proliferation detected by southern blot analysis. **Arch. Dermatol.**, 124:399.

Takatsuki K, 1989. Adult T cell leukemia (ATL): An overview. In: **"HTLV-1 and the nervous system"**, Alan R Liss, Inc., New York; p. 57.

Takigawa M, F Inoue, K Iwatsuki and M Yamada, 1988. Does adult Tcell leukemia/lymphoma belong to the cutaneous T cell lymphoma category? **J. Am. Acad. Dermatol.**, 18:379.

Uchiyama T, J Ydoi, K Sagawa, K Takatsuki and H Uchino, 1977. Adult T cell leukemia: clinical and hematological features of 16 cases. **Blood**, 50:481.

Van der Loo EM, GNP Van Muijen, WA Van Vloten, W Beens, E Scheffer and CJML Meijer, 1979. C-type virus-like particles specifically localized in Langerhans cells and related cells of skin and lymph node of patients with mycosis fungoides and Sézary's syndrome. A morphological and biochemical study. **Virchows Arch. B Cell Path.**, 31:193.

Waldmann TA, WC Greene and PS Sarin, 1984. Functional and phenotypic comparison of human T cell leukemia/lymphoma virus positive adult T cell leukemia with human T cell leukemia/lymphoma virus negative Sézary leukemia, and their distinction using antiTac monoclonal antibody identifying the human receptor for T cell growth factor. **J. Clin. Invest.**, 73:1711.

Watanabe T, M Seiki and M Yoshida, 1984. HTLV type I (US isolate) and ATLV (Japanese isolate) are the same species of human retrovirus. **Virology**, 133:238.

Whittemore AS, EA Holly, I-M Lee, EA Abel, RM Adams, BJ Nickoloff, L Bley, JM Peters and C Gibney, 1989. Mycosis fungoides in relation to environmental exposures and immune response: a case-control study. **J. Natl. Cancer Inst.**, 81:1560.

Wong-Staal F and RC Gallo, 1985. Human T lymphotropic retroviruses. **Nature**, 317:395.

Yamada Y, 1983. Phenotypic and functional analysis of leukemic cells from 16 patients with adult T cell leukemia/lymphoma. **Blood**, 61:192.

Yamaguchi K, H Nishimura, H Kohrogi, M Jono, Y Miyamoto and K Takatsuki, 1983. A proposal for smoldering adult T cell leukemia: a clinicopathologic study of five cases. **Blood**, 62:758.

Zackheim HS, 1981. Cutaneous T cell lymphomas. A review of the recent literature. **Arch. Dermatol.**, 117:295.

Zambruno G, L Mori, A Marconi, N Mongiardo, B De Rienzo, V Bertazzoni and A Giannetti, 1991. Detection of HIV-1 in epidermal Langerhans cells of HIV-1 infected patients using the polymerase chain reaction. **J. Invest. Dermatol.**, 96:979.

HTLV-1 PROVIRAL SEQUENCES IN CUTANEOUS CD30-POSITIVE T LARGE CELL LYMPHOMAS

Peter Kaudewitz*
Iannis Anagnostopoulos†
Michael Hummel†
Harald Stein†

*   Department of Dermatology
University of Munich
Germany

†   Steglitz Medical Center
Free University of Berlin
Berlin, Germany

Correspondence to: Dr. P. Kaudewitz, Department of Dermatology,
University Hospital, Frauenlobstrasse 9-11,
D-8000 Munchen, Germany

ABSTRACT

The goal of this study was to elucidate a possible implication of HTLV-1 in non-epidemic T cell lymphomas. Six patients with primary and secondary CD30$^+$ T large cell lymphomas, and four patients with small cell cutaneous T cell lymphomas (CTCL), were investigated for the presence of HTLV-1 related DNA sequences. Southern blot hybridization and enzymatic DNA amplification (PCR) revealed incomplete HTLV-1-specific sequences in all large cell lymphomas examined. In the small cell CTCL examined these sequences could not be detected. Our results suggest that HTLV-1 may be closely associated with a proportion of cutaneous T large cell lymphomas.

Basic Mechanisms of Physiologic and Aberrant Lymphoproliferation in the Skin
Edited by W.C. Lambert *et al.*, Plenum Press, New York, 1994

195

INTRODUCTION

The pathogenesis of nonendemic cutaneous T cell lymphoma is largely unknown. Several hypotheses have been put forward to explain the process of malignant transformation of dermotropic T cells. Among these, viral infection, specifically viral infection of Langerhans cells, was suggested over a decade ago (MacKie, 1981). The hypothesis that a virus may also be involved in the development of nonendemic T cell lymphoma has been revitalized by two important findings: First, antibodies against HTLV-1 related antigens are present in the serum of approximately 10% of patients with nonendemic CTCL (Saxinger et al., 1985, Lange-Wantzin, 1986). Second, the clinical and histological features of endemic HTLV-1-positive adult T cell lymphoma (ATL), especially of the so-called smoldering form, are similar, to a certain extent, to those observed in nonendemic CTCL (Takatsuki et al., 1982).

The percentage of HTLV-1 seropositive cases within larger series of patients with non-endemic CTCL varies from 1% (Gallo et al., 1983) to 12% (Lange-Wantzin et al., 1986). Although HTLV-1 seropositivity and HTLV-1 infection do not strictly correlate, the low proportion of positive patients with CTCL indicates that non-endemic CTCL is a heterogeneous group with respect to HTLV-1 involvement. The observed clinicopathologic spectrum of CTCL (Kaudewitz and Braun-Falco, 1991) allows the possibilty that only certain types of CTCL are associated with HTLV-1.

Most previous serologic studies have either concentrated on small cell variants of CTCL or failed to detail the clinicopathologic subtypes. We therefore searched for a possible involvement of HTLV-1 in a small series of cutaneous T large cell lymphomas with special emphasis on CD30-positive cases. Uncertainties of serologic detection methods to implicate HTLV-1 were overcome by the use of a molecular biologic approach to demonstrate presence of HTLV-1 proviral DNA sequences within tumor lesions of the patients.

MATERIALS AND METHODS

Ten patients with cutaneous T cell lymphoma were studied. Biopsies from lesional skin and one lymph node were bisected and one half was snap frozen in liquid nitrogen and stored at -70 C. The remaining half was fixed in formalin and processed for routine histological evaluation.

In 5 patients, the cutaneous infiltrate was composed of large tumor cells with some variaton in tumor cell morphology from case to case. In the remaining patients, the skin was predominantly infiltrated by small atypical lymphoid cells. Based on these findings, evaluated in conjunction with the clinical history and presentation, the diagnosis of mycosis fungoides was made in four of these cases and one patient was diagnosed as having Sézary syndrome. The diagnosis of classical mycosis fungoides was revised in one of the four cases after a six month clinical follow-up because of detection of endemic HTLV-1 in the home area of the patient

(Meytes et al., 1990). Staging of all patients was performed according to the recommendations of the EORTC cutaneous lymphoma study group. The clinical features of all of the patients are summarized in Table 1.

Immunophenotyping of skin infiltrates and lymph nodes were performed as described previously (Kaudewitz et al., 1989). High molecular weight DNA was extracted from skin and lymph node biopsies. Frozen tissue samples were crushed and digested with proteinase K in Tris buffer containig EDTA, NaCl and SDS. After phenol/chloroform extraction, 15 μg of DNA was digested to completion by the restriction enzymes, BamHI, EcoRI and HindIII, electrophoresed on an $>0.8\%$ agarose gel and transferred to a Hybond membrane. The size fractionated DNA was then hybridized with TCR β probe labelled with ^{32}P by the random primer DNA labelling method. The same blots were hybridized with complete HTLV-1 probe (p23-3i, obtained from Dr. R.C. Gallo) labelled by the same procedure. The membranes were washed under conditions of high stringency at 67°C for 40 minutes in a solution of 0.2x standard saline/citrate containing 0.1% SDS.

Table 1. Clinical features of CD30$^+$ large cell CTCL

Case	Age	Sex	Duration of disease	TNM stage	
1	51	F	2 months	Ia	$(T_1N_0B_0M_0)$
2	16	M	2 months	IIb	$(T_3N_0B_0M_0)$
3	50	F	1 month	IIb	$(T_3N_0B_0M_0)$
4	79	M	48 months	IIb	$(T_3N_0B_0M_0)$
5	63	M	168 months	IIb	$(T_3N_1B_0M_0)$
6	72	M	8 months	IVa	$(T_3N_3B_0M_0)$
7	67	F	240 months	IVa	$(T_3N_3B_0M_0)$
8	24	M	3 months	IVa	$(T_3N_3B_0M_0)$
9	35	F	60 months	IVa	$(T_3N_3B_1M_0)$
10	76	M	72 months	IVa	$(T_3N_3B_1M_0)$

DNA prepared from the HTLV-1 positive cell line Hut102 and from lymph node biopsies of T and B cell non-Hodgkin lymphomas was used as controls.

To further obtain evidence for a possible role of HTLV-1, especially in cutaneous T large cell lymphomas, 1 μg of DNA extracted from skin lesions was used for enzymatic amplification of HTLV-1 proviral sequences by PCR. The primer pair used recognized sequences located 391 base pairs apart in the pol gene of HTLV-1. They are complementary (primer coding sense 5'-

AACCCAGTATTCCCAGTTAA-3') to bases 2702-2721 and (primer anticoding sense 5'-AGAATGTCATCCATGTACTG-3') to bases 3074-3093 of the HTLV-1 genome. Twenty pmol of each primer was added to 10 μl of a buffer containing 50 mM KCL, 2.5 mM MgCl$_2$, 10 mM TRIS buffer (pH 8.3), 200 μM each dTNPs and 2.5 units Taq polymerase. After initial denaturation at 94°C for 5 minutes, 30 cycles of denaturation at 94°C for 1 minute, annealing at 57°C for 30 seconds and extension at 72°C for 30 seconds were carried out. An aliquot of each amplification product was analyzed by electrophoresis on a 2% agarose minigel stained with ethidium bromide. DNA from the HTLV-1-negative cell lines U937, U266, and L428 was used as negative controls.

In all cases analyzed for presence of HTLV-1-related DNA sequences, T cell antigen receptor (TCR) β chain configuration indicated a monoclonal T cell proliferation, shown by the presence of an additional band distinguishable from the germ line pattern. Based on this result, interpreted in conjunction with histological and clinical data, the cutaneous infiltrates analyzed are therefore regarded as cutaneous T cell lymphomas.

Evidence for the presence of HTLV-1 related DNA sequences in a proportion of these cases was first obtained from Southern blot hybridization (Figure 1). Five cases gave a positive hybridization result. In only one patient, however, could a band greater than 9 kb, indicating hybridization with the complete HTLV-1 genome, be detected. Despite the use of the EcoRI enzyme, which does not cleave within the proviral DNA sequence, the remaining four positive cases showed smaller bands, ranging from 4 to 6 kb.

In all five cases positive with Southern blot analysis, and in one additional case, an amplification product of the expected size could be obtained using PCR for the detection of pol sequences. Amplification of DNA from control cell lines and from the morphologicaly unsuspicious lymph node did not produce any DNA fragment detectable on agarose minigels (Figure 2).

These results indicate that, in a proportion of patients investigated, HTLV-1 related DNA sequences are detectable in lesional skin biopsies. This is similar to the results of serologic studies performed on a larger series of patients at the DNA level; HTLV-1 was also detectable in only a subgroup of cutaneous T cell lymphomas. It was therefore of interest to correlate the clinical, histological, and immunophenotypical features of our patients with results obtained from molecular biologic studies.

Except for one case, all patients presented with tumorous skin infiltrates at the time of biopsy. Among these, four patients also had coexisting patches and plaques. In five patients the initial skin lesions consisted of isolated or regionally grouped tumors of varying size that had developed during considerably brief intervals. One patient had erythroderma with more pronounced plaques in the axillary region.

Morphologically, the cutaneous infiltrates in patients with coexisting patches and plaques, or with erythroderma, were composed of small to medium-sized atypical cells with varying degrees of nuclear indentation and finely dispersed chromatin. A varying proportion of small atypical cells with hyperchromatic nuclei was regularly found (Figure 3). The types of atypical cells we have described completely infiltrated the dermis in a nodular growth pattern. In one patient, tumors coexisting with patches and plaques were found to be exclusively of large atypical cells that had rounded nuclei and prominent nucleoli.

Immunohistochemically, the vast majority of infiltrating cells in patients with coexisting patches and plaques was consistently found to express CD3, CD4, and T cell receptor β.

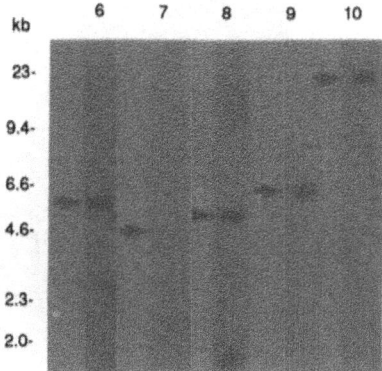

Figure 1. Southern blot analysis of the six cutaneous T cell lymphoma cases (6-10) that gave a positive hybridization result (arrowed) with the HTLV-1 probe labeled with (^{32}P)dCTP. The genomic DNA was digested with EcoRI. A band greater than 9 kb, thus representing copies of the complete HTLV-1 genome, was detected only in case 10. All other HTLV-1-positive cases showed smaller bands, probably stemming from defective HTLV-1. (reprinted from Anagnostopoulos et al., 1990).

Activation antigens, such as CD25 and CD30, were detectable on only a few intermingled cells, with the exception of one case in which the lesion was comprised entirely of CD30 positive tumor cells.

In each of these cases, the diagnosis of advanced stage mycosis fungoides was based on a combined assessment of clinical presentation, histomorphology, immuno-phenotype and T cell antigen receptor status. The case which presented with tumorous infiltrates composed primarily of CD30 positive large atypical cells was categorized as mycosis fungoides which had transformed into large cell anaplastic lymphoma. In those patients that had developed isolated or regionally grouped tumors, these tumors were composed of large atypical cells with abundant cytoplasm and rounded to kidney shaped nuclei with vesicular chromatin and one or multiple prominent nucleoli (Figure 4). Considerable numbers of small atypical cells were not detectable. In two of these cases the large atypical cells produced a rather monotonous histomorphological appearance, whereas in the remaining two the atypical cells were smaller, more pleomorphic and often multinucleated. These latter cases were categorized as CD30 positive cutaneous T large cell lymphoma. In the Kiel classification these correspond to large cell anaplastic lymphoma.

HTLV-1 related sequences were only detected in the large cell anaplastic CD30 positive type of cutaneous T cell lymphoma. In the small cell variants of mycosis fungoides and in the

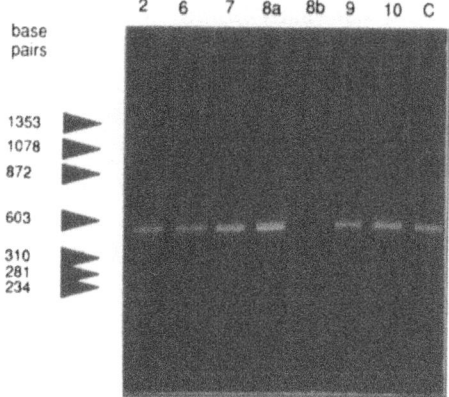

Figure 2. PCR DNA amplificates that could be detected with HTLV-1-specific primers in cases 2 and 6 to 10, as well as in the positive control (Lane C), which is DNA from the HTLV-1⁺ cell line, HUT102. Analysis was performed on 2% agarose gels stained with ethidium bromide. As indicated in the left-hand margin, ΦX174 DNA digested with HaeIII served as a standard. Two samples were investigated from case 8: one from the skin tumor (8a) and one from the uninvolved lymph node (8b). Only DNA from the skin tumor yielded an amplificate. (reprinted from Anagnostopoulos et al., 1990).

Sézary syndrome, no evidence for an implication of HTLV-1 could be obtained. Although the number of patients investigated is rather small, our results support the concept that HTLV-1 may be associated with certain types of CTCL, especially CD30 positive T large cell lymphoma.

DISCUSSION

The frequency of the observed association is as yet unclear. There is accumulating evidence for the presence of HTLV-1-related proviral sequences in a small proportion of patients with CTCL. D'Incan et al. (1990) described the detection of HTVL-1 retroviral sequences in a patient with mycosis fungoides. Hall and coworkers (1991) obtained a positive hybridization signal with complete HTLV-1 probe and EcoRI digested DNA from cultured peripheral blood B lymphocytes of a patient with CTCL. The band obtained, however, was considerably smaller than the expected 9 kb, similar to our results. When lesional skin biopsies were investigated by PCR for various HTLV-1-specific regions, these were demonstrable in all five patients. Only one patient contained sequences from all four major proviral regions and the pattern of detectable regions was different in each of the four remaining patients. Cultured peripheral blood

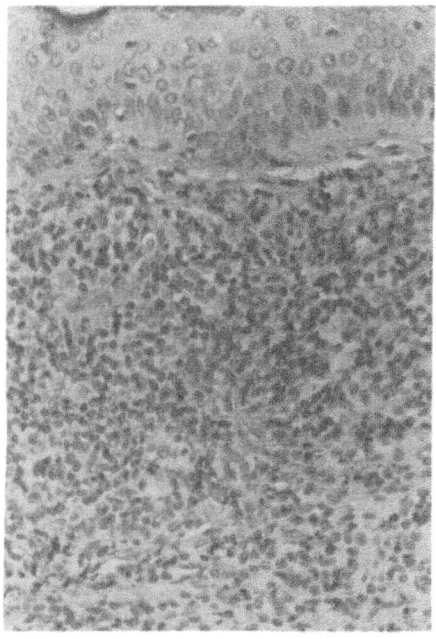

Figure 3. Small cell infiltrates in a HTLV-1-negative case of mycosis fungoides.

lymphocytes from patients with CTCL were also used by Zucker-Franklin (1991) to search for pol region proviral sequences. These were found in 3 of 9 patients. Other investigators completely failed to detect any HTLV-1-associated DNA fragments in 27 patients with CTCL (Chadburn et al., 1991). From the study of Hall et al., and from our work it may be concluded that integration of the complete proviral DNA is rarely found in non-endemic CTCL. Instead, fragments of varying size and from varying regions are detectable in an as yet undefined proportion of patients with CTCL. These findings have been interpreted to indicate the presence of truncated or deleted proviral sequences, most likely derived from HTLV-1 provirus. The

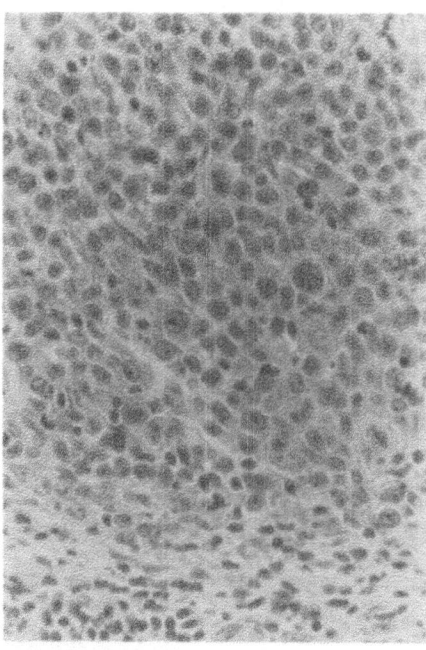

Figure 4. Large atypical tumor cells from a case positive for HTLV-1 proviral sequences.

precise nature of this virus remains to be determined. DNA sequence analysis of the hybridizing DNA fragment obtained by Hall et al. revealed large deletions and a number of single base pair mutations, thus further supporting the above conclusions.

Hall et al. (1991) also demonstrated that mutations in the expected HTLV-1-related sequences may occur. Although their extent is unclear, detection of such mutant sequences may become difficult when using HTLV-1 specific probes and may account for some of the negative cases reported. We currently have neither a sound pathogenic concept, nor definite treatment modalities, for CTCL. Continuing to search for an implicated viral agent may improve our position in both respects.

REFERENCES

Agnagnostopoulos I, M Hummel, P Kaudewitz, H Herbst, O Braun-Falco and H Stein, 1990. Detection of HTLV-1 proviral sequences in CD30-positive large cell cutaneous T cell lymphoma (Rapid Communication). **Am. J. Pathol.**, 137:1317.

Chadburn A, E Athan, R Wleczorek and DM Knowles, 1991. Detection and characterisation of human T cell lymphotropic virus type I (HTLV-1) associated T cell neoplasms in an HTLV-1 non endemic region by polymerase chain reaction, **Blood**, 77:2419.

D'Incan M, YJ Bignon, P Souteyrand, PH Roger, HN Rance and NB Dastugue, 1990. Polymerase chain reaction (PCR) detection of an HTLV-1 DNA sequence in the genome of cutaneous T cell lymphoma (CTCL) patients, **J. Invest. Dermatol.**, 94:393 (Abstr).

Gallo RC, VS Kalyanaraman, MG Sarngadharan, A Sliski, EC Vonderheid, M Maeda, Y Nakao, K Yamada, Y Ito, N Gutensohn, S Murphy, PA Bunn, D Catovsky, MF Greaves, DW Blayney, W Blattner, WF Jarrett, H zur Hausen, M Seligmann, JC Brouet, BF Haynes, BV Jegasothy, E Jaffe, J Cossman, S Broder, RI Fisher, DW Golde and M Robert-Guroff, 1983. Association of the human type C retrovirus with a subset of adult T cell cancers, **Cancer Res.**, 43:3892.

Hall WW, RC Liu, O Schneewind, H Takahasi, MH Kaplan, XX Riupe and A Vahlne, 1991. Deleted HTLV-1 provirus in blood and cutaneous lesions of patients with mycosis fungoides, **Science**, 253:317.

Kaudewitz P and O Braun-Falco, 1991. Malignant cutaneous lymphomas, In: RH Champion and RJ Pye, Eds., **Recent Advances in Dermatology**, Churchill Livingstone, Edinburgh, London.

Kaudewitz P, H Stein, U Dallenbach, F Eckert, K Bieber, G Burg and O Braun-Falco, 1989. Primary and secondary cutaneous Ki-1+ (CD30+) anaplastic large cell lymphomas, **Am. J. Pathol.**, 135:359.

Lange-Wantzin G, K Thomsen, NJ Nissen, C Saxinger and RC Gallo, 1986. Occurrence of human lymphotropic virus (type I) antibodies in cutaneous T cell lymphoma, **J. Am. Acad. Dermatol.**, 15:598.

MacKie R, 1981. Initial event in mycosis fungoides is viral infection of epidermal Langerhans cells. **Lancet**, ii:283.

Meytes D, B Schochat, H Lee, G Nadel, Y Sidi, M Cerney, P Swanson, M Shaklai, Y Kilim and M Elgat, 1990. Serological and molecular survey for HTLV-1 infection in a high-risk Middle Eastern group, **Lancet**, 336:1533.

Poiesz BJ, FW Ruszetti, VS Kalyanaraman and RC Gallo, 1981. Isolation of a new type C retrovirus (HTLV-1) in primary uncultured cells of a patient with Sézary T cell leukemia, **Nature**, 294:268.

Rattner L and BJ Poiesz, 1988. Leukemias associated with human T cell lymphotropic virus type I in a non-endemic region, **Medicine**, 67:401.

Saxinger WC, GL Wantzin, K Thomsen, M Hoh and RC Gallo, 1985. Occurrence of HTLV-1 antibodies in Danish patients with cutaneous T cell lymphoma, **Scand. J. Haematol.**, 34:455.

Takatsuki K, T Uchimaya, Y Ueshima, T Hattori, T Topibana, M Tsudo, Y Wano and J Yodoi, 1982. Adult T cell leukemia: Proposal as a new disease and cytogenic, phenotypic and functional studies of leukemic cells, **GANN Monograph. Cancer Res.**, 28:13.

von der Helm D, K von der Helm, G Burg, O Braun-Falco and F Deinhardt, 1988. Antikorper gegen HTLV-1 bei T lymphoproliferativen Erkrankungen der Haut, **Hautarzt**, 39:348.

Zucker-Franklin D, EE Coutavas, MG Rush and DC Zouzias, 1991. Detection of human T-lymphotrophic virus-like particles in cultures of peripheral blood lymphocytes from patients with mycosis fungoides, **Proc. Natl. Acad. Sci. USA**, 88:7630.

Yoshida T, M Kikuchi, K Oshima, M Takeshita, N Kimura, M Kozura and H Sato, 1989. Anti-human T cell lymphotropic virus type I antibody positive adult T cell leukemia/lymphoma with no monoclonal proviral DNA, **Cancer**. 64:2515.

PRESENCE OF EPSTEIN-BARR VIRAL DNA AND EBV LATENT GENE PRODUCTS IN HODGKIN AND NON-HODGKIN LYMPHOMA: HIGH EXPRESSION OF EBV-DNA SEQUENCES IN NON-HODGKIN LYMPHOMA WITH VARIABLE NUMBERS OF CD30-POSITIVE CELLS

C. J. L. M. Meijer[*]

P. Kanavaros[*]

N. N. Jiwa[*]

R. Willemze[†]

P. C. de Bruin[*]

J. M. M. Walboomers[*]

[*] Department of Pathology

[†] Department of Dermatology

Free University Hospital

Amsterdam, The Netherlands

Correspondence to: Dr. C.J.L.M. Meijer, Department of Pathology,

University Hospital, de Boelelaan 1117,

1081 HV Amsterdam, The Netherlands

INTRODUCTION

Epstein-Barr Virus (EBV) is a human DNA-gamma herpesvirus. The EBV genome consists of double stranded DNA of approximately 175 kb. It has two configurations: linear and episomal. The DNA consists of 4 internal repeats (IR 1-4) and the terminal repeat. IR1 is also known as the "large internal repeat". Furthermore, the genome has 5 unique domains (U 1-5). The DNA encodes for about 100 different genes, but expression of only a limited number of genes has been investigated in vitro and in vivo. Localization of the major latent genes on the EBV genome has been described elsewhere (Sample and Kieff, 1991). EBV has a particular propensity for infecting B lymphocytes. EBV is able to transform and induce cell proliferation

Basic Mechanisms of Physiologic and Aberrant Lymphoproliferation in the Skin
Edited by W.C. Lambert *et al.*, Plenum Press, New York, 1994

205

of these cells. Although about 80 - 100% of the adult population is infected by EBV, this primary infection is mainly asymptomatic. Several clinical entities have been associated with EBV, however; infectious mononucleosis and endemic Burkitt lymphoma are examples. Futhermore, particular forms of nasopharyngeal carcinoma, hairy leukoplakia in patients suffering from AIDS and B cell lymphoproliferative diseases in immuno-compromised patients, i.e., AIDS and transplant recipients, have been suggested to be associated with EBV. In non-immuno-compromised patients the pathogenesis of EBV related lymphoproliferative diseases is obscure. In the present study we survey data concerning the presence of EBV, at the DNA, RNA and protein levels, in Hodgkin and non Hodgkin lymphomas in non-immuno-compromised individuals and its possible role in the pathogenesis of this group of diseases.

MATERIALS AND METHODS

It is not our intention to describe all techniques used for demonstrating EBV at the DNA, RNA and protein level. Therefore one is referred to more specific studies (Hamilton-Dutoit et al., 1991; Masih et al., 1991; Brocksmith et al., 1990; Bashir et al., 1989; Ukara et al., 1990). Here we will discuss: (i) DNA detection methods: Southern blot (SB) analysis and the polymerase chain reaction (PCR); (ii) DNA/RNA in situ hybridization (DNA, RNA in situ hybridization, DISH, RISH); and (iii) Detection of EBV associated antigens by use of immunohistochemistry: Southern blot analysis has been used for two different purposes. First, before PCR became available, SB was used for detection of EBV genomic sequences in different lymphoproliferative disorders (Weiss et al., 1987). In nearly all studies the large internal repeat (BamHI W fragment) has been used. This sequence is normally present one to ten times in each viral genome. Furthermore, SB can be used for the detection of episomal EBV (clonal or non-clonal) or for the detection of linear genome (non-clonal). This is done by specific hybridization with the terminal repeat (XhoI 1.9 kb fragment) as a probe. As a very sensitive EBV-DNA detection method, the PCR can be used. This method has been applied by several authors; they were able to detect EBV genomic sequences in both non-Hodgkin (both B cell and T cell) and Hodgkin lymphomas (Weiss et al., 1989; Uhara et al., 1990; Kanavaros et al., 1992, 1993; Su et al., 1991). Because PCR is a non-morphological technique, no differentation can be made between the presence of EBV in neoplastic cells or in latently infected cells (Brocksmith et al., 1991). Although DISH, using the BamH1 W fragment, is probably less sensitive than PCR, it has the advantage that cells harboring EBV can be identified. Several authors have claimed that RISH using small EBV encoded RNA probes (EBER 1 and 2) is more sensitive than DISH. EBER 1 and 2 expression can be detected in both Hodgkin and non-Hodgkin lymphomas (Wu et al., 1990) and in certain nasopharyngeal carcinoma (Wu et al., 1991). At this moment it is not clear whether all lymphoproliferative disorders harboring the EBV genome express EBER 1 and 2. It is known that another EBV related disease, hairy leukoplakia, does not express EBER 1 (Gilligan et al., 1990). It has been supposed that EBER expression is down-regulated in lytic infections. The most important antigens of EBV are the Epstein Barr nuclear antigens (EBNA) 1 - 6, and the latent membrane proteins (LMP) 1 and 2, which are all latent antigens, the 'ZEBRA protein' (so called switch protein, turning a latent infection into a productive infection; the BZLF fragment) and the replicative antigens: the early antigens (EA) and viral capsid antigen (VCA). At this moment monoclonal antibodies against EBNA 2, LMP 1, ZEBRA, EA and VCA are available.

Relation of EBV and the Expression of Cellular Genes in vitro

EBV infections may cause major changes in the expression of cellular genes in vitro. A brief overview is given in Table 1.

Table 1. Relation between EBV and the expression of cellular genes in vitro

Function	Role of EBV Mediated by	References
- upregulation/induction of the activation marker, CD30	infection	Stein et al., 1985
- upregulation of the B cell activation marker, CD23	LMP/EBNA-2	Wang et al., 1987 Cordier et al., 1990
- upregulation of CD21 (the 'EBV receptor')	EBNA-2	Cohen et al., 1987 Cordier et al.,1990
- upregulation of certain cellular adhesion molecules, like LFA-1, ICAM-1 and LFA-3	LMP-1	Wang et al., 1988
- induction/upregulation of cellular (proto-)oncogenes:		
bcl-2	LMP-1	Henderson et al., 1991
c-myc	infection	Alfieri et al., 1991
c-fgr	EBNA-2	Knutson, 1990

Although the mechanisms are poorly understood, the LMP-1 and EBNA-2 seem to be involved in the upregulation of the B cell marker, CD21 (also known as EBV receptor) and B cell activation marker, CD23. Moreover, LMP-1 is also involved in the induction/upregulation of the proto-oncogene, bcl-2, whereas EBNA-2 increases the level of mRNA of c-fgr in vitro. It is unknown whether these mechanisms are important for in vivo infections.

In the present paper, the following techniques were used: PCR procedure: the PCR was performed on purified DNA of snap frozen tissue specimens. To see whether the suitable DNA was present, β globin PCR was performed using specific primers as described by Saiki et al (1985). The PCR mixture consisted of 15 ng purified DNA of clinical sample or the product of dewaxed tissue, 10 mM Tris HCl pH 9.6, 15 mM MgCl$_2$, 1.5 mM KCl, 1 mM dNTPs, 50 pM β globin or EBV specific primers and 1 unit Taq DNA polymerase (Perkin and Elmer, Emmeryville, California). Forty cycles of amplification were performed using a PCR processor (Biomed, Germany). Each cycle included a denaturation step (one minute at 95° C) and a primer annealing/extension step (three minutes at 60° C). After gel electrophoresis (20% of the sample), only the samples showing a strong band of 110 base-pairs were selected for the EBV-PCR. Primers of the BamHI W fragment (large internal repeat) of the EBS B95.8 strain were used. They span a length of 240 base-pairs and recognize at least 100 different EBV isolates (Jiwa and Gratama, personal communication). Primer A (sense) consisted of 5'-CTCTGGTAGTGATTTGGGCCC-3' and primer B (antisense) of 5-GTGAAGTCACAAACAAGCCC-3'. A third internal oligonucleotide was used for hybridization procedures.

DNA in situ hybridization Probes: a large internal repeat of 3.1 kb (BamHI W fragment) of the EBV B95.8 strain and a 5 kb EcoRI EBV fragment (Kreatech, Amsterdam) were biotinylated with Bio 11 dUTP (BRL, Gaitingburg) by random primer labeling. The DNA in situ hybridization protocol is described elsewhere (Merchenthaler et al. 1989; Mullink et al., 1989; 1992). Briefly: paraffin embedded material was deparaffinized. Peroxidases were blocked with 1% H$_2$O$_2$-methanol for 30 minutes and material was digested in 0.1% proteinase K in 0.05 mM Tris HCl pH 7.6 containing 5 mM EDTA for various times. Hybridization was performed using 1 ng probe/μl. Hybridization mixture consisted of 50% formamide, 2 times SSC, 10 times Denhart's solution, 10% dextran sulphate, 250 mg/ml sheared salmon sperm DNA. After hybridization, the biotinylated hybrid was detected by a multilayer immunohistochemical detection system, which consisted of a monoclonal anti-biotin antibody, a biotinylated goat anti-rabbit antibody followed by streptavidin HRP. The peroxidase was visualized by incubation for 5 minutes in 0.2 mg/ml DAB, 0.002% H$_2$O$_2$ and 0.07% NiCl$_2$ in 50 mM Tris HCl, pH 7.6. Nickel was finally silver enhanced as described elsewhere (Merchentaler et al., 1989; Mullink et al., 1992).

RESULTS AND DISCUSSION

Morbus Hodgkin

An association between Hodgkin disease and EBV has been suggested from different studies. First, patients with Hodgkin disease have increased titers of EBV-associated antigens

(Mueller, 1987). Second, there seems to be an increased risk of getting Hodgkin disease after mononucleosis infectiosa (Munoz et al., 1978). Moreover, several studies have shown that, in about half of cases, EBV-DNA sequences can be demonstrated in lymphoid tissues afflicted with

Table 2. EBV in Hodgkin disease, non-Hodgkin lymphomas and reactive lymphoid hyperplasia

	PCR+	DISH+L	MP+
CD30+ B-NHL (n=38)			
cb/cc	4/6	2/6	0/6
cb	21/26	14/23*	4/26
immunoblastic	2/2	2/2	1/2
LCAL	4/4	1/3	0/3
TOTAL	31/38 (82%)	19/34 (56%)	5/37 (14%)
CD30+ T-NHL (n=5)			
pleom M/L	4/4	2/4	1/4
LCAL	5/12	4/12	1/12
TOTAL	9/16 (56%)	6/16 (37.5%)	2/16 (20%)
CD30⁻ B NHL (n=22)			
cb/cc	2/6	0/6	0/6
immunocytoma polymorphic	1/5	1/5	0/5
cb pleomorphic	2/11	0/10	0/10
TOTAL	5/22 (22%)	1/21(5%)	0/21 (0%)
CD30⁻ T NHL (n=1)			
AILD	1/1	0/1	0/1
Hodgkin disease NS (n=25)	14/25 (56%)	10/19**	9/25 (36%)
Reactive lymphoid hyperplasia	12/50 (24%)	0/7	0/10

*3 EBV-PCR negative cases of cb and
**6 EBV PCR negative cases of Hodgkin disease were not tested for DISH CD30+ NHL: non-Hodgkin lymphomas with variable numbers of CD30+ cells. Only in large cell anaplastic lymphoma, 2-80% of the neoplastic cells showed CD30. EBV-DISH was never positive in EBV-PCR negative cases.

Hodgkin disease. Using DISH, several authors have shown that the EBV genome is mainly present in Reed-Sternberg cells and their mononuclear variants (Agnostopoulos et al., 1989; Weiss et al., 1989; Libetta et al., 1990; Mullink et al., 1992; Karameris et al. 1992). Recently, our group has confirmed these findings (Table 2, Jiwa et al., 1992). The strong association between the presence of EBV and Hodgkin disease suggests that EBV may have a pathogenic role in at least a number of Hodgkin cases. Recently, demonstration of LMP-1 in Reed-Sternberg cells and their mononuclear variants by Pallesen et al (1991; Table 2) has further strengthened this hypothesis. The exact way that EBV exerts its putative oncogenic role is unknown. It is widely accepted that EBV requires the C3-d receptor (CD21 antigen or a receptor which can be demonstrated by cross-reaction with the anti-CD21 antibody (Young et al., 1989; Thomas et al., 1989) in order to infect permissive cells. Therefore, it was not unexpected that we could demonstrate a relationship between the presence of EBV-DNA in Reed-Sternberg cells and CD21 antigen expression by these cells, although this finding was not absolute. Thus, 9 of 12 EBV positive cases of Hodgkin disease expressed the CD21 antigen, versus one of 12 EBV negative cases of Hodgkin disease. Whether the Reed-Sternberg cells and their precursors already expressed the CD21 antigen, by which EBV could infect these cells, or whether these cells expressed upregulated CD21 antigen after EBV infection, as can be shown in vitro, remains unsolved (Cohen et al., 1987; Cordier et al., 1990). The upregulation of CD30 by EBV in CD30 negative lymphoblastoid cell lines, and the immortalizing effect of LMP on EBV infected cells, argue for a pathogenic role for EBV in Hodgkin disease, since both CD30 and LMP-1 are expressed on Reed-Steinberg cells. Several observations argue for a limited role for EBV in the pathogenesis of Hodgkin disease, however:

i) In a recent study Coates et al. (1991) described for the first time the presence of EBV-DNA sequences in reactive lymphocytes in Hodgkin disease.

ii) Using a very sensitive RISH, Khan et al. (1992) were able to demonstrate the EBV-RNAs, EBER1 and EBER-2, not only in the Reed-Sternberg cells and their variants, but in some cases also in reactive lymphocytes.

iii) Secondary replication of EBV$^+$ cells is seen in settings of depressed immunity, a situation often encountered in Hodgkin disease.

iv) The high prevalence of EBV in Hodgkin disease at young (< 20 years) and old age (> 70 years) and the low prevalence of EBV in cases of Hodgkin disease at adult ages, which is the peak incidence of Hodgkin disease , also indicate that EBV is probably a pathogenic event only in a small number of Hodgkin disease cases (Jarrett et al., 1991).

In conclusion, the data indicate that EBV may have a pathogenic role in EBV$^+$ cases of Hodgkin disease, especially those where EBV is found by DISH exclusively in Reed-Sternberg cells and related variants. Alternatively, it seems likely that EBV latently infected reactive cells, in settings of immunodeficiency as encountered in Hodgkin disease, are secondarily activated to become blastoid cells and therefore may be a secondary phenomenon in Hodgkin disease.

Non-cutaneous Non-Hodgkin Lymphomas

Most studies on EBV in non-Hodgkin lymphomas (NHL) concentrate on the immunopheno-type, i.e., T or B cell type of these lymphomas (Agnostopoulos et al. 1991; Herbst et al., 1990; Su et al., 1991; Staal et al., 1991; Oshima et 1 1991). Here we will concentrate on the presence of EBV in cells with CD30 expression, for the following reasons:

i) As discussed above, EBV is mainly found in CD30$^+$ Reed-Sternberg cells and their variants.

ii) CD30 can be upregulated in vitro after infection with EBV (Stein et al. 1985). A strong association is found between the presence of EBV-DNA sequences on the one hand and brain lymphomas, endemic Burkitt lymphomas and nasal T cell lymphomas on the other (Hamilton-Dutoit et al., 1991; Harabuchi et al., 1990), both by PCR and DISH. In the other types of lymphoma, EBV-DNA sequences are found by PCR in 15 to 25 % of cases. Very recently, Herbst et al (1991) have shown that, in large cell anaplastic B cell lymphomas, EBV DNA sequences are present in 67% of cases, whereas in T-LCAL and LCAL of undetermined lineage the percentage of cases with EBV is 28% (Table 2). Our results are summarized in Table 2. The significance of these findings is difficult to estimate since in lymph nodes with hyperplasias about 15-25 per cent of the cells are also PCR-EBV$^+$ (Table 2). Using DISH we could demonstrate EBV genomic sequences in 60-80% of PCR-EBV positive NHL (Kanavaros et al., 1992). By contrast, in PCR-EBV$^+$ reactive lymph nodes, no DISH-EBV$^+$ signals could be obtained, indicating that the EBV-DNA copy number per cell is below the detection level of DISH. Probably some latently infected lymphocytes are demonstrated. Studies for EBV latent antigens, i.e., EBNA2 and LMP 1, reveal that only small percentages of NHL express these antigens. Others (Hamilton-Dutoit et al., 1992) found EBNA2 in one of 201 cases of NHL, whereas transformation associated EBV LMP-1 and -2 was found in 13 (6%) of the NHL investigated. Surprisingly, LMP expression was found in 10% of the peripheral T cell lymphomas, and in only 4 per cent of the B cell lymphomas, all of which were high grade. These findings suggest that the putative oncogenic role of EBV in sporadic NHL is small.

Non-Hodgkin Lymphomas with Variable Numbers of CD30$^+$ Cells (Non-large Cell Anaplastic Lymphoma)

The finding that in Hodgkin disease EBV is mainly present in Reed-Sternberg cells expressing the CD30 antigen, and the fact that EBV can upregulate CD30 expression in lymphoblastoid cell lines, have prompted us to investigate the presence of EBV in NHL with variable numbers of CD30$^+$ cells. These lymphomas include large cell anaplastic lymphomas (L CAL) of B cell, T cell or undetermined lineage with 2-80 percent CD30$^+$ cells as well as other types of lymphomas which show small groups of individual CD30$^+$ cells. In most of the latter lymphomas, the CD30[+] cells appeared to have developed secondarily in the course of the disease (secondary blast transformation). These lymphomas were selected for CD30 expression from a larger group of lymphomas (> 800) from the files of the comprehensive Cancer Centre Amsterdam and contained 5-30% CD30[+] cells (Kanavaros et al., 1992a; 1992b). By PCR we found an 80% prevalence of EBV genomic sequences in these CD30[+] non-LCAL lymphomas (Table 2). Using DISH we were able to confirm the presence of EBV in 56% of these cases.

EBV was present in neoplastic cells, which outnumbered CD30[+] cells (Kanavaros et al., 1992). The significance of the presence of EBV in CD30[+] non-LCAL lymphomas is not clear. First, it may well be that during lymphomagenesis a partial immune defect develops inducing secondary activation of EBV latently infected cells to blastoid cells expressing CD30. In favor of this notion is the low percentage of CD30[+] lymphomas expressing LMP-1and EBNA-2 (Oshima et al., 1990). Second, EBV may play a role in the pathogenesis of these lymphomas. Indirect support for this hypothesis can be provided from previous findings of clonality of EBV in the genome in B and T cell NHL. Recently, however, non-clonal EBV sequences have also been demonstrated in B and T NHL. Moreover, a recent study of Masih et al. has shown clonal EBV in hyperplastic lymph nodes (Masih et al., 1991). How EBV promotes malignancy is poorly understood, but EBV may promote malignant transformation by inducing activation of oncogenes such as bcl-2, c-fgr and myc. Support for this idea is obtained from previous studies reporting amplification and deregulation of the myc oncogene (Lacy et al., 1987) and induction of the bcl-2 oncogene in EBV infected B cell lines. Since these data (Lacy et al., 1987; Henderson et al., 1991) were obtained from in vitro studies, however, it is likely that other phenomena, such as a decrease in immune surveillance, may contribute to the in vivo emergence of lymphomas harboring EBV.

Cutaneous Versus Non-cutaneous CD30[+] Large Cell Anaplastic Lymphoma

Interestingly, although the number of B-LCAL was small, all four LCAL of B cell type were EBV[+] by PCR. Only one was EBV-DISH[+], indicating low copy numbers of EBV per cell in these lymphomas (Table 3). LMP and EBNA-2 could not be demonstrated. Similar findings were observed by Herbst et al. (1991). A much lower prevalence of EBV was present in LCAL of T cell type by PCR (5 of 16 cases tested:Table 3). In four cases, EBV could also be found by DISH and in one case LMP was present. Interestingly, all four primary cutaneous LCAL of T cell type were EBV negative. This observation has also been made by others (Anagnostopoulos et al., 1989). This seems important because primary cutaneous LCAL have a more favorable clinical course than their nodal counterparts (Bruin et al., 1992). Recently, we were also unable to detect EBV-DNA in five cases of lymphomatoid papulosis by PCR and DISH. Moreover, we could also not detect LMP-1 expression. These findings indicate that EBV does not play a role in the spectrum of primary cutaneous CD30[+] lymphoid proliferations as has been suggested by Messenger et al., (1981), Lee et al., (1990) and Slater (1991) in spite of increased antibody titers to EBV in lymphomatoid papulosis and cutaneous T cell lymphomas.

Table 3. EBV in CD30[+] large cell anaplastic lymphoma (LCAL).

	cases	PCR[+]	DISH[+]	LMP[+]
non cutaneous B-LCAL	4	4/4	1/3	0/3
non cutaneous T-LCAL	12	5/12	4/12	1/12
cutaneous LCAL	4	0/4	0/4	0/4

REFERENCES

Alfieri C, M Birkenbach, E Kieff, 1991. Early events in Epstein-Barr virus infection of human B lymphocytes. **Virology**, 181:595-608.

Anagnostopoulos I et al., 1989. Demonstration of monoclonal EBV genomes in HD and Ki-1 positive anaplastic large cell lymphoma by combined SB and ISH. **Blood**, 74: 810-816.

Bashir R, F Hochberg, RH Singer, 1989. Detection of Epstein-Barr virus by in situ hybridization. **Am. J. Pathol.**, 135: 1035-1044.

Brocksmith D, CA Angel, JH Pringle, I Lauder, 1991. Epstein-Barr viral DNA in Hodgkin's disease: Amplification and detection using the polymerase chain reaction. **J. Pathol.**, 165:11-15.

Coates PJ, G Slavin, AJ D'Ardenne, 1991. Persistence of Epstein-Barr virus in Reed-Sternberg cells throughout the course of Hodgkin's disease. **J. Pathol.**, 164:291-297.

Cohen JHM, E Fischer, MD Katatchkine, GM Lenoir, C Lefevre-Delvincourt, JP Revillard, 1987. Expression of CR1 and CR2 complement receptors following Epstein-Barr virus infection of Burkitt's lymphoma cell lines. **Scand. J. Immunol.**, 25:587-598.

Cordier M et al., 1990. Stable transfection of EBV nuclear antigen 2 in lymphoma cells containing the EBV P3HR1 genome induces expression of B cell activation molecules CD21 and CD23. **J. Virol.**, 64:1002-1013.

de Bruin PC, AL Noorduyn, P vd Valk, P v Heerde, PJ v Diest, MM vd Sandt, GJ Ossekoppele, CJLM Meijer, 1993. Non-cutaneous T cell lymphomas. Recognition of a lymphoma type (large cell anaplastic) with a relatively favorable prognosis. **Cancer**, in press.

Gilligan K, P Rajadurai, L Resnick, N Raab-Traub, 1990. Epstein-Barr virus small nuclear RNAs are not expressed in permissively infected cells in AIDS-associated leukoplakia. **Proc. Natl. Acad. Sci. USA**, 87:8790-8794.

Hamilton-Dutoit SJ, HJ Delecluse, M Raphael, G Lenoir, G Pallesen, 1991. Detection of Epstein-Barr virus genomes in AIDS related lymphomas: Sensitivity and specificity of in situ hybridization compared with Southern blotting. **J. Clin. Pathol.**, 44:676-680.

Hamilton-Dutoit SJ, G Pallesen, 1992. A survey of Epstein-Barr virus (EBV) gene expression in sporadic non-Hodgkin's lymphomas: Detection of EBV in a subset of peripheral T cell lymphomas. **Am. J. Pathol.**, in press.

Harabuchi Y, N Yamanaka, A Kataura et al, 1990. Epstein-Barr virus in nasal T cell lymphomas in patients with lethal midline granuloma. **Lancet**, 335:128-130.

Henderson S, M Rowe, C Gregory, D Croom-Carter, F Wang, R Longnecker, E Kieff, A Rickinson, 1991. Induction of bcl-2 expression by Epstein-Barr virus latent membrane protein 1 protects infected B cells from programmed cell death. **Cell**, 65:1107-1115.

Herbst H, G Niedobitek, M Kneba et al, 1990. High incidence of Epstein-Barr virus genomes in Hodgkin's disease. **Am. J. Pathol.**, 137(1):13-18.

Herbst H, F Dallenbach, M Hummel, G Niedobitek, T Finn, LS Young, M Rowe, N Muller-Lantzsch, H Stein, 1991. Epstein-Barr virus DNA and latent gene products in Ki-1 (CD30)-positive anaplastic large cell lymphomas. **Blood**, 78:2666-2673.

Jarrett RF, A Gallagher, DB Jones, FE Alexander, AS Krajewski, A Kelsy, J Adams, B Angus, S Gledhill, DH Wright, RA Cartwright, DE Onions, 1991. Detection of Epstein-Barr virus genomes in Hodgkin's disease: Relation to age. **J. Clin. Pathol.**, 44:844-848.

Jiwa NM, P vd Valk, H Mullink, W Vos, A Horstman, MM Maurice, DEM Oldeweghuis, JMM Walboomers, CJLM Meijer. 1992. Epstein-Barr virus DNA in Reed-Sternberg cells of Hodgkin lymphomas is frequently associated with CD21 (EBV receptor) expression. **Histopathology**, in press.

Kahn G, PJ Coates, RK Gupta, HP Kangro, G Slavin, 1992. Abstract Pathological Society of Great Britain and Ireland 118. **J. Pathol.**, in press.

Kanavaros J, NM Jiwa, P de Bruin, P vd Valk, LA Noorduyn, P van Heerde, R Gordijn, CJLM Meijer, 1992. High incidence of EBV genome in CD30 positive non-Hodgkin's lymphomas. **J. Pathol.**, 168:307-315.

Kanavaros J, M Jiwa, P vd Valk, J Walboomers, A Horstman, G Pallesen, CJLM Meijer, 1993. Expression of Epstein-Barr virus latent gene products and associated cellular activation and adhesion molecules in Hodgkin's disease and non-Hodgkin's lymphomas arising in non-immunocompromised individuals. **Human Pathol.**, in press.

Karameris A, P Kanavaros, 1992. Demonstration of Epstein Barr virus genome in neoplastic cells of Hodgkin's disease by in situ hybridization, in paraffin-embedded tissue using biotinylated probes. **Path. Res. Pract.**, 188:310-314.

Knutson J, 1990. The level of c-fgr RNA is increased by EBNA-2, an Epstein-Barr virus gene required for B cell immortalization. **J. Virol.**, 64:2530.

Lacy J, WP Summers, M Watson, PM Glazer, WC Summers, 1987. Amplification and deregulation of myc following Epstein-Barr virus infection of a human B cell. **Proc. Natl. Acad. Sci. USA**, 84:5838.

Lee PYP, M Charley, M Thorp, BV Jegasothy, JS Deng, 1990. Possible role of Epstein-Barr virus infection in cutaneous T cell lymphoma. **J. Invest. Dermatol.**, 95:309-312.

Libetta CM, JH Pringle, CA Angel, AW Craft, AJ Malcolm, I Lauder. Demonstration of Epstein-Barr viral DNA in formalin-fixed, paraffin-embedded samples of Hodgkin's disease. 1990. **J. Pathol.**, 161:255-260.

Masih A, D Weisenburger, M Duggan, J Armitage, R Bashir, D Mitchel, R Wickert, DT Purtilo, 1991. Epstein-Barr viral genome in lymph nodes from patients with Hodgkin's disease may not be specific to Reed-Sternberg cells. **Am. J. Pathol.**, 139(1):37-43.

Merchenthaler I, Stankovics, F Gallyas F, 1989. A highly sensitive one-step method for silver intensification of the nickel-diaminobenzidine end-product of peroxidase reaction. **J. Histochem. Cytochem.**, 37:1563-1565.

Messenger AG, TL Marshall, R Summerley, 1981. A case of lymphomatoid papulosis and systemic lymphoma. **Br. J. Dermatol.**, 104:77-82.

Mueller N. 1987. Epidemiologic studies assessing the role of the Epstein-Barr virus in Hodgkin's disease. **Yale J. Biol. Med.**, 60:321-327.

Mullink H, JMM Walboomers, TD Tadema et al., 1989. Combined immuno- and non-radioactive hybridocytochemistry on cells and tissue sections: Influence of fixation, enzyme pretreatment and choice of chromogen on detection of antigen and DNA sequences. **J. Histochem. Cytochem.**, 37:603-609.

Mullink H, W Vos, NM Jiwa et al, 1992. Application and comparison of silver intensification methods for the DAB and DAB-Ni endproduct of the peroxidase reaction after immunohistochemistry and in situ hybridisation. **J. Histochem. Cytochem.**, 40:495-504.

Munoz N, RJ Davidson, B Whitthof, JE Ericsson, G de The, 1978. Infectious mononucleosis and Hodgkin's disease. **Int. J. Cancer**, 22:10-13.

Oshima K, M Kikuchi, F Eguchi et al, 1990. Analysis of Epstein-Barr viral genomes in lymphoid malignancy using Southern blotting, polymerase chain reaction and in situ hybridization. **Virchows Archiv. B Cell Pathol.**, 59:383-390.

Pallesen G, SJ Hamilton-Dutoit, M Rowe, LS Young, 1991. Expression of Epstein-Barr virus latent gene products in tumour cells of Hodgkin's disease. **Lancet**, 1991:320-322.

Saiki RK, S Scharf, F Faloona, KB Mullis, T Horn, HA Ehrlich, N Arnheim, 1985. Enzymatic amplification of beta-globin genomic sequences and restriction site analysis for diagnosis of sickle cell anemia. **Science**, 230:1350-1354.

Sample C, E Kieff, 1991. Molecular basis for Epstein-Barr virus induced pathogenesis and disease. In: T Ooka, JW Sixby, Eds: **Seminars in Immunopathology**, Springer, vol. 13, pp. 133-146.

Slater D, 1991. Editorial: Epstein-Barr virus: An aetiological factor in cutaneous lymphoproliferative disorders? **J. Pathol.**, 165:1-4.

Staal S, R Ambinder, WE Beschorner et al., 1989. A survey of Epstein-Barr virus DNA in lymphoid tissue: Frequent detection in Hodgkin's disease. **Am. J. Pathol.**, 91:1-5.

Stein H, DY Mason, J Gerdes et al., 1985. The expression of the Hodgkin's disease associated antigen Ki-1 in reactive and neoplastic lymphoid tissue: Evidence that Reed-Sternberg cells and histiocytic malignancies are derived from activated lymphoid cells. **Blood**, 66:848-858.

Su IJ, HC Hsieh, KH Lin et al, 1991. Aggressive peripheral T cell lymphomas containing Epstein-Barr viral DNA: A clinicopathologic and molecular analysis. **Blood**, 77:799-808.

Thomas JA, DH Crawford, 1989. Epstein-Barr virus/complement receptor and epithelial cells. Letter to the Editor. **Lancet** ii, 449-450.

Uhara H, Y Sato, K Mukai, I Akao, Y Matsuno, S Furuya, T Hoshikawa, Y Shimosato, T Saida, 1990. Detection of Epstein-Barr virus DNA in Reed-Sternberg cells of Hodgkin's disease using the polymerase chain reaction and in situ hybridization. **Jpn. J. Cancer Res.**, 81:272-278.

Wang F, CDE Gregory, M Rowe, et al., 1987. Epstein-Barr virus nuclear antigen 2 specifically induces expression of the B cell activation antigen CD23. **Proc. Natl. Acad. Sci. USA**, 84:3452-3456.

Wang P, D Liebowitz, F Wang, C Gregory, A Richinson, R Larson, T Springer, E Kieff, 1988. Epstein-Barr virus latent infection membrane protein alters the human B lymphocyte phenotype: Deletion of the amino terminus abolishes activity. **J. Virol.**, 62:41-73.

Weiss LM, JG Strickeler, RA Warnke, DT Purtilo, J Sklar, 1987. Epstein-Barr viral DNA in tissues of Hodgkin's disease. **Am. J. Pathol.**, 129:86-91.

Weiss LM, LA Movahed, RA Warnke, J Sklar. 1989. Detection of Epstein-Barr viral genome in Reed-Sternberg cells of Hodgkin's disease. **N. Eng. J. Med.**, 320:502-506.

Wu TC, RB Mann, P Charache, SD Hayward, S Staal, BC Lambe, RF Ambiner. 1990. Detection of EBV gene expression in Reed-Sternberg cells of Hodgkin's disease. **Int. J. Cancer**, 46: 801-804.

Wu TC, RB Mann, JI Epstein, E McMahon, WA Lee, P Charache, SD Hayward, RJ Kurman, GS Hayward, RF Ambinder. 1991. Abundant expression of EBER 1 small nuclear RNA in nasopharyngeal carcinoma. **Am. J. Pathol.**, 138:1461-1469.

Young LS, CW Dawson, AB Rickson. 1989. Epstein-Barr virus/complement receptor and epithelial cells. Letter to the Editor. **Lancet** ii, 448-449.

INFLAMMATORY PRECURSORS OF MYCOSIS FUNGOIDES

W. Clark Lambert

Department of Laboratory Medicine and Pathology
Department of Dermatology
UMDNJ-New Jersey Medical School
Newark, NJ, U.S.A.

Correspondence to: Dr. W. C. Lambert,
Department of Laboratory Medicine and Pathology,
Room C-524 Medical Sciences Building,
UMDNJ-New Jersey Medical School,
Newark, NJ 07103-2714, U.S.A.

ABSTRACT

Evidence for and against the hypothesis that inflammatory dermatoses may progress to mycosis fungoides or Sézary syndrome is reviewed, and two cases which may represent examples of such a progression are presented. Arguments for and against the hypothesis that large plaque parapsoriasis, retiform parapsoriasis, or both, should be classified as mycosis fungoides are discussed. It is the author's opinion that large plaque parapsoriasis should not be classified as mycosis fungoides, because it may only represent one of several inflammatory dermatoses that may progress to MF, because cell marker studies show these lymphocyte populations to be different, because this would be inconsistent with other dermatologic nomenclature, in which other potentially pre-cancerous conditions are not diagnosed as cancer, and because further investigations may provide information which allows us to distinguish between those cases of large plaque parapsoriasis which are progressing to mycosis fungoides and those which are not.

Basic Mechanisms of Physiologic and Aberrant Lymphoproliferation in the Skin
Edited by W.C. Lambert *et al.*, Plenum Press, New York, 1994

217

INTRODUCTION

The hypothesis that a number of types of longstanding, recalcitrant dermatitis may, on occasion, give rise to mycosis fungoides has been put forward, based on clinical experience, by a number of authors for many years (Degos, 1953, Lambert, 1985; 1987; Lambert and Schwartz, 1988) and has been seemingly borne out by epidemiologic studies which show that many cases of mycosis fungoides had been previously diagnosed as having one of several inflammatory dermatoses, including atopic dermatitis, seborrheic dermatitis, and psoriasis, as well as large plaque parapsoriasis (Green et al., 1979). Moreover, there have been a number of individual reports of cases of mycosis fungoides or Sézary syndrome arising from inflammatory dermatoses, including atopic dermatitis (Abel et al., 1986; Lange-Vejlsgaard et al., 1989; Rajka and Winkelmann, 1984), allergic contact dermatitis resulting from occupational exposure (Cohen et al., 1980) and other types (Fransway and Winkelmann, 1988). Atopic dermatitis has also been associated with Hodgkin disease (Armlot and Green, 1978; Winkelmann and Rajka, 1983), which, in turn, may share certain etiopathologic factors with mycosis fungoides (Kadin, 1993; reviewed in Lambert, 1993; 1994).

The case for progression, in some cases, to mycosis fungoides is probably stronger for atopic dermatitis than for most other inflammatory dermatoses except for those in the parapsoriasis group (see below). Not only are clear-cut case reports available (see above) but also a plausible mechanism is readily presented by the fact that immunophenotypic studies have shown a very similar pattern of inflammatory cell types between the two diseases (Cooper, 1993), with, in particular, T_{H2} type CD4$^+$ T cells abundant in both mycosis fungoides and in lesional atopic skin (von der Heijden et al., 1991), and it has even been proposed that a monoclonal expansion of these cells may already be present in lesional skin in atopic dermatitis (den Otter et al., 1993). On the other hand, the case for occupationally acquired allergic contact dermatitis progressing to mycosis fungoides (Abel, 1990, Cohen et al., 1980) has been cast into doubt by two negative case-control studies (Tuyp et al., 1987; Whittemore et al., 1989). Of these two studies, the more convincing is that of Whittemore et al. (1989), who examined 174 cases of mycosis fungoides along with 294 controls in selected regions of California and Washington (State) in the U.S.A. Using sophisticated subject-selection and telephone interviewing techniques, the investigators found no positive correlation between exposure to chemicals or allergic contact dermatitis and relative risk of mycosis fungoides. They also did not find a statistically significant association between atopy (eczema, asthma, hay fever, or urticaria) and mycosis fungoides. However, since atopy is quite common in the general population, an association may be present which was not detected. Moreover, specific reports, such as that of Cohen et al. (1980), provide convincing evidence that in specific situations occupational dermatosis can progress to mycosis fungoides, and I have seen evidence of this as well in my own clinical experience (Lambert et al., in preparation). It may be that individual susceptibility pays a decisive role in whether an inflammatory dermatosis can progress to mycosis fungoides. Such individual differences in cancer susceptibility have now been well documented for other types of cancer, and I and others have proposed genetic models for surveillance genes (such as DNA repair genes) related to carcinogenesis in the general population to account for these differences (reviewed in Lambert and Lambert, 1992).

There are, indeed, a number of authors who do not accept the hypothesis that inflammatory dermatoses can progress to mycosis fungoides, and they make a strong argument for their position, based largely on the same evidence cited above in favor of this concept. These authors argue that whereas many cases of mycosis fungoides had earlier been diagnosed as having an inflammatory dermatosis, these may have actually been misdiagnoses, due simply to clinical and histologic resemblance of early stages of mycosis fungoides to inflammatory conditions (Edelson, 1980). This position is supported by the fact that whereas the spectrum of diseases included within the CTCL group are not rare, comprising altogether a condition about as common as Hodgkin disease (Chuang et al., 1990), there have been only a handful of well documented reports of dermatitis progressing to CTCL, and in some cases even those reports have only referred to a condition resembling an inflammatory dermatosis (reviewed above). Thus observed associations may have been fortuitous. The problem is well demonstrated by the report of Koch et al. (1987), who reported a series of patients, and discussed others from the files of their institution, in which mycosis fungoides began in childhood or adolescence. They noted that in many cases the patient had a prior diagnosis of atopic dermatitis, which is arguably in support of the above hypothesis that atopic dermatitis can progress to mycosis fungoides. They also noted, however, that in some of their cases diagnosed as atopic dermatitis there was little or no pruritus noted, whereas pruritus is a characteristic finding in atopic dermatitis, a finding that could be used as an argument against the hypothesis that atopic dermatitis can progress to mycosis fungoides.

If inflammatory dermatoses do, indeed, progress to mycosis fungoides or other forms of CTCL, then it would appear that the typical course is a gradual one, with features of the inflammatory disease gradually giving way to those of the CTCL. This would tend to make the fact that the disease was, indeed, originally inflammatory difficult to recognize at the end of this transformation, which is always the time point at which the progression is reviewed. Added to this is the fact that the patient is likely to be referred, particularly in the late stages of this progression, and the physician doing the evaluating, typically a consultant with special expertise in CTCL, is thus likely to see only the later stages of this slow progression from inflammatory dermatosis to CTCL, and therefore is very unlikely to have witnessed the early stages when the disease was more typical of the dermatosis. These influences would tend to obscure the progression of inflammatory dermatosis to mycosis fungoides in cases reported in the literature. It is thus important that physicians with well documented cases showing this progression report them, even though, individually, they may only represent sporadic case reports.

I now report two examples, on both of which I have only incomplete data, of progression of what appeared to have been a longstanding, recalcitrant dermatosis to unequivocal mycosis fungoides confirmed by biopsy.

CASE REPORTS

Case One

A Haitian female had been followed at UMDNJ-University Hospital with a diagnosis of atopic dermatitis since age seven. When I first saw her, at age 13, she had typical features of moderate to severe atopic dermatitis with lesions on the face, trunk and extremities. Pruritus was relatively mild, compared to the severity of her disease, but severe pruritus had been noted previously in her course. A complete blood count and other laboratory studies were within normal limits. Two brothers had asthma and hay fever (one each) and her mother and maternal grandmother had hay fever. Paternal family history was unavailable.

She was treated with fluorinated corticosteroids applied sparingly to lesional skin, together with generous application of emollient, several times per day. Facial lesions were similarly treated with non-fluorinated corticosteroids. The patient was advised to decrease the frequency of baths, which had been two or more per day, and to use only extremely mild soaps. An oatmeal preparation was also applied to the bath water and she was advised to apply the topical medications immediately upon completing her baths. Hydroxyzine, in doses titered to her individual level of efficacy and tolerance, was administered for pruritus.

The lesions improved but did not completely clear, and she was maintained on this regimen until age 16, when a gradual worsening of lesions on her extremities was noted. These lesions had become less pruritic and more indurated than previously. A biopsy of a lesion on her left arm was obtained; photomicrographs are shown in Figures 1 and 2. On basis of this biopsy, a diagnosis of atopic dermatitis with progression to mycosis fungoides was made. At this time, however the patient and her family returned to Haiti, and were lost to follow-up.

Case Two

A 72 year old caucasian male with a 40 year history of psoriasis vulgaris was seen in consultation, referred because of resistance to a treatment regimen that had been effective for many years. This regimen had consisted of a topical tar preparation applied with ultraviolet B light (Goeckermann system) applied two to three times per day at home by the patient. This treatment had been discontinued one month prior to my examination.

The patient's father and brother had both had psoriasis. He had been in good health except for heart disease treated with digoxin. He denied excessive use of ethanol and tobacco, although he used both in moderate amounts. The patient associated worsening of his lesions with moving from New Jersey to Florida six months prior to my examination.

Physical examination revealed a slightly to moderately obese man with 20 to 30% skin involvement with lesions varying from salmon colored plaques with a micaceous scale, typical

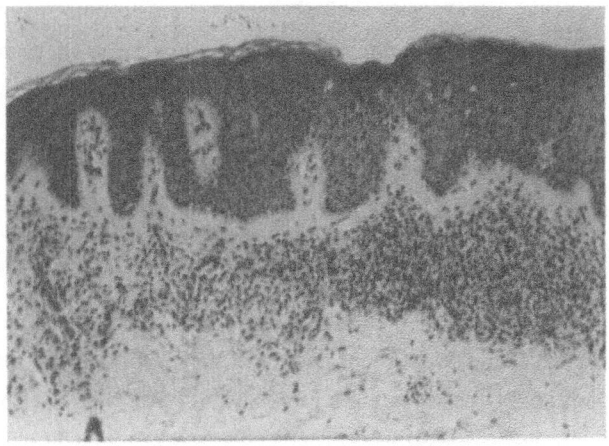

Figure 1. Case 1. Histologic changes typical of atopic dermatitis showing also atypical lymphocytes characteristics of mycosis fungoides.

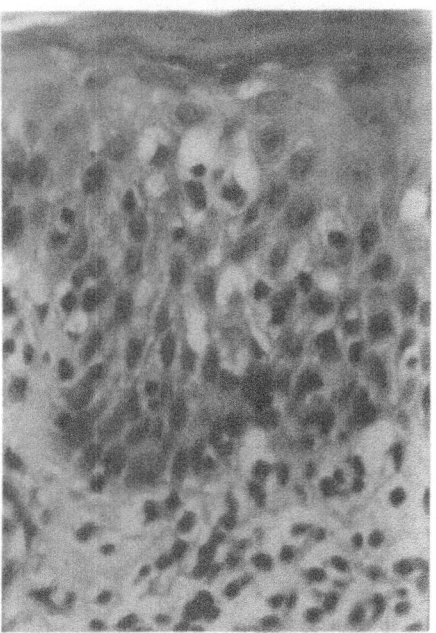

Figure 2. Higher power photomicrograph of the same section seen in Figure 1, showing a collection of unequivocally atypical lymphocytes diagnostic of mycosis fungoides.

of psoriasis vulgaris, to more dermatitic lesions with a fine scale. The gradations between these lesions were continuous in all areas. Lesions were present on the extensor aspects of the extremities, on the inferior aspects of the torso, and on the upper thighs and buttocks. The scalp was spared. Pitting was noted in all ten nails of the upper extremities but not on those of the lower extremities. The more dermatitic appearing lesions were mainly present on the torso, buttocks and thighs.

Biopsy of a lesion on the abdomen showed changes of both psoriasis vulgaris and mycosis fungoides (Figures 3 and 4), and were interpreted as progression of psoriasis to mycosis fungoides. Prior to initiation of treatment for the latter disorder, however, the patient died of myocardial infarction.

DISCUSSION

I believe that certain longstanding, recalcitrant inflammatory dermatoses can progress to mycosis fungoides, and that this progression is not rare, although it is uncommon. I also believe that this progression is grossly underreported, for the reasons given above. I wish to emphasize that these are opinions, not statements of fact. They are based on the data and on the literature reviewed above. I urge the reader not only to form his own opinion, but also to avoid any degree of certainty regarding that opinion not justified by the available data.

I will now address, as a separate discussion, the issue of whether certain diseases in the parapsoriasis group should be classified as a stage of mycosis fungoides.

SHOULD LARGE PLAQUE PARAPSORIASIS AND RETIFORM PARAPSORIASIS BE CLASSIFIED AS "PATCH STAGE OF MYCOSIS FUNGOIDES"?

Among dermatoses that have been considered to be inflammatory in nature, only certain of those in the parapsoriasis group have been noted to frequently progress to mycosis fungoides (Lambert, 1985; 1987; Lambert and Everett, 1981; Lambert and Schwartz, 1988). For this reason, some authors have chosen to re-classify large plaque parapsoriasis as "patch stage of mycosis fungoides" (Sanchez and Ackerman, 1979). I believe that this re-classification is unwise, but rather than attempt to influence the reader one way or the other, I would like to present what I believe is a fair representation of the case for both sides of this issue, so as to allow the reader to formulate his or her own opinion.

First, a few points regarding the nosology of the disorders that have been included within the group known as parapsoriasis need to be addressed. These diseases include pityriasis lichenoides [including pityriasis lichenoides et varioliformis acuta (synonyms: PLEVA; PLVA; Mucha-Habermann disease) and pityriasis lichenoides chronica], small plaque parapsoriasis [including the variant known as digitate dermatosis (Hu and Winkelmann), and, in turn, the variant of digitate dermatosis known as xanthoerythrodermia perstans (Radcliffe-Cocker)], large plaque parapsoriasis and retiform parapsoriasis (considered by some to be variants of large plaque parapsoriasis; Lambert and Everett, 1981; Lambert, 1987; Lambert and Schwartz, 1988). These entities appear to be unrelated, except as noted above, although a handful of cases of pityriasis lichenoides or lymphomatoid papulosis associated with large plaque parapsoriasis have been reported, and I have seen one example of this association as well. Only large plaque parapsoriasis and retiform parapsoriasis will be considered here; the association between

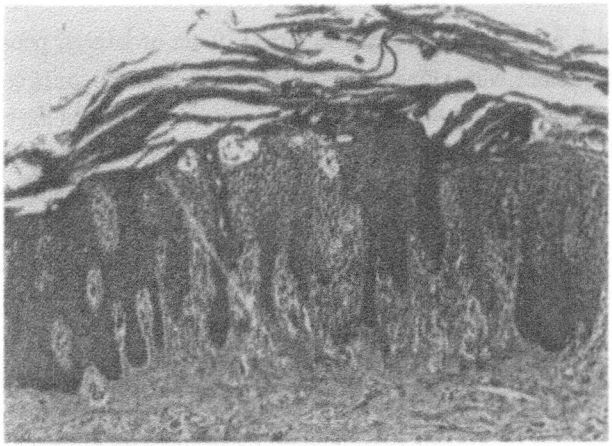

Figure 3. Case 2. Histologic changes typical of psoriasis vulgaris showing also atypical lymphocytes characteristics of mycosis fungoides.

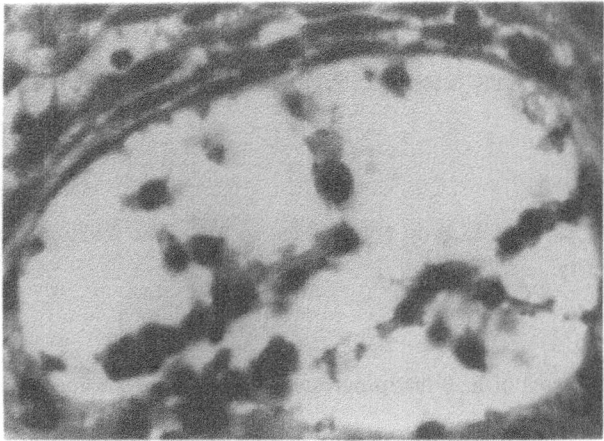

Figure 4. Higher power photomicrograph of the same section seen in Figure 3, showing a collection of uneqivocally atypical lymphocytes diagnostic of mycosis fungoides.

lymphomatoid papulosis and lymphoma is considered elsewhere in this volume (Whittaker, 1993). A recent claim that small plaque parapsoriasis is also to be considered a "patch stage of mycosis fungoides" (King-Ismael and Ackermann, 1992) is discussed below. I have also addressed this latter issue elsewhere (Lambert, 1992).

Large plaque parapsoriasis presents as large (10 cm or larger), poorly defined, often atrophic dermatitic lesions with a fine scale which tend to occur on areas covered by bathing trunks (i.e., buttock and inguinal region on men and women and also on the breasts of women) as well as the axillae. Retiform parapsoriasis, which is extremely rare, presents as widespread "net-like" or retiform atrophic lesions which affect much of the torso and sometimes proximal extremities. The recorded incidence of progression of the former disorder to mycosis fungoides is about 20 to 30% (Lambert and Everett, 1981), whereas the latter disorder consistently progresses to mycosis fungoides.

I have no objection to referring to retiform parapsoriasis as a stage of mycosis fungoides because of the high incidence (as best as can be recorded with the handful of cases reported) of progression to that disease. Since these lesions are not patches, however, it seems inappropriate to refer to them as a "patch stage" of anything.

The remainder of my discussion will address the issue of whether large plaque parapsoriasis (LPP) should be classified as "patch stage of mycosis fungoides" (PSMF). Each issue is given a separate heading, followed by the arguments for and against the hypothesis that LPP should be classified as PSMF.

HYPOTHESIS: LPP is PSMF

Argument in favor, 1: Many cases of LPP progress to mycosis fungoides (MF)

Arguments against:

1a. Many cases of LLP do not progress to MF. This fraction is probably the clear majority.

1b. Those cases of LLP that progress to MF often take many years or decades to do so.

1c. It appears that a number of longstanding (especially recalcitrant) dermatoses other than LLP (or retiform parapsoriasis) may also progress to MF. This may not be a rare event, and since these other dermatoses are much more common than LPP, the number of cases of MF arising from these other dermatoses may be significant. This entire issue is reviewed above.

1d. Progression of non-neoplastic disorders to cancer is well known to occur in other systems. These include: progression of hepatic cirrhosis to hepatocellular carcinoma, of schistosomiasis (*S. haematobium*) to bladder carcinoma, and of diverticulitis to multiple myeloma (reviewed in Lambert and Everett, 1981).

1e. Even if progression of LPP to MF were an extension or modification of the same process, the nosologic convention is <u>not</u> to name the precursor lesion a type of cancer. Thus actinic (solar) keratosis is not called squamous cell carcinoma, lentigo maligna is not called lentigo maligna melanoma, and cervical dysplasia is not called cervical carcinoma, even though each of these is known to progress in a percentage of cases to its corresponding type of cancer.

Argument in favor 2: Progression of LPP to MF, when it occurs, is a gradual process.

Arguments against:

2a. Inflammatory dermatoses other than LPP which progress to MF also appear to do so as a gradual process. (Reviewed above)

2b. Other entities, which are not called cancer, which progress to cancer do so as a gradual, continuous process. Examples: progression of actinic (solar) keratosis to squamous cell carcinoma; progression of lentigo maligna to lentigo maligna melanoma.

Argument in favor 3: Poikiloderma is a prominent component of both LPP and MF. Poikiloderma is especially likely to be seen in LPP which is progressing to MF.

Argument against

3. Poikiloderma is also a prominent component of a number of other dermatoses, such as those due to physical injury, photo-chemical injury, and collagen-vascular diseases. These dermatoses rarely, if ever progress to MF.

Argument in favor 4: Both LPP and MF contain T cells in their infiltrate. Some are atypical (Sézary cells) in cases of LPP progressing to MF.

Arguments against:

4a. T cells, particularly T_{H2} cells, are found in the infiltrate of atopic dermatitis as well as MF (reviewed above).

4b. $CD8^+$ T cells appear to be relatively more common than $CD4^+$ cells in lesional skin in most cases of LPP, compared to MF, in which CD4$^+$ cells usually predominate in lesioned skin.

4c. Sézary cells, or cells resembling Sézary cells, are also found in lesions and in blood of patients with other inflammatory dermatoses (Reviewed above).

Argument in favor 5: At least one dermatopathology laboratory has identified distinctive diagnostic changes in both MF and LPP.

Argument against:

5. That same laboratory has found the same changes in lesions of small plaque parapsoriasis (King-Ismael and Ackerman, 1992), which does not progress to MF. Therefore the criteria are invalid and should probably discarded, or used only to distinguish MF and LPP from certain specific diseases.

In addition to the above considerations regarding the nosology of LPP and MF, there are management considerations in classifying LPP as MF. As already pointed out, it is inconsistent to classify possibly pre-MF lesions as MF, when the same is not done for other potentially pre-cancerous lesions. Even if it turns out that all LPP cases are progressing, at whatever rate, towards MF, moreover, it seems to me to be inappropriate to classify patients as having MF who, in fact, have a prognosis quite different from that of patients with overt MF. On the other hand, if it turns out that in the future we are able to identify subsets of patients with LPP who do, and who do not, progress to MF, then many patients may have been classified as having cancer who, in fact, do not have cancer. Therefore, if all patients with LPP had been diagnosed as having MF, we would then have to modify our diagnoses as follows:

(i) "patch stage of MF, MF type", and

(ii) "patch stage of MF, non-MF type".

It seems to me that the nosology is confusing enough as it is. I therefore personally favor the concept that LPP is an entity which may progress to MF but which should not be classified as MF.

REFERENCES

Abel EA, 1990. Mycosis fungoides and occupational exposures. Is there an association? **Dermatol. Clinics.**, 8:169-171.

Abel EA, BJ Nickoloff, DM Shelby, W Watson and GS Wood, 1986. Tumor stage mycosis fungoides in a patient treated with long-term corticosteroids for asthma and atopic-like dermatitis. **J. Dermatol. Surg. Oncol.**, 12:1089-1093.

Amlot PL and AL Green, 1978. Atopy and immunoglobulin E concentrations in Hodgkin's disease and other lymphomas. **Br. Med. J.**, i:327.

Beer WE, 1992. Concomitance of psoriasis and atopic dermatitis. **Dermatology**, 184:265-270.

Belsito DV, TJ Flotte, HW Lim, RL Baer, J Thorbecke and I Gigli, 1982. Effect of glucocorticosteroids on epidermal Langerhans cells. **J. Exp. Med.**, 155:291-302.

Bendelac A, NTJ O'Connor, and MT Daniel, 1987. Non-neoplastic circulating Sézary-like cells in cutaneous T-cell lymphoma, **Cancer**, 60:980-986.

Bonvalet D, K Colau-Gohm, and S Belaich, 1977. Les differéntes formes du parapsoriasis en plaques. **Ann. Dermatol. Venereol.**, 104: 18-25.

Bunn PA, and SI Lamberg, 1979. Report of the Committee on Staging and Classification of Cutaneous T-Cell Lymphomas. **Cancer Treat. Rep.**, 63:725-728.

Cerroni L, J Smolle, and HP Soyer, 1990. Immunophenotyping of cutaneous lymphoid infiltrates in frozen and paraffin-embedded tissue sections. A comparative study. **J. Am. Acad. Dermatol.**, 22:405-413.

Chuang TY, D Su and SA Muller, 1990. Incidence of cutaneous T cell lymphoma and other rare skin cancers in a defined population. **J. Am. Acad. Dermatol.**, 23:254-256.

Cohen SR, KS Stenn, IM Braverman and GJ Peck, 1980. Mycosis fungoides: Clinicopathologic relationships, survival and therapy in 59 patients with observations on occupation as a new prognostic factor. **Cancer**, 46:2654-2666.

Cooper KD, 1992. Skin-infiltrating lymphocytes in normal and disordered skin: Activation signals and functional roles in psoriasis and mycosis fungoides-type cutaneous T-cell lymphoma. **J. Dermatol.**, 19:731-737.

Degos R, 1953. **Dermatologie**, Flemmarion, Paris.

Duncan SC and RK Winkelmann, 1978. Circulating Sézary cells in hospitalized dermatology patients. **Br. J. Dermatol.**, 99:171-178.

Edelson RL, 1980. Cutaneous T cell lymphoma: Mycosis fungoides, Sézary syndrome, and other variants. **J. Am. Acad. Dermatol.**, 2:89-106.

Everett MA, 1985. Early diagnosis of mycosis fungoides: Vacuolar interface dermatitis. **J. Cutan. Pathol.**, 12:271-278.

Fischermann AB, PA Bunn, Jr., JG Gucion, MJ Matthews and JD Minna, 1979. Exposure to chemicals, physical agents, and biologic agents in mycosis fungoides and the Sézary syndrome. **Cancer Treat. Rep.**, 63:591-596.

Fischer AA, 1987. Allergic contact dermatitis mimicing mycosis fungoides. **Cutis**, 40:19-21.

Fransway AF and RK Winkelmann, 1988. Chronic dermatitis evolving to mycosis fundoides: Report of four cases and review of the literature. **Cutis**, 42:330-335.

Greene MH, NA Daloger, SI Lamberg, CE Argyropoulos and JF Fraumeni, 1979. Mycosis fundoides: Epidemiologic observations. **Cancer Treat. Rep.**, 63:597-606.

Greene MH, HA Pinto, JA Kant, K Siler, EC Vonderheid, SI Lamberg and NA Dalager, 1982. Lymphomas and leukemias in the relatives of patients with mycosis fungoides. **Cancer,** 49:737-741.

Grosshans E, 1986. Le parapsoriasis en plaques. **Ann. Dermatol. Venereol.,** 113:865-867.

van der Heijden FL, EA Wierenga, JD Bos and ML Kapsenberg, 1991. High frequency of IL-4 producing CD4+ allergen-specific T lymphocytes in atopic dermatitis lesional skin. **J. Invest. Dermatol.,** 97:389-394.

Kadin ME, TH Davis, SP Balk, SP Newcom, S Cheititz, and J Massague, 1993. Mechanism for tumor progression in lymphomatoid papulosis: Hypothesis based on studies of tumor cell lines clonally derived from lymphomatoid papulosis. In: WC Lambert, B Giannotti and WA van Vloten, Eds. **Basic Mechanisms of Physiologic and Aberrant Lymphoproliferation in the Skin,** Plenum Press, New York, This Vol.

Koch SE, HS Zackheim, ML Williams, V Fletcher and PE LeBoit, 1987. Mycois fungoides beginning in childhood and adolescence. **J. Am. Acad. Dermatol.,** 17:563-570.

King-Ismael D and AB, Ackerman, 1992. Guttate parapsoriasis/digitate dermatosis (small plaque parapsoniasis) is mycosis fungoides. **Am J. Dermatolopathol.,** 14:518-530.

Lambert WC, 1984. Parapsoriasis. In T. Provost and E. Farmer, Eds. **"Current Therapy in Dermatology"** Philadelphia, B.C. Decker. pp. 16-22.

Lambert WC, l985. Premycotic eruptions. **Dermatol. Clin.,** 3:629-645.

Lambert WC, 1987. Parapsoriasis. In: T.B. Fitzpatrick, A.Z. Eisen, K. Wolff, I.M. Freedberg and K.F. Austen, Eds. **"Dermatology in General Medicine"** Third Ed., New York, McGraw-Hill, pp. 991-1006.

Lambert WC, 1992. Response to "Guttate parapsoriasis/digitate dermatosis (small plaque parapsoriasis) is mycosis fungoides". **Am. J. Dermatolopathol.,** 14:532-533.

Lambert WC, 1993. What is mycosis fungoides? A modest proposal. In: WC Lambert, B Giannotti and WA van Vloten, Eds. **Basic Mechanisms of Physiologic and Aberrant Lymphoproliferation in the Skin,** Plenum Press, New York, This Vol.

Lambert WC, 1994. The thymus bypass model: A new hypothesis for the etiopathogenesis of mycosis fungoides and related diseases. In Burg, G, Ed: **"Cutaneous Lymphomas",** **Dermatol. Clinics,** in press.

Lambert WC and MA Everett, 1981. The nosology of parapsoriasis. **J. Am. Acad. Dermatol.,** 5:373-395.

Lambert WC and MW Lambert, 1992. Co-recessive inheritance: A model for surveillance genes in higher eukaryotes. **Mutation Res.,** 273:179-192.

Lambert WC and RA Schwartz, 1988. Dermatitic precursors of mycosis fundoides. In: R.A. Schwartz, Ed., **"Skin Cancer: Recognition and Management",** Springer-Verlag, New York, pp. 152-161.

Lamberg SI, SB Green, DP Byar, JB Block, WE Clendenning, MC Douglass, EH Epstein, Jr., ZY Fuks, LE Golitz, AL Lorinz, EI McBurney, B Michel, HH Roenigk, Jr., EJ van Scott and EC Vonderheid, 1984. Clinical staging for cutaneous T-cell lymphoma. **Ann. Int. Med.,** 100: 187-192.

Lange-Vejlsgaard G, E Ralfkiaer, JK Larsen, N O'Connor and K Thomsen, 1989. Fatal cutaneous T cell lymphoma in a child with atopic dermatitis. **J. Am. Acad. Dermatol.**, 20:954-958.

Lazar AP, WA Caro, HH Roenigk, 1989. Parapsoriasis and mycosis fungoides: The Northwestern University experience, 1970 to 1985. **J. Am. Acad. Dermatol.**, 21:919-923.

Le Boit PE, 1986. Cutaneous lymphomas and their histopathologic imitators. **Semin. Dermatol.**, 5:322-333.

McMillan EM, 1985. Monoclonal antibodies and cutaneous T cell lymphoma. **J. Am. Acad. Dermatol.**, 12:102-104.

den Otter W, JW Koten, RA Maas and DJ der Kinderen, 1992. Are atopic disorders due to a TH2 clone? (letter), **Br. J. Dermatol.**, 128:102.

Rajka G and RK Winkelmann, 1984. Atopic dermatitis and Sézary syndrome. **Arch. Dermatol.**, 120:83-84.

Ralfkiaer E, KC Gatter, GL Wantzin, 1986. Immunohistological reactivity pattern of the anti-cutaneous T-cell lymphoma antibody BE2. **Br. J. Dermatol.**, 114:677-684.

Ralfkiaer E, GL Wantzin, DY Mason, K Hou-Jensen, H Stein and K Thomsen, 1985. Phenotypic characterization of lymphocyte subsets in mycosis fundgoides: Comparison with large plaque parapsoriasis and benign chronic dermatoses. **Am. J. Clin Pathol.**, 84:610-619.

Rijlaarsdam U, E Scheffer, CJ Meijer, 1991. Mycosis fungoides-like lesions associated with phenytoin and carbamazepine therapy. **J. Am. Acad. Dermatol.**, 24: 216-220.

Rowden G and MG Lewis, 1976. Langerhans cells: Involvement in the pathogenesis of mycosis fungoides. **Br. J. Dermatol.**, 95:665-672.

Sanchez JL and AB Ackerman, 1979. The patch stage of mycosis fungoides. Criteria for histologic diagnosis. **Am J. Dermatopathol.**, 1:5-26.

Sausville EA, JL Eddy, RW Makuch, 1988. Histopathologic staging at initial diagnosis of mycosis fungoides and the Sézary syndrome. **Ann. Intern. Med.**, 109:372-382.

Souteyrand P and M d'Incan, 1990. Drug-induced mycosis fungoides-like lesions. **Curr. Probl. Dermatol.**, 19:176-182.

Thivolet J and J Kanitakis, 1987. Les immunomarquages dans les lymphomes cutanes, **Rev. Prat.**, 37: 1457-1463.

Thomas I, SG Nychay, RA Schwartz, WC Lambert and CJ Janniger, 1993. The red face: Cutaneous lymphomas. In: A Rebora, Ed., **"The Red Face", Clinics Dermatol.**, 11:319-328.

Tosca AD, AG Varelzidis, J Economidou, 1986. Mycosis fungoides: Evaluation of immunohistochemical criteria for the early stages of the disease and differentiation between stages. **J. Am. Acad. Dermatol.**, 15:237-245.

Tuyp E, A Burgoyne, T Aitchison and R Mackie, 1987. A case-control study of possible causative factors in mycosis fungoides. **Arch. Dermatol.**, 123:196-200.

Weinstock MA and JW Horm, 1988. Mycosis fungoides in the United States. **JAMA**, 260:42-46.

Whittaker SJ, 1993. The pathogenesis of lymphomatoid papulosis. In: WC Lambert, B Giannotti and WA van Vloten, Eds. **Basic Mechanisms of Physiologic and Aberrant Lymphoproliferation in the skin.** Plenum Press, New York, This Vol.

Whittemore AS, EA Holly, IM Lee, EA Abel, RM Adams, BJ Nicholoff, L Bley, JM Peters and C Gibney, 1989. Mycosis fungoides in relation to environmental exposures and immune response: A case control study. **J. Natl. Cancer Inst.,** 81:1560-1567.

Winkelmann RK and G Rajka, 1983. Atopic dermatitis and Hodgkin's disease, **Acta Dermatovenereol. (Stockh.),** 63:176-177

THE HISTOLOGICAL SPECTRUM OF CUTANEOUS T-CELL LYMPHOMA

Neil Smith, F.R.C.P., F.R.C. Path.

Skin Tumour Unit
St. John's Institute of Dermatology
St. Thomas' Hospital
London, United Kingdom

Correspondence to: Dr. N. Smith, St. John's Inst. of Dermatology,
St. Thomas' Hospital, Lambeth Palace Road,
SE1 7EH London, England (U.K.)

ABSTRACT

The term, cutaneous T-cell lymphoma, has been used to describe a variant of T-cell lymphoma with primary manifestations in the skin. Recent progress in techniques such as immunohistochemistry and molecular biology (Wood et al., 1986) has shown that cutaneous T-cell lymphoma is a heterogenous group, with many clinicopathological subsets (Slater, 1991). The diagnostic criteria for certain specific forms of cutaneous T-cell lymphoma are reviewed with an emphasis on the light microscopic appearances. The following entities are described: mycosis fungoides, Sézary syndrome, pagetoid reticulosis, HTLV-1 associated T-cell lymphoma, and CD30 positive lymphoproliferative disorders.

INTRODUCTION

Cutaneous T-cell lymphoma is a term originally used by Lutzner et al. in 1975 to describe a group of cutaneous lymphomas with primary manifestations in the skin. These include Sézary syndrome and mycosis fungoides. The term has gained wide acceptance, but advances in lymphoma research, particularly with the development of tools such as immunohisto-

Basic Mechanisms of Physiologic and Aberrant Lymphoproliferation in the Skin
Edited by W.C. Lambert *et al.*, Plenum Press, New York, 1994

231

chemistry and modern molecular biological techniques, have shown that T-cell lymphomas that may present in the skin are a widely diverse group.

The various classifications of non-Hodgkin lymphomas which have been developed over the years, including the so-called working formulation, have all been based on the study of primary nodal lymphomas. The group of peripheral T-cell lymphomas that commonly present with skin involvement do not fit very satisfactorily into any of these classifications. The up-dated Kiel classification is perhaps the most suitable for the classification of cutaneous T-cell lymphomas, but even in this classification there are anomalies. Large cell anaplastic lymphoma (CD30 positive lymphoma) is classified as a high-grade lymphoma in the Kiel classification. It is known, however, that a group of lymphoproliferative disorders with skin manifestations that contain many large anaplastic (CD30 positive) cells may be associated with a good prognosis. The conditions, lymphomatoid papulosis and regressing atypical histiocytosis, often run a benign course for many years, and primary cutaneous large cell anaplastic lymphoma can also be associated with a reasonably good prognosis (Lindholm et al., 1989). Alternative classifications have been proposed for T-cell lymphomas affecting the skin (Kerl et al., 1991; Pinkus et al., 1990; Su et al., 1990).

The diagnosis of any form of cutaneous lymphoma is based, as with other conditions, on the patient's history, careful clinical examination and the results of laboratory and other investigations. Of all the ancillary investigations helpful in establishing the diagnosis of cutaneous lymphoma, skin biopsy is one of the most important. The skin is readily accessible and, in addition to light microscopic examination, various other studies, such as electron microscopy, immunohistochemistry, cytomorphometry (Rieger et al., 1989; Van der Loo et al., 1981), and DNA cytometry (Vogt et al., 1991) may yield valuable information. Modern molecular biological techniques, including determination of immunoglobulin and T-cell receptor gene rearrangements, may help to establish evidence of clonality even in early stage disease. In situ hybridization and the polymerase chain reaction method may help to establish a viral cause for some malignant lymphoproliferative conditions. A viral etiology has already been established for adult T-cell lymphoma/leukemia.

Light microscopy still remains a simple and very useful tool in the delineation of the various subsets of cutaneous T-cell lymphomas. In the remainder of this chapter I will discuss the characteristic histopathological features of a selection of T-cell lymphomas that may present with skin lesions.

MYCOSIS FUNGOIDES

Mycosis fungoides is one of the commonest lymphomas to present to the dermatologist, and, in the early stages, may be quite difficult to diagnose histologically. It is most important that a biopsy is taken from an appropriate site, where the skin lesion is typical of the eruption as a whole. Old or regressing lesions or lesions that have been modified by topical treatment should be avoided. It is useful, in early stage disease, to take several biopsies from different types of skin lesions. The light microscopic appearance of mycosis fungoides depends on various factors.

First, the clinical pattern of mycosis fungoides is reflected in the histology. Lesions that appear to the clinician as psoriasiform may show elongation of rete ridges. Lesions that clinically have poikilodermatous features may show histologically epidermal atrophy and telangiectasia, and lesions which appear granulomatous may show the presence microscopically of histiocytes and epithelioid cells.

The second factor affecting the histological appearance of mycosis fungoides is the stage of the disease. Obviously, advanced tumour stage disease will have different histological appearances, and indeed a different immunohistochemical profile, from that of very early patch stage disease.

Third, lesions that have been treated with topical preparations, such as corticosteroids or nitrogen mustard, or lesions that have been excoriated or lichenified by the patient, will show secondary histological changes.

Despite the variability of the histology of mycosis fungoides, related to the factors described above, the following criteria are the most reliable for making the diagnosis (Everett, 1985; Nickoloff, 1988; Sanchez and Ackerman, 1979).

(i) A band-like upper dermal infiltrate of mononuclear cells in the papillary dermis.

(ii) Some degree of epidermotropism wlth mononuclear cells colonizing the overlying epidermis. Although great attention has been given in the literature to the presence of collections of mononuclear cells within the epidermis (so-called Pautrier microabscesses), in fact single cell colonization of the epidermis, particularly of the lower layers, is very much more common. The mononuclear cells within the epidermis are often surrounded by a clear halo which probably represents a processing artefact.

(iii) The areas of the epidermis colonized by mononuclear cells show a relative absence of spongiosis unless there has been some secondary eczematous change.

(iv) Under high power examination, usually a number of lymphocytes in the dermis and within the epidermis show some degree of cytological and nuclear atypia. The nuclei of a proportion of lymphocytes may be hyperchromatic and show a convoluted or cerebriform morphology. The number of distinctly atypical cells present within lesions of mycosis fungoides, however, is very variable and obviously atypical cells may on occasion be hard to find. Special techniques, such as the use of interference contrast microscopy or the examination of plastic-embedded material, may make it easier for the histopathologist to detect characteristic abnormalities of the mononuclear cell nuclei.

In early stage mycosis fungoides the epidermis may be thickened, sometimes mimicking psoriasis, or may show some degree of atrophy, particularly in forms of mycosis fungoides where the clinical appearance is that of poikiloderma. The degree of epidermotropism of mononuclear cells is very variable and is most marked in the variant of cutaneous T-cell lymphoma known as pagetoid reticulosis, which will be discussed later.

Another variable feature is the presence of other cell types within the dermal infiltrate, particularly the presence of histiocytes and eosinophils. Eosinophils and histiocytes may be fairly numerous in some varieties of cutaneous T-cell lymphoma. The significance of this particular pattern of infiltrate compared with a predominantly mononuclear cell pattern is uncertain.

Histopathological changes occur in more advanced plague stage and tumour stage mycosis fungoides. The most important differences between advanced stage disease and early stage disease are:

> (i) The tendency for the dermal infiltrate to extend deeper into the dermis and subcutaneous tissues and to lose its epidermotropism. Because of this, advanced stage mycosis fungoides may be difficult to distinguish from some other forms of cutaneous lymphoma, including cutaneous B-cell lymphoma.

> (ii) The proportion of cytomorphologically atypical cells in the infiltrate is much greater in advanced stage disease when compared with early patch stage mycosis fungoides. Increasing numbers of lymphocytes with large and hyperchromatic nuclei may be seen as well as immunoblasts and cells resembling Sternberg-Reed cells that may express the CD30 phenotype.

> (iii) Antigen loss and the acquisition of inappropriate antigens may be seen by mononuclear cells in the later stages of mycosis fungoides.

The histological differential diagnosis of mycosis fungoides in its various stages includes the following:

Actinic reticuloid or chronic actinic dermatitis. In this condition, atypical mononuclear cells may be seen both in the dermal infiltrate and colonizing the epidermis. Spongiosis, however, may also be seen and changes of lichenification are frequently present. The dermal infiltrate is often more polymorphic than normally seen in early stage mycosis fungoides, with the presence of mononuclear cells, histiocytes, eosinophils, plasma cells and large stellate cells, sometimes referred to as Montgomery giant cells, that are normally an indication of chronicity. In addition there may be signs of solar elastosis of dermal connective tissue.

Drug eruptions. Reactions to various systemic drugs can produce histology similar to that seen in some malignant lymphomas. Epidermotropism, however, is not usually a marked feature and eosinophils may be seen in the infiltrate.

Among the drugs that may, on occasion, give rise to pseudolymphomatous tissue reactions are various anticonvulsants, such as phenytoin (Welykyj et al., 1990), silicilates and phenylbutazone.

Insect bites and parasitic infestations. The histology of certain insect bite reactions may consist of a dense granulomatous and lymphocytic dermal infiltrate with mild to moderate cytological atypia and, frequently, the presence of eosinophils. Persistent reactions to scabies can show similar histological features for a long time after the original infestation.

Syphilis. The histology of the cutaneous lesions of secondary syphilis include, in common with cutaneous T-cell lymphoma, a bandlike infiltrate of mononuclear cells and histiocytes in the upper dermis, together with some degree of exocytosis of cells into the overlying epidermis. The presence of a significant proportion of plasma cells in the infiltrate, and any evidence of endarteritis, should alert the pathologist to the possibility of this diagnosis.

Capillaritis. The various forms of capillaritis and pigmented purpuric eruption that occur in the skin may show, histologically, an upper dermal perivascular and confluent infiltrate in which a proportion of the lymphocytes may be large and hyperchromatic. In addition, there is normally evidence of red cell extravasation and deposition of hemosiderin pigment. Some swelling of the endothelial cells of small papillary dermal blood vessels may also be seen.

Melanocytic disorders. Occasional examples of epidermotropic mycosis fungoides and pagetoid reticulosis may show collections of hyperchromatic cells, often with a peripheral halo, both singly and in groups, near the epidermodermal junction and within the epidermis. These features can produce a superficial resemblance to malignant melanoma in situ or dysplastic nevi. Because of the loss of certain lymphocyte and T-cell antigens by the mononuclear cells colonizing the epidermis, these cells may erroneously be interpreted as melanocytes.

Other lymphoproliferative diseases. Many other lymphoproliferative diseases of the skin, both benign, such as lupus erythematosus and Jessner lymphocytic infiltrate, and those probably representing a low-grade form of lymphoma but tending to have a chronic course, such as lymphomatoid papulosis and regressing atypical histiocytosis, may be mistaken, on occasion, for mycosis fungoides. Close correlation between the clinical and histopathological features in these cases is required for accurate diagnosis.

Immunohistochemistry of mycosis fungoides

Immunophenotypic analysis of both fresh, frozen and paraffin-embedded tissue can be a helpful aid in the diagnosis of many forms of cutaneous T-cell lymphoma. The increased availability of new and reliable labels that can be used on paraffin-processed material has greatly increased the value of immunophenotyping (Cerroni et al., 1990; Dreno et al., 1990). Rationalization of the nomenclature used to describe different mononuclear cell antigens (the CD or cluster of differentiation system) has also significantly helped communication between individual workers in this field. In mycosis fungoides the proliferating mononuclear cells are most frequently of the CD4 phenotype. Moreover, most commonly they are the helper inducer phenotype (CD45RA⁻, CDw29⁺) (Sterry and Mielke, 1989). In certain cases of mycosis fungoides and other cutaneous T-cell lymphomas, such as pagetoid reticulosis (MacKie and Turbitt, 1984), lymphomatoid granulomatosis and Sézary syndrome, however, the CD8 (suppressor/cytotoxic) phenotype has been expressed. The exact significance of a CD8 variant of cutaneous T-cell lymphoma is uncertain; some workers have suggested a more favorable outcome in CD8 positive lymphoma when compared with CD4 positive variants of mycosis fungoides whereas in other cases there has been a very aggressive course with fatal outcome (Agnarsson et al., 1990). Michie et al (1990) have drawn attention to the discordant expression of antigens between intraepidermal and intradermal T-cells in mycosis fungoides in a small number of cases and recently Sterry and Hauschild have recorded the loss of leucocyte common antigen (CD45) in some forms of pagetoid reticulosis. Variable antigen expression has also been noted in epidermotropic and non-epidermotropic T-cell clones (Shiohara et al., 1989). It is also known that the antigenic phenotypic profile of both intraepidermal and dermal mononuclear cells in mycosis fungoides varies depending on the stage of the disease.

SÉZARY SYNDROME

Sézary syndrome (Wieselthier et al., 1990) is normally regarded as a variety of cutaneous T-cell lymphoma in which patients are erythrodermic and suffer from troublesome pruritus. In the blood of these patients, atypical T-lymphocytes, with characteristic light microscopic and ultrastructural appearances, are seen. These cells are known as Sézary cells. Other clinical features that may be present include generalised peripheral lymphadenopathy, skin edema and pigmentation, hyperkeratosis of the palms and soles and nail dystrophy. Unfortunately, however, the diagnostic criteria for Sézary syndrome are not precise and the term is used by different workers to include different groups of patients. Patients with "benign" forms of erythroderma, such as erythrodermic psoriasis, drug reactions and erythrodermic eczema, may have circulating Sézary cells. Winkelmann has suggested that a figure of 1,000 Sézary cells per mm³ in the peripheral blood should form one of the diagnostic criteria for the diagnosis. In the Skin Tumour Unit at the St. John's Institute of Dermatology, we use the clinical criteria of pruritus and erythroderma plus the hematological criterion of more than 1,000 circulating Sézary cells per mm³. Even using these criteria, it is quite likely that we are dealing with a heterogenous population, some patients possibly having a form of non-malignant lymphoproliferative disease, such as photosensitive eczema. A further problem is the subjectivity of the diagnosis of Sézary cells on a routine blood film. There is wide inter- and even intra-observer variation in Sézary cell counts on blood films, and, even using modern automated methods, the small cell variant of Sézary syndrome may well be missed. Attempts have been made to differentiate the "benign" from genuinely "malignant forms of Sézary syndrome and the phenotype of the circulating Sézary cell has been suggested as a useful diagnostic marker. Unfortunately, further experience has shown this technique to be of limited value.

Histopathology of Sézary syndrome

The histopathological features described for early stage mycosis fungoides can also be seen in Sézary syndrome. There is frequently a band-like upper dermal mononuclear cell infiltrate, which may be quite dense. Normally, a proportion of cells in the infiltrate show hyperconvoluted and atypical nuclei; ultrastructural observations and cytomorphometry may aid in detecting these cells. In the author's experience, epidermotropism is much less frequently seen than in classic plaque stage mycosis fungoides, and histopathological features of eczema, such as spongiosis, may be superimposed on the histopathology of the Sézary syndrome, itself, making a differentiation from other causes of erythroderma very difficult. Holdaway and Winkelmann (1974) described three patterns of histopathology in patients with the diagnostic criteria of Sézary syndrome. These were termed "dermal lymphocytic reticulosis, dermal reticulosis" and "lymphoma". It seems likely however, that there is a spectrum of changes that may be seen in patients with Sézary syndrome. Sentis, Willemze and Scheffer (1986) have emphasised the difficulty in separating the histopathology of Sézary syndrome from other conditions.

PAGETOID RETICULOSIS

Woringer and Kolopp originally described the case of a 13 year-old boy with an erythematosquamous, polycyclic lesion on the forearm which gradually increased in size over a period of six years. The histology of a skin biopsy from the lesion showed a striking picture, with psoriasiform hyperplasia of the epidermis, extensive colonization of the epidermis by mononuclear cells and a relatively cell-poor dermal infiltrate. Since then there have been numerous similar reports under the titles of "Woringer-Kolopp disease", "pagetoid reticulosis" and "epidermotropic reticulosis". The clinical characteristics of most of these cases have been those of a slowly-growing, scaly, erythematous plaque, usually on an acral site occurring over a long period of time. There has been a very satisfactory response, in most cases, to relatively low doses of radiotherapy, and in the original reported cases there was no evidence of systemic involvement.

Histopathologically, all cases have shown the histological features described above and, although in the early reports there was some uncertainty as to the nature of the cells colonizing the epidermis, lymphocytes, Merkel cells and histiocytes all having their advocates, there seems now no doubt that pagetoid reticulosis is a variety of cutaneous T-cell lymphoma. Wood and colleagues have shown evidence of T-cell clonality in cases of pagetoid reticulosis and have also commented on the T-cell antigen deficiencies of the intraepidermal component. Sterry and Hauschild have contrasted the loss of the leucocyte common antigen marker in cases of localized pagetoid reticulosis with those of so-called disseminated pagetoid reticulosis of the Ketron-Goodman type (Sterry and Hauschild, 1991). It may well be that the Ketron-Goodman type of disseminated pagetoid reticulosis is nothing more than generalized mycosis fungoides with marked epidermotropism, and that the term, pagetoid reticulosis, is best reserved for those cases where there is a solitary, slowly growing plaque, typically on an acral site. Occasional cases have been reported, however, where the classical picture of localized pagetoid reticulosis has eventuated in a more widespread and disseminated form of the condition.

ADULT T-CELL LYMPHOMA/LEUKEMIA (HTLV-1 ASSOCIATED LYMPHOMA)

Although this form of lymphoma is, in many cases, a systemic disease rather than a primary cutaneous lymphoma, skin manifestations may be the first sign of the disorder and skin lesions are seen in approximately 50% of cases. Although this form of lymphoma/leukemia was first described from Japan by Uchyama and colleagues in 1977, it was not until 1980 that an association between this form of lymphoma and the retrovirus which has become known as HTLV-1, was made. It is interesting that the patient from whom the retrovirus was first isolated was thought clinically to have a form of mycosis fungoides. The clinical features of HTLV-1 associated lymphoma are now well recognized. Skin lesions are common and they vary considerably in their morphology. Plaques, nodules and papules, and ulcerated tumors have all been described, as well as erythrodermic forms. Lymphadenopathy and enlarged liver and spleen may be frequently seen, and hypercalcemia, with osteolytic bone lesions, is also a prominent feature. Although when atypical cells are present in the blood the clinical course is normally an aggressive one, with death within six months to two years, it is possible for skin involvement to precede systematization of the disease by many years (Tonkin et al., 1990).

The histology of skin lesions from HTLY-1 associated lymphoma mirrors the variability of skin lesions. The histology in most cases is characterized by a heavy dermal cellular infiltrate composed of atypical mononuclear cells with a variable admixture of small lymphocytes, histiocytic cells, eosinophils and plasma cells. A predominantly granulomatous type of pattern, with histiocytes and multinucleate giant cells may be seen in a minority of cases. The pattern of the dermal infiltrate may be nodular or diffuse; angiocentric and angiodestructive variants have been described.

Epidermotropism is only positive in about half of skin biopsies, and interstitial arrangement of atypical lymphoid cells in rows between collagen bundles (an "Indian file" pattern) is seen in about 75% of cases. High power examination reveals, in a proportion of cases, large lymphoid cells with scanty cytoplasm, sometimes exhibiting in fixed tissue sections a scalloped margin and a mosaic-like arrangement, with cells fitting closely together. Other phenotypic variations are commonly seen, but the multi-lobulated cell often identified in the peripheral blood is rarely seen in histological sections. In most cases of HTLV-1 associated lymphoma, the phenotype of the cell is that of a CD4 positive helper lymphocyte, but several variants have been described, including a case where there was a dual cell population with both helper/inducer cells and suppressor/cytotoxic cells also present.

The isolation of human retroviruses and developments in molecular techniques, allowing determination of clonal integration of viral DNA from lymphoma tissue samples, has opened up exciting new horizons. There is mounting evidence that various forms of cutaneous lymphoma may be etiologically related to viruses similar to the HTLV-1 virus (Anagnostopoulos et al., 1990; Hjelle, 1991).

LYMPHOMATOID PAPULOSIS, REGRESSING ATYPICAL HISTIOCYTOSIS, LARGE CELL ANAPLASTIC LYMPHOMA AND THE CD30 POSITIVE PHENOTYPE

Since Macauley first described the condition of lymphomatoid papulosis, the clinical picture, of widespread scattered papular and necrotic skin lesions that arise in crops and undergo spontaneous resolution, has become well recognized. The histology of lymphomatoid papulosis often consists of a relatively wedge-shaped infiltrate in the upper and mid-dermis involving the epidermis and containing a large number of atypical mononuclear cells, some resembling the cells seen in mycosis fungoides and others larger, with prominent nucleoli, resembling imnunoblasts or Reed-Sternberg cells. It is this atypia which differentiates patients with lymphomatoid papulosis from those with pityriasis lichenoides, although it is likely that both conditions are at separate ends of the same spectrum. Despite the sometimes dramatically atypical cytology of the cellular infiltrate in lymphomatoid papulosis, the clinical course of the disease, in the majority of patients, remains a benign one with recurrent crops of lesions occurring over a long period of time. A number of patients, however, do, after a period of years, go on to develop a more aggressive lymphoma, and it seems likely that lymphomatoid papulosis, itself, is a form of low-grade T-cell lymphoma.

Considerable progress was made in the histopathology of lymphomatoid papulosis by Willemze, when he described two different patterns seen in biopsies from skin lesions; the so-called "type A" pattern, where large pleomorphic histiocytoid cells with relatively pale nuclei and prominent eosinophilic nucleoli are seen, and the "type B" pattern, in which small cerebriform mycosis fungoides-type cells are more plentiful. Although, in many cases, mixed patterns of infiltrate are seen there does seem to be some correlation between the light microscopic appearances from biopsies and evidence of clonality as derived from immuno-globulin and T-cell receptor gene rearrangement studies (Whittaker et al., 1991).

In 1982, Flynn described two patients with cutaneous lesions that also underwent spontaneous regression where the histology showed evidence of epidermotropism, some degree of epidermal hyperplasia and a markedly atypical cellular component in the underlying infiltrate.

Although the condition was termed "regressing atypical histiocytosis", subseguent evidence has suggested this, too, is a form of T-cell proliferation.

The recognition of the CD30 (Ber H2, Ki-1) antigen, originally considered to be specific for the Reed-Sternberg cells of Hodgkin disease, but now thought to be an activation marker present in many forms of T-cell, B-cell and null cell lymphomas, has further increased our appreciation of the spectrum of cutaneous lymphomas. CD30 positivity may be seen in a proportion of cases of lymphomatoid papulosis (particularly those with a type A histological pattern), some forms of regressing atypical histiocytosis, and, of course, in the so-called large cell anaplastic lymphoma. Reference has already been made to the apparent discrepancy of large cell anaplastic lymphoma of nodal origin being in the high-grade malignancy group of the Kiel classification, when there is a relatively benign course of some large cell anaplastic lymphomas that present in the skin. There seems little doubt that the CD30 label marks a wide variety of tumors, and, at present, other criteria are needed. In the second edition of their monograph on non-Hodgkin lymphomas, Leonard and Feller divide CD30 positive non-Hodgkin lymphomas into large cell anaplastic lymphomas of primary and secondary type and CD30 positive lymphomas of variable morphology. Time is needed to determine whether this classification will prove to be a useful one.

CONCLUSION

From the above discussion of histopathological features that may be seen in a variety of T-cell lymphomas that affect the skin, it can be seen that the spectrum of cutaneous T-cell lymphoma is indeed a wide one. Other forms of T-cell lymphoma that affect the skin and could have been included are angiotropic lymphoma of T cell type, angioinmunoblastic lymphade-nopathy, lymphomatoid granulomatosis, granulomatous slack skin disease, multilobulated lymphoma, and Lennert's lymphoma. It is clear from the contributions to this book that we have made important and rapid advances in recent years in our understanding of physiological and aberrant lymphoproliferation in the skin. One of the most important reguirements for continued progress is close cooperation between the clinician, the pathologist and the basic scientist. With continued co-operation our increased understanding of the nature and course of the many forms of cutaneous lymphoma will allow us to select more rational and specific forms of therapy for our patients.

REFERENCES

Agnarsson BA, EC Vonderheid and ME Radin, 1990. Cutaneous T cell lymphoma with suppressor/cytotoxic (CD8) phenotype: Identification of rapidly progressive and chronic subtypes. **J. Am. Acad. Dermatol.**, 22:569.

Anagnostopoulos I, H Hunmel, P Kaudewitz, H Herbst, O Braun-Falco and H Stein, 1990. Detection of HTLV-1 proviral sequences in CD30-positive large cell cutaneous T-cell lymphomas. **Am. J. Pathol.**, 137:1317.

Cerroni L, J Smolle, HP Soyer, A Hartinez Aparicio, and H Kerl, 1990. Immunophenotyping of cutaneous lymphoid infiltrates in frozen and paraffin-embedded tissue sections: A comparative study. **J. Am. Acad. Dermatol.**, 22:405.

Dreno B, B Bureau, J-F Stalder, and P Litoux, 1990. HY7 monoclonal antibody for diagnosis of cutaneous T cell lymphoma. **Arch. Dermatol.**, 126:1454.

Everett MA, 1985. Early diagnosis of mycosis fungoides: vacuolar interface dermatitis. **J. Cutan. Pathol.**, 12:271.

Hjelle B, 1991. Human T-cell leukaemia/lymphoma viruses. **Arch. Pathol. Lab. Med.**, 115:440.

Holdaway DR and RR Winkelmann, 1974. Histopathology of Sézary syndrome. **Mayo Clin. Proc.**, 49:541.

Kerl H, L Cerroni and G Burg, 1991. The morphologic spectrum of T-cell lymphomas of the skin: A proposal for a new classification. **Semin. Diag. Pathol.**, 8:55.

Lindholm JS, DR Barron, ME Williams and SN Swerdlow, 1989. Ki-1-positive cutaneous large cell lymphoma of T cell type: Report of an indolent subtype. **J. Am. Acad. Dermatol.**, 20:342.

Lutzner HA, R Edelson, P Schein, I Green, C Kirkpatrick and A Ahmed, 1975. Cutaneous T-cell lymphomas: The Sézary syndrome, mycosis fungoides, and related disorders. **Ann. Intern. Med.**, 83:534.

MacKie RM and ML Turbitt, 1984. A case of Pagetoid reticulosis bearing the T cytotoxic suppressor surface marker on the lymphoid infiltrate: Further evidence that pagetoid reticulosis is not a variant of mycosis fungoides. **Br. J. Dermatol.**,110:89.

Michie SA, EA Abel, RT Hoppe, RA Warnke, and GS Wood, 1990. Discordant expression of antigens between intraepidermal and intradermal T cells in mycosis fungoides. **Am. J. Pathol.**, 137:1447.

National Cancer Institute Sponsored Study of Classification of Non-Hodgkin's Lymphomas, 1982, Summary and description of a working formulation for clinical usage. **Cancer**, 49:2112.

Nickoloff BJ, 1988. Light-microocopic assessment of 100 patients with patch/plague stage mycosis fungoides. **Am. J. Dermatopathol.**, 10:469.

Pinkus GS, CJ O'Hara and JW Said, 1990. Peripheral/post-thymic T-cell lymphomas: A spectrum of disease. **Cancer**, 65:971.

Rieger E, J Smolle, S Hoedl, F-M Juettner, and H Kerl, 1989. Morphometrical analysis of mycosis fungoides on paraffinembedded sections. **J. Cutan. Pathol.**, 16:7.

Sanchez JL and AB Ackerman, 1979. The patch stage of mycosis fungoides. **Am. J. Dermatopath.**, 1:5.

Sentis HJ, R Willemze and E Scheffer, 1986. Histopathologic studies in Sézary syndrome and erythrodermic mycosis fungoides: A comparison with benign forms of erythroderma. **J. Am. Acad. Dermatol.**, 15:1217.

Shiohara T, N Morlya, C Gotoh, J Hayakawa, X Saizawa, H Yagita and M Nagashima, 1989. Differential expression of lymphocyte function-associated antigen 1 (LPA-1) on epidermotropic and non-epidermotropic T-cell clones. **J. Invest. Dermatol.**, 93:804.

Slater DN, 1991. Cutaneous lymphoproliferative disorders: an assessment of recent investigative techniques. **Br. J. Dermatol.**, 124:309.

Sterry W and V Mielke, 1989. CD4+ cutaneous T-cell lymphomas show the phenotype of helper/inducer T cells (CD45RA-, CDw29+). **Br. Invest. Dermatol.**, 93:413.

Sterry W and A Hauschild, 1991. Loss of leucocyte common antigen (CD45) on atypical lymphocytes in the localized but not disseminated typo of Pagetoid reticulosis. **Br. J. Dermatol.**, 125:238.

Su I-J, Y-C Wu, Y-C Chen, H-C Hsieh, A-L Cheng, C-H Wang and ME Kadin, 1990. Cutaneous manifestations of post-thymic T cell malignancies: Description of five clinicopathologic subtypes. **J. Am. Acad. Dermatol.**, 23:653.

Tonkin RS, GJS Rustin and FJ Paradinas, 1990. HTLV-1 associated T-cell lymphoma in a patient with a 10 year history of nonepidermotrophic T-cell skin infiltrates. **Clin. Oncol.**, 2:354.

Van der Loo EM, WA Van Vloten, CJ Cornelisse, E Scheffer and CJLM Meijer, 1981. The relevance of morphometry in the differential diagnosis of cutaneous T-cell lymphomas. **Br. J. Dermatol.**, 104:257.

Vogt T, W Stolz, O Braun-Falco, P Raudewitz, F Eckert, W Abmayr, R Dummer and G Burg, 1991. Prognostic significance of DNA cytometry in cutaneous malignant lymphomas. **Cancer**, 68:1095.

Welykyj S, R Gradini, J Nakao and M Massa, 1990. Carbamazeplne induced eruption histologically mimicking mycosis fungoides. **J. Cutan. Pathol.**, 17:111.

Whittaker S, N Smith, R Russell Jones and L Luzzatto, 1991. Analysis of, and T-cell receptor genes in lymphomatoid papulosis: Cellular basis of two distinct histologic subsets. **J. Invest. Dermatol.**, 96:791.

Wieselthier JS and HK Koh, 1990. Sézary syndrome: Diagnosis, prognosis, and critical review of treatment options. **J. Am. Acad. Dermatol.**, 22:381.

Wood GS, LM Weiss, RA Warnke and J Sklar, 1986. The immunopathology of cutaneous lymphomas: Immunophenotypic and immunogenotypic characteristics. **Semin. Dermatol.**, 5:334.

CUTANEOUS T-CELL LYMPHOMA:
CLUES TO DIAGNOSIS IN EARLY LESIONS

Marco Santucci

Institute of Morbid Anatomy and Histopathology
University of Florence
Florence, Italy

Correspondence to: Dr. M. Santucci, Ist. di Anat. e Pathol.,
University degli Studi, Viale GB Morgagne 85,
I-50134 Florence, Italy

ABSTRACT

The correct identification of cutaneous T-cell lymphomas and their differentiation from both inflammatory dermatoses and reactive lymphoid hyperplasias represent a vexing problem when dealing with the initial phases of a lymphomatous process. Even advanced diagnostic techniques, like immunophenotyping, quantitative DNA cytophotometry, and molecular genetic analysis, have proven to be unsuitable for solving the problem; thus, light microscopy remains the basic, gold standard diagnostic procedure. In order to make a definite diagnosis of lymphoma from early lesions, the most important and cardinal feature is the presence of lymphocytes with extremely convoluted (cerebriform), medium-large-sized (7-9 μm) nuclei (medium-large cerebriform cells), singly or in clusters in the epidermis and in discrete collections in the dermis. Additional histologic features are: (i) epidermotropism, manifested as single cells lining up along the basal keratinocytes near the dermal-epidermal junction; (ii) tendency of medium-large cerebriform cells within the epidermis to congregate and seemingly to touch one another; (iii) absence of spongiotic microvesiculation; (iv) little or no edema of the papillary dermis; slight to moderate fibrosis in some cases; and (v) a tendency of the dermal infiltrate, which as a rule is rather monomorphous in composition, to assume a lichenoid configuration.

INTRODUCTION

The correct identification of cutaneous T-cell lymphomas (CTCL) and their proper differentiation from both inflammatory dermatoses and reactive lymphoid hyperplasias quite often represent a vexing problem, especially when dealing with the initial phases of a lymphomatous process. The absence of reliable morphoarchitectural criteria for the distinction between reactive and early neoplastic cutaneous lymphoid infiltrates reflects the often profoundly different ideas of experts on what is the histologic picture of early lesions of CTCL.

Even advanced and experimental diagnostic techniques, like immunophenotyping (Ralfkiaer, 1991), quantitative DNA cytophotometry (Everett, 1986), and molecular genetic analysis (LeBoit and Parslow, 1987; Bignon and Souteyrand, 1990; Volkenandt et al., 1991), have proven to be unsuitable in solving the problem; this is due to the absence of aberrant immunophenotypes or of abnormal content of DNA, or the paucity of monoclonal cells so as to be undetectable by DNA analysis in these early phases. Thus, the light-microscopic diagnosis of early CTCL remains the basic, gold standard, procedure.

Many authorities have stated that in the very initial lymphomatous stages a specific diagnosis of CTCL cannot be made (Lever and Schaumburg-Lever, 1987), since early lesions show a non-specific dermatitis (Montgomery, 1967) or the histologic changes are in many ways similar to those observed in eczematoid dermatitis and neurodermatitis (Graham et al., 1972). Therefore, more reliance has to be placed on the clinical picture than on the histologic appearance to identify them (Samman, 1966), since the clinical picture may be more suggestive than the histopathologic picture (Caro, 1978). At present, it is considered probable that the lymphomatous disorder evolves through a multistage process with an initial reactive polyclonal proliferation, finally transforming into a clonal malignancy (Slater, 1987).

These statements do not automatically imply that identification of the early phases of the disease is always impossible. For this purpose, at times, the critical feature for histologic diagnosis has been identified as the presence of an increased number of mononuclear cells (not necessarily atypical) distributed singly or in small collections within an epidermis devoid of spongiotic microvesiculation (Sanchez and Ackerman, 1979); or neoplastic cells have been reported to be identifiable by their nuclei which have an oval, irregular outline, hyperchromasia and slightly larger size when compared to a small mature lymphocyte (Freeman, 1986); or the basic requisite for the diagnosis has been claimed to reside in the identification of a characteristic cell with a convoluted nucleus (mycosis cell, Lutzner cell or Sézary cell) (Reed, 1986). At times, the diagnosis has been based on the contemporaneous presence of both cytologic characteristics and the numerical representation of the atypical cells in the infiltrates (Reed, 1986). Finally, it has even been stated that the histoarchitectural pattern (i.e., vacuolar interface dermatitis), and not the cytologic characteristics, is the crucial and cardinal feature in differential diagnosis in the earliest phases of the lymphomatous process (Everett, 1985).

The aim of this investigation was to test the diagnostic utility of the currently published histologic criteria for the differentiation of early lesions of CTCL and their simulants (Sanchez and Ackerman, 1979; Everett, 1985; Jones, 1986; Nickoloff, 1988; Burg and Kaudewitz, 1990; LeBoit and Epstein, 1990; King-Ismael and Ackerman, 1992; Rijlaarsdam and Willemze, 1991; Burg et al., 1992), and to focus on those which proved to be the most useful in properly differentiating these conditions.

MATERIALS AND METHODS

The case materials used in this investigation were collected by the E.O.R.T.C.- B.M.F.T. Cutaneous Lymphoma Project Group (chaired by Professor Günter Burg), and was provided by representatives from 19 European Centers (Antwerp (B), Barcelona (E), Bordeaux (F), Créteil (F), Florence (I), Gent (B), Giessen (D), Graz (A), Groningen (NL), Hamburg (D), Hannover (D) Copenhagen (DK), Innsbruck (A), Leuven (B), Milan (I), Salzburg (A) Utrecht (NL), Villejuif (F), and Würzburg (D)) participating in the E.O.R.T.C. Symposia on the Histopathology of Early Mycosis Fungoides Lesions which were held in Gent in May 1989 and in Würzburg in September 1990.

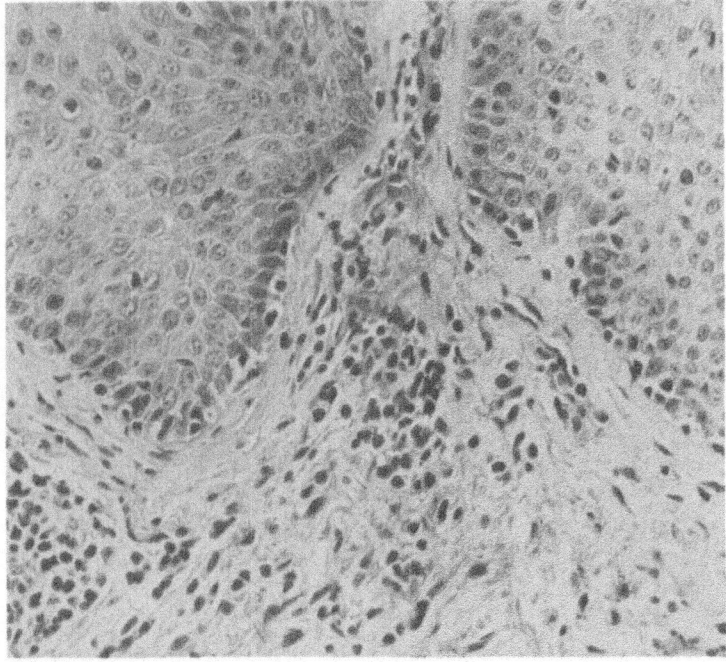

Figure 1. Medium-large cerebriform cells -- separated from the surrounding keratinocytes by clear spaces giving them the appearance of haloed cells and resembling melanocytes -- infiltrate the epidermis in a somewhat linear configuration at the basal level. In the dermis, medium-large cerebriform cells are present in discrete collections.

The referring physicians were asked to contribute cases in which histologic material from the very beginning of the disease was available, irrespective of whether or not initial biopsies were considered diagnostic for lymphoma. The material consisted of a series of 32 cases (for a total number of 73 slides). All cases had complete clinical information (i.e., age of lesions, staging, treatment and duration of the disease) and follow-up data. In these cases, the diagnosis of lymphoma was unequivocally established by clinical events (i.e., later development of plaques and/or nodules) and/or indubitable histologic findings. For this study, slides representative of the initial phases of the lymphomatous process were considered to be those obtained from patients with stage IA disease (limited plaques, papules or eczematous patches covering less than 10% of the skin surface).

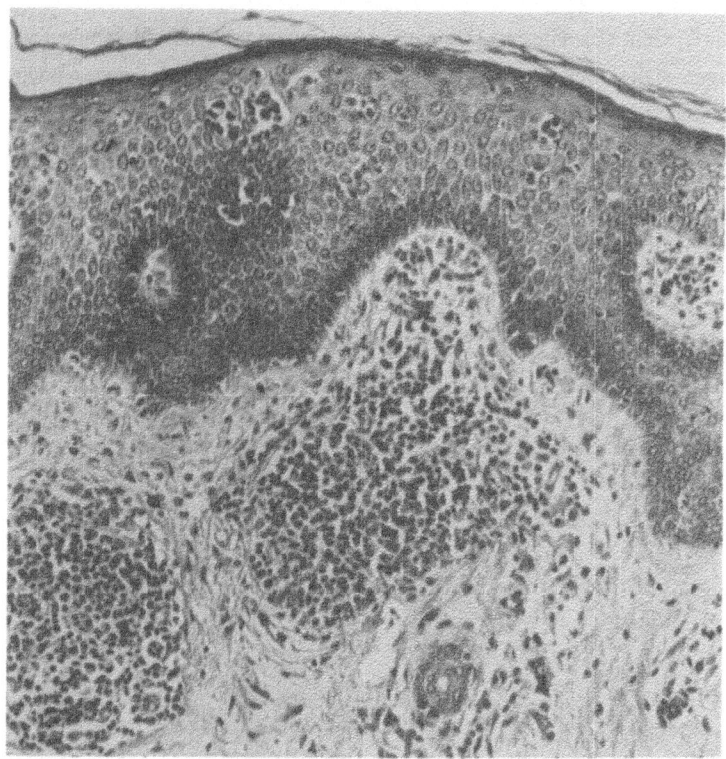

Figure 2. Medium-large cerebriform cells infiltrate the epidermis, which is mostly normal in morphologic configuration, mainly in tiny groups, and are found in the papillary dermis in discrete collections. Plasma cells, eosinophils, and macrophages are conspicuously absent.

Twenty-four slides from 18 patients fulfilled the above-mentioned criteria. The remaining 49 slides were considered to be representative of non-initial disease. In addition, 13 slides of eczematous or psoriasiform simulators of CTCL were blindly and randomly mixed with the contributed cases as negative controls.

All specimens had been routinely processed and stained by the hematoxylin and eosin and the Giemsa stains.

Currently published histologic criteria (morphology, number, arrangement, distribution, and position of epidermal infiltrating lymphoid cells; pattern and composition of the dermal infiltrate; and possible concomitant epidermal and/or dermal changes) for the differentiation of early lesions of CTCL and their eczematous, lichenoid, or psoriasiform simulators were tested for their diagnostic utility in properly distinguishing these conditions. For this study, four diagnostic categories were used: (i) definite lymphoma (i.e., lymphoma without any doubt), (ii) probable

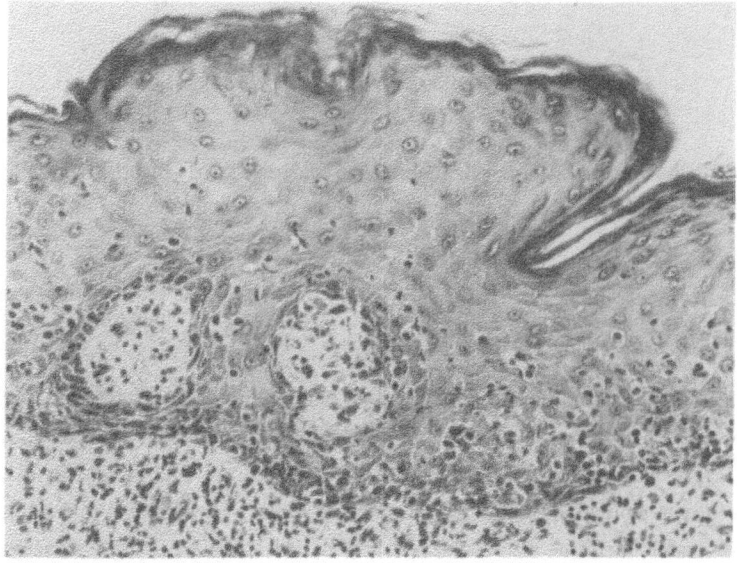

Figure 3. Neoplastic cells infiltrate the epidermis mainly as single cells. Note that their size is approximately the same as that of surrounding keratinocytes.

lymphoma (i.e., a diagnosis of lymphoma cannot be confidently made), (iii) possible lymphoma (i.e., a diagnosis of lymphoma cannot be confidently excluded), and (iv) non-lymphoma (i.e., non-lymphoma without any doubt).

HISTOPATHOLOGIC FEATURES OF EARLY CTCL LESIONS

The histomorphology of early lesions has been found to vary according to the clinical picture and duration of lesions prior to the biopsy, so that three main aspects can be identified, as follows (Figures 1-6):

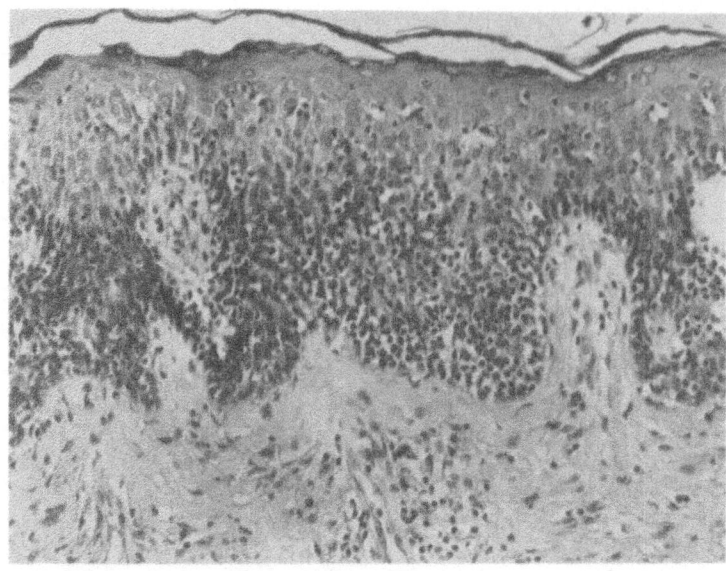

Figure 4. Medium-large cerebriform cells infiltrate the epidermis across almost its entire breadth, with a prevalence for the lower portion. Note the paucity of the dermal infiltrate.

The histologic picture of the **most initial early lesions** -- clinically represented by orange-pink discolored patches without significant alterations in their surfaces -- is that of a superficial perivascular lympho(histio)cytic infiltrate, sometimes with lichenoid foci, that may obscure the dermal-epidermal interface. Lymphoid cells with roundish-to-oval, convoluted nuclei approximately the same size as the nuclei of basal keratinocytes are always found within the epidermis -- and sometimes in the epithelium of adnexa -- mostly singly, but also in tiny collections, with few if any Langerhans cells and no significant cytopathic changes in the surrounding keratinocytes. The single lymphoid cells are often separated from the surrounding keratinocytes by clear spaces, giving them the appearance of <u>haloed cells</u>. Cells that are indubitably atypical are not usually observed within the dermal infiltrate, but lymphoid cells with medium-large-sized (*), roundish, highly convoluted nuclei (i.e., medium-large cerebriform cells) are consistently present mixed with smaller cerebriform cells, small lymphocytes, and non-phagocytizing histiocytes. Plasma cells, eosinophils, and macrophages are absent from the dermal infiltrate. The epidermis is mostly normal in morphologic configuration. As a rule, there is no spongiotic microvesiculation; conversely, widened intercellular spaces with stretched intercellular bridges are often present. The papillary dermis is usually normal without evidence

---

(*) A medium-sized nucleus has a diameter of 5-9 μ, a large one 10-12 μ, and a small-sized nucleus less than 5 μ (Suchi et al, 1987). The terminology "medium-small" and "medium-large" derives from the need to separate into two groups the broad range of medium size when speaking of cerebriform cells and therefore, conventionally, medium-large sized is 7-9 μ and medium-small 5-7 μ.

of edema; the superficial vascular plexus is normal or slightly dilated, without extravasated erythrocytes.

Intermediate early lesions -- clinically represented by brown-red discoloration patches with clinical features of atrophy and sometimes scaling -- show a deep as well as superficial perivascular lympho(histio)cytic infiltrate, not infrequently in a lichenoid array in the papillary dermis. Medium-large cerebriform cells are consistently found within both the epidermis -- usually singly as haloed cells, or in small groups -- and the dermis, in discrete collections. When haloed lymphoid cells are apposed to basal and lower level keratinocytes in a somewhat linear configuration on the epidermal side of the dermal-epidermal junction, they can resemble, and be mistaken for, melanocytes. Dyskeratotic keratinocytes may be scattered within the epidermis. Plasma cells, eosinophils, and neutrophils are absent from the dermal infiltrate. Conversely, melanophages, siderophages, and telangiectases are often found in the papillary dermis, which is often markedly thickened by coarse collagen fibers associated with an increased number of stellate fibroblasts. The epidermis is usually thinned with obliteration of the rete ridges and dermal papillae. The cornified layer is altered by laminated and/or compact orthokeratosis or by foci of parakeratosis. Lymphoid cells in the epidermis are sometimes a little larger than the infiltrating cells in the dermis, and their nuclei may be clearly atypical (large cerebriform and/or pleomorphic cells) in a small minority of cases.

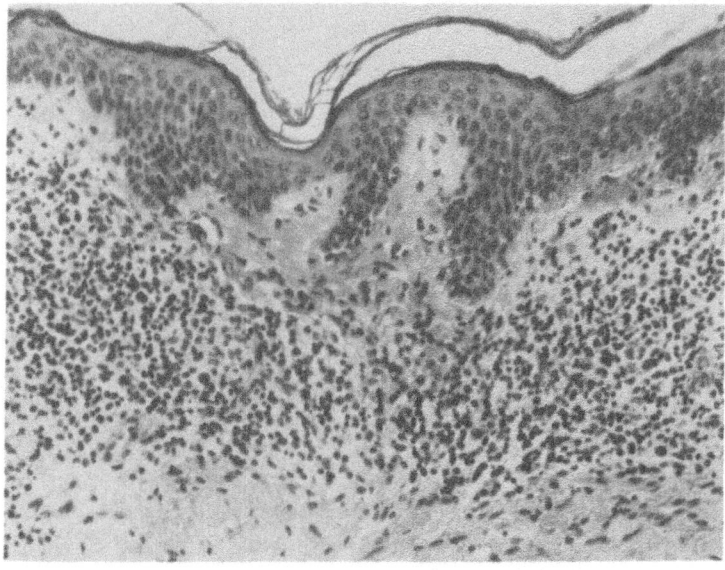

Figure 5. The epidermis is unaffected by the neoplastic proliferation. Medium-large and large cerebriform cells are arranged in a band-like fashion in the upper dermis.

Finally, the **most advanced early lesions** -- clinically characterized by slightly elevated, pink-to-purple in color, scaly, irregularly shaped plaques -- histologically reveal moderately dense lympho(histio)cytic infiltrates around the blood vessels of the superficial and deep plexa.

The infiltrating cells fill a widened papillary dermis and are arranged in a band-like configuration. Significant numbers of large cerebriform cells are consistently found within the epidermis, singly or in collections of different sizes and shapes, not infrequently mixed with medium and large pleomorphic lymphocytes. Dyskeratotic keratinocytes are quite often present in the epidermis, especially if it is riddled by cerebriform or pleomorphic lymphocytes. The epidermis is usually psoriasiform, with ortho- or parakeratotic scales. Sclerotic collagen is often found between the dermal band-like infiltrate and the overlying epidermis. Cerebriform and pleomorphic lymphocytes are present in significant numbers in the dermal infiltrate mixed with inflammatory cells, especially plasma cells and eosinophils. The more long-standing the lesion, the more conspicuous is the reactive inflammatory infiltrate and the more numerous the atypical lymphocytes.

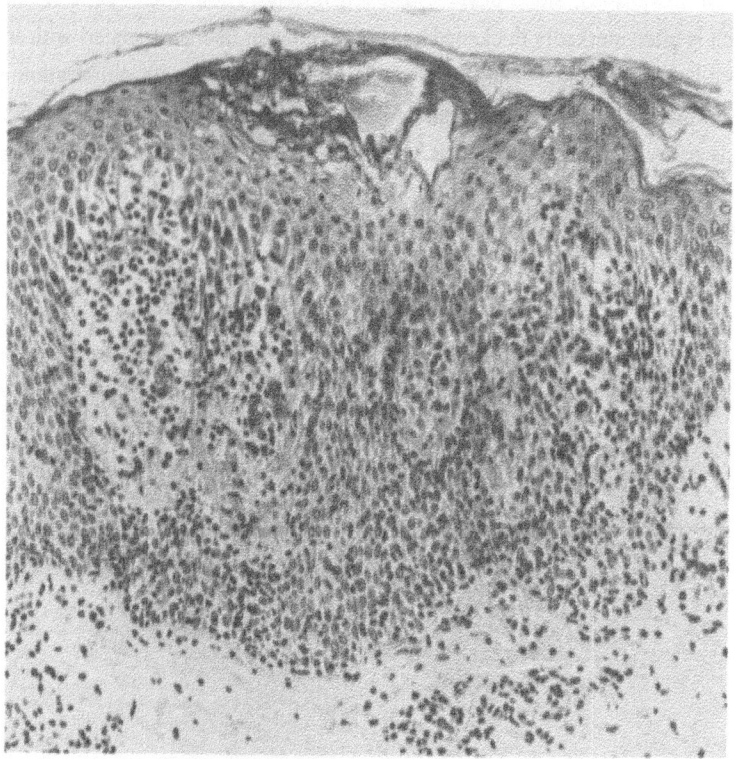

Figure 6. Despite the presence of spongiotic microvesiculations, this lesion characterized by a spongiotic lichenoid pattern is clearly diagnostic of lymphoma, due to the presence of significant numbers of medium-large cerebriform cells.

RESULTS AND COMMENT

The results obtained by the author using the abovementioned histomorphologic criteria are reported in Table 1.

Table 1. Results of the Histologic Investigation*

	Proportion of lesions read as lymphoma		
	Early Lesions	Non-Initial Lesions	Control Cases
Definite Lymphoma	77.0%	85.7%	-
Probable Lymphoma	14.7%	10.2%	-
Possible Lymphoma	8.3%	4.1%	15.4%
Non-Lymphoma	-	-	84.6%

(*) Evaluation of the reproducibility of the histologic diagnosis and of the inter- and intra-observer agreement goes beyond the scope of the present paper and will be considered in detail in another article.

It is worth noting that the specificity was quite excellent; using strict histologic criteria, no control case was read as probable or definite lymphoma. Therefore, it is possible to avoid overdiagnosing.

Conversely, sensitivity (i.e., correct identification of lymphoma as lymphoma and of non-lymphoma as non-lymphoma) showed less excellent values. Astonishingly, it was similar among the three groups. The observed sensitivities for early lymphomatous lesions (75%) or simulators of CTCL (84.6%) can be considered good, especially in light of the difficulties of the diagnostic problem and of the claimed impossibility of consistently identifying early lesions and differentiating them from CTCL simulators by histopathology alone. The observed sensitivity (85.7%) for non-initial lymphomatous lesions is less understandable, and some comments are due.

A possible explanation for this disappointing sensitivity for non-initial lymphomatous lesions can be found in the very nature of cutaneous lymphoid infiltrates, in which there is an admixture of nuclear size and shape, and the assessment of lymphocyte morphology is often quite difficult. This is especially true when proper fixation of specimens has not been performed and/or thin, well-stained sections are not available, as was not infrequently the case in the present investigation due to the heterogeneous sources of the referred material. Fine cytologic distinctions are much more difficult to evaluate in the skin than in lymph nodes, largely because of a greater tendency toward evident artefactual distortions, such as nuclear shrinkage, hyperchromatism, distortion of the nuclear contour, and excessive crowding or separation of cells. When the technical quality of slides is less than optimal, the unequivocal identification of medium -large cerebriform cells -- that only rarely are indubitably atypical -- may not always be possible; this points up the utmost importance of technical quality when dealing with lymphoproliferative disorders. This is confirmed by the relatively high percentage of the non-initial lymphomatous lesions read as probable lymphoma (10.2%), that, if added to the percentage read as definite lymphoma, raises the total percentage to a more reasonable value of 95.9% for non-initial lesions, and to 91.7% for early lesions. In our opinion, these total sensitivities represent a very good result, based on histomorphology alone.

Finally -- and this consideration applies to all fields of pathology -- not every lesion present in a given patient with a neoplastic disease necessarily represents the "principal" pathologic process; this is especially true in cutaneous specimens where the occurrence of a variety of idiopathic lesions is well known. Therefore, we have to consider the possibility of the contemporaneous presence in these patients of non-neoplastic (? drug-induced, ? paraneoplastic, ? allergic) lesions which, if confused with the specific ones on clinical grounds and thus errone-ously biopsied, would introduce a bias into the overall results.

CONCLUSIONS

Cutaneous T-cell lymphomas are incredibly protean and exceptions may be found to almost every statement that has been written about them (LeBoit, 1991). Irrespective of the fact that in a specific single lesion it is theoretically possible to find any morphologic pattern, it is important to remember -- whatever the disorder is -- that some features are very frequently found as opposed to others that are quite rare, and that some features are pathognomonic as opposed to others which, although typical, may also be seen in other disorders.

With this in mind, in order to make a definite diagnosis of lymphoma from early lesions -- irrespective of the type and/or age of the lesion -- the most important and cardinal feature is the presence of medium-large-sized lymphocytes with extreme nuclear convolutions (medium-large cerebriform cells), singly or in clusters in the epidermis and in discrete collections in the dermis. We must stress the crucial importance of the presence of significant numbers of medium-large cerebriform cells, especially at the dermal level, since occasional and/or sparse cells, variably mixed with a polymorphous cellular infiltrate, are not infrequently seen in a variety of cutaneous inflammatory disorders, including many simulants of CTCL (Freeman, 1986; Nickoloff, 1988).

In our experience, the number (few or many), arrangement (singly or in nests), distribution (across the entire breadth of the epidermis, in several discrete areas, confined to a single focus, or in a somewhat linear configuration at the basal-suprabasal level), and position (whether in the upper part as well as in the lower portion of the epidermis) of epidermal cerebriform cells; the pattern and composition of the dermal infiltrate; and possible concomitant epidermal and/or dermal changes are not cardinal elements for the diagnosis of CTCL. On the other hand, additional histologic features that can help in differentiating early lymphomatous lesions from their spongiotic, lichenoid, or eczematous simulators are: (i) presence within the epidermis of mononuclear cells with nuclei roughly the same size as those of surrounding keratinocytes; (ii) epidermotropism manifested as single cells lining up along the basal keratinocytes on the epidermal side of the dermal-epidermal junction; (iii) tendency of mononuclear cells within the epidermis to congregate and seemingly to touch one another; (iv) mononuclear cells high in the granular zone and even in the cornified layer; (v) absence of spongiotic microvesiculation (what appears at first glance to be a spongiotic lichenoid dermatitis, on a more thorough examination will probably reveal an early lymphomatous lesion); (vi) little or no edema of the papillary dermis in the most initial early lesions; fibrosis in the thickened papillary dermis in intermediate and advanced, early lesions; and (vii) a dermal infiltrate with a tendency to a lichenoid configuration which as a rule is rather monomorphous in composition in initial and intermediate early lymphomatous lesions. Finally, features that are indicative of clear-cut disease (e.g., typical Pautrier's collections or clearly atypical lymphoid cells), which, unfortunately are only seldom, if ever, observed in the initial phases of the disease, obviously -- when present -- supply additional valuable help in this highly difficult diagnostic task.

ACKNOWLEDGEMENTS

A significant part of this work was performed during sabbatical furloughs Marco Santucci spent at the Klinik und Poliklinik fur Hautkrankheiten der Universitat Würzburg (D) directed by Professor Günter Burg.

REFERENCES

Bignon YL and P Souteyrand, 1990. Genotyping of cutaneous T-cell lymphomas and pseudolymphomas, In: WA van Vloten, R Willemze, G Lange Vejlsgaard and K Thomsen, Eds. **Cutaneous Lymphoma, Current Problems in Dermatology**, vol. 19 (H Honigsmann, Ed:), Karger, Basel.

Burg G and P Kaudewitz, 1990. Where are we today in the diagnosis of cutaneous lymphoma?, In: WA van Vloten, R Willemze, G Lange Vejlsgaard and K Thomsen, Eds., **Cutaneous Lymphoma, Current Problems in Dermatology**, vol. 19 (H Honigsmann, Ed.), Karger, Basel, 1990.

Burg G, M Santucci, AC Feller and É Szabó, 1992. Diagnostic problems in minimal lymphoproliferative skin infiltrates. **Am. J. Dermatopathol.**, 14:74.

Caro WA, 1978. Biopsy in suspected malignant lymphoma of the skin. **Cutis**, 21:197.

Everett MA, 1985. Early diagnosis of mycosis fungoides: Vacuolar interface dermatitis. **J. Cutan. Pathol.**, 12:271.

Everett MA, 1986. Questions to the Editorial Board and Other Authorities. **Am. J. Dermatopathol.**, 8:536.

Freeman RG, 1986. Questions to the Editorial Board and Other Authorities. **Am. J. Dermatopathol.**, 8:536.

Graham JH, Johnson WC, and Helwig EB, 1972. **Dermal Pathology**, Harper & Row, Hagerstown, MD.

Jones RE, 1986. Questions to the Editorial Board and Other Authorities. **Am. J. Dermatopathol.**, 8:536.

King-Ismael D and AB Ackerman, 1992. Guttate parapsoriasis/digitate dermatosis (small plaque parapsoriasis) is mycosis fungoides. **Am. J. Dermatopathol.**, 14:518.

LeBoit PE and TG Parslow, 1987. Gene rearrangements in lymphoma. Applications to dermatopathology, **Am. J. Dermatopathol.**, 9:212.

LeBoit PE, and Epstein BA, 1990. A vase-like shape characterizes the epidermal-mononuclear cell collections seen in spongiotic dermatitis. **Am. J. Dermatopathol.**, 12:612.

LeBoit PE, 1991. Variants of mycosis fungoides and related cutaneous T-cell lymphomas. **Semin. Diagn. Pathol.**, 8:73.

Lever WF, and G Schaumburg-Lever, 1987. **Histopathology of the Skin**, 6th ed., JB Lippincott Co., Philadelphia.

Montgomery H, 1967. **Dermatopathology**, Harper & Row, New York.

Nickoloff BJ, 1988. Light-microscopic assessment of 100 patients with patch/plaque-stage mycosis fungoides. **Am. J. Dermatopathol.**, 10:469.

Ralfkiaer E, 1991. Immunohistological markers for the diagnosis of cutaneous lymphomas. **Semin. Diagn. Pathol.**, 8:62.

Reed R, 1986. Questions to the Editorial Board and Other Authorities. **Am. J. Dermatopathol.**, 8:536.

Rijlaarsdam U and R Willemze, 1991. Cutaneous pseudo-T cell lymphomas. **Semin. Diagn. Pathol.**, 8:102.

Slater DN, 1987. Recent developments in cutaneous lymphoproliferative disorders. **J. Pathol.**, 153:5.

Samman PD, 1972. The natural history of parapsoriasis en plaques (chronic superficial dermatitis) and prereticulotic poikiloderma. **Br. J. Dermatol.**, 87:405.

Sanchez JL and AB Ackerman, 1979. The patch stage of mycosis fungoides. Criteria for histologic diagnosis. **Am. J. Dermatopathol.**, 1:5.

Suchi T, K Lennert, L-Y Tu, M Kikuchi, E Sato, AG Stansfeld, and AC Feller, 1987. Histopathology and immunohistochemistry of peripheral T cell lymphomas: A proposal for their classification. **J. Clin. Pathol.**, 40:995.

Volkenandt M, HP Soyer, H Kerl and JR Bertino, 1991. Development of a highly specific and sensitive molecular probe for detection of cutaneous lymphoma. **J. Invest. Dermatol.**, 97:137.

MORPHOLOGIC AND PROGNOSTIC FEATURES OF ADVANCED MYCOSIS FUNGOIDES

Helmut Kerl
Lorenzo Cerroni
Stefan Hoedl

Department of Dermatology
University of Graz
Graz, Austria

Correspondence to: Dr. H. Kerl, Department of Dermatology,
University of Graz, Auenbruggerplatz 8,
A-8036 Graz, Austria

ABSTRACT

Mycosis fungoides (MF) is a cutaneous T cell lymphoma (CTCL) of low grade malignancy, characterized by the proliferation of small to medium sized cells with cerebriform nuclei. Many patients show, in the advanced stages of the disease, progression to a large cell lymphoma (LCL). In this study, biopsies of tumors from 36 patients with advanced MF were examined for cytomorphologic evidence for transformation into LCL. The findings were: 44.4% of these cases showed no evidence of transformation; only classical MF with small to medium sized cells with cerebriform nuclei were seen. 13.9% showed T-immunoblastic lymphoma, with predominance of cells with round to oval nuclei and prominent, centrally located nucleoli. 25.0% showed medium sized and large T cells with pleomorphic nuclei. 5.6% showed large anaplastic T cell lymphoma with cytomorphologic features of large anaplastic and immunoblastic cells and cells resembling Reed-Sternberg cells. 11.1% showed unclassified LCL, characterized by large cells with features of pleomorphic cells and immunoblasts. Immunohistochemical investigations revealed aberrant patterns of antigen expression (loss of one or more pan-T cell antigens or simultaneous presence of activation and proliferation-associated antigens). Clusters of B lymphocytes were found in about one-third of these cases. Analysis of overall survival from time of first biopsy diagnostic of MF showed a statistically significant difference between patients with non-transformed MF versus those in which transformation to LCL had occurred (ten-year survival, 46.6% versus 11.1%; $p < 0.02$).

Basic Mechanisms of Physiologic and Aberrant Lymphoproliferation in the Skin
Edited by W.C. Lambert *et al.*, Plenum Press, New York, 1994

255

INTRODUCTION

Mycosis fungoides (MF) is a low-grade malignant T cell lymphoma of the skin, which is characterized by a slow progression with prolonged survival. Histology of early lesions reveals a band-like infiltrate in the superficial dermis with epidermotropism of single lymphocytes and/or collections of cells (so-called Pautrier "microabscesses") in the epidermis. In tumor lesions, the infiltrate is usually dense, nodular or diffuse, involves the entire dermis down to the subcutaneous fat, and may lose its epidermotropic features. Cytomorphologically, MF is characterized by the proliferation of small- to medium-sized cells with cerebriform nuclei and immunophenotypic features of T-helper lymphocytes (CD3+, CD4+, CD8-). In several studies, however, sequential biopsies have shown histologic transformation to a large cell lymphoma (LCL) (Buechner et al., 1979, Catterall et al., 1983, Cerroni et al., 1992, Dmitrowsky et al., 1987, Kerl et al., 1991, Ralfkiaer et al., 1989, Salhany et al., 1988, Scheen et al., 1984, Tykocinsky et al., 1984, van der Putte et al., 1984, Yanagihara et al., 1984). This finding is usually associated with more aggressive biological behavior and rapidly fatal outcome (Dmitrowsky et al., 1987, Greer et al., 1990, Salhany et al., 1988). In this article we review the clinical, histopathological, and immuno-histochemical features of cutaneous lesions from 36 patients with advanced MF.

CLINICAL FEATURES OF CUTANEOUS LESIONS OF ADVANCED MYCOSIS FUNGOIDES

Clinical features of cutaneous tumors in MF patients were variable. Thirty-two patients with MF presented with nodules and tumors on preexisting eczematous patches and plaques or on unaffected skin. The lesions were often ulcerated. The color varied from reddish-brown to deeper hues of red, including violet. Three patients with Sézary syndrome developed numerous papules, nodules and tumors in the late stages of the disease. One patient with disseminated pagetoid reticulosis (Ketron-Goodman type) presented with ulcerated plaques and nodules on the trunk and upper extremities.

HISTOPATHOLOGIC FEATURES OF TUMOR INFILTRATES

A major problem in the classification of the tumor infiltrates of advanced MF is the admixture of different cells. It may be difficult to distinguish the neoplastic clone of cells from the "normal" reactive infiltrate. In addition, neoplastic cells with different cytomorphologic features may be present within the same infiltrate, thus making a correct classification of these cases difficult.

Based upon the cytomorphologic features of the neoplastic infiltrate, five different types of lymphoma were recognized in the advanced stages of MF in this study:

i)   predominance of small- to medium-sized cells with cerebriform nuclei ("classical" type MF) (16 cases);

ii) predominance of cells with cytomorphologic features of T immunoblasts (T-immunoblastic lymphoma) (5 cases);

iii) predominance of cells with cytomorphologic features of medium- and large-sized pleomorphic cells (T medium- and large-cell pleomorphic lymphoma) (9 cases);

iv) predominance of cells with cytomorphologic features of large anaplastic cells (T large cell anaplastic lymphoma) (2 cases); and

v)   predominance of large cells showing cytomorphologic features of pleomorphic cells and immunoblasts (unclassifiable large cell lymphoma) (4 cases).

Architectural patterns

Cutaneous tumors of MF revealed dense, diffuse or nodular infiltrates involving the entire dermis and frequently the subcutaneous fat. Adnexal structures were invaded, and in some cases totally destroyed, by the neoplastic cells. Although it is generally thought that epidermotropism is not found in the advanced lesions of MF, we could observe the presence of single lymphocytes or collections of cells within the epidermis in more than 60% of tumor-stage lesions of MF, regardless of cytomorphologic features of the neoplastic infiltrates. High endothelial venules were usually numerous within the infiltrate.

Cytomorphologic features

Tumor-stage lesions of **"classical"** MF (16 cases, 44.4%) were characterized by cytologically small- and medium-sized atypical cells with complex folded nuclear membranes ("cerebriform" cells, Lutzner cells). Histopathological features of MF and Sézary syndrome were similar. A distinction between cerebriform cells and small and medium pleomorphic cells that can also be found in adult T cell leukemia/lymphoma is, in our opinion, impossible. Cerebriform and pleomorphic cells probably represent the same cell type morphologically, which apparently develops in response to some types of antigen.

In **T-immunoblastic lymphoma** (5 cases, 13.9%) (Figure 1) the cells were large, with round, oval, or slightly irregular vesicular nuclei and in most cases only one, usually centrally located, prominent nucleolus. The cytoplasm was basophilic or pale stained.

T medium- and large-cell pleomorphic lymphoma (9 cases, 25.0%) (Figure 2) presented with an infiltrate characterized by medium- or large-sized cells with pleomorphic

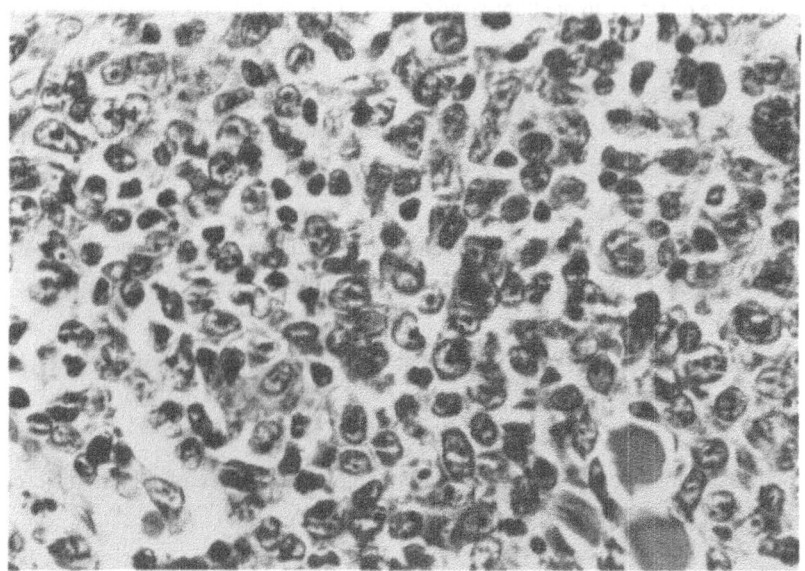

Figure 1. MF with transformation into T-immunoblastic lymphoma. Immunoblasts with round or oval nuclei and prominent, centrally located nucleoli are seen.

nuclei. Designations that have been used to describe the nuclear irregularities of the pleomorphic cells include maple-leaf, walnut seed-like, jelly fish appearence, banana bunch appearance, embryo-like, and others. Many nuclei were lobulated, twisted, or cerebriform. The cytoplasm was pale gray with Giemsa staining.

Pleomorphic lymphoma has been described in patients with adult T cell leukemia/lymphoma (ATLL), associated with HTLV-1 infection (Maeda et al., 1989). MF patients developing T medium- and large-cell pleomorphic lymphoma, however, do not have a T lymphotropic virus type 1 infection.

In **T large cell anaplastic lymphoma** (2 cases, 5.6%) (Figure 3) the infiltrate was composed of large cells with rounded or irregularly shaped nuclei containing one or more prominent nucleoli. The weakly eosinophilic or pale cytoplasm was abundant. The tumor cells of large cell anaplastic lymphoma may, in some instances, resemble histiocytes. In other cases, a carcinoma-like or sarcoma-like appearance may be seen (Chan et al., 1989). Frequently, giant cells and binucleated cells with features of Reed-Sternberg cells are found. Most of the tumor cells express the activation antigen Ki-1/BerH2 (CD30) (Stein et al., 1985).

Unclassifiable T large cell lymphoma (4 cases, 11.1%) was characterized by the admixture of more than one large cell type, most often pleomorphic cells and immunoblasts. None of the cell types predominated within the infiltrate, thus rendering a precise classification impossible. A correct classification of T large cell lymphoma occurring in MF patients may also be hampered by technical problems (i.e., bad fixation).

IMMUNOHISTOCHEMICAL FEATURES OF TUMOR INFILTRATES

Cutaneous tumors of MF revealed similar immunohistochemical characteristics, irrespective of the cytomorphological features of the neoplastic cells. Partial loss of one or more T cell-associated antigens (CD2, CD3, CD5) was found in most cases (Ralfkiaer et al., 1985). In some cases the cells retained the T-helper cell phenotype observed in the patch/plaque-stage lesions, whereas in other cases the cells showed an aberrant pattern of antigen expression

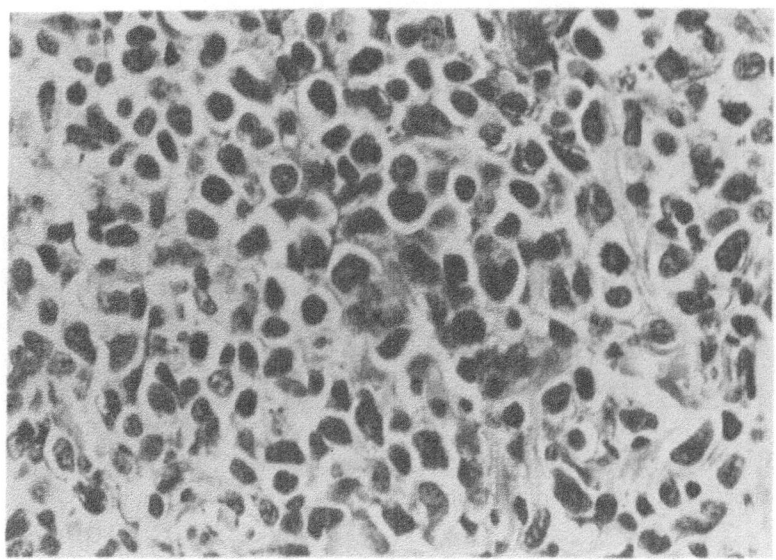

Figure 2. MF with transformation into T medium- and large-cell pleomorphic lymphoma. The infiltrate is predominantly composed of medium- and large-sized pleomorphic lymphocytes.

(CD4$^+$/CD8$^+$ or CD4$^-$/CD8$^-$). Activation markers (CD25, CD71, HLA-DR) were generally positive. CD30 (Ki-1/BerH2) expression could be found in both of our cases with cytomorphologic features of large cell anaplastic lymphoma, and in a variable number of cells in two cases of T-immunoblastic lymphoma and in two cases of "non-transformed" MF. Expression of CD30 by neoplastic cells in diseases other than large cell anaplastic lymphoma has been previously reported (Ralfkiaer et al., 1989). Proliferation markers (PCNA/cyclin, Ki-67) were expressed by a variable number of cells in both transformed and non-transformed tumors. A variable proportion of monocyte/macrophages was marked by Mac387, CD11b, CD11c and CD68. T-zone Histiocytes (Langerhans cells, interdigitating reticulum cells) revealed a positive reaction with CD1 and anti-S100 antibodies in most cases.

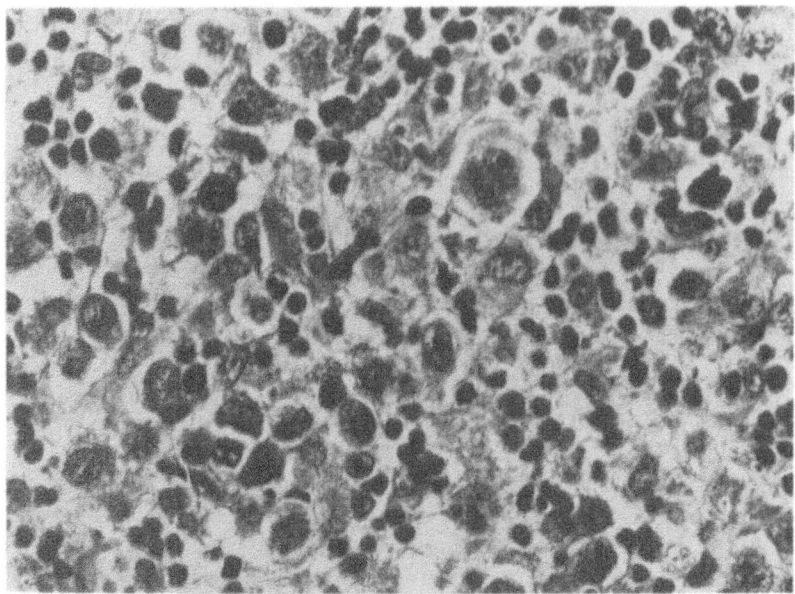

Figure 3. MF with transformation into large cell anaplastic lymphoma. Large anaplastic, immunoblastic, and Reed-Sternberg-like cells are present.

Interestingly, clusters of B cells (CD19$^+$, CD20$^+$) formed a distinct compartment in 30.6% of tumor-stage lesions of MF. Similar findings have been previously described in MF patients (Cerroni et al., 1992, van der Putte et al., 1989). The aggregates were of small size and usually located at the base of the infiltrate. In one case, dendritic reticular cells were detectable within the B cell clusters, indicating the presence of fully developed germinal centers.

Adhesion molecules LFA-1 (CD11a/CD18) and ICAM-1 (CD54) are expressed by the majority of the neoplastic cells in tumor infiltrates of both "classical" type and LCL-MF (Cerroni et al., 1992). We could not demonstrate any association between LFA-1 or ICAM-1 expression and prognosis in MF patients.

PROGNOSIS

LCL developing in the advanced stages of MF are associated with an aggressive biological behavior and short survival (Kerl et al., 1986, Vonderheid et al., 1981). Although primary cutaneous Ki-1⁺ lymphoma has been reported to have a favorable prognosis (Beljaards et al., 1989), Ki-1⁺ large cell anaplastic lymphoma occurring in the advanced stages of MF bears a bad prognosis, with an aggressive course and short survival. In a recent study on "non-transformed" tumor-stage MF compared with LCL-MF, we could correlate the shorter survival time of patients with LCL-MF with an earlier onset of tumors, (i.e., with a shorter time between first biopsy diagnostic of MF and tumor-stage development (Cerroni et al., 1992). In fact, ten-year survival rates after onset of tumors were not statistically different (23.0% for non-trans-

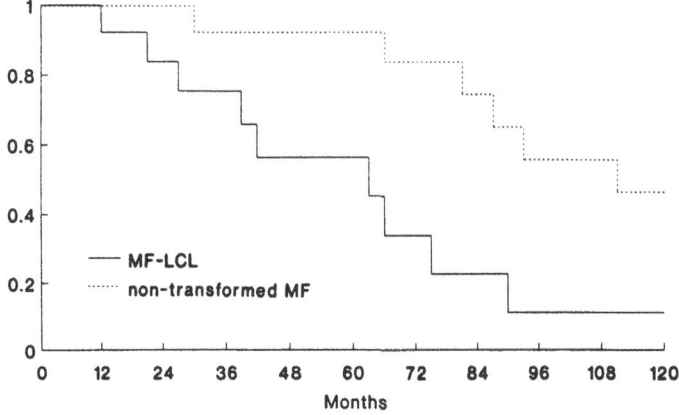

Figure 4. Survival from first diagnostic biopsy. Non-transformed MF, broken line; LCL-MF, full line. The differences between the two groups are statistically significant (p < 0.02).

formed tumor-stage MF, 11.1% for LCL-MF-patients, p > 0.05), whereas overall survival from first biopsy diagnostic of MF showed a statistically significant difference between the two groups (ten-year survival rate, 46.6% and 11.2%, respectively, p < O.02) (Figure 4). These data suggest that the more aggressive course of LCL-MF is not due to biologic properties acquired after large cell conversion, but is likely to be ascribed to features of the neoplastic cells already present at the onset of MF.

Our study indicates that: i) MF and CTCL are heterogenous, and thus that the term, CTCL, is an oversimplification; ii) MF-patients with LCL have a poor prognosis; and iii) recognition of LCL occurring in MF should provide a better assessment of future therapeutic approaches.

REFERENCES

Beljaards RC, CJLM Meijer, E Scheffer et al., 1989. Prognostic significance of CD30 (Ki-1/Ber-H2) expression in primary cutaneous large-cell lymphomas of T cell origin. A clinicopathologic and immunohistochemical study in 20 patients. **Am. J. Pathol.,** 135:1169-1178.

Buechner S and T Rufli, 1979. Manifestation eines malignen Lymphoms von hohem Malignitaetsgrad in Spaetstadium der Mycosis fungoides. **Dermatologica**, 159:125-131.

Catterall MD, BJ Addis, JL Smith and PE Coode, 1983. Sézary syndrome: Transformation to a high grade T cell lymphoma after treatment with cyclosporin A. **Clin. Exper. Dermatol.**, 8:159-169.

Cerroni L, E Rieger, S Hoedl and H Kerl, 1992. Clinicopathologic and immunologic features associated with transformation of mycosis fungoides to large cell lymphoma. **Am. J. Surg. Pathol.**, 16:543-552.

Chan JKC, CS Ng, PK Hui, TW Leung, ESF Lo, WH Lau and LJM McGuire, 1989. Anaplastic large cell Ki-1 lymphoma. Delineation of two morphological types. **Histopathology**, 15:11-34.

Dmitrovsky E, MJ Matthews, PA Bunn et al., 1987. Cytologic transformation in cutaneous T cell lymphoma: A clinicopathologic entity associated with poor prognosis. **J. Clin. Oncol.**, 5:208-215.

Edelson RL, 1975. Cutaneous T cell lymphomas. Perspective. (NIH Conference) **Ann. Intern. Med.**, 83:548-552.

Greer JP, KE Salhany, JB Cousar et al., 1990. Clinical features associated with transformation of cerebriform T cell lymphoma to a large cell process. **Hematol. Oncol.**, 8:215-227.

Kerl H, S Hoedl, J Smolle and K Konrad, 1986. Classification and prognosis of cutaneous T cell lymphomas. **Z. Hautkr.**, 61:63-67.

Kerl H, L Cerroni, and G Burg, 1991. The morphologic spectrum of T cell lymphomas of the skin: A proposal for a new classification. **Semin. Diag. Pathol.**, 8:55-61.

Maeda K and M Takahashi, 1989. Characterization of skin infiltrating cells in adult T cell leukaemia/lymphoma (ATLL): Clinical, histological and immunohistochemical studies on eight cases. **Br. J. Dermatol.**, 121:603-612.

Ralfkiaer E, G Lange Wantzin, DY Mason, K Hou-Jensen, H Stein and K Thomsen, 1985. Phenotypic characterization of lymphocyte subsets in mycosis fungoides. **Am. J. Clin. Pathol.**, 84:610-619.

Ralfkiaer E, K Thomsen, N Agdal, K Hou-Jensen and G Lange Wantzin, 1989. The development of Ki-1-positive large cell non-Hodgkin's lymphoma in pagetoid reticulosis. **Acta. Derm. Venereol (Stockh)**, 69:206-211.

Salhany KE, JB Cousar, JP Greer, TT Casey, JP Fields and RD Collins, 1985. Transformation of cutaneous T cell lymphoma to large cell lymphoma. A clinicopathologic and immunologic study. **Am. J. Pathol.**, 132:265-277.

Scheen SR, PM Banks and RK Winkelmann, 1984. Morphologic heterogeneity of malignant lymphomas developing in mycosis fungoides. **Mayo. Clin. Proc.**, 59:95-106.

Stein H, DY Mason, J Gerdes et al., 1985. The expression of the Hodgkin's disease associated antigen Ki-1 in reactive and neoplastic lymphoid tissue: Evidence that Reed-Sternberg cells and histiocytic malignancies are derived from activated lymphoid cells. **Blood**, 66:848-858.

Suchi T, K Lennert, LY Tu et al., 1987. Histopathology and immunohistochemistry of peripheral T cell lymphomas: A proposal for their classification. **J. Clin. Pathol.**, 40:995-1015.

Tykocinski M, R Schinella and A Greco, 1984. The pleomorphic cells of advanced mycosis fungoides. An ultrastructural study. **Arch. Pathol. Lab. Med.**, 108:387-391.

van der Putte SCJ, J Toonstra, HC van Prooyen, RA de Weger and JAM van Unnik, 1984. Sézary syndrome with early immunoblastic transformation. **Arch. Dermatol. Res.**, 276:17-26.

van der Putte SCJ, J Toonstra and DF van Wichen, 1989. B cells and plasma cells in mycosis fungoides. **Am. J. Dermatopathol.**, 11:509-516

Vonderheid EC, DW Tam, WC Johnson, EJ van Scott and PE Wallner, 1981. Prognostic significance of cytomorphology in the cutaneous T cell lymphomas. **Cancer**, 47:119-125.

Yanagihara ET, JW Parker, PR Meyer, MJ Cain, F Hofman and RJ Lukes, 1984. Mycosis fungoides/Sézary's syndrome progressing to immunoblastic lymphoma. A T cell lymphoproliferation with both helper and suppressor phenotypes. **Am. J. Clin. Pathol.**, 81:249-257.

PRIMARY CUTANEOUS CD30 (Ki-1) POSITIVE LARGE CELL LYMPHOMAS: DEFINITION AND DIFFERENTIAL DIAGNOSTIC ASPECTS

Rein Willemze*†
Peter Kaudewitz‡
Emilio Berti*⁺
Raffaele Gianotti*⁺
Rob C. Beljaards*†
Chris J.L.M. Meijer*†

* Department of Dermatology
† Department of Pathology
  Free University Hospital
  Amsterdam, The Netherlands

‡ Department of Dermatology
  University of Munich
  Munich, Germany

⁺ Department of Dermatology
• IRCS
  University of Milan
  Milan, Italy

Correspondence to: Prof. Dr. R. Willemze, Department of Dermatology,
University Hospital, de Boelelaan 1117,
1081 HV Amsterdam, The Netherlands

ABSTRACT

Recent studies have suggested that primary cutaneous CD30 (Ki-1) positive T-large cell lymphomas represent a distinct type of cutaneous lymphoma with a favorable prognosis. Here

Basic Mechanisms of Physiologic and Aberrant Lymphoproliferation in the Skin
Edited by W.C. Lambert *et al.*, Plenum Press, New York, 1994

265

the results of recent studies aimed to define this new type of cutaneous lymphoma more precisely are presented. The importance of differentiating these lymphomas from other CD30⁺ lymphoproliferative disorders that may occur in the skin is emphasized. Recent evidence suggesting that these primary cutaneous CD30⁺ large cell lymphomas are closely related to lymphomatoid papulosis is discussed.

INTRODUCTION

In 1982, Schwab et al. described the monoclonal antibody Ki-1, raised against the Hodgkin disease cell line, L428. It was first considered to react selectively with Hodgkin and Reed - Sternberg cells in Hodgkin disease, and with occasional non-neoplastic cells, in perifollicular areas in reactive lymph nodes and tonsils. Subsequent studies demonstrated that this Ki-1 (CD30) antigen is also expressed by activated T and B cells and by certain large cell lymphomas (LCL) of both T cell, B cell and indeterminate phenotypes (Stein et al., 1985; Kadin et al., 1986; Agnarsson et al., 1988; Chott et al., 1990; Bitter et al., 1990). These lymphomas have characteristic histologic features, including an anaplastic cytology, cohesive growth pattern, partial involvement of lymph nodes with frequent infiltration of lymph node sinuses, and interstitial fibrosis. Because of their distinctive histologic features, these lymphomas have been accepted as a distinct morphologic entity, designated as anaplastic large cell lymphoma (Stein et al., 1985; Suchi et al., 1987). More recently, these lymphomas have also been termed Ki-1 or CD30 positive (large cell) lymphoma (Kadin et al., 1986: Chott et al., 1990; Bitter et al., 1990). Use of the term Ki-1 positive lymphoma has caused confusion, however, as it soon turned out that the CD30 antigen may also be expressed on malignant lymphomas that do not have the characteristic features of anaplastic large cell lymphomas. Therefore, in recent studies distinction has been made between anaplastic and non-anaplastic subtypes of CD30 positive large cell lymphomas (Piris et al., 1990).

PRIMARY CUTANEOUS CD30 POSITIVE LARGE CELL LYMPHOMA: DEFINITION OF A NEW TYPE OF CUTANEOUS LYMPHOMA

In recent years it has been firmly established that the CD30 positive LCL described in lymph nodes can also present primarily in the skin (Beljaards et al., 1989; Berti et al., 1989; Kaudewitz et al., 1989; Sterry et al., et al, 1989; Lindholm et al., 1989, Banerjee et al., 1991). Recognition of these primary cutaneous CD30 positive LCL has been facilitated by the availibility of Ber-H2, an antibody that recognizes a formalin-resistant epitope of the CD30 antigen, and which can thus be used retrospectively on (stored) paraffin-embedded material (Schwarting et al., 1989). As for their nodal counterparts, these primary cutaneous CD30⁺ LCL have been defined variously on the basis of morphological (anaplastic cytology) and/or immunophenotypical criteria (expression of CD30 antigen), and designated accordingly as "anaplastic large cell lymphoma" or as "Ki-1⁺" or "CD30⁺ large cell lymphoma". At two recent workshops that were aimed to achieve concensus on the definition and terminology of these lymphomas, clinical, histological and immunophenotypical data of 47 primary cutaneous CD30⁺ LCL from five different European centers were analyzed. All patients met the following criteria: (i) predominance (>75%) or large clusters of CD30⁺ blast cells in the initial skin biopsy, (ii) no evidence of lymphomatoid papulosis (LyP), (iii) no history of, or concurrent, LyP, mycosis fungoides (MF) or other type of (cutaneous) lymphoma, and (iv) no extracutaneous localization at presentation. In this study, no differences were found in clinical presentation or prognosis between anaplastic and non-anaplastic CD30⁺ LCL, i.e., between CD30⁺ LCL with and CD30⁺ LCL without the characteristic morphology of anaplastic cells (Beljaards et al., 1993). For that reason, the term "primary cutaneous CD30⁺ LCL" rather than "anaplastic large cell lymphoma", is preferred.

Clinically, most patients with this type of cutaneous lymphoma present with solitary or localized skin lesions that may consist of one to several papules, nodules or small tumors or a huge, often ulcerating, tumor. Uncommonly, patients present with several scattered nodular skin lesions that are not confined to one anatomical area. Remarkably, in some patients the skin lesions have a tendency to resolve spontaneously. Histologically, these lymphomas are characterized by the presence of dense, non-epidermotropic infiltrates of large CD30⁺ tumor cells. Characteristically, these cells show round, oval or irregularly shaped nuclei, one or several prominent, often eosinophilic, nucleoli and abundant cytoplasm (anaplastic cytology). Multinucleated cells, including Reed-Sternberg cells, may be present. In a minority of cases, the CD30⁺ tumor cells do not show the characteristic features of anaplastic cells, and might be classified morphologically as pleomorphic or immunoblastic large cell lymphoma (non-anaplastic cytology). In most cases the tumor cells show a cohesive growth pattern. Inflammatory cells, mainly small lymphocytes, occasional histiocytes and eosinophils are generally found at the periphery of these infiltrates.

Immunophenotypically, most primary CD30⁺ LCL have an aberrant CD4⁺ T-cell phenotype with variable loss of pan-T cell antigens. They strongly express CD30 and other activation antigens, and are often reactive with antibodies against the high cutaneous lymphocyte antigen (HECA 452) (Noorduyn et al., 1992), but generally do not express CD15 (Leu-M1) and epithelial membrane antigen (EMA) (Beljaards et al., 1991). It is important to note that, on paraffin sections, staining for leukocyte common antigen may be negative in these CD30⁺ lymphomas (Beljaards et al., 1991).

In patients with solitary or localized skin disease, radiotherapy is the preferred mode of treatment. Systemic polychemotherapy, generally CHOP-like courses, is only warranted in those rare patients that have more generalized skin lesions at presentation, or in patients developinq extracutaneous disease. Initial therapy generally results in complete remission. Relapses are frequently seen, however, not uncommonly in the same skin area and with the same morpholoqy as the initial skin lesion. Although approximately 25% of patients with this type of lymphoma are destined to develop extracutaneous disease, generally involvement of peripheral lymph nodes, available data suggest that these primary cutaneous CD30⁺ large cell lymphoma have a favorable prognosis (see Table 1).

Table 1. Comparison between primary cutaneous CD30$^+$ and CD30$^-$ large cell lymphomas (LCL)

	CD30$^+$ LCL	CD30$^-$ LCL
Number	47	22
M/F ratio	1.5:1	1.8:1
Age, median	60	69
range	2-95	23-89
Extent of skin lesions		
-solitary/localized	42	5
-generalized	5	17
current status		
- complete remission	36	3
- alive with disease		3
- died of lymphoma	4	15
- died of unrelated disease	6	1
Survival median (months)	38	16
range (months)	3-126	1-48

* Beljaards et al., 1993

† Data derived from the registry of the Dutch Cutaneous Lymphoma Working Group

DIFFERENTIAL DIAGNOSIS OF PRIMARY CUTANEOUS CD30 POSITIVE LARGE CELL LYMPHOMA

The primary cutaneous CD30$^+$ large cell lymphomas, as defined above, must be differentiated from other, both CD30$^+$ and CD30$^-$, lymphoproliferative disorders in the skin. The following groups can be distinguished:

1. Primary Cutaneous CD30 Negative T-Large Cell Lymphomas

CD30$^+$ LCL are part of a much broader group of primary cutaneous large cell lymphomas of T cell origin. These primary cutaneous T large cell lymphomas, which constitute approximately 80% of all CTCL other than MF/SS, represent an extremely heterogeneous group, both clinically, histologically and immunophenotypically. In recently published classifications for peripheral T-cell lymphomas, three groups of T-large cell lymphomas are distinguished: pleomorphic, medium-sized and large cell subtype, immunoblastic subtype and large cell anaplastic subtype (Suchi et al., 1987; Stansfeld et al., 1988). In previous studies, we have demonstrated that differentiation between these morphologic subgroups is often difficult, and that the reproducibilty and clinical (prognostic) significance of this new classification is limited (Beljaards et al., 1989). In the same study, a clear-cut relationship was found between expression of CD30 antigen and clinical behavior and prognosis. In contrast to the CD30[+] LCL described above, primary cutaneous T-large cell lymphomas, in which no or only a few scattered tumor cells expressed CD30 antigen, generally presented or rapidly developed more generalized skin lesions, and had a much worse prognosis, than the CD30[+] LCL. A recent evaluation of 22 patients with such a primary cutaneous CD30[-] T-large cell lymphoma provides further support for this conclusion (see Table 1). Statistical analysis showed that not only CD30 expression, but also age, extent of skin lesions at the time of presentation and mode of initial therapy had a significant effect on survival. These studies also demonstrated, however, that CD30 expression is by far the most important prognostic criterion for this group of primary cutaneous T-large cell lymphomas (Beljaards et al., unpublished observations). These data indicate that any large cell lymphomas of T-cell origin, irrespective of the morphology of the neoplastic cells, should always be investigated for CD30 expression.

2. Skin Manifestations of Primary Noncutaneous CD30[+] Large Cell Lymphomas

CD30[+] LCL may develop de novo in the skin, but can also represent a manifestation of a CD30[+] LCL that has developed primarily at extracutaneous sites. Since, in published reports, distinction between primary and secondary cutaneous CD30[+] LCL is not always made, the frequency of skin involvement in primarily extracutaneous CD30[+] LCL is not precisely known. In recent years, a number of differences between the primary cutaneous CD30[+] LCL and primary noncutaneous CD30[+] LCL has emerged. Primary cutaneous CD30[+] LCL are usually of T-cell or, in some cases, of null cell origin; they are often reactive with HECA-452, but generally do not express epithelial membrane antigen (EMA). By contrast, primary non-cutaneous CD30[+] LCL may be of T-cell, B-cell or null cell origin, and are generally EMA[+] (Fujimoto et al., 1988; Delsol et al., 1988; Piris et al., 1990), but HECA-452 negative (Noorduyn et al., 1992). Whereas primary node-based CD30[+] LCL are often associated with a specific translocation involving chromosomes 2 and 5 [t(2;5)(p23;q35)], this translocation has not yet been reported in primary cutaneous CD30[+] LCL (Bitter et al., 1990). With respect to the clinical differences, previous studies have suggested a high incidence of Ki-1 lymphomas in children and adolescents (Kadin et al., 1986; Chott et al., 1990)). Available data indicate, however, that primary cutaneous CD30[+] LCL, without concurrent extracutaneous disease, is rare in patients under 20 years of age (Beljaards et al., 1993). The most important difference is the favorable prognosis of patients with a primary cutaneous CD30[+] LCL, which contrasts with the poor prognosis generally ascribed to patients with a primary, node-based CD30[+] LCL (Chott et al., 1990; Chan et al., 1989). An exception must be made for CD30[+] LCL occurring in children, which have a good prognosis. Because of the differences outlined above, it is important that future studies make a distinction between primary cutaneous and primary noncutaneous CD30[+] LCL.

3. CD30+ Large Cell Lymphomas Secondary to Other Types of Cutaneous T-Cell Lymphoma

Previous studies have suggested that CD30+ LCL that develop from another type of cutaneous T cell lymphoma (CTCL), such as MF or LyP, generally have a poor prognosis (Kaudewitz et al., 1989; Sterry et al., 1989). In a recent study on 14 patients, however, with a CD30+ LCL that developed from preexistent LyP, it appeared that only those patients that developed systemic CD30+ LCL had a poor prognosis (Beljaards and Willemze, 1992). Six of 10 patients that developed systemic CD30+ LCL died of systemic lymphoma one to 72 months (median, 3 months) after diagnosis. LyP patients that developed CD30+ LCL limited to the skin, however, ran a favorable clinical course. All five patients were in complete remission at the time of publication, with a median survival of 36 months (range 12-180 months) after diagnosis. Similar studies on CD30+ LCL developing from preexistent MF are necessary before final conclusions can be made on the prognosis of this particular group of patients. Until then, distinction should be made between CD30+ LCL that develop de novo in the skin and CD30+ LCL that develop from another type of CTCL.

4. LYMPHOMATOID PAPULOSIS

Differentiation between primary cutaneous CD30+ LCL and LyP is generally not difficult. Clinically, LyP is characterized by the continous waxing and waning of predominantly papular skin lesions and a prolonged, but essentially benign course. Recent studies suggest that the risk for an individual LyP patient to develop systemic lymphoma is less than 5% (Beljaards and Willemze, 1992). Histologically, LyP type A lesions show a dense inflammatory infiltrate, often containing many neutrophils and/or eosinophils, with variable numbers of scattered CD30+ blast cells (Willemze et al., 1982; Kadin et al., 1985; Kaudewitz et al., 1986). Large clusters of CD30+ cells in a cohesive growth pattern are generally not found (see below). Despite the clinical and histologic differences outlined above, there is increasing evidence that primary cutaneous CD30+ LCL and LyP are closely related conditions. This conclusion is based on the cytomorphologic and immunophenotypical similarities between the large atypical cells in the LyP type A lesions and the neoplastic cells of the CD30+ LCL, the observation that both conditions have a favorable prognosis and the tendency, although to a variable degree, to resolve spontaneously, development of a (systemic) CD30+ LCL in patients with well-established LyP and the existence of borderline cases. Two groups of borderline cases can be distinguished. First, some patients may show recurrent self-healing skin lesions, that, on histologic examination, show the characteristic features of a CD30+ LCL, i.e. cohesive sheets of CD30+ blast cells with few or no admixed inflammatory cells. Such cases, for which we have proposed the term "LyP, diffuse large cell type", may have a somewhat increased risk to develop a CD30+ LCL, as compared with patients with classical LyP (Beljaards and Willemze, 1992). The second group of borderline cases includes patients who present with one or several large tumors that have histologic features characteristic of LyP type A. Some of these patients may show spontaneous regression. Similar cases have been designated as regressing a typical histiocytosis (RAH). In previous studies we have demonstrated that the clinical presentation and course of such cases is similar to that of patients with a primary cutaneous CD30$^+$ LCL (Beljaards et al., 1993). We therefore agree with other investigators that this ill-defined term should be avoided.

The overlapping clinical and histologic features suggest that the primary cutaneous CD30$^+$ LCL and LyP represent a continuous spectrum of CD30$^+$ lymphoproliferative disorders (Willemze and Beljaards, 1993). One may even wonder whether future studies should still make a distinction between the different subgroups within this spectrum. Notably, cases of LyP have already been included in recently published series of CD30$^+$ LCL (Chan, et al., 1989: Banerjee, et al., 1991). Because of the differences in clinical behavior, however, in particular, the frequency of spontaneous regression and the risk of developing systemic lymphoma, and consequently differences in the extent of staging procedures and therapy required, we feel that it is still important to make a distinction between these conditions. Future studies should be focused, above all, on the mechanisms involved in the spontaneous remission observed in LyP as well as a proportion of the CD30$^+$ LCL. The results of such studies will not only enhance our understanding of the pathogenic relationship between both conditions, but may also result in new therapeutic strategies for this group of diseases.

REFERENCES

Agnarsson BA and ME Kadin, 1988. Ki-1 positive large cell lymphoma. A morphologic and immunologic study of 19 cases. **Am. J. Surg. Pathol.** 12:264.

Banerjee SS, J Heald and M Harris, 1991. Twelve cases of Ki-1 positive anaplastic large cell lymphoma of the skin. **J. Clin. Pathol.** 44:119.

Beljaards RC, CJLM Meijer, E Scheffer, J Toonstra, WA van Vloten, SCJ van der Putte, ML Geerts and R Willemze, 1989. Prognostic significance of CD30 (Ki-1/Ber-H2) expression in primary cutaneous large-cell lymphomas of T-cell origin: A clinicopathologic and immunohistochemical study in 20 patients. **Am. J. Pathol.**, 135:1169.

Beljaards RC, CJLM Meijer, E Scheffer, P van der Valk and R Willemze, 1991. Differential diagnosis of cutaneous large cell lymphomas using monoclonal antibodies in paraffin embedded skin biopsies. **Am. J. Dermatopathol.**, 13:342.

Beljaards RC, P Kaudewitz, E Berti, R Gianotti, C Neumann, R Rosso, M Paulli, CJLM Meijer and R Willemze, 1993. Primary cutaneous CD 30+ positive large cell lymphoma: Definition of a new type of cutaneous lymphoma with a favorable prognosis. An European multicenter study of 47 patients. **Cancer**, 71:2097.

Beljaards RC and R Willemze, 1992. The prognosis of patients with lymphomatoid papulosis associated with other types of malignancies. **Br. J. Dermatol.**, 126:5g6.

Berti E, R Gianottit and E Alessi, 1989. Primary anaplastic large cell lymphoma of the skin. **Dermatologica**, 178:225.

Bitter MA, WA Franklin, RA Larson, TW McKeithan, CM Rubin, MM Le Beau, JK Stephans and JW Vardiman, 1990. Morphology in Ki-1 (CD30) positive non-Hodgkin lymphomas is correlated with clinical features and the presence of a unique chromosomal abnormality, t(2:5)(p23;q35). **Am. J.Surg.** Pathol., 14:305.

Chan JK, CS Ng, PK Hui, TW Leung, ESF Lo, WH Lau and LJ McGuire, 1989. Anaplastic large cell Ki-1 lymphoma. Delineation of two morphological types. **Histopathol.**, 15:11.

Chott A, K Kaserer, I Augustin, M Vesely, R Heinz, W Oehlinger, H Hanak and T Radaszkiewicz, 1990. Ki-1 positive large cell lymphoma. A clinicopathologic study of 41 cases. **Am. J. Surg. Pathol.**, 14:439.

Delsol S, T Al Saati, KC Gatter, J Gerdes, R Schwarting, P Caveriviere, F Rigal-Huguet, A Robert, H Stein and DY Mason, 1988. Coexpression of epithelial membrane antigen (EMA), Ki-1, and interleukin-2 receptor by anaplastic large cell lymphomas. Diagnostic value in so called malignant histiocytosis. **Am. J. Pathol.**, 130:59.

Fujimoto J, JI Hata, E Ishii, N Kiyokawa, S Tanaka, Y Morikawa, K Shimizu and H Hajikano, 1988, et al. Ki-1 lymphomas in childhood: Immunohistochemical analysis and significance of epithelial membrane antigen (EMA) as a new marker. **Virchows Archiv. A. Pathol. Anat. Histopathol.**, 412:30.

Kadin ME, D Sako, N Berliner, W Franklin, B Woda, M Borowitz, K Ireland, A Schweid, Ph Herzog, B Lange and R Dorfman, 1986. Childhood Ki-1 lymphoma presenting with skin lesions and peripheral lymphadenopathy. **Blood**, 68:1042.

Kadin M, K Nasu, D Sako, J Said and E Vonderheid, 1985. Lymphomatoid papulosis. A cutaneous proliferation of activated helper T cells expressing Hodgkin disease associated antigens. **Am. J. Pathol.**, 119:315.

Kaudewitz P, H Stein, G Burg, DY Mason and O Braun-Falco, 1986. Atypical cells in lymphomatoid papulosis express the Hodgkin cell associated antigen Ki-1. **J. Invest. Dermatol.**, 86:350.

Kaudewitz P, H Stein, F Dallenbach, F Eckert, K Bieber, G Burg and O Braun-Falco, 1989. Primary and secondary cutaneous Ki-1+ (CD30+) anaplastic large cell lymphomas. **Am. J. Pathol.**, 135:359.

Lindholm JS, DR Barron, ME Williams and SH Swerdlow, 1989. Ki-1 positive cutaneous large cell lymphomas of T-cell type; Report of an indolent subtype. **J. Am. Acad. Dermatol.**, 20:342.

Noorduyn LA, RC Beljaards, ST Pals, P van Heerde, T Radaszkiewicz, R Willemze and CJLM Meijer, 1992. Differential expression of the HECA-452 antigen (cutaneous lymphocyte associated antigen, CLA) in cutaneous and non-cutaneous T-cell lymphomas. **Histopathology**, 21:59.

Piris M, DC Brown, KC Gatter and D Mason, 1990. CD30 expression in non-Hodgkin lymphoma. **Histopathology**, 17:211.

Schwab U, H Stein, J Gerdes, H Lemke, H Kirchner, M Schaadt and V Diehl, 1982. Production of a monoclonal antibody specific for Hodgkin and Sternberg-Reed cells of Hodgkin's disease and a subset of normal lymphoid cells. **Nature**, 299:65.

Schwarting R, J Gerdes, H Durkop, B Falini, S Pileri and H Stein, 1989. Ber-H2, a new anti-Ki-1 (CD30) monoclonal antibody directed at a formol-resistant epitope. **Blood**, 74:1678.

Stansfeld AG, J Diebold, Y Kapanci, G Kelenyi, K Lennert, O Mioduszewska, H Noel, F
Rilke, G Sundstrom, JAM van Unnik and D Wright, 1988. Updated Kiel classification for
lymphomas. **Lancet**, i, 292.

Stein H, DY Mason, J Gerdes, N O'Connor, J Wainscoat, G Pallesen, K Gatter, B Falini, G
Delsol, H Lemke, R Schwarting and K Lennert, 1985. The expression of
Hodgkin disease associated antigen Ki-1 in reactive and neoplastic lymphoid tissue.
Evidence that Reed Sternberg cells and histiocytic malignancies are derived from actIvated
lymphoid tissue. **Blood**, 66:812.

Sterry W, B Korte and C Schubert, 1989. Pleomorphic T-cell lymphoma and large cell
anaplastic lymphoma of the skin. **Am. J. Dermatopathol.**, 11:112.

Suchi T. Lennert, LY Tu, M Kikuchi, E Sato, AG Stansfeld and AC Feller, 1987. Histopathology and immunohistochemistry of peripheral T cell lymphomas: A proposal for their
classification. **J. Clin. Pathol.**, 40:995.

Willemze R, CJLM Meijer, WA van Vloten and E Scheffer, 1982. The clinical and
histological spectrum of lymphomatoid papulosis. **Br. J. Dermatol.**, 107:131.

Willemze R and RC Beljaards, 1993. Spectrum of primary cutaneous CD30 (Ki-1)- positive
lymphoproliferative disorders. Guidelines for management and treatment. **J. Am. Acad.
Dermatol.**, 28:973.

ANALYSIS OF CLINICAL, HISTOPATHOLOGIC AND IMMUNOPATHOLOGIC PARAMETERS IN ERYTHRODERMIC VARIANTS OF CUTANEOUS T-CELL LYMPHOMA WITH IMPLICATIONS FOR STAGING

Eric C. Vonderheid, M.D.*

Gary R. Kantor, M.D.*

Edward C. Pequignot, M.S.†

Stuart R. Lessin, M.D.‡

Peter C. Nowell, M.D.˙

J. Bruce Elfenbein, M.D.**

Kathleen Kerrigan, R.N., M.S.*

Marshall E. Kadin, M.D.⁗

* Division of Dermatology
† Department of Neoplastic Disease
Hahnemann University
Philadelphia, PA, U.S.A.

‡ Department of Dermatology
˙ Department of Pathology and Laboratory Medicine
University of Pennsylvania
Philadelphia, PA, U.S.A.

⁗ Department of Pathology
Beth Israel Hospital
Harvard Medical School
Boston, MA, U.S.A.

** Department of Pathology
Temple University Health Sciences Center
Philadelphia, PA, U.S.A.

Correspondence to: Dr. E. C. Vonderheid, Division of Dermatology, Mailstop 478
Hahnemann University, Broad and Vine Streets,
Philadelphia, PA 19102, U.S.A.

Basic Mechanisms of Physiologic and Aberrant Lymphoproliferation in the Skin
Edited by W.C. Lambert *et al.*, Plenum Press, New York, 1994

275

ABSTRACT

In a 5-year interval (1984 to 1989), 32 patients with erythroderma caused by cutaneous T-cell lymphoma (CTCL) were evaluated in the Cutaneous Lymphoma Center at Hahnemann University. These patients were classified further as erythrodermic mycosis fungoides (E-MF) or Sézary syndrome (SS) on the basis of quantitative counts of Sézary cells on peripheral blood smears, and the two groups were compared using multiple clinical, histopathologic, and immunopathologic findings obtained at the time of presentation. Apart from differences related to leukemic involvement, statistically significant differences between the two subgroups of erythrodermic CTCL were found for the frequency of (i) documented lymph node involvement, (ii) a marked degree of tumor cell pleomorphism in skin biopsy specimens, and (iii) complete response to treatment lasting more than 6 months. The prognostic importance of these clinical and pathologic parameters was also determined by univariate analysis using the entire data set. The individual variables identified as possibly being associated with a favorable prognosis included (i) younger age of the patient, (ii) long duration of disease prior to study, (iii) 15 or fewer Sézary cells per 100 lymphocytes [the definition of the E-MF clinical subtype], (iv) presence of epidermal edema, (v) a dermal infiltrate composed predominantly of small lymphocytes, (vi and vii) absence of CD71 and CD30 positive tumor cells in the skin, and (viii) complete response to treatment. These variables were then entered into a Cox model for multivariate analysis. The patient's age, clinical subtype of erythrodermic CTCL, presence or absence of tumor cells expressing the transferrin receptor (CD71, T9) in the skin, and response to treatment were the variables that correlated best with survival. The results of this study suggest that the differences between E-MF and SS are related more to degree of tumor burden than to etiopathogenesis. In addition, demonstration of blood involvement by quantitative Sézary cell counts is useful to define at least two prognostic groups within the erythrodermic CTCL spectrum and should be adopted for staging purposes.

INTRODUCTION

The term, cutaneous T-cell lymphoma (CTCL), was introduced in 1975 to encompass closely related malignant T-cell lymphoproliferative disorders whose clinical manifestations first appear in the skin (Lutzner et al., 1975). The CTCL spectrum includes two major presentations, mycosis fungoides (MF) and Sézary syndrome (SS), which are sometimes referred to as aleukemic and leukemic expresions of CTCL, respectively (Schein et al., 1975). Other investigators have argued that the histopathologic features of SS are distinctive and suggest that SS should be separated from MF (Imai et al., 1986; Scheffer et al., 1986). Thus, the precise nosologic designation of MF, particularly those patients who present with generalized erythroderma without evidence of blood involvement, is uncertain, and terms such as pre-Sézary syndrome and erythrodermic MF (E-MF) have been used to describe such patients (Winkelmann et al., 1984; Sentis et al., 1986).

In a prior publication (Vonderheid et al., 1985), we reported that quantitative counts of atypical lymphocytes with cerebriform nuclei (Sézary cells) on routine blood smears provided both diagnostic and prognostic information for patients with erythrodermic CTCL. Specifically, we found that leukemic involvement was usually confirmed by concurrent cytogenetic analysis of the blood when the proportion of Sézary cells exceeded 15% of the lymphocytes. This smear criterion of blood involvement was subsequently adopted in our center as presumptive evidence for the diagnosis of SS in the appropriate clinical setting. However, since high numbers of Sézary-like cells can occur in actinic reticuloid (Neild et al., 1982; Toonstra et al, 1985; Chu et al., 1986) and certain drug reactions (Rosenthal et al., 1982), additional studies need to be done to confirm the diagnosis.

To better understand the relationship between SS and the aleukemic erythrodermic variants of CTCL (herein referred to as E-MF), we have compared a large number of clinical and pathologic findings obtained on patients classified into E-MF and SS groups on the basis of quantitative Sézary cell counts. Our findings indicate that E-MF and SS are part of a spectrum of erythrodermic CTCL and that the differences between these two subsets are related to the magnitude of the tumor burden.

METHODS

During the interval from January 1984 through February 1989, all patients referred for evaluation to the Cutaneous Lymphoma Center at Hahnemann University had skin biopsy specimens from representative lesions processed for routine histopathology and for immunopathology. Of this group, 179 patients were diagnosed to have CTCL, of which 32 (18%) presented with generalized or nearly generalized erythroderma. Four of these patients also had evidence of scattered infiltrated plaques superimposed on the erythroderma and one patient had a solitary 2 cm diameter tumor with superficial ulceration on the left thigh; this lesion was shown to be a secondary type of Ki-1 lymphoma and was not used for comparative analysis of pathologic findings.

The erythrodermic CTCL patient population consisted of 22 males and 10 females (median age 70 years, range 36 to 87 years). These patients were classified further into the E-MF group or SS group depending on whether the proportion of lymphocytes with cerebriform nuclei (Sézary cells) in the lymphocyte population on peripheral blood smears was $\leq$ 15% or > 15%, respectively (Vonderheid et al., 1985). In addition to quantitative Sézary cell counts, most patients were studied for evidence of leukemic T-cells using one or more special techniques: electron microscopy (28 patients), immunophenotyping of lymphocyte subsets (25 patients), cytogenetics (23 patients), and Southern blot analysis for rearrangement of the beta chain portion of the T-cell receptor (TCR) gene (18 patients). The results of these special studies are presented in Table 1. Since quantitative morphometry was not performed, electron microscopy was considered positive only if lymphocytes with markedly convoluted nuclei were observed. The methods used for chromosome and Southern blot analysis are given elsewhere (Nowell et al., 1982; Rook et al., 1991). A serologic test for human T-lymphotropic virus, type 1 (HTLV-1) was obtained in 25 patients and was negative except for an equivocally positive result in one patient from Spain (patient MR).

Information concerning each patient was extracted from the medical record for subsequent analysis. The clinical parameters included the age, race, and sex of the patient, the date of initial evaluation at our center, the estimated total duration of disease manifestations, the date that the diagnosis of CTCL was initially suggested on a diagnostic test (usually a skin biopsy), the size (diameter) and extent (number of regions) of palpable lymphadenopathy, the presence or absence of liver or spleen enlargement, and evidence of visceral involvement. In addition to the erythrodermic appearance of the skin, the presence of poikiloderma, follicular mucinosis, or ulceration was recorded. The staging evaluation routinely included a chest roentgenogram and computed tomography of the abdomen and pelvis. Of the 24 patients with palpable lymphadenopathy, a lymph node biopsy was obtained in 18 patients, and lymphomatous involvement, as manifested by effacement of nodal architecture by tumor cells, was present in 9 (50%) specimens, all of whom had SS. Hepatomegaly was present in three patients with E-MF and in one patient with SS and splenomegaly was present in two patients with SS. The follow-up interval for patients in this study ranged from one to 85 months (median 33 months) and the median survival was 60 months.

The skin biopsy specimens from one or more representative areas of involved skin were bisected and processed for histopathology and immunopathology as previously described (Nasu et al., 1985). The routine skin sections were reviewed to confirm that histopathologic features diagnostic for CTCL (29 patients) or highly suggestive of CTCL (three patients) were present. In addition, the following histologic parameters were recorded on each case: general appearance of the epidermis (normal, atrophic, psoriasiform, irregular acanthosis), the pattern of dermal infiltrate (patchy, superficial diffuse, patchy or diffuse with involvement of the reticular dermis), the predominant size of lymphocytes (small cell, intermediate cell, mixed cell, large cell), degree of pleomorphism of lymphocytes (relative numbers of cells with large hyperchromatic nuclei) in the dermal infiltrate, degree of epidermotropism (relative numbers of atypical cells in the epidermis), the presence or absence of single cells along the basal layer of the epidermis, Pautrier microabscesses, parakeratosis, spongiosis, interface change, Grenz zone formation, ulceration, atypical cells invading follicular structures (folliculotropism), follicular mucinosis, mitotic count of one or more per high power field, immunoblasts, Reed-Sternberg-like cells, granuloma formation, eosinophils, and plasma cells. Likewise, the corresponding immunopathology sections were reviewed and the tumor cell immunophenotype was recorded as positive, negative, or equivocal for the Pan T-cell antigens (antibody used) CD2 (OKT11), and CD3 (Leu4), CD4 (Leu3), CD5 (Leu1), CD8 (Leu2), and the majority T-cell antigen CD7 (3A1). In addition, the level of expression of activation/proliferation markers on the tumor cells was determined for HLA-DR, CD25 (Tac), CD71 (T9), and CD30 (Ki-1) antigens according to the following scale: none or rare positive cells (negative), few to 19% positive cells (slight), 20% to 49% positive cells (moderate), and 50% or more positive cells (marked). These results are presented in Tables 2 and 3.

For statistical analysis of data, Student's t-test and the log rank test were used to compare mean and median values for quantitative variables of the E-MF and SS subgroups, respectively. Fisher's exact test was used to compare proportions because of the small sample size involved. Log rank and Gehan tests were used to detect survival differences between groups. The Cox proportionate hazards model was used to test for variables which have prognostic significance. BMDP statistical software was used for the analysis.

RESULTS

Comparison of Erythrodermic Subsets

Patients with the erythrodermic form of CTCL were classified as E-MF (aleukemic erythrodermic CTCL) and SS (leukemic CTCL) on the basis of quantitative Sézary cell results on initial blood smears obtained at the time of presentation to our center (Table 1). The total leukocyte count (WBC) was not significantly different between the E-MF and SS groups (median 8,400/mm^3 versus 9,400/mm^3, respectively), but significant differences were observed for the percentage of lymphocytes (median 15% versus 29%, $p < 0.01$), absolute lymphocyte counts (median 1,344/mm^3 versus 2,760/mm^3, $p < 0.05$), and the CD4/CD8 ratio (median 2.8 versus 5.6, $p < 0.05$). Also, Sézary cells with diameters $> 14\mu$m were observed only on smears from 9 patients with SS ($p < 0.005$). In the E-MF group, concurrent chromosome analysis showed an abnormal T-cell clone in the blood in none of the 6 patients studied, with the possible exception of one patient (patient HM) who had 3 of 65 metaphases with an identical karyotype: 51, XY, +Xq-, +3, +8, +9, +18. This patient subsequently achieved a sustained complete response following extracorporeal photopheresis. Conversely, in the SS group, a chromosomally abnormal clone was present in 12 of 17 patients studied (Table 1). More recently, cryopreserved peripheral blood lymphocytes from some of these patients have been analyzed for rearrangement of the beta-chain portion of the T-cell receptor gene (TCR). None of the 6 patients studied in the E-MF group showed evidence of a T-cell clone versus 9 of 11 patients studied in the SS group (Table 1). However, one patient (patient GB) in the E-MF group was shown to have a T-cell clone by TCR analysis, but not by cytogenetics, on a specimen obtained nine months after initial evaluation when the quantitative Sézary count had increased from 0% to 19%. One other patient (patient DT) has also shown evidence on blood smears of progression from E-MF to SS, but confirmatory studies are not available. Thus, these data indicate that quantitative Sézary cell counts provide a reasonably reliable method to screen for the presence or absence of circulating neoplastic T-cells in erythrodermic CTCL patients.

Table 1. Initial Hematologic Results on Patients with Erythrodermic Cutaneous T-Cell Lymphoma.

Pt	Diagnosis	WBC /%Lymph	Sézary Count	EM*	CD4/8 Ratio	Cytogenetics	TCR
CA	E-MF	7,100/ 2	0	—	2.7	ND	G
GB	E-MF	7,600/ 35	0	—	2.9	ND	ND
MB	E-MF	7,100/ 29	0	ND	3.3	ND	ND
JB	E-MF	12,500/ 24	9	—	ND	Normal	ND
JG	E-MF	8,400/ 15	0	—	ND	Normal	G
TH	E-MF	9,600/ 14	3	ND	ND	Normal	G
IJ	E-MF	8,800/ 11	0	—	3.3	ND	ND
CL	E-MF	13,800/ 10	13	—	2.2	Normal	G
HM	E-MF	6,900/ 15	11	ND	ND	Clone**	ND
PM	E-MF	6,200/ 27	0	—	2.0	ND	G
AM	E-MF	11,500/ 11	10	ND	ND	ND	ND
FR	E-MF	5,200/ 16	0	+	2.3	ND	G
DT	E-MF	12,200/ 49	8	—	9.7	Normal	ND
ECl	SS	18,100/ 51	27	—	2.5	Clone	R
FC	SS	5,200/ 25	46	+	0.2***	Normal	G
ECu	SS	28,000/ 27	51	+	18.2	Clone	R
SE	SS	12,000/ 23	42	+	4.5	Clone	ND
CF	SS	18,800/ 43	59	—	14.7	Clone	ND
HG	SS	5,400/ 35	30	—	2.7	Normal	R
EH	SS	10,300/ 55	83	+	9.0	Clone	R
LH	SS	10,200/ 25	20	+	4.9	Normal	R
MH	SS	7,500/ 25	28	+	5.1	Normal	R
TM	SS	6,900/ 40	16	+	ND	ND	G
MM	SS	7,100/ 29	25	+	5.0	Normal	R
ER	SS	7,400/ 15	31	+	9.3	Clone	ND
GR	SS	9,400/ 42	28	+	ND	Clone	ND
WR	SS	35,000/ 82	43	+	84.0	Clone	R
MR	SS	5,300/ 17	44	+	6.9	ND	G
JS	55	5,100/ 23	43	+	1.8	Clone	ND
JT	SS	11,000/ 34	22	—	6.0	Clone	R
DW	SS	9,300/ 26	24	+	4.6	Clone	ND
RW	SS	13,400/ 47	15	—	8.7	Clone	ND

Abbreviations: ND = not done; R = rearranged; G = germline

* Electron microscopy indicated as positive (+) if lymphocytes with markedly convoluted nuclei present, negative (-) if not present.

** 3 of 65 cells had an identical abnormal karyotype.

*** Reversal of CD4/CD8 ratio confirmed.

Table 2. Skin Histopathologic Findings in Patients with Erythrodermic Cutaneous T-cell Lymphoma.

Parameter Studied	E-MF (n=13)	SS (n=19)
General Epidermal Appearance*		
Normal	1	3
Atrophic	0	1
Psoriasiform	4	9
Irregular acanthosis	8	5
Epidermotropism		
Slight	1	3
Moderate	5	8
Marked	7	8
Single cells at basal layer	8	10
Pautrier microabscesses	8	16
Parakeratosis	9	13
Spongiosis	12	15
Interface change	9	13
Pattern of Infiltrate		
Patchy	5	6
Diffuse superficial	7	13
Superficial and deep	1	0
Lymphocyte predominance		
Small cell	12	12
Intermediate cell	1	6
Mixed	0	1
Lymphocyte pleomorphism		
Slight	4	5
Moderate	7	3
Marked	2	11
Reed-Sternberg-like cells	2	4
Mitotic count > one/HPF	0	3
Granuloma formation	4	3
Eosinophils	7	6
Plasma cells	7	9

* One case of SS not studied

To determine whether E-MF and SS are part of a spectrum of erythrodermic CTCL or separate disease entities, detailed comparison between the two groups was made using multiple parameters other than hematologic findings. The ages of patients in the two subsets did not differ significantly (median age 73 years, range 46 to 83 years for E-MF and median age 66 years, range 36 to 87 years for SS, p> 0.3).

Statistically significant differences in clinical and staging results were found for the frequency of lymph node involvement (0/6 E-MF versus 9/12 SS, p< 0.005), stage IV disease (0/13 E-MF versus 9/19 SS p< 0.005), and complete response to treatment lasting more than 6 months (4/13 E-MF versus 0/19 SS, p< 0.05). No difference was apparent for sex or race, the size and extent of lymphadenopathy, total duration of disease (median 39 months for E-MF versus 30 months for SS, p> 0.4), time from first pathologic evidence of disease to referral (median 5 months for E-MF versus 6 months for SS, p> 0.3), and the follow-up time (median 33 months for E-MF versus 32 months for SS). Thus, the major clinical differences between the two subsets of erythrodermic CTCL pertain to the greater magnitude of tumor involvement in SS compared to E-MF.

Similarly, the frequency of multiple histopathologic and immunopathologic findings were compared for the two subsets of erythrodermic CTCL. The only histopathologic parameter that was statistically different was to a marked degree of tumor cell pleomorphism in 11 of 19 patients with SS compared to two of 13 E-MF patients (p< 0.05). An additional histopathologic variable that approached statistical significance was the more frequent occurrence of small lymphocytes predominating in the dermal infiltrate in 12 of 13 E-MF patients versus 12 of 19 SS patients (p=0.07). Differences between E-MF and SS were even less apparent with skin immunopathologic findings. An aberrant tumor cell phenotype, i.e., the loss of one or more mature T-cell markers, CD2, CD3, CD4, CD5 or CD7, was present in 20 patients with CTCL without a significant difference in the frequency in the two subsets (p> 0.3). Tumor cell aberrancy was attributed mostly to the deficient expression of CD7 (19 patients) compared to CD5 (5 patients), CD2 (4 patients), CD4 (2 patients), and CD3 (one patient). One patient with E-MF (patient PM) had an unusual suppressor T-cell phenotype that was CD8$^+$, CD2$^-$, CD5$^-$, and CD7$^-$. No difference was found between E-MF and SS for these individual antigens, but E-MF patients were more likely to show a loss of two or more mature T-cell markers (5 of 7 patients) compared to SS (2 of 13 patients) when aberrancy was present (p< 0.05).

Since CTCL may represent, in some instances, an expansion of a CD4$^+$, CD7$^-$ cell normally present in small numbers in the peripheral blood (Matutes et al, 1983), the loss of the CD7 marker may be more apparent than real, and may not have the same biologic significance as a loss of another mature T-cell marker. Consequently, analysis also was performed for tumor cell aberrancy other than CD7, again with no difference found between E-MF and SS (p> 0.3). In addition, the level of expression of activation/proliferation markers by tumor cells in the skin were compared. No significant difference was found for the activation markers HLA-DR (p> 0.4), CD25 (p> 0.2), or CD30 (p> 04). However, it is worth noting that 5 of 19 patients with SS had more than 20% of the tumor cells positive for CD71 (transferrin receptor), a marker of cell proliferation, compared to none of the E-MF patients (p= 0.07). This finding suggests that

Table 3. Skin Immunopathologic Findings in Patients with Erythrodermic Cutaneous T-cell Lymphoma.

Parameter Studied	E-MF (n=13)	SS (n=19)
Aberrancy of CD2	2	2
CD3	1	0
CD4	2	0
CD5	4	1
CD7	6	13
CD25		
Negative	3	2
Slight	6	12
Moderate	4	4
Marked	0	1
CD71*		
Negative	3	5
Slight	9	9
Moderate	0	5
Marked	0	0
HLA-DR		
Negative	2	2
Slight	3	5
Moderate	2	5
Marked	6	7
CD30		
Negative	11	13
Slight	2	4
Moderate	0	1
Marked	0	1

* One case of E-MF not studied for CD71

a higher proportion of tumor cells may be undergoing proliferation in the skin in SS than in E-MF.

Prognostic Implications

Treatment for almost all patients with erythrodermic CTCL consisted of a systemic regimen alone (10 patients) or combined with a some type of topical therapy (20 patients). One patient with E-MF (patient PM) received topical treatments only (methoxsalen photochemotherapy, topical mechlorethamine) and one patient with SS (patient SE) elected not to receive any treatment because of mild symptomatology and stable course. The most common systemic regimens administered consisted of an alkylating drug (chlorambucil, 21 patients; cyclophosphamide, 3 patients), often combined with prednisone, and also extracorporeal photopheresis with or without low doses of interferon alfa (13 patients). Other systemic agents used were methotrexate (7 patients), and isotretinoin (6 patients). The topical treatments included applications of mechlorethamine hydrochloride (20 patients), methoxsalen photochemotherapy (5 patients), or total skin electron beam (4 patients). A complete response to treatment was recorded at some time during follow-up in only 6 patients (4 with E-MF, 2 with SS), but the remission was sustained for more than 6 months only in the 4 patients with E-MF. At the time of last contact, 8 of the 13 (62%) patients in the E-MF group were alive compared to 6 of 19 (32%) patients in the SS group (p= 0.09). The median survival of E-MF patients was > 80 months compared to 32 months for patients with SS (p> 0.1, Figure 1).

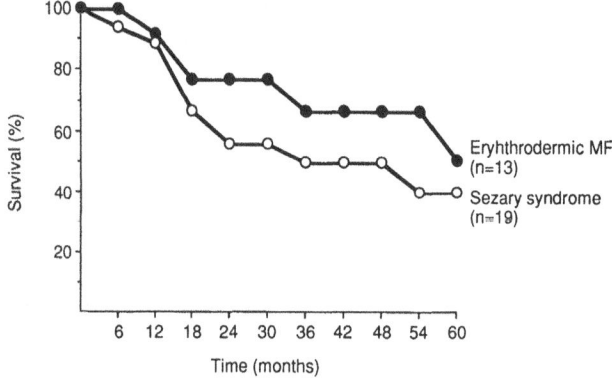

Figure 1. Survival curves show that patients classified as erythrodermic mycosis fungoides (E-MF) have a better prognosis than patients with Sézary syndrome (SS) using a quantitative Sézary cell count of ≤ 15% as the criterion for separation. However, the difference between the two curves is not statistically significant (p= 0.13) presumably due to the small number of patients in each group.

To determine which, if any, clinical or pathologic parameter had prognostic significance in erythrodermic CTCL, each variable was subjected initially to univariate analysis using the combined patient data set with survival as the dependant variable. The stringency of the test was set at p< 0.15 for screening purposes. Of note, the presence or absence of lymph node involvement, defined as effacement of nodal architecture (or N-rating), and stage III versus IV were parameters that showed no apparent difference in survival patterns in this analysis (p > 0.3 and p > 0.4, respectively). The variables that were associated with a relatively favorable prognosis included younger age, relatively long duration of disease prior to study, Sézary cell count of $\leq$ 15% (which defines the E-MF subset), epidermal edema (spongiosis), predominance of small lymphocytes in the dermal infiltrate, absence of CD71 and CD30 antigen expression by tumor cells, and a complete response to treatment. These variables were entered as covariates into the Cox regression model for stepwise multivariate analysis. The variables that were selected as being associated with adverse survival were advanced patient age (p < 0.005), failure to achieve a complete response to treatment (p < 0.05), presence of CD71$^+$ cells in the dermal infiltrate (p = 0.07), and a quantitative Sézary cell count exceeding 15% (p = 0.1). Moreover, comparison of MFCG stage III and IV and clinical groups E-MF and SS in the model indicated that only the clinical grouping based on Sézary cell count was significantly related to survival (p < 0.04).

DISCUSSION

In a 5-year interval the erythrodermic form of CTCL represented 18% of the 179 patients with CTCL who presented to our center. The majority (19 of 32) of these patients had evidence of leukemic involvement by quantitative Sézary cell count and therefore can be classified as SS (Wieselthier and Koh, 1990). Compared to patients with absent or small numbers of Sézary cells on smears (our definition of E-MF), patients with SS (i) have a greater degree of lymphocytosis, usually accompanied by a larger ratio of T-helper to T-suppressor (CD4/CD8) cells, (ii) are more likely to have evidence of a T-cell clone in the blood by chromosome or Southern blot analysis, (iii) have lymph nodes that are more likely to show effacement of nodal architecture when biopsied, thus indicating a higher stage of disease using the current MFCG staging system, (iv) show a more marked degree of tumor cell pleomorphism in skin specimens, and (v) are less likely to achieve a sustained complete response to treatment. In addition, there is evidence that SS differs from E-MF in the predominant size of the atypical lymphocytes (larger in SS) and proportion of proliferating transferrin receptor positive (CD71$^+$) tumor cells (higher in SS) in the dermal infiltrate.

These findings can be attributed to differences in the degree of tumor burden in these two subsets of erythrodermic CTCL rather than to a difference in etiopathogenesis. According to this concept, SS occurs in those patients with a relatively higher rate of tumor cell proliferation in the skin (and possibly extracutaneous sites as well), resulting in the observed morphologic and immunophenotypic differences in the skin and release of larger numbers of such cells into the blood, where they can be demonstrated on blood smears. In addition, the presence on smears of Sézary cells with large diameter, which occurred only in patients with SS in this series, also may reflect release of such cells from the skin or other sites since marked pleomorphism of tumor cells was more often observed in SS than in E-MF. More careful studies are needed in the future to clarify the possible relationship between the cytology of Sézary cells in skin and blood.

If our interpretation is correct that E-MF and SS are part of a spectrum of erythrodermic CTCL, then one would expect E-MF to evolve into SS as part of its natural history and SS to assume the appearance of E-MF during successful treatment. In this series, two patients (patients GB, DT) developed smear criteria of SS during follow-up and the presence of a neoplastic clone was confirmed by Southern blot analysis in one. Similar observations have been made by Buechner and Winkelmann (1983) in patients classified as pre-SS. Moreover, treatment often decreases the number of Sézary cells in the skin and blood to levels used to define E-MF, but we have presented no data to state whether blood cytogenetics or Southern blot studies revert to normal, although we have observed this in other patients.

The opinion that SS should be distinguished from classic MF on the basis of histopathology (Imai et al., 1986; Scheffer et al., 1986) is not addressed in this study. However, we have observed several patients with classic MF who subsequently developed typical manifestations of SS as well as occasional patients with SS who had evidence of atypical lymphocytes in the blood prior to developing erythroderma (unpublished observations). This anecdotal experience leads us to believe that SS and classic MF are closely related lymphoproliferative disorders of mature T-cells and that their nosologic relationship is analogous to that for chronic lymphocytic leukemia and well-differentiated lymphocytic lymphoma.

With the recent availability of the Southern blot technique, which is at least a 10-fold more sensitive way to detect clonal or oligoclonal T-cell populations than smears or cytogenetics, some cases of erythrodermic CTCL that do not have large numbers of Sézary cells or abnormal chromosomes will be shown to have a detectable, presumably malignant T-cell clone in the blood, thereby broadening the SS definition (Weiss et al., 1989; Bakels et al., 1991). It is conceivable that even more sensitive molecular genetic probes using the polymerase chain reaction may detect clonality in the blood of all or nearly all patients with erythrodermic CTCL (Lessin et al., 1991; Volkenandt et al., 1991). In this situation, the diagnostic importance of quantitative Sézary cell counts as a method to detect blood involvement will diminish in importance, but the prognostic significance will likely remain, since it is a measure of tumor burden.

Patients with erythrodermic CTCL are recognized to have a relatively poor prognosis compared to patients with other forms of CTCL, e.g., classic mycosis fungoides. This perception is reflected in a widely adopted staging system based on the tumor-node-metastasis (TNM) format in which erythroderma is assigned a T_4 skin rating (Bunn and Lamberg, 1979). Consequently, all patients with erythrodermic CTCL are placed in stage III ($T_4 N_{0-1} M_0$), IVa ($T_4 N_{3-4} M_0$), or IVb ($T_4 N_{0-4} M_1$). However, the status of the peripheral blood (B-rating) is not used for staging because no concensus could be reached at the workshop regarding the criteria to be used to designate the presence of blood involvement or the prognostic implications of such a finding. However, subsequent work by us (Vonderheid et al., 1985) and others (Willemze et al.,1983; Schechter et al., 1987) has shown that blood involvement is apt to be present when the proportion of Sézary cells in the lymphocyte population is about 20%. In addition, the present study indicates that quantitative Sézary cell counts also have prognostic implications, as shown by survival analysis, and may be useful for staging purposes (B-rating). The median survival rate for patients with more than 15 Sézary cells per 100 lymphocytes (herein classified as SS) is about half that for patients with fewer Sézary cells on blood smears (Figure 1).

In addition to the number of Sézary cells, the size of the Sézary cells may provide prognostic information. In a previous study (Vonderheid et al., 1985), we reported that the proportion of large Sézary cells (15 to 20 μm diameter) within the Sézary cell population actually correlated better with survival than Sézary cell counts. Subsequently, Schechter et al., (1987) also observed that patients with a "mixed cell" cytology (smears with > 20% Sézary cells with > 11 μm diameter) had a significantly worse survival than those with predominantly small Sézary cells. Although not addressed in this study, these observations lead us to suggest that quantitative Sézary cell counts may be used to define three prognostic groups within the erythrodermic CTCL spectrum: a low count group corresponding to E-MF, a high count small cell group corresponding to the small cell variant of SS, and a high count mixed or large cell group corresponding to the classic variant of SS. Moreover, we propose that a quantitative Sézary cell count of 20% be adopted as the criterion for the B-rating in the MFCG staging system and be given importance equal to that of the N-rating. Thus, a patient with erythrodermic CTCL with more than 20% Sézary cells on quantitative count will be staged as IVa ($T_4N_{0-3}B_1M_0$) until future prospective studies determine the relative merits of the grading of lymph node histopathology vis-a-vis cytologic assessment of positive smears. For example, the finding of a large cell immunoblastic lymphoma in a lymph node of a patient undergoing cytologic transformation to a high grade lymphoma may not be reflected in blood smear findings and may therefore have independent significance (Dmitrovsky et al., 1987; Salhany et al., 1988; Vonderheid et al., 1991).

Finally, in addition to the prognostic implications of Sézary cells, a number of other variables have been reported to be associated with survival in patients with erythrodermic CTCL, including the patient's sex (Winkelmann and Linman, 1973), race (Weinstock and Horm, 1988), age and duration of disease (Vonderheid et al., 1985), and histopathologic findings in lymph node specimens (Vonderheid et al., 1992). In the present study, univariate analysis of skin related factors also suggested a possible association with epidermal edema (spongiosis), the predominant size of lymphocytes in the dermal infiltrate, expression of the proliferation marker CD71 (transferrin receptor) and activation marker CD30 (Ki-1 antigen) by tumor cells, and a complete response to treatment. Multivariate analysis showed that age, leukemic involvement, and treatment response were the covariates that correlated most significantly with survival. However, because of the small number of patients available, the power of the statistical analysis was limited and these observations need to be confirmed with a larger number of patients.

ACKNOWLEDGEMENTS

This study was supported by the Leonard and Ruth Levine Skin Research Foundation, American Cancer Society Grant CD-62577, Council for Tobacco Research, USA, Inc. No. 2630R2, VA Career Development Award NIH R29-CA 55017, NIH CA 42232, and the Lester I. Conrad Research Foundation.

REFERENCES

Bakels V, JW van Oostveen, RLJ Gordijn, JMM Walboomers, CJLM Meijer, and R Willemze, 1991. Diagnostic value of T-cell receptor beta gene rearrangement analysis on peripheral blood lymphocytes of patients with erythroderma. **J. Invest. Dermatol.**, 97:782.

Buechner SA and RK Winkelmann, 1983. Pre-Sézary erythroderma evolving to Sézary syndrome. **Arch. Dermatol.**, 119:285.

Buechner SA and RK Winkelmann, 1983. Sézary syndrome. **Arch. Dermatol.**, 119:979.

Bunn PA Jr. and SI Lamberg, 1979. Report of the committee on staging and classification of cutaneous T-cell lymphomas. **Cancer Treat. Rep.**, 63:725.

Chu AC, D Robinson, JLM Hawk, R Meachum, NF Spittle and NP Smith, 1986. Immuno-logic differentiation of the Sézary syndrome due to cutaneous T-cell lymphoma and chronic actinic dermatitis. **J. Invest. Dermatol.**, 86:134.

Dmitrovsky E, MJ Matthews, PA Bunn, GP Schechter, RW Makuch, CF Winkler, J Eddy, EA Sausville and DC Ihde, 1987. Cytologic transformation in cutaneous T cell lymphoma: A clinicopathologic entity associated with poor prognosis. **J. Clin. Oncol.**, 5:208.

Imai S, G Burg and O Braun-Falco, 1986. Mycosis fungoides and Sézary's syndrome show distinct histomorphological features. **Dermatologica**, 173:131.

Johnson SC, DJ Cripps and DH Norback, 1979. Actinic reticuloid: A clinical, pathologic and action spectrum study. **Arch. Dermatol.**, 115:1078.

Lessin SR, AH Rook and G Govera, 1991. Molecular diagnos of cutaneous T-cell lymphoma: Polymerase chain reaction amplification of T-cell antigen receptor beta-chain gene rearrange-ments. **J. Invest. dermatol.**, 96:299.

Lutzner M, R Edelson, P Schein, I Green, C Kirkpatrick and A Ahmed, 1975. Cutaneous T-cell lymphomas: The Sézary syndrome, mycosis fungoides and related disorders. **Ann. Intern. Med.**, 83:S34.

Matutes E, D Robinson, M O'Brien, BF Haynes, H Zola, and D Catovsky, 1983. Candidate counterparts of Sézary cells and adult T-cell lymphoma-leukemia cells in normal peripheral blood: An ultrastructural study with the immunogold method and monoclonal antibodies. **Leuk. Res.**, 7:787.

Nasu K, J Said, EC Vonderheid, J Olerud, D Sako and M Kadin, 1985. Immunopathology of cutaneous T-cell lymphomas. **Am. J. Pathol.**, 119:436.

Neild VS, JLM Hawk, RAJ Eady and JJ Cream, 1982. Actinic reticuloid with Sézary cells. **Clin. Exp. Dermatol.**, 7:143.

Nowell PC, JB Finan and EC Vonderheid, 1982. Clonal characteristics of cutaneous T-cell lymphomas: Cytogenetic evidence from blood, lymph nodes and skin. **J. Invest. Dermatol.**, 78:69.

Rook AH, MB Prystowsky, M Cassin, M Boufal and SR Lessin, 1991. Combined therapy for Sézary syndrome with extracorporeal photochemotherapy with low-dose interferon alfa therapy. **Arch. Dermatol.**, 127:1535.

Rosenthal CJ, CA Noguera, A Coppola and SN Kapelner, 1982. Pseudolymphoma with mycosis fungoides manifestations, hyperresponsiveness to diphenylhydantoin, and lymphocyte disregulation. **Cancer**, 49:2305.

Salhany KE, JB Cousar, JP Greer, TT Casey, JP Fields and RD Collins, 1988. Transformation of cutaneous T cell lymphoma to large cell lymphoma. **Am. J. Pathol.**, 132:265.

Schechter GP, EA Sausville, AB Fischmann, F Soehnlen, E Joyce, M Matthews, AF Gazdar, J Guccione, D Munson, R Makuch and PA Bunn, Jr, 1987. Evaluation of circulating malignant cells provides prognostic information in cutaneous T cell lymphoma. **Blood**, 69:841.

Scheffer E, CJLM Meijer, WA van Vloten and R Willemze, 1986. A histologic study of lymph nodes from patients with the Sézary syndrome. **Cancer**, 57:2375.

Schein PS, JS MacDonald and R Edelson, 1975. Cutaneous T-cell lymphoma. **Cancer**, 38:1859.

Sentis HJ, R Willemze and E Scheffer, 1986. Histopathologic studies in Sézary syndrome and erythrodermic mycosis fungoides. A comparison with benign forms of erythroderma. **J. Am. Acad. Dermatol.**, 15:1217.

Toonstra J, H van Weelden, FHJ Gmelig Meyling, SC van der Putte, SI Schiere and H Bart de la Faille, 1985. Actinic reticuloid simulating Sézary syndrome: Report of two cases. **Arch. Dermatol. Res.**, 277:149.

Volkenandt M, HP Soyer, H Kerl and JR Bertino, 1991. Development of a highly specific and sensitive molecular probe for detection of cutaneous lymphoma. **J. Invest. Dermatol.**, 97:137.

Vonderheid EC, LW Diamond, S-M Lai, F Au, and MA DellaVecchia, 1992. Lymph node histopathology in cutaneous T-cell lymphoma: A prognostic classification system based on morphologic assessment. **Am. J. Clin. Pathol.**, 97:121.

Vonderheid EC, EL Sobel, PC Nowell, J Finan, M Helfrich and D Whipple, 1985. Diagnostic and prognostic significance for Sézary cells in peripheral blood smears from patients with cutaneous T-cell lymphoma. **Blood**, 66:358.

Weinstock MA and JW Horm, 1988. Population-based estimate of survival and determinants of prognosis in patients with mycosis fungoides. **Cancer**, 62:1658.

Weiss LM, GS Wood, E Hu, EA Abel, RT Hoppe and J Sklar, 1989. Detection of clonal T-cell receptor gene rearrangements in the peripheral blood of patients with mycosis fungoides/Sézary syndrome. **J. Invest. Dermatol.**, 92:601.

Wieselthier JS and HK Koh, 1990. Sézary syndrome: Diagnosis, prognosis, and critical review of treatment options. **J. Am. Acad. Dermatol.**, 22:381.

Willemze R, WA van Vloten, J Hermans, MJM Damsteeg and CJLM Meijer, 1983. Diagnostic criteria in Sézary's syndrome: A multiparameter study of peripheral lymphocytes in 32 patients with erythroderma. **J. Invest. Dermatol.**, 81:392.

Winkelmann RK, SA Ruechner and JL Diaz-Perez, 1984. Pre-Sézary syndrome. **J. Am. Acad. Dermatol.**, 10:992.

Winkelmann RK and JW Linman, 1973. Erythroderma with atypical lymphocytes (Sézary syndrome). **Am. J. Med.**, 55:192.

A SCORING SYSTEM BASED ON DIFFERENTIALLY WEIGHTED CRITERIA FOR ESTABLISHING A STANDARDIZED THRESHOLD FOR THE DIAGNOSIS OF EARLY MYCOSIS FUNGOIDES

Kevin D. Cooper, M.D.
Immunodermatology Unit
Department of Dermatology
University of Michigan
Ann Arbor, Michigan U.S.A.

Correspondence to: Dr. K. Cooper, Deparment of Dermatology,
University of Michigan School of Medicine, R5538 Kresge I, Box 0530,
Ann Arbor, MI 48109, U.S.A.

ABSTRACT

The threshold for the early diagnosis of the mycosis fungoides form of cutaneous T cell lymphoma (MF-CTCL) is indistinct, and varies from center to center, because there is no "gold standard" for this diagnosis. Neither the clinical nor the histologic features allow all cases to be diagnosed in the early patch/plaque forms of the disease. Adjunctive tests of high specificity but low sensitivity are now coming into increasing clinical use; these appear to have value in making this diagnosis. A scoring system is now proposed that standardizes the threshold for the diagnosis of MF-CTCL in its early stages. Scores are assigned according to the strength of clinical morphology (2 point maximum), distribution (2 point maximum), and histology (3 point maximum) with regard to likelihood of MF-CTCL. A threshold of 5 points is defined as the inclusion point. Additional points (2 points each, up to a maximum of 4 points) can be gathered in support of the diagnosis if highly specific adjunctive tests (i.e., Pan T cell marker discordance, T cell receptor gene rearrangement, Sézary cells in the blood, elevated nuclear contour index, or aneuploidy) are positive. It is proposed that application of standardized threshold criteria to characterize patients entered into studies of pathogenesis, diagnosis, therapy, or prognostication will standardize Stage I MF-CTCL patients, allowing better comparisons of

Basic Mechanisms of Physiologic and Aberrant Lymphoproliferation in the Skin
Edited by W.C. Lambert *et al.*, Plenum Press, New York, 1994

291

studies executed at different centers, and will homogenize patient entry into multi-center protocols.

INTRODUCTION

A standardized threshold for making an early diagnosis of the mycosis fungoides form of cutaneous T cell lymphoma (MF-CTCL) remains problematic, despite the advent of adjunctive techniques (Payne et al., 1986; Weiss et al., 1989; Weiss et al., 1985; Lindae et al., 1988; van Vloten et al., 1985; Vonderheid, 1989) and careful cataloging of characteristic histologic features (Nickoloff, 1988). The problem arises because clinicians recognize an early form of MF-CTCL, with characteristic morphology and body distribution, at a point in time when the histologic features may be nonspecific or merely suggestive; conversely, histopathologists can recognize clearly diagnostic features of MF-CTCL in skin lesions demonstrating clinical morphology that is not specific for MF-CTCL. However, both inter- and intra-rater variability in the early histologic diagnosis of MF-CTCL is high, even among highly experienced dermatopathologists (Burg, 1993). Thus, neither the clinical presentation nor the histologic picture serves as a "gold standard" by which all cases can be consistently diagnosed in the early patch/plaque forms.

A number of adjunctive tests have been developed that are fairly specific for the diagnosis of MF-CTCL. Whereas, if positive, this is considered strong evidence for the diagnosis, they are only rarely positive in early lesions (Vonderheid, 1989). Criteria such as aneupoidy (Hagedorn et al., 1977; Ralfkiaer et al., 1989; van Vloten et al., 1974), an elevated nuclear contour index (Lutzner et al., 1968; Simon, 1987; Meyer et al., 1977; Payne et al., 1986), loss of pan T cell markers (Buechner et al., 1984; van der Putte et al., 1988; Schmoeckel et al., 1979; Lutzner et al., 1968; Chu et al., 1984; Verga et al., 1991), extremely elevated CD4:CD8 ratios (Vonderheid et al., 1987), diffuse epidermal HLA-DR expression (Verga et al., 1991) or the presence of clonal T cell proliferation by detection of distinct T cell receptor gene rearrangements (TCRGR) (Ralfkiaer et al., 1987; Weiss et al., 1985; Weiss et al., 1989) have been found to be fairly specific for MF-CTCL if present, but are of insufficient sensitivity to routinely detect characteristic abnormalities in a clinicopathologically non-diagnostic situation. Consequently, there is currently no single diagnostic test that can be used to diagnose early forms of MF-CTCL.

The blurriness of the border between subthreshold and threshold MF-CTCL results in significant variations between centers with regard to patient inclusion criteria in studies of pathogenesis, diagnosis, therapy and prognosis. Although the TNM staging system has been useful in comparing survival of patients with clearly established disease from different centers, direct comparisons of data emanating from different centers regarding early MF-CTCL is currently difficult because of varying subjective inclusion criteria from center to center. Thus, establishment of clinical, pathologic and laboratory features that can be used to objectively define inclusion criteria would be extremely useful in multi-center investigations and in comparisons of investigations of early stage disease between different centers.

Clinicians often make the diagnosis of MF-CTCL based upon a constellation of clinical, histologic and adjunctive data. However, the process is poorly defined and varies significantly between clinicians and centers that publish on MF-CTCL. As with other complex diseases, such as systemic lupus erythematosus (SLE) and atopic dermatitis, important criteria can be identified and given relative weights in a scoring system. This paper proposes a scoring system that standardizes the threshold for the early diagnosis of MF-CTCL. Studies utilizing such a scoring system will have more homogeneous and comparable patients, particularly in the TNM Stage I group. More general use of these objective criteria may also reduce the use of controversial terms for precursor lesions used by clinicians to denote their high degree of clinical suspicion in the face of equivocal histology.

The criteria chosen emphasize those utilized intuitively by clinicians in the diagnosis; weight is given to morphology, distribution and histology. If sufficient points are not generated by the clinico-pathologic criteria, additional points can be added if highly specific adjunctive tests are positive. With the development of additional tests and prospective statistical validation of the scoring system, additional modifications will undoubtedly be needed, however. The proposed system, based on initial analysis of patients in our database, appears to be of sufficiently high specificity and sensitivity to be of immediate use.

Relative weighting and choice of diagnostic criteria

Five points are needed in the proposed system to achieve the diagnosis of early MF-CTCL (Table 1). A classical case would score 5 points on clinico-pathologic features alone. Because characteristic morphology and distribution both play a strong role in determining the degree of certainty of the diagnosis, both are given numerical values in the scoring system. Early plaques demonstrating classical morphology (poikiloderma atrophicans vasculare (P.A.V.), scaling poikiloderma, multiple, well demarcated tumid scaling plaques, or leonine facies) would score two points. If the lesions are present primarily in a classical distribution (buttocks, upper thighs, upper inner arms, inframammary area, or lower trunk), an additional two points is added, bringing the score to four. Many clinicians would be willing to make a clinical diagnosis of MF-CTCL in a number of such cases. Although the degree of certainty in such cases is high, however, it is not absolute. For this reason, at least one other criterion point is needed to reach the diagnostic threshold of 5 points in the scoring system. For instance, a biopsy that is at least suggestive of the diagnosis, or a positive, highly specific, adjunctive test (as defined below) would add sufficient points to make the diagnosis.

The assignment of two points to lesions with classical clinical morphology gives weight to the increased degree of clinical certainty that is engendered if such lesions are present. Classical morphology alone is not diagnostic, however, so less than 5 points is assigned as a maximum score for this parameter. In other cases, the morphology may only be consistent with a diagnosis of MF-CTCL, such as the occurrence of scaling dermatitic patches or plaques (either eczematous or psoriasiform). This reduced clinical certainty would then be recognized by the

Table 1. Differentially weighted criteria for a standardized diagnostic threshold in MF-CTL[1].

Score	0	1	2	3	Total
Clinical and Pathologic data:					
Clinical morphology	Non-typical (non-scaling lesions)	Consistent: Scaling dermatitis erythroderma, or alopecia mucinosa	Classical: PAV[2], leonine facies, or well demarcated tumid plaques		a: _____
Clinical distribution	Non-typical	Consistent: Extremities, head or upper trunk, in addition to classical distribution	Classical: Buttocks, lower trunk, thighs, upper inner arms, and inframammary areas		b: _____
Histology	Non-specific inflammatory changes	Suggestive changes, or atypical lymphocytes present	Consistent or probable changes for CTCL present	Diagnostic changes present	c: _____

A = Subtotal, Clinical and Pathologic data (= a+b+c):　　　_____

Adjunctive data:

Pan T marker loss (CD2, 3, or 5)	0(?,or<2)	1(?,see text)	≥ 2		d: _____
TCRGR[3]	—		+		e: _____
NCI[4]>11.5	—		+		f: _____

294

Table 1. Continued

Score	0	1	2	3	Total
Aneuploidy	−		+		g: ____
Peripheral blood Sézary cells > 15%	−		+		h: ____

B = Subtotal, Adjunctive data (maximum = 4) (= d+e+f+g+h): ____

Total, Clinical, Pathologic and Adjunctive data (= A+B): ____
(≥5 = MF-CTCL)

1. Exclusions: B Cell lymphoma, pleomorphic or large cell lymphomas, or any (non CTCL) specific diagnosis
2. PAV, Poikiloderma atrophicans vasculare
3. TCRGR, T cell receptor gene rearrangement
4. NCI, Nuclear contour index = $P / \sqrt{a}$ (nuclear perimeter / $\sqrt{}$nuclear area)

provision of only one point. Macular dyspigmentation or nonscaling, erythematous lesions, with even larger differential diagnoses, would not generate a point.

Similarly, because distribution is fairly specific for the diagnosis, if it is classical, predominance of lesions on the buttock, upper thighs, lower trunk, upper inner arms and infra-mammary areas provides 2 points. A distribution that does not include these areas has no specificity for MF, and carries no point value. In cases with a generalized distribution that includes the classical areas but also involves extensor surfaces, the head and neck, or the upper trunk, the degree of clinical certainty is reduced, although MF may be entertained in the differential diagnosis. This distribution is therefore consistent, and a single point is assigned. Thus, a case of atopic dermatitis or psoriasis may involve a classical area (ie., buttocks) but also usually involves a nonclassical area as well, resulting in a single point. Psoriasis, atopic dermatitis, chronic dermatitis, and drug eruptions typically only generate 2-3 points in this system; without histologic and/or specific test confirmation, the 5 point threshold is not reached.

Although histologic features characteristic of MF-CTCL have been identified, the relative specificity and weight of these features have not been agreed upon, and the pathologist utilizes a constellation of features on the slide to estimate whether it is of high or low likelihood that the features represent MF-CTCL. Generally, each pathologist communicates his degree of certainty with some sort of scale of terms such as: diagnostic of MF, probable MF, consistent with MF, suggestive of MF or atypical lymphocytic infiltration. Otherwise, a description of a nonspecific dermatitis (spongiotic, psoriasiform, delayed type hypersensitivity reaction, etc.), is provided if the probability is felt to be extremely low. Increased certainty on the part of the pathologist is recognized in the scoring system with increased points. Until a standardized scoring system for histologic diagnosis of MF-CTCL is agreed upon, this 0-3 scale may vary somewhat in its application to terminology utilized by different pathologists. Because diagnostic histology is the strongest single parameter, the number of histologic points assigned is 3. Assignment of a value less than 5, however, means that histologically diagnostic MF-CTCL must be confirmed either by consistent clinical features or by an adjunctive test. This prevents the occasional false-positive histology from automatically labelling a patient with a diagnosis of lymphoma, if there is no other supporting clinical or adjunctive data.

On the other hand, a diagnostic biopsy in the face of either classical morphology or a classical distribution alone would provide the 5 points necessary for diagnosis. Histology in a patient with a typical distribution only requires consistent morphology (e.g., nonspecific dermatitis) to reach 5 points. Thus, even without the use of adjunctive criteria, the consistency of the diagnostic threshold is facilitated and can be standardized between centers.

Although the scoring system can tolerate their entry, it is preferable to exclude from this analysis cases with diagnoses of B cell lymphoma, pleomorphic or large cell lymphomas, or other (non CTCL) specific diagnoses (such as pityriasis lichenoides et varioliformis acuta or lymphomatoid papulosis). Sézary syndrome patients with consistent histology will breach the 5 point threshold for diagnosis. Generalized erythroderma, which is not specific for CTCL, provides 1 point on distribution and one point on morphology. Therefore, Sézary patients with nonepidermotropic atypical histology (one point) will require a positive adjunctive test to breach threshold. This can be from blood as well as from skin, so that > 15% Sézary cells, a positive blood T cell receptor gene rearrangement, or discordant pan T cell marker expression on blood cells would be diagnostic.

Adjunctive Criteria

Each of the chosen criteria are highly specific, but not particularly sensitive if performed on early lesions of MF-CTCL (Vonderheid, 1989). That is, a negative result does not rule out the disease, but a positive result is strongly indicative of disease. Thus, each test, if positive, provides 2 points. Only a few clinicians use more than two or three of these tests simultaneously on a routine basis. Even if one does, however, the maximum number of possible adjunctive test points would be limited to 4. This precludes a diagnosis of MF-CTCL in the unlikely instance of lesions with marked aneuploidy, a positive TCRGR, and loss of pan T cell markers, but absolutely no clinical or pathological support for the diagnosis.

On the other hand, a patient with a consistent dermatitis (1 point) in a classical distribution (2 points) and only suggestive histology (1 point), would be diagnosed as MF-CTCL if a TCRGR were present. Similarly, a classical plaque (2 points) in an atypical location (0 points) and only consistent histology (2 points) would require confirmation by an adjunctive test (2 points) to breach the diagnostic threshold. Thus, although classical Worringer-Kollop disease would breach the threshold (morphology = 2, histology = 3), less classical, unilesional cases would not be included unless an adjunctive test were positive.

It is assumed that the immunophenotype analysis is performed on frozen lesional tissue utilizing antibodies that detect the truly pan T cell markers, CD2, CD3, and CD5. Discordantly low expression of two or more markers would constitute a positive test. Discordantly low expression of a single marker could be argued to constitute a single point, but the variability of immunophenotype staining makes such reliance somewhat difficult. Similarly, it could be argued that a very high CD4:CD8 ratio, a discordantly low representation of the $CD7^+$ T cell subset, or diffuse epidermal HLA-DR expression should constitute a point. Detailed analysis will be needed to verify the reproducibility, specificity, and value of these possible criteria in such a scoring system.

The T cell receptor gene rearrangement method is assumed to involve Southern Blot hybridization of DNA extracted from either lesional skin, blood or lymph node. The system also assumes the use of probes for the alpha or beta chain of the T cell receptor. As more sensitive tests are developed, specificity and sensitivity values will have to be reverified. Similarly, tests for nuclear contour index and aneuploidy are assumed to conform to published methodology.

CONCLUSION

A scoring system that standardizes a threshold for the diagnosis of early MF-CTCL using differentially weighted criteria is presented. It is hoped that the advent of more sensitive tests will obviate the need for such a system. Furthermore, retrospective and prospective evaluation of patients included and excluded in relation to ultimate diagnostic outcome is needed, and is underway at our institution. In the interim, however, this system is less subjective than the current situation (although most clinicians already intuitively weigh these various diagnostic features). Most importantly, application of a system such as this to characterize patients entered into studies of pathogenesis, diagnosis, therapy, or prognostication will standardize Stage I MF-CTCL patients for better comparisons of studies executed at different centers, and will homogenize multi-center protocols, much like the reporting of TNM stage or lesion stage has improved comparisons of later stages of MF-CTCL (Lamberg et al., 1979).

ACKNOWLEDGEMENTS

The author wishes to thank Drs. Zsuzsanna Bata-Csorgo, Kefei Kang, Margaret Terhune, Robert Tigelaar, Richard Edelson and Willem A. van Vloten for their helpful, specific suggestions that have been incorporated into the scoring system.

REFERENCES

Burg G, SA Buechner, RK Winkelmann and PM Banks, 1984. T cells and T-cell subsets in mycosis fungoides and parapsoriasis: A study of 18 cases with anti-human T-cell monoclonal antibodies and histochemical techniques. **Arch. Dermatol.**, 120:897-905.

Chu A, J Patterson, C Berger, E Vonderheid and R Edelson, 1984. In situ study of T-cell subpopulations in cutaneous T-cell lymphoma: Diagnostic criteria. **Cancer**, 54: 2414-2422.

Hagedorn M and G Kiefer, 1977. DNA content of mycosis fungoides cells. **Arch. Dermatol. Res.**, 258:127-134.

Lamberg SI, SB Green, DP Byar et al., 1979. Status report of 376 mycosis fungoides patients at 4 years: Mycosis Fungoides Cooperative Group. **Cancer Treat. Rep.**, 63:701-707.

Lindae ML, EA Abel, RT Hoppe and GS Wood, 1988. Poikilodermatous mycosis fungoides and atrophic large plaque parapsoriasis exhibit similar abnormalities of T-cell antigen expression. **Arch. Dermatol.**, 124: 366-372.

Lutzner MA and HW Jordan, 1968. The ultrastructure of an abnormal cell in Sézary's syndrome. **Blood**, 31:719-726.

Meyer CJ, AW van Leeuwen, EM van der Loo, LB van de Putte and WA van Vloten, 1977. Cerebriform (Sézary like) mononuclear cells in healthy individuals: A morphologically distinct population of T cells. Relationship with mycosis fungoides and Sézary's syndrome. **Virchows Arch.**, [B], 25:95-104.

Nickoloff BJ, 1988. Light-microscopic assessment of 100 patients with patch/plaque-stage mycosis fungoides. **Am. J. Dermatopathol.**, 10:469-477.

Payne CM, TM Grogan and PJ Lynch, 1986. An ultrastructural morphometric and immunohistochemical analysis of cutaneous lymphomas and benign lymphocytic infiltrates of skin: Useful criteria for diagnosis. **Arch. Dermatol.**, 122: 1139-1154.

Ralfkiaer E, NTJ O'Connor, J Crick, GL Wantzin and DY Mason, 1987. Genotypic analysis of cutaneous T-cell lymphomas. **J. Invest. Dermatol.**, 88:762-765.

Ralfkiaer E, JK Larsen, IJ Christensen, K Thomsen and GL Wantzin, 1989. DNA analysis by flow cytometry in cutaneous T-cell lymphomas. **Br. J. Dermatol.**, 120:597-605.

Schmoeckel C, G Burg and O Braun-Falco, 1979. Quantitative analysis of lymphoid cells in mycosis fungoides. Sézary's syndrome and parapsoriasis en plaques. **Arch. Dermatol. Res.**, 264:17-28

Simon GT, 1987. The value of morphometry in the ultrastructural diagnosis of mycosis fungoides. **Ultrastruct. Pathol.**, 11:687-691.

van der Putte SCJ, J Toonstra, DF van Wichen, JAM van Unnick and WA van Vloten, 1988. Aberrant immunophenotypes in mycosis fungoides. **Arch. Dermatol.**, 124: 373-380.

van Vloten WA, P van Duijn and A Schaberg, 1974. Cytodiagnostic use of Feulgen-DNA measurements in cell imprints from the skin of patients with mycosis fungoides. **Br. J. Dermatol.**, 91:365-371.

van Vloten WA and R Willemze, 1985. New techniques in the evaluation of cutaneous T-cell lymphoma. **Dermatol. Clin.**, 3:665-667.

Verga M and IM Braverman, 1991. The use of immunohistologic analysis in differentiating cutaneous T-cell lymphoma from psoriasis and dermatitis. **Arch. Dermatol.**, 127:1503-1510.

Vonderheid E, 1989. Diagnostic methods for cutaneous T Cell lymphoma. In: S. A. Muller, Ed: **Parapsoriasis**, Rochester: Mayo Foundation, pp. 83-94.

Vonderheid EC. E Tan, EL Sobel, E Schwab, B Micaily and BV Jegasothy, 1987. Clinical implications of immunologic phenotyping in cutaneous T cell lymphoma. **J. Am. Acad. Dermatol.**, 17:40-52.

Weiss LM, E Hu, GS Wood et al., 1985. Clonal rearrangements of T-cell receptor genes in mycosis fungoides and dermatopathic lymphadenopathy. **N. Engl. J. Med.**, 313:539-544.

Weiss LM, GS Wood, E Hu, EA Abel, RT Hoppe and J Sklar, 1989. Detection of clonal T-cell receptor gene rearrangements in the peripheral blood of patients with mycosis fungoides/Sézary syndrome. **J. Invest. Dermatol.**, 92:601-604.

CUTANEOUS B-CELL LYMPHOMA: A SALT-RELATED TUMOR?

Marco Santucci*
Nicola Pimpinelli†

* Institute of Morbid Anatomy and Histopathology
† Dermatology Clinic II
University of Florence
Florence, Italy

Correspondence to: Prof. M. Santucci, Istituto di Anatomia e Istologia Patologica, Università di Firenze, Viale GB Morgagni 85, I-50134 Florence, Italy

ABSTRACT

Patients with cutaneous involvement by non-Hodgkin B-cell lymphomas can be divided into three groups: those presenting with cutaneous disease alone (primary lymphomas, PL), those presenting with concurrent cutaneous and extracutaneous disease (concurrent lymphomas, CL), and those presenting with extracutaneous disease who subsequently develop skin involvement (secondary lymphomas, SL). In our experience, PL and CL almost always demonstrate nonagressive clinical behavior and have an overall benign prognosis (1.6% and 14.3% mortality rates, respectively), with a quite good response to treatment (93.7% and 100% complete remission rates, respectively), while SL quite often present an aggressive course (28.5% complete remission and 71.4% mortality rates). Histomorphologically, no significant difference exists between PL and CL in the histoarchitectural pattern, topography, depth of invasion, or cellular composition of the infiltrate, neoplastic cells being reminiscent of the whole spectrum of morphologies presented by parafollicular B-cells. In PL and CL, all of these parameters are usually related to the age and growth rate of lesions. In contrast, in SL no such correlation exists; more frequently the infiltrate is bottom-heavy, and neoplastic cells involve the deep dermis and subcutis. Close analogies between PL and CL are similarly present in the immuno-

Basic Mechanisms of Physiologic and Aberrant Lymphoproliferation in the Skin
Edited by W.C. Lambert *et al.*, Plenum Press, New York, 1994

301

phenotype of neoplastic cells: they express CD19, CD20, and CD22 while consistently lacking CD10 and CD5 antigens. In SL, conversely, neoplastic cells almost always express CD10 and/or CD5 antigens. Concerning adhesion molecules and homing receptors, PL and CL are characterized by absent/weak expression of LFA-1 (CD11a/CD18) and CD44 antigen (Hermes-3 homing receptor) on the one hand, and by strongly positive staining for LECAM-1 (Leu-8 antigen) in B-cells on the other hand; SL, however, present an almost opposite staining profile. The similar, typical clinical presentation and course, and the homogeneous morphoimmunologic features of PL and CL favor the conjecture of a single nature and similar origin for these lymphoproliferative disorders, which possibly represent different expressions of the same spectrum of disease, namely tissue-/organ-associated lymphoid tissue derived B-cell lymphomas, making them quite different from SL. Moreover, the existence of CL supports speculation regarding the existence of subtle interactions, the intimate natures of which are presently unknown, between local immune systems and the general immune system.

INTRODUCTION

The spread of non-Hodgkin lymphoma is not predictable. The disease may be unifocal in origin, but widespread dissemination is frequent. While the multifocal origin of the nodal lymphomas is well known, data on non-Hodgkin lymphomas occurring in multiple extranodal sites are sparse. In addition, an ill-understood preferential involvement of specific extranodal sites is seen in some of these neoplasms (Advani et al., 1990). The reason for this tropism is not clear, but it has been considered likely that it is closely linked to the homing process regulated by homing receptors on lymphoid cells and ligands on high endothelial venules (Picker et al., 1988; Streeter et al., 1988). The skin represents one of the most important extranodal sites.

Patients with cutaneous involvement by non-Hodgkin B-cell lymphoma can be divided into three groups: those presenting with cutaneous disease alone (i.e., primary lymphomas, PL), those presenting with concurrent cutaneous and extracutaneous disease (i.e., concurrent lymphomas, CL), and those presenting with extracutaneous disease who subsequently develop skin involvement (i.e., secondary lymphomas, SL).

In the present study, we investigated CL and SL, comparing their clinicopathologic, histomorphologic, and immunologic profile with that of a large series (83 cases) of PL already reported by our group (Santucci et al., 1991), with the aim of identifying similarities and differences existing among primary, concurrent, and secondary cutaneous B-cell lymphomas. The rather uniform characteristics of PL and CL give a hint to a similar origin for these lymphoproliferative disorders from tissue-/organ-associated lymphoid tissue.

MATERIALS AND METHODS

Patient Selection

The files of the Institute of Morbid Anatomy and Histopathology of the University of Florence (Italy) concerning lymphoproliferative disorders were reviewed and 19 cases of B cell lymphoma with concurrent or secondary cutaneous localization were extracted. Crucial criteria for the selection of cases were: i, presence of both cutaneous and extracutaneous lesions; ii, expression of B-cell restricted antigens by neoplastic cells; and iii, light chain monoclonal restriction or surface immunoglobulin (SIg)- negative staining by neoplastic cells. Due to a lack of available detailed clinical information and/or material useful for immunohistochemical phenotyping, five cases were discarded, and the present investigation was thus performed on seven cases of CL and seven cases of SL, plus the 83 cases of PL already reported by our group (Santucci et al., 1991), data from which will be briefly recapitulated.

In all patients who entered this study, extensive and careful staging procedures -- described elsewhere in detail (Pimpinelli et al., 1989; 1990) -- have been performed.

Patient Samples

Several skin biopsies were performed on all patients. Skin samples were obtained from lesions with different dimensions, ages, and growth rates. Furthermore, biopsies of lymph nodes (15 patients), soft tissues (2 patients), and nasopharynx (Waldeyer's ring) (1 patient) have been performed.

Each cutaneous specimen -- obtained under local anesthesia with carbocaine 2% by incisional biopsy or, in a minority of cases, by 4/6-mm punch biopsy -- was divided into 3 parts and processed for light and electron microscopy and immunohistochemistry, respectively.

Light Microscopy

The specimens were fixed in Duboscq-Brasil or in buffered formalin liquids for 12-24 hours, routinely processed, and embedded in Paraplast Plus with a melting temperature of $+56°C$ (Monoject Scientific Inc., Athy, Co. Kildare, Ireland). Four-to six-μm-thick sections were stained with hematoxylin and eosin, periodic acid-Schiff (PAS)-reaction, Giemsa and reticulin stains.

Electron Microscopy

Material for ultramicroscopic investigation was cut into one mm^3 blocks, quickly fixed for 3-6 hours at $+4°C$ in 2.5% glutaraldehyde in 0.1 M sodium cacodylate buffer (pH 7.4), and post-fixed for one hour at $+4°C$ in 1% osmium tetroxide in 0.1 M veronal acetate buffer (pH

7.4). The tissue blocks were stained en bloc by immersion in 2% uranyl acetate in pure alcohol; dehydration was done in graded ethanol-water solutions, diaphanization in propylene oxide, and embedding in epoxy resin (Araldite, Serva Feinbiochemica, Heidelberg, Germany). Polymerization was allowed to occur in Beem 00 capsules overnight at +80°C in an embedding oven.

Semi-thin sections, 0.5-1 μm in thickness, were cut from each block and stained with toluidine blue and eosin-erythrosin (Biagini et al., 1973). Ultra-thin serial sections, cut at 40-60 nm with the use of a diamond knife (Diatome Ltd., Bienne, Switzerland), were stained with uranyl acetate and lead citrate and examined in a Philips 410 LS transmission electron microscope at 100 kV accelerating voltage.

Immunohistochemistry

Immunohistologic studies were performed either on 4 μm paraffin sections or on 6 μm cryostat sections. Tissue sections were stained using either an immunoperoxidase (Hsu et al., 1981) or the alkaline phosphatase anti-alkaline phosphatase (APAAP) (Cordell et al., 1984) method. The monoclonal antibodies used are listed in Table 1.

Cryostat sections were obtained from quickly frozen tissue samples embedded in OCT medium (Miles Laboratories, Naperville, IL) and stored at -70°C until sectioned. Multiple serial sections were cut for each block, air dried for 12-24 hours, fixed in acetone for 10 minutes at room temperature, air dried again, and stored at -20°C until immunohistochemical staining.

A semiquantitative evaluation of the immunohistochemical reactions was performed by counting the number of stained cells in a total number of 100 cells in 5 consecutive microscopic fields at x400, and the mean values were calculated and recorded. Only cells in which the nucleus was in the microscopic plane of section were counted.

Statistical Analysis

The Kaplan and Meier technique (Kaplan and Meier, 1958) was used to determine the estimated probabilities of survival, computed from the time of diagnosis. Differences between groups were tested by the variance analysis test (Kruskal and Wallis, 1952).

RESULTS

Clinical Findings

In the PL group, there were 51 male and 32 female patients (male-to-female ratio, 1.6:1); the age at the first examination ranged from 22 to 88 years (mean, 55 years; median, 58 years).

Table 1. Antibody Panel

Antibody	Cluster Designation	Source
Leu-12	CD19	BD
B1	CD20	CC
B2	CD21	CC
Leu-14	CD22	BD
T11	CD2	CC
T3	CD3	CC
OKT4	CD4	OD
OKT8	CD8	OD
Leu-1	CD5	BD
OKT6	CD1a	OD
Leu-8	NA	BD
anti-LFA-1 α	CD11a	DP
anti-LFA-1 β	CD18	DP
anti-CD44	CD44	@
anti-ICAM-1	CD54	Φ
IL-2 r.	CD25	BD
HLA-DR	NA	BD
C3b r.*	CD35	DP
Ki-1	CD30	DP
Ber-H2I	CD30	DP
DRC-1	NA	DP
anti-NGFR (clone 20.4)	NA	§
J5	CD10	BD
Leu-M3	CD14	BD
Leu-M5	CD11c	BD
OKM1	CD11b	OD
ORT9	CD71	OD
Ki-67	NA	DP
L26I	CD20	DP
MB2I	NA	BI
LN1I	CDw75	BI
LN2I	CD74	BI
LN3I	NA	BI
UCHL-1I	CD45RO	DP
anti-CD3I	CD3	DP
MT1I	CD43	BI
MT2I	CD45RA	BI
anti-k*	NA	BD
anti-lambda*	NA	BD
anti-gamma	NA	BD
anti-μ	NA	DP
anti-δ	NA	DP

* Tested on both frozen and paraffin sections. I Tested on paraffin sections only. NA: not assigned.

BD: Becton & Dickinson, Mountain View, CA; CC: Coulter Clone, Sheffield, UK; OD: Ortho Diagnostic Systems, Raritan, NJ; DP: Dakopatts, Copenhagen, Denmark; BI: Biotest AG, Dreieich, Germany; @: kind gift of Prof. E. Berti, Milan, Italy; Φ: kind gift of Dr. S. Ferrone, New York, NY; §: kind gift of the Immunology Laboratories of the Dept. of Pediatrics, University of Florence, Medical School, Florence, Italy.

For predominant immunoreactivity see Chan et al., 1988, and Knapp et al., 1989.

In the CL group, there were five male and two female patients (male-to-female ratio, 2.5:1); the age at the first examination ranged from 22 to 78 years (mean, 55 years; median, 56 years). In the SL group, there were four male and three female patients (male-to-female ratio, 1.3:1); the age at the first examination ranged from 15 to 72 years (mean, 53 years; median, 58 years).

In the CL group, four patients presented with nodal involvement, two patients with soft tissue involvement, and one patient with nasopharyngeal (Waldeyer's ring) involvement. In the SL group, all patients presented with nodal involvement.

All patients presented with cutaneous red to violaceous nodules, plaques, or tumors of variable age and size. In the PL group, 72 patients had lesions confined to a rather circumscribed area of the skin, with a noticeable predilection for the back (44.6%) and the head (25.3%); in the remaining 11 patients, nodular cutaneous and subcutaneous lesions involved noncontiguous anatomic regions. In the CL group, six patients presented with isolated (five patients) or multiple (one patient) lesions confined to a rather circumscribed area of the skin: trunk (three patients), head (one patient), neck (one patient), and forearm (one patient). In the remaining patient, the lesions were disseminated over the trunk and limbs. In all cases, the lesions had slowly grown over 6-12 months. In the SL group, cutaneous lesions were disseminated in five patients; they were characterized by rapid growth (1-2 months) in six patients.

Blood-cell count, morphology and immunologic phenotyping of circulating mononuclear cells, and serum immunoglobulin quantitation were unremarkable in all patients except for a single case, affected by PL, who presented a mild hypogammaglobulinemia.

Treatment and Clinical Evolution

In the PL group, at presentation, 61 patients were treated with local orthovolt radiotherapy, in two cases preceded by reductive surgical excision. Nine patients were treated by surgical excision only. Due to the diffuse involvement of non-contiguous anatomic sites, eight patients were treated with short chemotherapy courses -- CVP (cyclophosphamide, vincristine, prednisone) or CVP-Bleomycin regimens (CVP-like regimens plus bleomycin) (Norton and Simon, 1977; Rossi Ferrini et al., 1978) -- in one case associated with local orthovolt irradiation, and two patients with α-2b-recombinant interferon (Intron-A, Schering Co., Kenilworth, NJ). Finally, three patients were treated with oral corticosteroids due to their refusal of any other therapeutic regimen. For further details on the PL group, see Santucci et al., 1991. In the CL group, five patients were treated with chemotherapy courses (CVP or CVP-Bleomycin regimens); the remaining two patients were treated by surgical excision of the soft tissue mass, followed by local orthovolt irradiation of cutaneous lesions. In the SL group, all patients were treated with chemotherapy courses: CHOP (cyclophosphamide, adriamicin, vincristine, prednisone) or COP-BLAM (cyclophosphamide, vincristine, prednisone, bleomycin, adriamicin, methotrexate) (Rossi Ferrini et al., 1978) associated with radiotherapy in three patients.

In the PL group, 78 patients (94%) went into complete remission; in the CL group, all patients went into complete remission; while in the SL group, this result was obtained in only two (28.5%) patients.

The disease-free period ranged from 2 to 100 months (median, 16 months) in the PL group; from 6 to 12 months (median, 10 months) in the CL group; and was 12 and 14 months (median, 13 months), respectively, in the two patients in the SL group.

Data on follow-up were available for 65 out of the 83 patients affected with PL, and for all patients affected by CL or SL. In both PL and CL groups, only one patient died of the disease, while in the SL group five out of seven patients died (1.5%, 14.3% and 71.4% mortality rates, respectively). The survival curves are depicted in Figure 1. With the variance analysis test, the two-year-survival differences between the PL or CL group and the SL group were highly significant (p=0.006).

Histologic Features

Histologic slides were reviewed without clinical information and the following parameters investigated:

Histoarchitectural pattern of the infiltrate. This was referred to as nodular (patchy), diffuse, or mixed (nodular + diffuse) (Santucci et al., 1987; 1991). The nodular pattern is not related to the presence of neoplastic or reactive follicles or germinal centers, and is characterized by discrete perivascular and/or periadnexal circular compartmentalizations of the infiltrate, resulting in lymphoid nodules of various sizes. In the diffuse pattern, discrete aggregates of infiltrating cells are no longer identifiable; the dermal collagen is permeated by a cellular infiltrate which is often rather uniformly dense throughout the involved dermis, completely overrunning and destroying the adnexa, and other times it shows a variable density, being sparse in some areas. Finally, the mixed pattern is characterized by the contemporaneous presence of histologic features of both nodular and diffuse patterns. Cases in which lymphoid nodules showed more or less evident phenomena of coalescence of cellular aggregates were also recorded as showing a mixed growth pattern.

Topography and depth of invasion of the infiltrate, and its amount. For this investigation, the reticular dermis was divided into three portions -- upper, mid, and lower -- each of them accounting for approximately one third of the entire dermal thickness. To record the topography of the cellular infiltrate, its upper and lower limits were taken into account. Since the loose connective tissue around skin appendages forms a functional unit with the papillary dermis, cellular infiltrates extending downwards exclusively at the periphery of the adventitial dermis around cutaneous appendages were considered as involving the upper dermis, only.

Cellular composition of the neoplastic infiltrate, and its histologic subtype. They were classified according to the Working Formulation for Clinical Usage (1982). Specifically, a case was classified as small cleaved cell (SCC) lymphoma when the estimated percentage of large cells was less than 25%; as mixed small and large cell (MC) lymphoma if the estimate for large cells was between 25% and 50%; and, finally, as large cell (LC) lymphoma if the percentage of large cells was more than 50%.

Amount and composition of the non-neoplastic cellular infiltrate

These data were recorded for each specimen and then matched with age and growth rate of lesions, and with their immunologic profile. A synthesis of the clinicopathologic correlations is reported below.

Lesions were categorized according to their age as follows: those aged less than 3 months were recorded as young lesions; those aged more than 12 months as old lesions; and those aged between 3 and 12 months as intermediate-aged lesions. Conversely, we used the terms early and late referring to the growth rate of lesions. Specifically, early lesions were represented by small, long-standing and slowly developed papules, plaques or nodules, being either young, intermediate-aged, or old; late lesions were represented by rapidly developed (i.e., lesions which doubled their size in less than 1 month) nodules or tumors, irrespective of their age.

In both PL and CL, the nodular histoarchitectural pattern was characteristic of young lesions, having been observed only very rarely in specimens taken from intermediate to old lesions; in this instance, large nodular aggregates of lymphoid cells were juxtaposed throughout the dermis without significant coalescence phenomena. The diffuse pattern was typical of old lesions, having been observed in only a few specimens taken from lesions less than 12 months old. The mixed pattern was not characteristic of any specific age of lesion, having been almost the most frequently observed. Neoplastic follicles were never observed; conversely, in intermediate to old, slowly developed lesions, we often found variable numbers of irregular or serpiginous reactive lymphoid follicles, containing irregularly shaped germinal centers more often showing the absence of "tingible body" macrophages or lacking the typical zonal architecture. Neoplastic cells formed broad, confluent strands external to follicular cortices or the other cell collections described above, in a fashion reminiscent of a parafollicular/interfollicular pattern (Nathwani et al., 1992). In SL, quite frequently the infiltrate was bottom-heavy, and neoplastic cells diffusely involved deep dermis and subcutis.

Regarding the topography of the lymphoid infiltrate, in all groups of lymphomas, the papillary dermis was constantly spared and a distinct Grenz-zone always resulted, except in specimens taken from ulcerated, tumorous lesions. In PL and CL, a certain correlation was found between the amount of infiltrate, its deepest extension, and the age and growth rate of lesions. In young early lesions, the infiltrate was generally inconspicuous and more often limited to the superficial portion of the reticular dermis, sometimes in a band-like fashion. Conversely, in intermediate to old and late lesions, a deeper involvement was the rule, and in the majority of old and late lesions the dermis and subcutis were infiltrated and almost entirely obscured by large numbers of neoplastic cells. These findings are contrary to the statement that in malignant cutaneous lymphoid infiltrates the involvement is never primarily localized to the upper dermis, and that the superficial aspects of the dermis are never diagnostic of lymphoma. In SL, conversely, no specific correlation was identified.

In PL and CL, the cellular composition of lymphoid infiltrates was highly variable, and neoplastic cells showed a range of appearance reminiscent of the whole spectrum of morphologies presented by parafollicular B-cells (Isaacson and Spencer, 1987; Sheibani et al., 1988; Lennert and Feller, 1992; Nathwani et al., 1992), with variable numbers of admixed small lymphocytes, plasma and lymphoplasmacytoid cells, polymorphonuclear granulocytes, and histio-

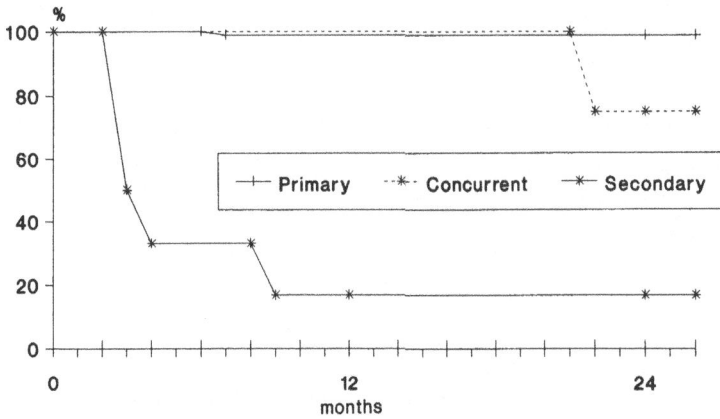

Figure 1. Estimated probabilities of survival from the time of diagnosis. Two-year-values show highly significant differences between the PL or CL group and the SL group (p=0.006).

cytes. The relative quantity of each cell morphology was highly variable both in different specimens from the same patient and different areas of the same specimen. SCC lymphoma was by far the least frequently observed subtype, and found exclusively in young early lesions, followed in frequency by MC and LC lymphoma. The cytomorphological categories showed a certain correlation with age and growth rate of lesions. In young lesions, it was typical to find a SCC lymphoma, even though a MC lymphoma represented the most frequent occurrence. In intermediate and old lesions a predominance of LC lymphomas was observed. Finally, in rapidly developed lesions, a LC lymphoma was almost always found. Characteristically, when a portion of a long-standing lesion had grown rapidly, a different morphologic type was quite often found in the two portions of the lesion; a MC lymphoma was more frequently observed in the long-standing, slowly enlarged portion, while a LC lymphoma was constantly found in the rapidly developed part. In early lesions, as opposed to what we observed in late lesions, variable numbers of cells with evident plasmacytic differentiation were frequently found. They did not generally show significant pleomorphism. Nonetheless, in some sections, there appeared to be a morphologic continuum between plasma cells or lymphoplasmacytoid cells and neoplastic cells; in these instances, a light chain monoclonal restriction was almost always documented. No differences in the evolution of the disease were identified in the patients we studied in relation to the histologic subtype.

In SL, the cell morphology was that of blast cells with abundant clear to eosinophilic cytoplasm, and a nucleus often having marked indentations and folds and slightly to moderately hypertrophic nucleoli. Specifically, neoplastic cells resembled large anaplastic centrocytes, centrocytoid cells, multilobulated cells, centroblasts, and immunoblasts; a marked pleomorphism of tumor cells was sometimes evident. The growth pattern was more often cohesive. An evident mitotic activity was observed only when there were consistent numbers of large, non-cleaved, centroblast- and/or immunoblast-like cells.

In PL and CL, neoplastic cells sometimes presented a skin appendage epidermotropism. The lymphocyte appendageal association was typically observed in both the ductal portion of eccrine sweat glands and the pilo-sebaceous units, the latter being involved at the sebaceous gland and/or the hair follicle isthmus level. In addition, tumor cells quite often showed more or less evident phenomena of invasion of the adventitia and endothelium of small vessels of the dermal vascular plexa; nerve entrapment, permeation of perineural spaces, or actual invasion of nerves; and/or infiltration of arrectores pilorum muscles.

In PL and CL, the non-neoplastic, reactive cellular infiltrate was variable, and often its actual amount could not be evaluated without immunologic assessment. The reactive infiltrate was more prominent in perivascular areas of the upper dermis; sometimes it was evident even in its mid- and deep portions. The vessels surrounded by reactive infiltrates had features of high endothelial venules, often showing an arborizing pattern and thickened basement membranes containing PAS-positive material. The reactive infiltrate was less conspicuous in old lesions in comparison to young ones, and in rapidly enlarged lesions in comparison to slowly developed ones. Furthermore, in specimens in which a portion of a long-standing lesion had grown rapidly, a dramatic difference in the amount of reactive infiltrate was observed between the two parts of the lesion, being virtually absent in the rapidly developed part in comparison to the slowly enlarged portion. In SL, conversely, a reactive cellular infiltrate was always virtually absent.

Relapses presented histologic features indistinguishable from those of primary lesions.

Submicroscopic Features

In PL and CL, even from the submicroscopic point of view, infiltrating cells appeared to be composed of a mixture of various cell types, the relative quantity of which was highly variable, depending on histologic subtype. Phagocytosing histiocytes; polymorphonuclear granulocytes; plasma and lymphoplasmacytoid cells; small- to medium-sized cerebriform T-lymphocytes; and accessory, interdigitating (IRCs) and dendritic (DRCs) reticulum cells were recognized and were admixed with the predominant medium- to large-sized neoplastic cell population.

Neoplastic cells, despite an evident morphologic variability, often showed some common, peculiar features. Tumor cells had an irregular cell contour, sometimes with short processes, more frequently with highly villous and intertwined cell membranes, due to which they were in contact with other neoplastic cells and DRCs. Nuclei were sometimes roundish, but more often grooved, infolded or irregularly indented, convoluted or multilobated, with a moderate to slight quantity of marginated heterochromatin. In the markedly irregular nuclei, multiple, generally inconspicuous to moderately hypertrophic nucleoli were observed, whereas the roundish or less irregular nuclei contained one or two prominent nucleoli. Cytoplasms were always abundant, and contained a moderate to large quantity of diffuse mono-/polyribosomes and, occasionally, small lipid droplets. Cytoplasmic organelles were often polarized towards the nuclear grooves and folds, and consisted of large mitochondria, some vesicles of smooth endoplasmic reticulum, a few dense-core primary lysosomes, and sometimes a pronounced Golgi zone and a well developed rough endoplasmic reticulum which, in some cells, appeared as cisternae parallel to the cell surface, with occasional inclusions of proteinaceous material inside them. No ribosome-lamella complexes were found.

Immunologic Findings

In PL and CL, CD19$^+$, CD20$^+$, CD22$^+$, LECAM-1(Leu-8)$^+$, HLA-DR$^+$, CD10$^-$, CD5$^-$, LFA-1 (CD11a/CD18)$^{(+)/-}$, CD44 (Hermes-3 homing receptor)$^{(+)/-}$, SIg$^+$ monoclonal/-neoplastic B-cells were found admixed with variable numbers of DRC-1$^+$, CD35$^+$, CD21$^{+/-}$, NGFR$^+$, CD14$^-$ DRCs. Variable numbers of reactive T-cells and CD1a$^+$ dendritic cells were found, with a CD4/CD8 ratio varying from 1:1 to 1:3. In SL, CD19$^+$, CD20$^+$, CD22$^+$, LECAM-1$^-$, HLA-DR$^+$, CD10$^{(+)/-}$, CD5$^{(+)/-}$, LFA-1 (CD11a/CD18$^+$, CD44$^+$, SIg$^+$ monoclonal/- neoplastic B-cells were found.

Concerning the immunoarchitecture of the lesions, three prototypical patterns were identified. The first one -- typical of young, early lesions of PL and CL -- was characterized by an evident, focal clustering of B-cells and DRCs (mainly located in the upper-mid reticular dermis), this resulting in a rather distinct compartmentalization of B- and T-cells. In these clusters, DRCs were loosely arranged in ill-defined meshworks with blurred and radiating contours, and they skipped the nodule centers in a centrifugal fashion. In the remaining areas of cell proliferation, B- and T-cells and their accessory cells were intermingled, with an overwhelming preponderance of T-cells (most of which expressed CD25 antigen). Macrophages were constantly few and sparse. Cells expressing CD71 and Ki-67 antigens were relatively few and exclusively found in B-cell clusters. The second pattern characteristic of non-young, slowly developed lesions of PL and CL was characterized by a quite uniform admixture of B-cells, T cells, and their respective accessory cells, without a distinct compartmentalization. Macrophages were constantly few and sparse. Cells expressing CD71 and Ki-67 antigens were few and sparse. In the third pattern -- typical of late lesions of PL and CL, and of all lesions of SL -- B-cells were always the large majority of infiltrating cells and they were quite often SIg. Reactive T cells were always few and sparse. Scattered macrophages were also found. The large majority of infiltrating cells expressed CD71 and Ki-67 antigens.

No significant differences in immunopathologic profile, as documented in both frozen and embedded tissue, were seen between primary and relapsing lesions. Concerning SIg, a uniform expression of light chains was more often documented in different lesions in the same patients.

COMMENT

Concerning demography, no significant difference was found among the three groups of patients, all types of lymphomas involving elderly patients. In PL and CL, a male prevalence was observed. All patients presented with nodules, plaques, or tumors of variable age and size. In the large majority of patients affected with PL and CL, the lesions were confined to a rather circumscribed area of the skin, with a noticeable predilection for the trunk and to a lesser extent for the head.

Histomorphologically, no significant difference was seen between PL and CL in the histoarchitectural pattern, topography, depth of invasion, or amount of the infiltrate. The mixed pattern was most frequently observed, followed in frequency by the diffuse, with the nodular least frequent. Similarly, no difference was observed between PL and CL in the cellular composition of the infiltrate, neoplastic cells showing a range of appearances reminiscent of the whole spectrum of morphologies presented by parafollicular B-cells. We never observed neoplastic follicles; conversely, in slowly developed lesions older than 6 months, we often found reactive lymphoid follicles. In PL and CL, all of these parameters were found to be related to the age and growth rate of lesions. In SL, conversely, no such specific correlation was found. The infiltrate was more frequently bottom heavy, and neoplastic cells involved the deep dermis and subcutis. We never observed reactive lymphoid follicles.

Close analogies between PL and CL were similarly observed in the immunophenotype of neoplastic cells, which were characterized by the absence of expression of CD10 and CD5 antigens. In SL, conversely, neoplastic cells almost constantly expressed CD10 and/or CD5 antigens. In addition, both PL and CL often presented, especially in young-early lesions, a peculiar follicular-like lesional immunoarchitecture, with an evident clustering and compartment-alization of B-cells and NGFR+ CD14- DRCs, which were surrounded by T-cell areas.

Concerning adhesion molecules and homing receptors, PL and CL were characterized on the one hand by absent/weak expression of LFA-1 and CD44 antigen, and on the other hand by positive staining for LECAM-1 in B-cells, while SL presented an almost opposite staining profile.

Primary and concurrent lymphomas almost constantly showed non-aggressive clinical behavior and had a benign overall prognosis, with a quite good response to treatment, while SL quite often showed with an aggressive course. Therefore, at present, the identification of morphologic subgroups has no clinical, therapeutic and/or prognostic relevance.

CONCLUSIONS

The morphologic features of PL have long supported a follicular-center-cell origin for these lymphomas, despite immunologic and genotypic evidence (i.e., negative staining for CD5 and CD10 antigens and absence of bcl-2 gene rearrangement) against this thesis. Conversely, the contemporaneous presence of lesions showing different cytologic aspects in the same patients supports a holistic concept, namely, that these aspects belong to one and the same type of cell. Recently, this thesis has been supported by morphometric studies (Gianotti and Montaperto, 1992) which demonstrated the presence of a unimodal population composed of cells with morphometric features that cannot be labeled as centrocytes nor as centroblasts or immunoblasts. A different key for the interpretation of the morphologic picture may be furnished by the fact that these aspects are consistent with those of so called centrocyte-like cells, monocytoid cells, immature sinus histiocytes, or parafollicular B-cells as we confirmed by electron microscopy, identifying cells with active nucleoli, a few strands of ergastoplasm, a relatively well developed Golgi apparatus and small, electron-dense lysosomes. This different interpretation might better account for the rather benign clinicopathologic behavior of PL and CL, which is similar to that presented by MALT-lymphomas and parafollicular (monocytoid) B-cell lymphomas of lymph nodes.

We feel that the typical clinical presentation and course, and the homogeneous -- even if amply variable -- morphoimmunologic features of primary and concurrent cutaneous B-cell lymphomas favor the conjecture of a peculiar, and possibly single, nature and similar origin for these lymphoproliferative disorders, probably linked to a specific cell type with peculiar homing features (i.e., constitutive cells retain a specific homing pattern and have a very low tendency to recirculate), and/or related to a peculiar behavior of the tissue-/organ associated lymphoid tissue. In our opinion, in fact, PL and CL represent different expressions of the same spectrum of disease (namely, tissue-/organ-associated lymphoid tissue derived B-cell lymphomas), and we believe that the existence of CL -- which are characterized from the onset by the contemporaneous presence of cutaneous and extracutaneous involvement -- supports speculation about the existence of subtle interactions, the intimate natures of which are presently unknown, between local immune systems and the general immune system.

ACKNOWLEDGEMENTS

The authors thank Umberto M. Reali, M.D., Head of the Division of Plastic Surgery, University of Florence Medical School, for having performed the statistical evaluations contained in this article.

This work was in part supported by grants from the Italian Ministries of Public Education, and of University and Scientific and Technologic Research.

REFERENCES

Advani SH, RS Iyer, R Gopal, CN Nair, T Saika, KA Dinshaw, PA Kurkure and SK Pai, 1990. Multifocal extranodal lymphomas: An expression of homing phenomenon. **Oncology**, 47:334.

Biagini G, C Scala, MM Bragaglia, P Borsetti and R Laschi, 1973. Technical improvements for ultrastructural investigation in routine pathology. **J. Submicrosc. Cytol.**, 5:271.

Chan JKC, CS Ng and PK Hui, 1988. A simple guide to the terminology and application of leucocyte monoclonal antibodies. **Histopathology**, 12:461.

Cordell JL, B Falini, WN Erber, Ak Ghosh, Z Abdulaziz, S MacDonald, KAF Pulfond, H Stein and DY Mason, 1984. Immunoenzymatic labelling of monoclonal antibodies using immune complexes of alkaline phosphatase and monoclonal antialkaline phosphatase (APAAP complexes). **J. Histochem. Cytochem.**, 32:219.

Gianotti R and C Montaperto, 1992. Morphometric study of primary cutaneous germinal center cell lymphomas. **Cancer**, 70:1905.

Hsu SH, L Raine and H. Fanger H, 1981. Use of avidinperoxidase complex (ABC) in immunoperoxidase techniques. A comparison between ABC and unlabeled antibody (PAP) procedures. **J. Histochem. Cytochem.**, 29:1349.

Kaplan EL and P Meier, 1958. Nonparametric estimation from incomplete observations. **Am. Stat. Ass. J.**, 53:457.

Knapp W, B Dörken, P Rieber, RE Schmidt, H Stein and AEG Kr von dem Borne, 1989, CD Antigens 1989. **Am. J. Pathol.**, 135:420.

Kruskal WH and WA Wallis, 1952. Use of ranks in one criterion variance analysis. **Am. Stat. Ass. J.**, 47:583.

Isaacson PG and J Spencer, 1987. Malignant lymphoma of mucosaassociated lymphoid tissue. **Histopathology**, 11:445.

Lennert K and AC Feller, 1992. **Histopathology of non-Hodgkin's lymphomas** (based on the updated Kiel classification), 2nd edition, Springer-Verlag, Berlin.

Nathwani BN, RL Mohrmann, RK Brynes, CR Taylor, ML Hansmann and K Sheibani, 1992. Monocytoid B-cell lymphomas: An assessment of diagnostic criteria and a perspective on histogenesis. **Hum. Pathol.**, 23:1061.

Norton L and R Simon, 1977. Tumor size, sensitivity to therapy and design of treatment schedules. **Cancer Treat. Rep.**, 61:1307.

Pimpinelli N, M Santucci, A Bosi, S Moretti, C Vallecchi, A Messori and B Giannotti, 1989. Primary cutaneous follicular centre-cell lymphoma: A lymphoproliferative disease with favourable prognosis. **Clin. Exp. Dermatol.**, 14:12.

Pimpinelli N, M Santucci, P Carli, M Paglierani, A Bosi, S Moretti and B Giannotti, 1990. Primary cutaneous follicular center cell lymphoma: Clinical and histological aspects, In: WA van Vloten, R Willemze, G Lange Vejlsgaard and K Thomsen, Eds:, **Cutaneous Lymphoma, Current Problems in Dermatology**, vol. 19 (H. Honigsmann ed.), Karger, Basel.

Picker LJ, LJ Madeiros, LM Weiss, RA Warnke and EC Butcher, 1988. Expression of lymphocyte homing receptor antigen in non-Hodgkin's lymphoma. **Am. J. Pathol.**, 130:496.

Rossi Ferrini P, G Bellesi and A Bosi, 1978. La chemioterapia dei linfomi non-Hodgkin, In: A Cajozzo, Ed., **Le Malattie Limfoproliferative**, Libreria Clemenza, Palermo.

Santucci M, N Pimpinelli, S Moretti, R Bondi and B Giannotti, 1987. Primary cutaneous follicular center cell lymphoma of the back (Crosti's reticulohistiocytoma): Comparison between early and late lesions, abstract 12, presented at the **8th International Dermatopathology Colloquium**, Barcelona, Spain, October 8-10.

Santucci M, N Pimpinelli and L Arganini, 1991. Primary cutaneous B-cell lymphoma: A unique type of low-grade lymphoma. **Cancer**, 67:2311.

Sheibani K, JS Burke, WG Swartz, A Nademanee and CD Winberg, 1988. Monocytoid B-cell lymphoma: Clinicopathologic study of 21 cases of a unique type of low grade lymphoma. **Cancer**, 62:1531.

Streeter PR, EL Berg, BT Rouse, RF Bargatze and EC Butcher, 1988. A tissue specific endothelial cell molecule involved in lymphocyte homing. **Nature**, 331:45.

The non-Hodgkin's lymphoma pathologic classification project: National Cancer Institute sponsored study of classifications of non-Hodgkin's lymphomas. Summary and description of a Working Formulation for clinical usage, 1982. **Cancer**, 49:2112.

PROLIFERATION ACTIVITY IN SKIN LESIONS OF MYCOSIS FUNGOIDES: PROGNOSTIC AND PATHOPHYSIOLOGIC IMPLICATIONS

Peter Kaudewitz
Rolf-Markus Szeimies

Department of Dermatology
University of Munich
Munich, Germany

Correspondence to: Dr. P. Kaudewitz, Department of Dermatology,
University Hospital, Frauenlobstrasse 9-11,
D-8000 Munchen 2, Germany

ABSTRACT

Proliferative activity of infiltrating mononuclear cells in cutaneous infiltrates was assessed in mycosis fungoides using the monoclonal antibody, Ki-67. The Ki-67 determined growth fraction was found to correlate with TNM stage, type of skin lesion, and predominant cytologic type of atypical infiltrating cells. When the distribution of Ki-67-positive cells was analyzed, no preferential localization of proliferating cells was evident. These results indicate that proliferative activity in mycosis fungoides may be useful as an additional prognostic parameter. The distribution of Ki-67-positive cells does not support the concept that proliferation of atypical T cells is restricted to certain compartments of the skin.

INTRODUCTION

Proliferative activity is an important biologic parameter of neoplastic tissue. A variety of different methods are available to determine the growth fraction in a given tumor. Some of

Basic Mechanisms of Physiologic and Aberrant Lymphoproliferation in the Skin
Edited by W.C. Lambert *et al.*, Plenum Press, New York, 1994

317

these, such as flow cytometry, require the desintegration of tumor tissue to obtain single cell suspensions. For others, such as incorporation of radiolabelled thymidine, the tissue under investigation must be processed in a way that is not amenable to routine application. Alternatively, expression of certain nuclear antigens correlates well with the proliferative state of cells in situ and these antigens can be demonstrated immunohistochemically by appropriate antibodies (Tan, 1982). These should work, with reproducable staining properties, under routine laboratory conditions.

Such qualities have been demonstrated for the antibody, Ki-67, in a number of immunohistochemical studies (Gerdes et al., 1984; Ralfkiaer et al., 1986). Ki-67 is directed against a human nuclear antigen present in both normal and malignant proliferating cells. This antigen is expressed in G_1, S, G_2, and mitosis but not in G_0 (Gerdes et al., 1984). The number of Ki-67 positive cells determined immunohistochemically on cryostat sections has been demonstrated to correlate well with histological grading of malignancy. Individual values within histologically defined tumor grades have shown a wide variation, however (Vollmer et al., 1986; Lelle et al., 1987; Kaudewitz et al., 1989). Thus, assessment of Ki-67 positive cells might help to establish a refined prognosis in individual cases.

A positive correlation of Ki-67 determined growth fraction and grade of malignancy has also been demonstrated for nodal non-Hodgkin lymphomas (Gerdes et al., 1987). In cutaneous lymphomas, especially in those that cannot be regarded as mere equivalents of nodal lymphomas, such studies are lacking. Among primary cutaneous lymphomas, mycosis fungoides is the most important entity, with a wide variety of clinical and histological presentations. We therefore investigated the possible correlation of the Ki-67 determined growth fraction in a given skin infiltrate with TNM stage, type of skin lesion (patch, plaque, or tumor) and predominant cytomorphological type of infiltrating cells. Immunohistochemical demonstration of Ki-67-positive cells in situ also allows one to address the question of whether their distribution follows any discernible pattern. It has been hypothesized that atypical T cells in the skin in mycosis fungoides proliferate in response to external stimuli provided by the local microenvironment. Distinct compartments, particularly the epidermis, have been attributed to produce such mediators, whereas it has been suggested that the dermis is inactive in this respect (Nickoloff et al., 1990). Identification of the distribution pattern of proliferating cells should clarify the question of whether localization of infiltrating cells within any distinct compartment of the skin is associated with different proliferative activity.

MATERIALS AND METHODS

Skin biopsies from 44 patients (TNM stage Ia and Ib: n = 11; IIa and IIb: n = 16; IV: n = 17) were investigated. The type of skin lesion available for investigation was classified as patch in 19 patients, plaque in 16 and tumor in 9 patients. The predominant cytomorphological cell types were grouped into small cell (i.e., size of a normal lymphocyte), seen in 20 patients, small to medium sized (i.e., up to twice the size of a normal lymphocyte), seen in 14 patients, and medium to large cell (i.e., more than two times the size of a normal lymphocyte) in 10 patients. The infiltrating cells were attributed to one of these categories according to the predominant cell type (i.e. more than 50% of atypical cells) assessed on hematoxylin and eosin stained paraffin sections. Cryostat sections were stained with Ki-67 using the alkaline phosphatase-anti-alkaline phosphatase (APAAP) method as described previously (Kaudewitz et al., 1989). The number of Ki-67 positive cells was calculated as the percentage of positive cells after counting 500 mononuclear infiltrating cells. Statistical analyses were performed using the two-tailed Student t test.

RESULTS

The results are given in Table 1 (TNM stage), Table 2 (type of infiltrate), and Table 3 (cell type). No statistically significant difference in the number of Ki-67 positive cells could be detected between patch and plaque lesions or between TNM stages I and II. The number of proliferating cells was significantly lower in patch and plaque lesions when compared to tumorous infiltrates, however, and in lesions in TNM stage I or II when compared to those in stage IV. When small cell infiltrates were assessed in comparison to medium and large cell infiltrates, all three cytologic types differed significantly in the number of Ki-67-positive cells.

Within the different categories investigated, the individual values for Ki-67 positive cells varied considerably. In patients where multiple biopsies were available, the proliferative activity differed according to the morphologic and histologic type of the lesion, but was approximately the same in morphologically and histologically similar lesions. The number of biopsies from such patients was too small, however, to obtain Ki-67 values for statistical analysis.

No obvious compartimentalization of Ki-67-positive cells could be observed. When intraepidermal T cells were present in larger amounts their growth fraction was equal to that of dermal infiltrating cells (Figure 1). Proliferating cells did not localize preferentially within the epidermis, but rather in all cases were also detectable in the dermal compartment (Figure 2). On the other hand, large numbers of Ki-67-negative mononuclear cells, clearly distinguishable from keratinocytes, were observed in the epidermis (Figure 3). Loss of epidermotropism, with proliferative activity restricted to the dermal compartment, was seen in advanced stages (Figure 4).

DISCUSSION

Assessment of proliferation activity in mycosis fungoides does not reveal preferential localization within the various compartments of the skin. Our observations do not support the hypothesis that only distinct compartments of the skin produce a special lymphokine profile to

Table 1. Percentage of Ki-67 positive cells, correlation with TNM stage.

TNM stage	Ia,Ib	IIa,IIb	IV
Number of biopsies	11	16	16
Mean	8.3	8.5	21.7
S.D.	8.0	6.6	13.4
S.E.M.	2.4	1.7	3.2

Statistical Analyses:

Ia, Ib vs. IIa, IIb	n.s.
Ia, Ib vs. IV	$p < 0.0005$
IIa, IIb vs. IV	$p < 0.0005$

Table 2. Percentage of Ki-67 positive cells, correlation with type of infiltrate.

Type of infiltrate	Patch	Plaque	Tumor
Number of biopsies	19	16	8
Mean	7.4	12.7	28.2
S.D.	6.2	7.7	14.7
S.E.M.	1.4	1.9	4.9

Statistical Analyses:

Patch vs. Plaque	n.s.
Patch vs. Tumor	$p < 0.0001$
Plaque vs. Tumor	$p < 0.0001$

induce proliferation of infiltrating cells.

The only reported type of cutaneous T cell lymphoma with almost exclusive intraepidermal localization of Ki-67-positive cells is pagetoid reticulosis (Kaudewitz et al., 1987; Wood et al., 1988). In this rare condition, however, atypical cells are virtually absent in the dermis and thus proliferative activity of such cells cannot be expected within the dermal compartment.

In situ assessment of proliferating cells in mycosis fungoides, as performed in the present study, cannot distiguish between normal and malignant proliferating T cells. At present, no

Table 3. Percentage of Ki-67 positive cells, correlation with the predominant infiltrating cell type.

Cytologic findings (Cell Size)	Small	Small/medium	Medium/large
Number of biopsies	20	14	10
Mean	5.6	13.3	30
S.D.	2.2	8.3	10.8
S.E.M.	0.5	2.2	3.4

Statistical Analyses:

Small vs. Small/medium	$p < 0.0001$
Small vs. Medium/large	$p < 0.0001$
Small/medium vs. Medium/large	$p < 0.0001$

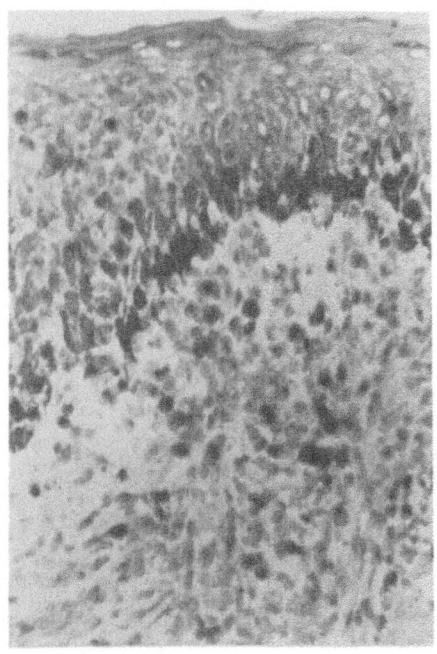

Figure 1. Both dermal and intraepidermal proliferation of infiltrating cells, demonstrated by positive staining with antibody Ki-67.

reliable method is available to perform such a distinction in situ. Even histomorphologic assessment, especially in the initial stages, fails in this respect. On the other hand, proliferative activity of other cellular components of the infiltrate does not interfere with that of infiltrating T cells. It has been shown that monocytic cells do not proliferate within the dermis.

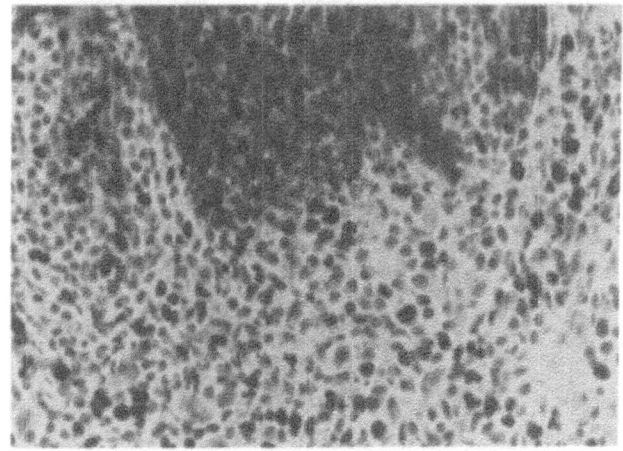

Figure 2. Considerable proliferative activity of dermal infiltrating cells.

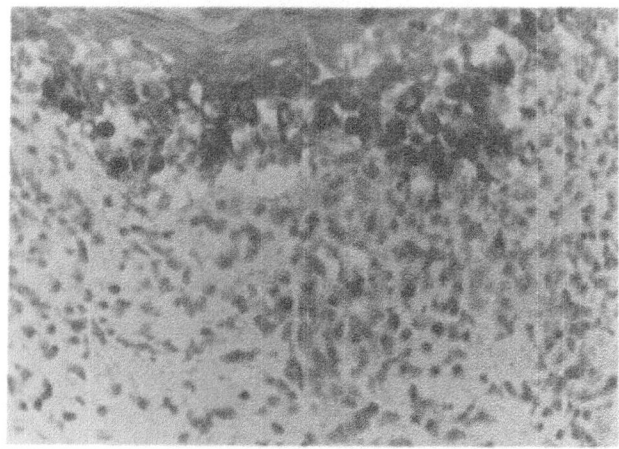

Figure 3. Large numbers of Ki-67-negative intraepidermal T cells with occasional Ki-67-positive dermal T cells.

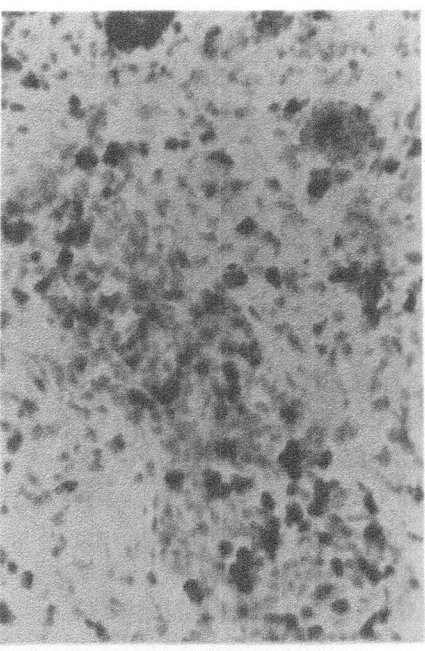

Figure 4. High proliferative activity of dermal infiltrating cells in advanced stage of mycosis fungoides.

As in other neoplasms, the number of Ki-67 positive cells in mycosis fungoides correlates with the clinical and morphologic grade of malignancy. It is possible that the wide variation of individual values observed within a given stage or type of lesion may be used to identify patients with a risk for rapid progression. The present study does not allow conclusions about the prognostic value of Ki-67 determined growth fraction when assessed as an independent parameter, however. Only larger series of biopsies, studied in conjunction with clinical course, can address this question. At present, observations in other types of cutaneous T cell lymphoproliferative disorders, such as lymphomatoid papulosis (Kaudewitz et al., 1985), with an extremely high growth fraction of atypical cells and a clinically benign course, warrant caution in concluding that proliferative activity is directly equivalent to malignant potential.

REFERENCES

Gerdes J, F Dallenbach and K Lennert, 1984, Growth fractions of malignant Non-Hodgkin Lymphomas (NHL) as determined in situ with the monoclonal antibody Ki-67. **Hematol. Oncol.**, 2:365.

Gerdes J, H Lemke, H Baisch, HH Wacker, U Schwab and H Stein, 1984. Cell cycle analysis of a cell proliferation associated human nuclear antigen defined by the monoclonal antibody Ki-67. **J. Immunol.**, 1333:1710.

Gerdes J, H Stein, S Pileri, MT Rivano, M Gobbi, E Ralfkiaer, KM Nielsen, G Pallesen, H Bartels, G Palestro and G Delsol, 1987. Prognostic relevance of tumor cell growth fraction in malignant non-Hodgkin's lymphomas. **Lancet** ii:448.

Kaudewitz P, H Stein, G Burg, DY Mason and O Braun-Falco, 1985. Atypical cells in lymphomatoid papulosis express the Hodgkin cell associated antigen Ki-1. **J. Invest. Dermatol.**, 86:350.

Kaudewitz P, G Burg, G Majiewski, J Gerdes, R Schwarting and O Braun-Falco, 1987. Cell populations in pagetoid reticulosis: An immunological study using cell activation associated monoclonal antibodies. **Acta. Derm. Venereol.**, 67:24.

Kaudewitz P, O Braun-Falco, M Ernst, M Landthaler, W Stolz, and J Gerdes, 1989. Tumor cell growth fractions in human malignant melanomas and the correlation to histopathologic tumor grading. **Am. J. Pathol.**, 134:1063.

Kaudewitz P, H Stein, F Dallenbach, F Eckert K Bieber, G Burg and O Braun-Falco, 1989. Primary and secondary cutaneous Ki-1+ (CD30+) anaplastic large cell lymphomas. **Am. J. Pathol.**, 135:359.

Lelle RJ, W Heidenreich, G Stauch and J Gerdes, 1987. The correlation of growth fraction with histologic grading and lymph node status in human mammary carcinoma. **Cancer**, 59:83.

Nickoloff BJ and EM Griffiths, 1990. Intraepidermal but not dermal T lymphocytes are positive for a cell cycle-associated antigen (Ki-67) in mycosis fungoides. **Am. J. Pathol.**, 136:261.

Ralfkiaer E, H Stein, J Bosq, KC Gatter, N Ralfkiaer, GL Wantzin and D.Y. Mason, 1986. Expression of a cell cycle associated nuclear antigen (Ki-67) in cutaneous lymphoid infiltrates. **Am. J. Dermatopathol.**, 8:37.

Tan EM, 1982. Autoantibodies to nuclear antigens (ANA). Their immunobiology and medicine. **Adv. Immunol.**, 33:167.

Vollmer E, A Roessner, J Gerdes, W Mellin, H Stein, S Chong-Schachel and E. Grundmann, 1986. Improved grading of bone marrow tumors with the monoclonal antibody Ki-67. **Cancer Res. Clin. Oncol.**, 112:281.

Wood GS, ML Weiss, CH Hu, E Abel, RT Hoppe, RA Warnke and J. Sklar, 1988. T cell antigen deficiencies and clonal rearrangements of T cell receptor genes in pagetoid reticulosis (Woringer-Kolopp disease). **N. Engl. J. Med.**, 318:164.

ERYTHRODERMIC ACTINIC RETICULOID

J. Toonstra*
A.H. Preesman*
S.C.J. van der Putte†
W.A. van Vloten*

* Department of Dermatology
† Department of Pathology
  University Hospital
  Utrecht, The Netherlands

Correspondence to: Dr. J. Toonstra or Dr. W. A. van Vloten,
Department of Dermatology, University Hospital, Heidelberglaan 100,
3584 CX Utrecht, The Netherlands

INTRODUCTION

Actinic reticuloid (AR) is a severe photodermatosis occurring in elderly male patients. It is part of the spectrum of chronic actinic dermatitis (CAD) (Norris and Hawk, 1990). A diagnosis of AR should only be made when all the following three criteria are present: (i) either persistently infiltrated skin on light-exposed areas or generalized erythroderma; (ii) photosensitivity to a wide range of wavelengths, including UV-B, UV-A and part of the visible spectrum; and (iii) on histologic examination, a dermal infiltrate with presence of atypical lymphocytes.

Erythroderma is not rare in AR. In the original series of ten patients described by Ive et al., at least six had episodes of erythroderma (Ive et al., 1969). Literature on erythrodermic AR, however, is very scarce. In particular, its resemblance to the Sézary syndrome (SS), an erythrodermic variant of cutaneous T-cell lymphoma (CTCL), has led to different opinions, such as: AR with Sézary cells (Neild et al, 1982), AR with progression into SS (Zugermann et al., 1980) and use of the term SS for erythrodermic forms of both CTCL and CAD (Chu et al., 1986).

Basic Mechanisms of Physiologic and Aberrant Lymphoproliferation in the Skin
Edited by W.C. Lambert *et al.*, Plenum Press, New York, 1994

325

In this chapter we present the clinical and histopathological data of ten patients with erythrodermic AR who were studied in our department.

CLINICAL FEATURES

All patients were elderly or middle-aged men with a generalized erythroderma. In several patients skin infiltration was more accentuated on exposed areas such as the face and dorsal parts of the hands. Loss of scalp hair as well as palmoplantar hyperkeratosis and onychodystrophy could be observed, especially in those patients with long-lasting erythroderma. In one patient large, bizarre patches of hyperpigmentation were present on both the trunk and arms and legs. (Figure 1a,b).

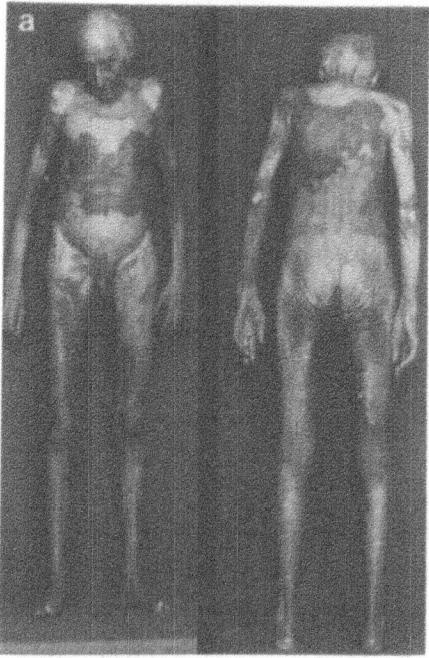 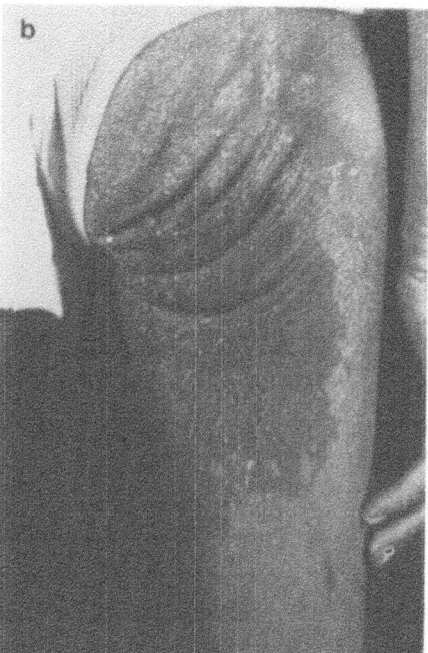

Figure 1. (a) Bizarre patches of hyperpigmentation on trunk and extremities in erythrodermic actinic reticuloid. (b) Close-up of superior aspect of right leg.

The duration of the erythroderma varied from 7 months to 6 years. Seasonal fluctuations were usually absent. Several patients had a marked erythroderma which was equally severe in summer and winter.

The range of photosensitivity is summarized in Table 1.

Table 1. Clinical and laboratory findings in 10 patients with erythrodermic actinic reticuloid.

Patient/ Sex	Age at time of diagnosis	Duration of erythroderma prior to diagnosis	Range of photosensitivity	CD4/CD8 ratio skin lymphocytes	CD4/CD8 ratio blood lymphocytes[1]	mean NCI blood[¶¶]	% cells with NCI> 6.5
1/M	52	2 years	UVB,UVA, violet/blue	>1	3	5.0	11
2/M	49	7 months	UVB,UVA, violet/blue green, orange/red	<1	0.3	6.5	48
3/M	80	6 years	UVB,UVA*	ND	2.6	5.3	21
4/M	62	1 year	UVB,UVA, violet/blue	<1	1.7	5.2	14
5/M	63	4 years	UVB,UVA*	<1	0.6	6.0	30
6/M	68	6 years	UVB**	<1	ND	5.9	30
7/M	53	10 months	UVB,UVA, violet/blue green	<1	1	5.0	12
8/M	75	1 year	UVB,UVA, violet/blue green	<1	1	5.7	25
9/M	63	2 years	UVB,UVA, violet/blue	<1	1	5.8	25
10/M	69	2 years	UVB,UVA, violet/blue green, orange/red	<1	0.5	6.3	46

[1] Normal values CD4/CD8 ratio in blood: 1.1-2.5
[¶¶] Mean value of Nuclear Contour Index (= P/√a, minimal value 3.54)
* Not possible to test the wavelengths of the visible light separately
** Sensitive for combination of UV-A plus visible light

LIGHT MICROSCOPY

Biopsies from lesional skin on exposed areas showed acanthosis, focal parakeratosis and no or only slight spongiosis. Exocytosis of lymphocytes was a common finding, sometimes leading to Pautrier-like microabcesses, mimicking mycosis fungoides (Figure 2). Dense dermal infiltrates of lymphocytes and histiocytes, sometimes extending into the subcutaneous fat, were present in the majority of patients. In a few patients a band-like infiltrate in the upper dermis could be observed.

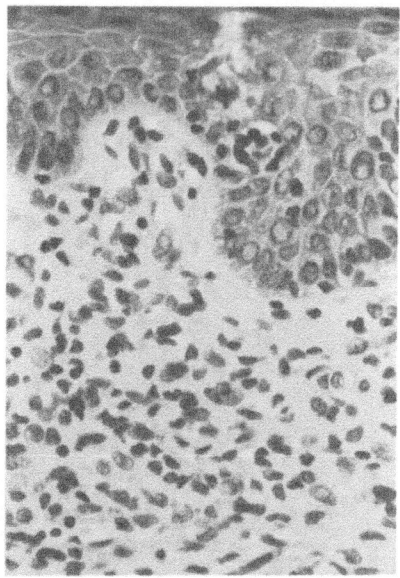

Figure 2. Detail of dermal infiltrate in actinic reticuloid, showing Pautrier-like microabscesses.

The infiltrate consisted mainly of lymphocytes with increased nuclear indentation in combination with varying numbers of plasma cells and eosinophils in most cases. The upper dermis revealed fibrosis with, characteristically, many stellate multinucleated fibroblasts (dendrocytes) in most patients.

Peripheral blood lymphocytes with increased nuclear indentation were found in all patients (Table 1) but counts were high in patients with a broad spectrum of photosensitivity.

ELECTRON MICROSCOPY

The cerebriform mononuclear cells (CMC), both in the dermal infiltrates and in isolated peripheral blood lymphocytes, were better demonstrated in semithin and ultrathin sections (Figure 3).

Lymphoid cells with a nuclear contour index (NCI; defined as perimeter/√area of the nucleus) of more than 6.5 were present in all patients with mean values between 11% and 48% (Table 1).

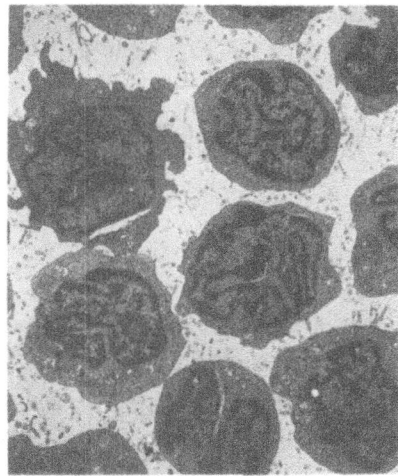

Figure 3. Isolated blood lymphocytes with increased nuclear indentation.

IMMUNOHISTOLOGY

In all patients the dermal infiltrates showed a predominance of T-cells with only sporadic B-cells. Remarkable was the fact that in nearly all patients the majority of the infiltrate expressed a suppressor phenotype (Table 1). The highest numbers of CD8$^+$ cells were observed in patients with long lasting erythroderma and severe photosensitivity, with values up to 90%. This remained a rather constant finding during the follow-up period. Even after several weeks of hospitalization in a darkened room a reversed CD4/CD8 ratio was still present.

CD1$^+$ cells were reduced in number in the epidermis and were present in small or large clusters in the upper dermis. Large numbers of histiocytes/macrophages (CD6$^+$) were present in small or large clusters in the upper and mid-dermis.

A conspicuous finding in several patients was the presence of IgE$^+$ dendritic cells within the infiltrates, roughly correlating with elevated serum IgE titers.

Peripheral blood lymphocytes also showed a predominance of suppressor (CD8$^+$) cells in many patients, although less often than in the skin (Table 1). The highest counts were again found in the most sensitive patients. With improvement of the clinical picture there was a tendency to normalization of the CD4/CD8 ratio.

COURSE AND PROGNOSIS

AR usually runs a chronic course. However, with appropiate therapy the erythrodermic state is reversible. Although the term "reticuloid" suggests a resemblance to malignant lymphoma, no clear progression to malignancy has been reported to date. A few patients have been reported with a malignant lymphoma but in our opinion these are only coincidental (Jenson and Sneddon, 1970; Thomson, 1977; Perrot et al., 1978; Frain-Bell, 1982).

One of the patients described here died of myeloid leukemia, but again this seemed to be only coincidental.

THERAPY

Avoidance of exposure to light and confinement to a darkened room gives improvement, but also leads to a severe rebound reaction after re-exposure to light. Proven contact allergens must be avoided. Effective treatment modalities are PUVA therapy (Hindson, et a;l., 1985) or tolerance induction therapy with UVB (Toonstra, et al., 1989). Azathioprine, often in combination with prednisone, has proven to be effective in several patients (Leigh and Hawk, 1984). Recently, cyclosporin has been reported to give excellent results (Toonstra et al., 1989; Norris et al., 1989). In two of our patients a rapid and complete clearance of the skin could be observed in a relatively short period of time with cyclosporine in a dosage of 3 mg/kg/day.

DISCUSSION

Erythroderma is not rare in actinic reticuloid (AR). In particular, its clinical and histopathological resemblance to Sézary syndrome (SW) has led to confusing opinions (Neild et al., 1982; Zugermann et al., 1980; Chu et al., 1986). Of importance in discriminating between these disorders, the dermal infiltrate in AR almost always has a $CD8^+$ predominance whereas SS is a $CD4^+$ lymphoma (Broder et al., 1976). AR is often associated with a reversed $CD4^+/CD8^+$ ratio of peripheral blood lymphocytes. Therefore, in erythrodermic patients who cannot be photo(patch) tested, a reversed $CD4^+/CD8^+$ ratio in the blood is highly suggestive for a diagnosis of AR.

Circulating blood lymphocytes with increased nuclear indentation can be found in both AR and SS. These cells are not specific for these diseases, but can rather be found in a variety of benign conditions, although in low concentrations (Duncan and Winkelmann, 1978). Numbers higher than 20% have been reported as a reliable criterion for a diagnosis of SS (Willemze et al., 1983). Seven of the patients described here had numbers higher than 20% (Table 1), thus showing an overlap with SS. Similar results were reported by Chu et al (4-70% Sézary cells; Chu et al., 1986) and Haynes et al (26% Sézary cells; Haynes et al., 1984).

In one of the patients in our series, large bizarre-shaped areas of hyperpigmentation were observed. Ive et al., (1990) also reported an erythrodermic AR patient with irregularly shaped, densely pigmented patches on the trunk (Ive et al., 1969). Recently, widespread vitiliginous depigmentation has been reported in two patients with AR (Von den Driesch et al., 1992). These authors suggested that the CD8$^+$ epidermotropic lymphocytes are responsible for cytotoxic destruction of melanocytes, leading in turn to depigmentation. Hypopigmented areas in AR have also been reported by others (Haynes et al., 1984; Galosi et al., 1982; Kaidbey and Messenger, 1984).

In conclusion, erythrodermic variants of AR should not be confused with SS; they are totally different entities. Immunohistochemical analysis of a skin biopsy or of peripheral blood lymphocytes in erythrodermic patients can provide important clues for a definitive diagnosis, allowing appropriate therapy to be started as soon as possible.

REFERENCES

Broder S, RL Edelson, MA Lutzner et al., 1976. The Sézary syndrome. A malignant proliferation of helper T-cells. **J. Clin. Invest.**, 58:1297-1306.

Chu AC, D Robinson, JLM Hawk et al., 1986. Immunologic differentiation of the Séary syndrome due to cutaneous T-cell lymphoma and chronic actinic dermatitis. **J. Invest Dermatol.**, 86:134-137.

Duncan SC and RK Winkelmann, 1978. Circulating Sézary cells in hospitalized dermatology patients. **Br. J. Dermatol.**, 99:171-178.

Frain-Bell W, 1982. Photosensitivity dermatitis and actinic reticuloid. **Semin. Dermatol.**, 1:161-168.

Galosi A, E Hölzle, G Plewig et al., 1982. PUVA-Therapie bei chronisch-persistierenden Lichtreaktion. **Hautarzt**, 33:657-661.

Haynes HA, JD Bernhard and RW Gange, 1984. Actinic reticuloid: Response to combination treatment with azathioprine, hydroxychloroquine, and prednisone. **J. Am. Acad. Dermatol.**, 10:947-952.

Hindson C, J Spiro and A Downey, 1985. PUVA-therapy of chronic actinic dermatitis. **Br. J. Dermatol.**, 113:157-160.

Ive FA, IA Magnus, RP Warin et al., 1990. "Actinic reticuloid"; A chronic dermatosis associated with severe photosensitivity and the histological resemblance to lymphoma. **Br. J. Dermatol.**, 81:469-485.

Jensen NE and IB Sneddon, 1970. Actinic reticuloid with lymphoma. **Br. J. Dermatol.**, 82:287-291.

Kaidbey KM and JL Messenger, 1984. The clinical spectrum of the persistent light reactor. **Arch. Dermatol.**, 120:1441-1448.

Leigh IM and JLM Hawk, 1984. Treatment of chronic actinic dermatitis with azathioprine. **Br. J. Dermatol.**, 110:691-695.

Neild VS, JLM Hawk, RAJ Eady et al., 1982. Actinic reticuloid with Sézary cells. **Clin. Exp. Dermatol.**, 7:143-148.

Norris DG, RDR Camp and JLM Hawk, 1989. Actinic reticuloid: Response to cyclosporine. **J. Am. Acad. Dermatol.**, 21:307-308.

Norris PG and JLM Hawk, 1990. Chronic actinic dermatitis. A unifying concept. **Arch. Dermatol.**, 126:376-378.

Perrot H, M Frionnet, C Frances et al., 1978. Sarcome ganglionaire généralisé au cours de l'évolution d'une actino-réticulose. **Ann. Dermatol. Venereol.**, 105:33-34.

Thomsen K, 1977. The development of Hodgkin's disease in a patient with actinic reticuloid. **Clin. Exp. Dermatol.**, 2:109-113.

Toonstra J, CJM Henquet, H van Weelden et al., 1989. Actinic reticuloid. A clinical, photo biologic, histopathologic and follow-up study of 16 patients. **J. Am. Acad. Dermatol.**, 21:205-214.

Von den Driesch P, M Fartasch and OP Hornstein, 1992. Chronic actinic dermatitis with vitiligo-like depigmentation. **Clin. Exp. Dermatol.**, 17:38-43.

Willemze R, CB de Graaf-Reitsma, J Cnossen et al., 1983. Characterization of T-cell sub populations in skin and peripheral blood of patients with cutaneous T-cell lymphomas and benign inflammatory dermatoses. **J. Invest. Dermatol.**, 80:60-66.

Zugermann C, D Beeaff and HH Roenigk, Jr., 1980. Photosensitivity and Sézary syndrome. **Cutis**, 25:495-499.

MORPHOMETRIC STUDY OF PRIMARY CUTANEOUS GERMINAL CENTER CELL LYMPHOMAS

Raffaele Gianotti*
Carlo Montaperto†

* First Department of Dermatology
IRCCS
Ospedale Maggiore
University of Milan
Milan, Italy

† First Institute of Pathology
University of Milan
Milan, Italy

Correspondence to: Dr. R. Gianotti, Department of Dermatology I,
University of Milan, Via Pace 9,
I-20122 Milan, Italy

ABSTRACT

The mixed small and large cell type of non-Hodgkin lymphoma (NHL) of the lymph node is associated with the most extreme degree of histological interobserver non-reproducibility. Histopathological examination of primary cutaneous germinal center cell (PCGCC) lymphomas of mixed cell subtype points out these difficulties. In order to morphometrically characterize PCGCC lymphomas, we have employed an image analyzer IBAS 2000 (Zeiss Kontron) to study seventeen centroblastic/centrocytic and centroblastic follicular and/or diffuse primary cutaneous lymphomas. The data obtained reveal morphometric differences in neoplastic cells between the follicular and diffuse patterns. In the follicular neoplasms, the cells tend to be smaller, more cleaved and more monomorphic than those observed in the diffuse forms. In all the follicular

Basic Mechanisms of Physiologic and Aberrant Lymphoproliferation in the Skin
Edited by W.C. Lambert *et al.*, Plenum Press, New York, 1994

333

and diffuse cases examined, we have observed a unimodal population, indicating the absence of a clear-cut differentiation between centroblasts and centrocytes. Furthermore, the presence of a consistent broad intermediate population means that there is a continuum of area size and nuclear profile between centrocytes and centroblasts.

INTRODUCTION

Among the groups of primary cutaneous lymphomas originating from the germinal center are the B-cell neoplasms that more commonly affect the skin. In most PCGCC lymphomas, cytological features show a mixed population of cells varying in size from small elements with an indented nucleus to larger ones, some of which have a multilobulated vesicular nucleus, others a round nucleus with multiple nucleoli.

As has been reported for NHL of mixed small and large cell type of the lymph node (Metter et al., 1985), estimation of the proportion of lymphoid cells in the mixed cell subtype of NHL proves difficult. This is probably due to the inability of the human eye to assess small, but significant differences in size and configuration of lymphocytic nuclei (Metter et al., 1985; Hall et al., 1985). These difficulties are greater in the histopathological evaluation of primary cutaneous germinal center lymphomas. The centroblasts may show multilobulation and elongation of the nucleus (banana shape), making a quantification of the various cellular subtypes and clear cut differentiation from cleaved cells difficult. This has caused a number of problems for dermatopathologists and pathologists in applying both the Working Formulation (The NHL Pathology Project, 1982) and the Kiel classification (Gerard-Marchand et al., 1974), created for lymph node neoplasms, to PCGCC lymphomas. In fact, some authors (Willemze et al., 1987) have suggested that one should classify the cutaneous form as a germinal center cell lymphoma, without specifying the cytotype.

The aim of our study was to identify the cell populations in PCGCC lymphomas employing morphometric analysis in order to evaluate whether it is possible to differentiate the neoplastic cell type by quantifying the various subsets.

MATERIALS AND METHODS

Materials

Seventeen biopsy specimens of PCGCC lymphomas obtained from fifteen patients were examined. All the biopsy specimens had been histologically classified as centroblastic/centrocytic lymphomas or centroblastic lymphomas of follicular and/or diffuse subtype prior to entry into the study. Immunological techniques had also been employed to demonstrate the B-cell phenotype in all cases; gene rearrangement analysis had been used in 11 cases to confirm the B-cell clonal population (Berti et al., 1988; Delia et al., 1989).

Morphometric analysis was performed using the following instruments: an image analyzer IBAS 2000 (Zeiss Kontron, Munich, West Germany), an automated Zeiss microscope, an A/D device interfaced for automatic focusing and movement of the stage, a controller for monochromatic device MPC64 (Zeiss Kontron, West Germany) and a Panasonic camera VW-50 CCD (Panasonic, Japan) to convert the microscopic image for digitalization and analysis.

Methods

Biopsy specimens fixed in Bouin's solution and embedded in paraffin were sectioned and stained with the Feulgen-Coleman reaction. In order to morphometrically characterize the PCGCC lymphomas, we considered the area, the perimeter and the form factor of nuclei of the neoplastic cells. The form factor (Form PE) (Ricco et al., 1989) is a numeric value to indicate the tendency to circularity of the measured object. This is obtained by the following formula: $4 \times 3.1415 \times area/perimeter^2$. The form factor value shows a range between 0 and 1.0 (Form PE=1 for a circle and <1 for elliptical and irregular structures.) To obtain a threshold to differentiate morphometrically the centroblasts from the centrocytes, a case of primary cutaneous centroblastic lymphoma (18th control case) and a case of primary cutaneous centrocytic lymphoma (2nd control case) were examined with an oil immersion objective at 100x and monochromatic light of 540nm wavelength. The neoplastic areas and the cells were chosen by one of us (RG). The area and the perimeter of 100 centroblasts and 100 centrocytes were measured. The obtained parameters were analyzed by Student t-Test (STT), Wilcoxon test (WT) and the normal distribution of goodness fit (NDGF) by using a software package by Lotus (Lotus development Corporation, 1986), Microstat (Ecosoft Inc, 1984). On the basis of the means and standard deviations (SDs), we established that 93 cells for each examined specimen were representative at 95% confidence limits. This pilot study enabled us to establish the cut-off values of $25\mu^2$ for the area, 0.74 for the Form PE and 20.60μ for the perimeter between the two groups of cells. Among the three parameters so obtained, we decided to keep the $25\mu^2$ area as the cut-off parameter to discriminate the two populations of cells because the Form PE and the perimeter showed an overlap of values between the two pilot control cases (Figure 1).

The data of this pilot study enabled us to consider as centrocytes the cells under the cut-off of $25\mu^2$ and as centroblasts the ones above the cut-off.

In the second stage of our work, all the specimens were examined, randomly measuring 100 neoplastic cells for each specimen and choosing the follicular area for measurement in the follicular/diffuse lymphomas. The same technical procedure and statistical analysis used for the pilot study were employed.

RESULTS

We performed a statistical elaboration of the data for different patterns of growth and for single cases.

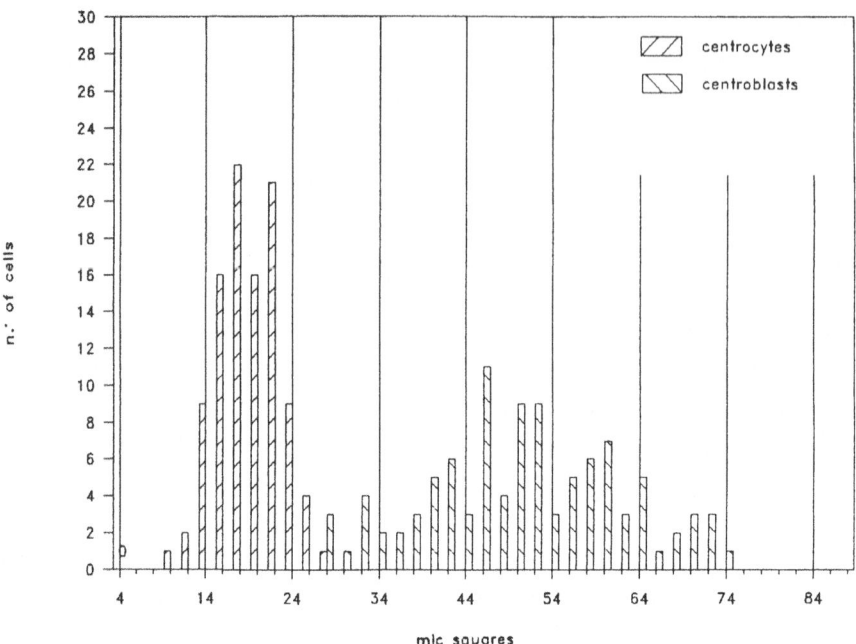

Figure 1. Pilot study: Frequency distribution of nuclear areas of centrocytes and centroblasts.

The follicular/diffuse lymphomas had a mean nuclear area of $26.48 \pm 7.03 \mu^2$, a nuclear perimeter of $23.59 \pm 3.20 \mu$, a form PE of 0.61 ± 0.08 and an average percentage below the cut-off value of $73\% \pm 7$ (Table 1). The diffuse lymphomas showed a mean nuclear area of $36.07 \pm 8.13 \mu^2$, a nuclear perimeter of $25.35 \pm 2.3 \mu$, a form PE of 0.71 ± 0.06 and a mean pecentage below the cut-off value of $40\% \pm 8\%$ (Table 1). Mean and standard deviation analysis of these values indicates significant differences in the cell populations in follicular and diffuse lymphomas. In the follicular group, the mean nuclear area varied from a minimum value of $22.98 \mu^2$ (Case 5) to a maximum value of $31.37 \mu^2$ (Case 6), which corresponds to a difference of 36% between the extremes (Figure 2). The nuclear perimeter showed a minor variability from 21.95μ (Case 5) to 24.86μ (Case 6), a difference of 13%. The Form PE varied from 0.65 (Cases 4,6 and 7) to 0.50 (Case 2), corresponding to a difference of 30%. This indicates that an increase in the perimeter is related to an increase in the area, as expected. The lowest percentage of cells below the cut-off limit observed in the follicular group was 61%.

In the diffuse lymphoma group, the mean nuclear area ranged from a minimum value of $25.45 \mu^2$ (Case 11) to a maximum of $46.40 \mu^2$ (Case 15) with a difference of 80% between them (Figure 3), the perimeter varied from $22.91 \mu^2$ (Case 11) to 27.21μ (Case 15) with a difference of 18%, while the Form PE ranged from 0.62 (Case 11) to 0.81 (Cases 15 and 9) with a difference corresponding to 33%. In this diffuse group, the highest percentage of cells below the cut-off was 64%. These data indicate that the highest degree of variability in diffuse

Table 1. Morphometric values of lymphocyte nuclei.

Follicular/diffuse lymphomas:

Case	Area		Perimeter		Form P.E.		Percentage
	Mean	S.D.	Mean	S.D.	Mean	S.D.	under cutoff
1	24.51	8.03	22.81	3.90	0.60	0.08	76
2	23.37	6.54	24.41	3.30	0.50	0.08	81
3	25.61	7.41	23.43	4.20	0.60	0.09	73
4	29.41	9.09	23.98	4.30	0.65	0.12	67
5	22.98	6.07	21.95	3.70	0.61	0.10	83
6	31.37	10.13	24.86	4.90	0.65	0.11	61
7	28.13	9.47	23.61	4.70	0.65	0.11	69
Mean	26.48	7.03	23.59	3.20	0.61	0.08	73

Diffuse lymphomas:

Case	Area		Perimeter		Form P.E.		Percentage
	Mean	S.D.	Mean	S.D.	Mean	S.D.	under cutoff
8	32.70	10.13	25.61	2.90	0.65	0.09	53
9	45.40	12.11	26.83	2.10	0.81	0.08	18
10	33.20	9.03	23.72	3.20	0.76	0.10	32
11	25.45	8.66	22.91	3.70	0.62	0.10	64
12	35.80	9.14	24.54	4.30	0.76	0.10	39
13	34.70	10.73	26.97	3.90	0.61	0.10	45
14	31.90	10.32	24.32	4.20	0.70	0.11	57
15	46.40	12.81	27.21	3.10	0.81	0.09	17
16	39.60	8.73	25.98	4.30	0.70	0.09	33
17	35.50	8.07	25.42	3.80	0.71	0.09	37
Mean	36.07	8.13	25.35	2.30	0.71	0.06	40

Statistical Analysis:

$t = 29.94$	$t = 13.19$	$t = 29.43$	$t = 5.38$
$p < 0.001$	$p < 0.001$	$p < 0.001$	$p > 0.05$

S.D., * Standard deviation; t, Student t-test score

lymphomas, compared with the follicular ones, is in their nuclear area, while the perimeter and the Form PE of the two types of lymphomas have the same variability. NDGF statistical analysis performed on the data obtained from the distribution of all values in each group showed that the populations were normal at confidence limits of 95%.

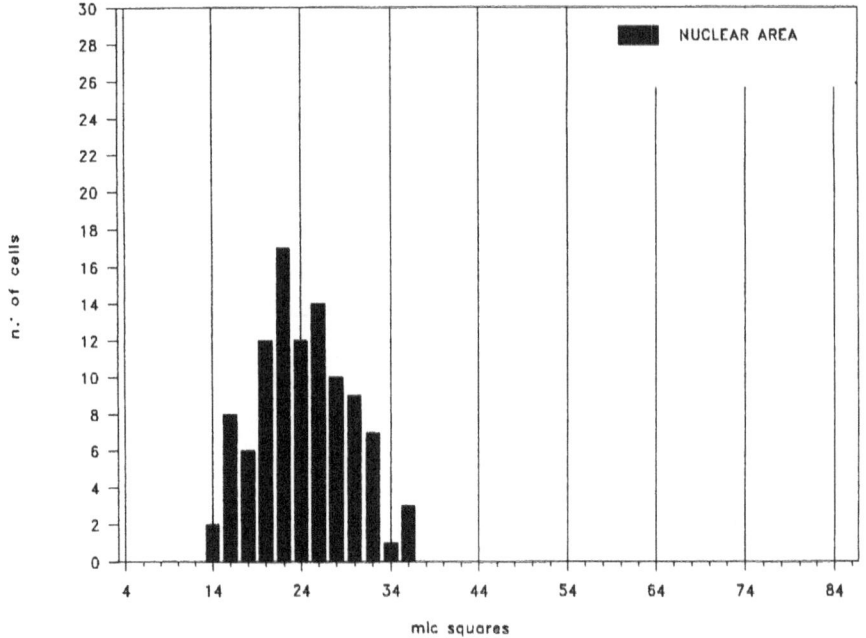

Figure 2. Frequency distribution of nuclear areas in a follicular case (#5).

The WT test, performed on all of the parameters, did not show a significant difference between any of the single groups (p > 0.05). On the other hand, the STT test performed between the follicular group and the diffuse group showed significant differences (p < 0.001) for area, perimeter and Form PE.

All the frequency histograms of the examined parameters (Area, Perimeter and Form PE) in the cases studied fit into a unimodal distribution.

Analysis of measurements in the distribution diagram of each examined specimen has shown the constant presence of a cell population in the neighborhood of the cut-off area. This was observed in each specimen independently, whether from the follicular or the diffuse histopathological pattern (Figures 4 and 5).

DISCUSSION

The rules for segregating cutaneous lymphomas of germinal center cell origin in any of the widely used classification of NHL have not been substantiated by experimental application. Metter et al. (1985) illustrated the variability and subjectivity of the criteria used by pathologists in deciding which lymphocytes are considered large and small or cleaved and non-cleaved.

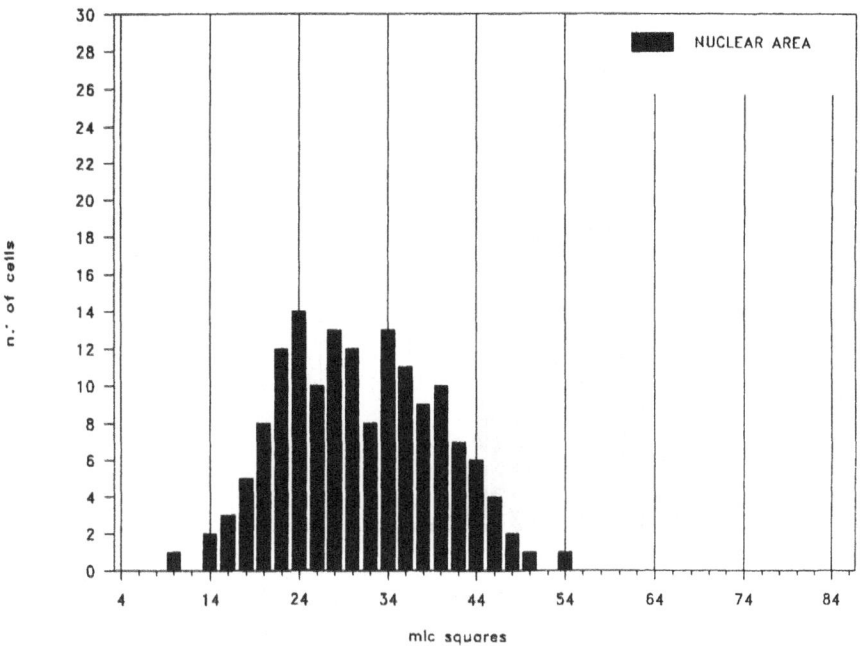

Figure 3. Frequency distribution of nuclear areas in a diffuse case (#8).

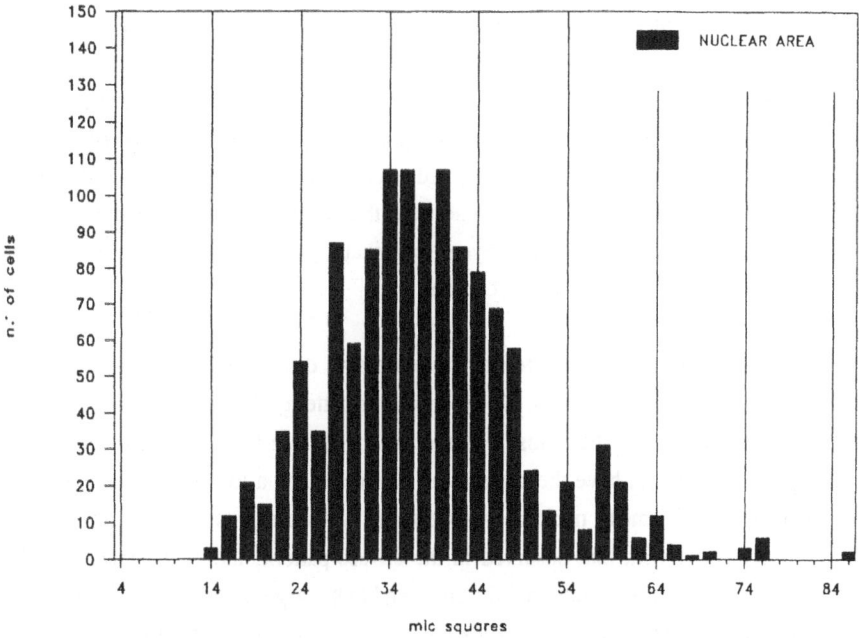

Figure 4. Frequency distribution of nuclear areas in all the diffuse cases.

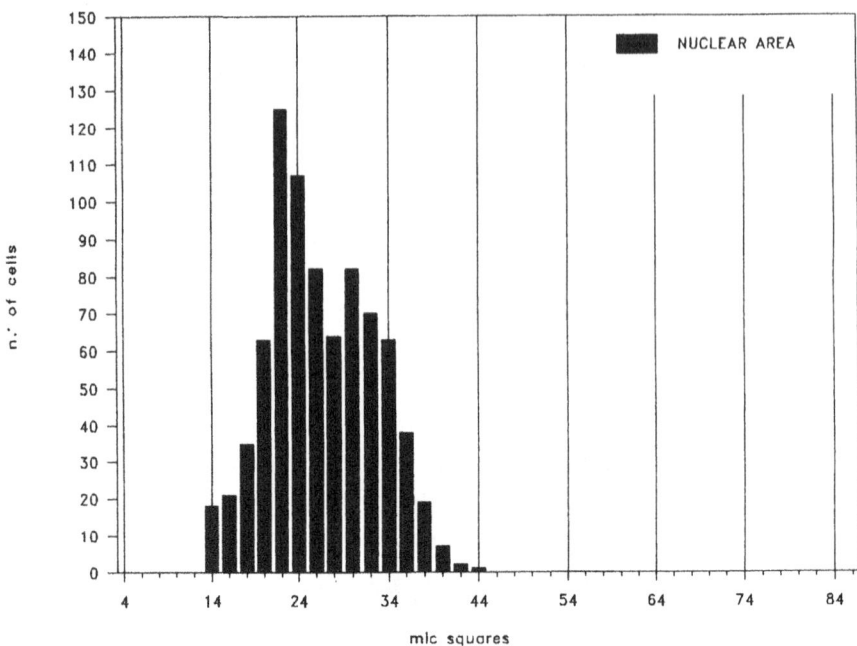

Figure 5. Frequency distribution of nuclear areas in all the follicular cases.

The range of 26% to 61% in interobserver reproducibility reported for mixed small and large cell types of NHL in the lymph nodes (Metter et al., 1985; Woodruff et al., 1981; Velez-Garcia et al., 1983) points up the difficulties of the human eye in assessing significant differences in size and configuration of lymphocyte nuclei when an evaluation of a single cell, and not a comparison, is required. In skin, the great variability of forms and indentations of the same kinds of cells probably depends on cutaneous homing that differs from that of the lymph node. In fact, it is significant to note the observed overlapping in the values of Form PE and perimeter, and not in the values of area, in choosing the centrocytes and centroblasts for the pilot study. This means that the observer's eye discriminated the two populations of cells more on the basis of size than on irregularity of contour.

The data obtained from our study reveal morphometric differences in the neoplastic cells between the two groups of proliferations. In the follicular pattern, all the proliferating cells tend to be smaller and more cleaved than those observed in the diffuse form. In fact, they have an inferior mean nuclear area but have the same mean perimeter and a lower value of mean Form PE. The increment of the mean nuclear area between the two extremes inside the follicular group is low if compared with that observed in the diffuse pattern, indicating marked cellular monomorphism. In the diffuse lymphoma, the cells tend to be larger and show a high variability of cellular area between the extremes, indicating a pleomorphism of the infiltrate. As the difference in the area (80% difference between the extremes) is not associated with a similar difference in the perimeter or by a decrease in the Form PE, we could expect a low percentage of cleaved cells in the lymphocyte population of the diffuse lymphoma.

Analyzing the data obtained in the two different patterns of proliferation, we predicted that we would find a high number of centrocytes in the more follicular lymphomas and a predominant population of centroblasts in the more diffuse areas. In reality, a variety of analyses of the morphometric data always indicated a unimodal population. This means that there is a continuum of area size and of nuclear profiles from round and irregular to complexly shaped. In fact, the consistent differences observed between the distribution diagrams of each examined specimen and those extrapolated from the pilot study indicate the presence of a wide cell population with intermediate morphometric features that cannot be properly labelled, and make a clear-cut morphometrical differentiation between centroblasts and centrocytes difficult. This does not mean that a certain percentage of nuclei in cutaneous germinal center cell lymphoma is not distinctly irregular in contour, deeply indented (cleaved) or large and round (centroblasts), especially in the diffuse monomorphic proliferation. These results underline the considerable overlap of lymphocyte nuclear parameters between the mean subtype of cells in cutaneous mixed small and large cell lymphomas. This might lead the pathologist to a misinterpretation in the quantification and differentiation of the cells due to the lack of a clear-cut distinction between centroblasts and centrocytes.

The complexity of lymphocyte populations in terms of nuclear size, form and chromatin organization suggest that the use of morphometric analysis in support of light microscopy should be recommended in the classification of NHL of mixed cell type.

REFERENCES

Berti E, E Alessi and R Caputo, 1988. Reticulohistiocytoma of the dorsum. **J. Am. Acad. Dermatol.**, 19:259.

Delia D, MG Borrello and E Berti, 1989. Clonal immunoglobulin gene rearrangements and normal T-cell receptor, bcl-2, and c-myc genes in primary cutaneous B-cell lymphomas. **Cancer Res.**, 49:4901.

Gerard-Marchand R, I Hamlin and K Lennert, 1974. Classification of non-Hodgkin's lymphomas. **Lancet**, 2:406.

Hall TL and YS Fu, 1985. Application of quantitative microscopy in tumor pathology. **Lab. Invest.**, 53:5.

Metter GE, BN Nathwani and JS Burke, 1985. Morphological subclassification of follicular lymphoma: Variability of diagnoses among hematopathologists: A collaborative study between the repository center and pathology panel for lymphoma clinical studies. **J. Clin. Oncol.**, 3:25.

Ricco R, G De Benedictis and T. Lettini T, 1989. Non-Hodgkin's lymphoma diagnosis aided by the S.A.M. system. **Path. Res. Pract.**, 185:719.

The Non-Hodgkin's lymphoma Pathologic Classification Project, 1987. National Cancer Institute sponsored study of classification of non-Hodgkin's lymphomas: Summary and description of a Working Formulation for clinical usage. **Cancer**, 49:2112.

Velez-Garcia E, J Durant and R Gams, 1983. Results of a uniform histopathologic review system of lymphoma cases. A ten-year study from the Southeastern Cancer Study Group. **Cancer**, 52:675.

Willemze R, CJLM Meijer and HJ Sentis, 1987. Primary cutaneous large cell lymphomas of follicular center cell origin. **J. Am. Acad. Dermatol.**, 16:518.

Woodruff RD, 1981. Reviewing histologic diagnosis of lymphoma: Comparison of original and review diagnoses in 269 cases. **Arch. Pathol. Lab. Med.**, 105:573.

BCL-2 GENE REARRANGEMENT AND PROTEIN EXPRESSION IN PRIMARY CUTANEOUS B CELL LYMPHOMAS

F. Pezzella*
M. Santucci†
A. Neri‡
D. Trecca‡
M. Jones*
E. Berti#

* Department of Hematology
  John Radcliffe Hospital
  Oxford, England

† Institute of Morbid Anatomy and Histopathology
  University of Florence
  Florence, Italy

‡ Institute of Medical Science
# First Department of Dermatology
  University of Milano
  Milan, Italy

Correspondence to: Dr. E. Berti, Department of Dermatology I,
University of Milan, Via Pase 9,
I-20122 Milan, Italy

ABSTRACT

Primary cutaneous B cell lymphomas (CBCLs) have been recently identified on the basis of their clinical, histological, phenotypic and genotypic features. CBCLs usually show a slow

Basic Mechanisms of Physiologic and Aberrant Lymphoproliferation in the Skin
Edited by W.C. Lambert *et al.*, Plenum Press, New York, 1994

343

progression with a benign evolution in most cases. Cytological features vary from small lymphocytic to large cell lymphomas. Phenotypic and genotypic data provide evidence for clonal proliferation of mature B lymphocytes. The aim of our study was to analyze the occurrences of bcl-2 gene rearrangement and protein expression in a large series of CBCLs, including many follicular lymphomas. Our results show that only 60% of the CBCLs are positive for bcl-2 protein. Interestingly enough, the small cell lymphomas were all strongly stained, whereas 60% of the large cell lymphomas were negative. Furthermore, only one of 20 follicular CBCLs analyzed showed bcl-2 rearrangement using probes for the major breakpoint region (pFL-1). The pattern of bcl-2 expression observed in primary cutaneous lymphomas, and the absence of bcl-2 gene rearrangement, suggest a similarity between these tumors and MALT B cell lymphomas.

INTRODUCTION

Within the group of extranodal non-Hodgkin lymphomas (NHL), the primary cutaneous low grade B-cell lymphomas represent a recently described pathological entity.

An unusual presentation of this condition was first described in 1951 by Crosti and colleagues (Berti et al., 1988), who thought it had a histiocytic origin. It was therefore called "reticulo-histiocytoma of the dorsum" or "Morbus Crosti" (Crosti disease). This clinical entity was then investigated by other groups, who demonstrated its B lymphocytic clonal origin and postulated that these lymphomas originate from B-follicles, on the ground that they are composed of medium and large sized cells of irregular shape, similar to those present in lymph node germinal centers (Berti et al., 1988; Pimpinelli et al., 1989; Willemze et al., 1987a; 1987b). Recently, two additional series have been reported, consisting of 50 and 60 primary cutaneous B-cell lymphomas, respectively, clearly showing an extreme variability in both clinical and cytological features (Berti et al., 1991; Santucci et al., 1991).

An interesting phenotypic result has been the negative or weak expression reported for the CALLA/CD10 antigen, which is characteristically only present in nodal follicular lymphomas, as well as irregular expression of antigens characteristic of the mantle zone cortex cells (Berti et al., 1991). In all cases investigated, molecular studies have shown rearrangement of heavy chain and/or light chain genes of immunoglobulins, but in none of the cases has rearrangement of the bcl-2 proto-oncogene, which occurs in the majority of nodal follicular lymphomas, been found (Delia et al., 1989). Other authers (Volkenand et al., 1992) have recently reported similar findings describing a series of 14 B cell cutaneous lymphomas in which only one had the 14;18 translocation. These two findings bring closer together cutaneous low grade B cell lymphomas and mucosa associated lymphoid tissue (MALT) B cell lymphomas. The latter were recently described and characterized; and it is now known that MALT lymphomas originate from mantle zone B cells (Isaacson et al., 1989).

The aims of the present study were to obtain a more complete picture of the bcl-2 proto-oncogene rearrangement, by investigating a greater number of cases, and to evaluate the expression of the bcl-2 protein, in a group of 66 patients affected by cutaneous low grade B cell lymphoma. A phenotypic characterization was carried out in all cases using paraffin sections and in 44 cases also using frozen tissue.

MATERIALS AND METHODS

Paraffin Embedded Tissue

Either formalin (35 cases) or Bouin (31 cases) fixed tissue sections, obtained from the files of the First Department of Dermatology, University of Milan, and the Institute of Morbid Anatomy and Histopathology, University of Florence, were stained with hematoxylin and eosin (H&E) and by immunohistochemical techniques.

Frozen Tissue

Specimens were frozen, immediately after biopsy, in Freon 22 which was cooled in liquid nitrogen, and stored at -80° C. In this way it was possible to study the complete immunophenotype of 44 cases of cutaneous low grade B cell lymphoma. Suitable DNA for Southern blotting was obtained in 20 of 44 cases.

Immunohistological Staining

Immunophenotyping was carried out with the antibodies described in Table 1. Bcl-2 expression was investigated by using anti bcl-2 monoclonal antibodies 100 and 124.

Immunohistological staining was performed on both formalin-fixed and cryostat sections using the alkaline-phosphatase-anti-alkaline phosphatase (APAAP) procedure as previously described (Cordell et al., 1984).

DNA Isolation and Genomic Southern Blot Analysis

High molecular weight DNA was extracted from the same lymphoma biopsies used for immunophenotypic analysis, a portion (20 μg) digested to completion with 3-5 units/μg of the appropriate restriction enzymes (BamHl, EcoRl, HindIII, Sacl or PstI; Biolabs, Beverly, MA, and Amity PG, Buckingham, UK), size-fractionated on 0.6-1.4% agarose gel by electrophoresis, transferred onto Gene Screen Plus filters (NEN, Boston, MA), and hybridized with the indicated DNA probes.

Table 1. Antibodies employed for immunophenotype definition.

On paraffin-embedded tissue	On cryostat sections
CD3	CD21
CD20 (L26)	CD22
CD45 Ra (F811-13)	DRC1
CD45 Ro (UCHL-1)	CD69
	KB61
	CD1c
	anti IgD
	Leu 8

Bcl-2 was analyzed with the 1.5 kilobase HindIII Eco RI insert from pFL1 detecting the major t(14;18) breakpoint cluster regions on chromosome 18.

RESULTS

A detailed presentation of our results is provided in Table 2.

Immunophenotype Characterization

Paraffin Embedded Tissue: In all cases, the immunophenotype was investigated on paraffin embedded material. The antibodies L26 (CD20) and F/811-13 (CD45RA) allowed localization of B-cell areas; This was particularly important in cases where there was a large number of infiltrating "reactive" T lymphocyte as shown by UCHL1 (CD45RO) and anti CD3 antibodies (since normal T lymphocytes are also positive for the presence of the bcl-2 protein).

Frozen Tissue: A total of 44 cases were investigated on cryostat sections. The antibody T015 (CD22) has shown a strong positive reaction in all cases examined. The anti CD21 (1F8) antibody stained 23 (52%) of the 44 cases studied. The anti-DRC-1 antibody demonstrated the presence of dendritic cells, such as those present in lymphoid follicles, in variable numbers, in 25 of 38 cases analyzed (65%). The anti-IgD antibody was found to give positivity in 13 of 34 (38%), the antibody KB61 in 10 of 31 (32%), and the anti-CD1c antibody (clone L161) in 9 of 26 (34%) cases examined. The antibody Leu-8 showed positive results in 18 of 36 cases (50%). These data demonstrate that the cutaneous B-cell lymphomas show a marked degree of phenotypic heterogeneity.

Table 2. Immunostaining for the bcl-2 protein and rearrangement of the bcl-2 gene in 44 cases of B cell cutaneous non-Hodgkin lymphoma.

Case No.	Kiel Class	W.F.	bcl-2 Staining		Staining Note	bcl-2 Gene
			Lymphoma	GC*		
C-1[1]	cb/cc	D	Neg	Neg		G
C-1[2]	FL/D	D	Neg	Neg		G
T-2[1]	cb/cc	?	Mix	-		
T-2[2]	cb/cc	D	Mix	-		
Z-3[1]	cb/cc	?	NW	-		G
Z-3[2]	?	?	Neg	Neg		
DG-4	?	?	Neg	Neg		
E-5	?	?	Mix	-	Large C[+]	
T-6	?	?	Mix	Neg		
N-7	?	?	NW	-		G
21-8	cc/cll	?	Pos	-		
22-9	cb/cc (?)	?	Neg	-	Few C[+]	
12-10	cc/cll	?	Pos	-		
1-11[1]	cb/cc (?)	?	Mix	-		
1-11[2]	cll	A	Pos	-		
1-11[3]	cll	A	Pos	-		
1-11[4]	cll	A	Pos	-		
1-11[5]	cb/cc	F	Mix	-		
2-12[1]	cc/cll	?	NW	-		
2-12[2]	cll	A	Pos	-		
3-13[1]	cb/cc	?	Pos	-	Poor M.	
3-13[2]	cll	A	Pos	-		
3-13[3]	cc	F	Pos	-		
M-14	cb/cc/FL	C	Pos	Pos	React. (?)	
14-15	cb/cc/FL	C	Mix	Neg	React. (?)	
Ca-16	cb/cc/FL/D	D	Neg	-		
C0-17[1]	cb/cc/FL/D	D	Mix	Neg	Small C[+]	
C0-17[2]	cb/cc	F	Pos	-		G
P-18	cb/cc/FL/D	D	Neg	-		G
B-19	cb/cc/FL	D	Neg	-		G
TR-20	cb/i/sc	E	Mix	Neg		
BE-21	cc/sc	E	Pos	-		R
X1-22[1]	cc/sc	E	Pos	-		
X1-22[2]	cc/sc	E	Mix	-		
4-23[1]	cc/sc	E	NW	NW	Poor St.	

Case No.	Kiel Class	W.F.	bcl-2 Staining		Staining Note	bcl-2 Gene
			Lymphoma	GC*		
4-23[2]	cc/sc	E	NW	-	Poor St.	
4-23[3]	cc	E	Mix (?)	-	Poor St.	
6-24	cc (?)	E	Mix	Neg	React. (?)	
20-25	cc	E	Pos	-	Poor St.	
25-26	cc/i (?)	E	Pos	Neg		
26-27	cc	E	Pos	-		
28-28	cc	E	Mix	-		
24-29	cb/cc	E	Pos	-		
X2-30[1]	cb/cc	E	NW	-	Poor St.	
X2-30[2]	cb/cc	E	Pos (?)	-	Poor St.	
9-31	cb/cc	E	NW	-		
4-32[1]	cb/cc	E	Pos (?)	-	Poor St.	
X4-32[2]	cb/cc	F	Neg	-		
X3-33[1]	cb/cc	F	NW	-	Poor Cs.	
X3-33[2]	cb/cc	F	Pos (?)	-	Poor Cs.	
PE-34[1]	cb/cc	F	Neg	-		G
PE-34[2]	cc	G	Neg	-		G
35-35	cb/cc	E	Pos	-		G
10-36	cb/cc	E	Mix	-	Small C[+]	
15-37	cb/cc	E	Mix	-	Small C[+]	
G-38	cb/cc	F	Neg	-		
V-39	cb/cc	F	Pos	-		
18-40	cb/cc	F	NW	-		
23-41	cb/cc	F	Mix	-		
11-42	cb/cc	F	Mix	-		
13-43	cb/cc	F	Mix	-		
7-44	cb/cc	F	Mix	-		
M0-45[1]	cb/cc	G	Neg	-		G
M0-45[2]	cb/cc	G	Neg	-		G
M0-45[3]	cb/ML	G	Neg	-		G
M0-45	cb/ML	G	Neg	-		G
RU-46[1]	cb/cc	G	Mix	-		G
RU-46[2]	cb/cc	G	Mix	-		G
RU-46[3]	cb/cc	G	Mix	-		G
PA-47	cb/cc	G	Mix	-		G
ZA-48	ML	G	Neg	-		
5-49	ML	G	NW	-		

continued

Table 2. continued.

Case No.	Kiel Class	W.F.	bcl-2 Staining		Staining Note	bcl-2 Gene
			Lymphoma	GC*		
M-50	cc/ML	G	Mix	-	Less +	
29-51[1]	cc/ML	G	Neg	-		
29-51[2]	cb/ML	G	Neg	-		
P-52	ML	G	Neg	-		G
A-53	cb/cc/ML	G	Neg	-		G
19-54	cc	G	NW	-		
8-55	cb/cc	G	Neg	-	Giant C+	
5-56[1]	cb/cc	G	Neg	-		
5-56[2]	LC	G	Neg	-	Poor St.	
5-56[3]	cb/cc	G	Neg	-		
BR-57[1]	LC	G	Neg	-		G
BR-57[2]	LC	G	Neg	-		G
16-58	cb/ML	G	Neg	-		
17-59	cb/cc	G	Neg	-		
27-60	cb/cc/ML	G	NW	-		
61-61	LC	G	Neg	-		
GA-62	cc	G	Neg	-		G
BO-63	LC	G	Neg	-		G
BV-64	cb	G	Neg	-		G
A-65	cb/cc/ML	G	Neg	-		G
C0-66	LC	G	Neg	-		G

*Germinal center-like structure

W.F. = Working Formulation; bcl-2 Prot. = bcl-2 protein; bcl-2 R. = Rearrangement; Mix = Mixed; NW = Not Working; C = Cells; Poor M. = Poor Morphology; React. = Reactive; Poor St. = Poor Staining; Poor Cs. = Poor Counterstaining; Kiel Classification: cll = chronic lymphocytic leukemia; FL = Follicular; ML = Mantle Zone; D = Diffuse; cc = centrocytic; cb = centroblastic; i = intermediate; LC = Large Cell. Superscript numbers refer to successive biopsies (first, second, etc.) obtained from the same patient.

BCL-2 Expression

Detailed results obtained from the study of the expression of bcl-2 protein are shown in Table 2. Successful staining was obtained on 81 specimens (55 first biopsies and 26 relapsies).

A diagnostic definition according to Kiel and the Working Formulation classifications was made in 47 of 55 first biopsies (Table 3).

From analysis of the data it can be seen that, on 47 biopsies, bcl-2 protein was negative in 16 (34%), with a mixed pattern in 13 (27.5%) and positive in 18 (38.5%) cases.

Moreover (Table 3), it can be observed that all of the cases characterized by proliferation of small cells were positive, whereas 16 of 27 (60%) either large or small and large cell lymphomas did not express bcl-2 protein, 7 (26%) had a mixed pattern in which the "large" cells were negative, the "small" cells being positive, and only in 4 cases (15%) were large neoplastic cells uniformly positive.

From 15 patients, 26 biopsies of relapses were examined but only slight differences in the results were found for each single case over a period of time, such as giving a mixed pattern instead of a positive reaction and vice versa.

In 10 cases it was not possible to reach a diagnostic definition using the Working Formulation (Table 2).

Germinal center-like structures, with highly proliferating cells demonstrated by positivity with Ki-67 antibody, were observed in 9 of the 55 first biopsies; in all but one case these structures were bcl-2 negative.

Southern Blot Analysis

There was no evidence for rearrangenent of the bcl-2 gene in 19 of the 20 cases studied using the pFL-1 probe.

The only confirmed positive case (N° 21, Table 2 and Figure 1) simultaneously developed superficial and visceral lymph nodal involvement.

DISCUSSION

The negative staining for CD10/CALLA and the absence of rearrangement in the bcl-2 proto-oncogene in CBCL has been confirmed in this study. These results not only fail to support the hypothesis that the majority of these lymphomas originate from the germinal center but also exclude the possibility, raised by other studies, of grouping these lymphomas with nodal follicular lymphomas, which show consistent expression of CD10/CALLA and, in 80% of cases, of bcl-2 protein. We have also confirmed the expression of some lymphocytic antigens (KB61, CD1c, IgD, Leu8, CD21), characteristic of the mantle zone cortex B lymphocytic subsets, in a variable percentage from 32 to 52 %, and, in approximately 65% of cases, the presence, within areas of proliferation, of reticular dendritic cells of the follicle, in these lymphomas.

Moreover, in most of primary cutaneous B-cell lymphomas characterized by proliferation of large centroblast-like cells, the protein, bcl-2, was not expressed, unlike follicular and diffuse lymphomas (Pezzella et al., 1990). The histological types in our series vary from the small lymphocytic to the multilobulated large cell lymphoma; it was not even possible to classify 10 cases, since the cellular morphology of the lymphoid elements in the skin appears particularly prone to "artefacts".

These findings suggest that primary cutaneous B cell lymphomas exhibit heterogeneity both in their phenotype and in their histological appearance. The histological type, the phenotypic characteristics and the absence of bcl-2 gene rearrangement appear to suggest a similarity between primary cutaneous and mucosa-associated lymphoid tissue (MALT) B cell lymphomas. Furthermore, Isaacson et al., (1991) have recently published a study of the bcl-2 protein expression in MALT lymphomas, demonstrating that it is present in slowly proliferating tumor cells outside the colonized follicles, whereas the ones inside, with a high rate of proliferation, were negative.

Table 3. Bcl-2 protein expression in 47 diagnostic biopsies of primary cutaneous B cell non-Hodgkin lymphomas classified according to Kiel and Working Formulation nomenclatures

Diagnosis Kiel (WF)	Negative bcl-2	Mixed bcl-2	Positive bcl-2	Total
small cells, n.o.s.			2	2
small lymphocytes (A)			2	2
FL, cb/cc (C)		1	1	2
FL, cb/cc (D)	3			3
small, cc(E)		3	5	8
small, cb/cc (E)		2	4	6
small and large, cb/cc (F)	1	4	2	7
large, cb/cc (G)	4	2	1	7
large, cc (G)	4	2	1	7
large, cb (G)	2		1	3
multilobulated (G)	2			2
large cells, n.o.s. (G)	1			1
TOTAL	16	13	18	47

n.o.s. = not otherwise specified

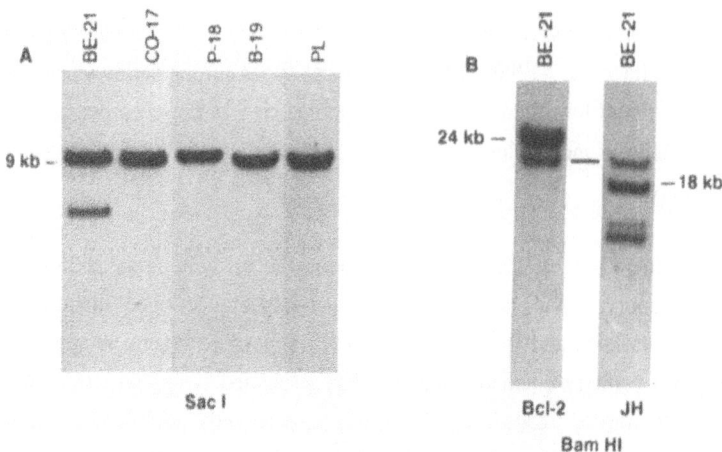

Figure 1. Bcl-2 gene rearrangement analysis of genomic DNAs from cutaneous B-cell lymphomas. Panel A: Sac 1-digested cellular DNAs probed with a genomic fragment specific for the breakpoint cluster region of the Bcl-2 gene (PFL-1 probe). Panel B: DNA from case BE-21 was digested with Bam H1 restriction enzyme and the filter was subsequently hybridized to PFL-1 and JH probes; the co-migrating fragment is indicated by the dash between lanes. PL: normal placental DNA. Germ line bands are indicated by dashes.

In our series it can also be seen that in 10 cases germinal center-like structures were present and in all but one of them the bcl-2 protein was not expressed. This finding further supports the proposed similarity between cutaneous and MALT B cell lymphomas.

Finally, we have confirmed that bcl-2 protein expression in lymphomas (Pezzella, 1990) is not a marker for bcl-2 gene rearrangement (which was absent in 19 of the 20 cases analyzed).

ACKNOWLEDGEMENT

The authors thank Doctor DY Mason for his stimulating suggestions.

REFERENCES

Berti E, E Alessi and R Caputo, 1991. Reticulohistiocytoma of the Dorsum (Crosti's Disease) and Other B-Cell Lymphomas. **Seminars in Diagnostic Pathology**, 8:82-90.

Berti E, E Alessi, R Caputo, R Gianotti, D Delia, and P Vezzoni, 1988. Reticulohistiocytoma of the dorsum. **J. Am. Acad. Dermatol.**, 19:259-272.

Cordell JL, B Falini, WN Erber, AK Ghosh, Z Abdulaziz, S MacDonald, KAF Pulford, H Stein, and DY Mason, 1984. Immunoenzymatic labelling of monoclonal antibodies using immune complexes of alkaline phosphatase and monoclonal anti-alkaline phosphatase (APAAP complexes). **J. Histochem. Cytochem.**, 32:219-229.

Delia D, MG Borrello, E Berti, MA Pierotti, D Biassoni, R Gianotti, E Alessi, MG Rivietti, R Caputo, and G Della Porta, 1989. Clonal immunoglobulin gene rearrangements and normal T-cell receptor,bcl-2 and c-myc genes in primary cutaneous B-cell lymphomas. **Cancer Res.**, 49:49014905.

Isaacson PG, A Dogan, SK Price, and J Spencer, 1989. Immunoproliferative small intestinal disease: An immunohistochemical study. **Am. J. Surg. Pathol.**, 13:1023-33.

Isaacson PG, AC Wotherspoon, TC Diss, LX Pan, 1991. bcl-2 expression in lymphomas. **Lancet**, 337:175-76.

Pezzella F, AGD Tse, JL Cordell, KA Pulford, KC Gatter, and DY Mason, 1990. Expression of the bcl-2 oncogene protein is not specific for the 14;18 chromosomal translocation. **Am. J. Pathol.**, 137:225-231.

Pimpinelli N, M Santucci, A Bosi, S Moretti, C Vallecchi, A Messori and B Giannotti, 1989. Primary cutaneous follicular center-cell lymphoma: A lymphoproliferative disease with favourable prognosis. **Clin. Exp. Dermatol.**, 14:12-19.

Santucci M, N Pimpinelli and L Arganini, 1991. Primary cutaneous B-cell lymphoma: A unique type of low-grade lymphoma. Clinicopathologic and immunologic study of 83 cases. **Cancer**, 67:2311-2326.

Volkenadt M, L Cerroni, E Rieger, HP Soyer, O Koch, R Wienecke, J Atzpodien, JR Bertino and H Kerl, 1992. Analysis of the 14;18 translocation in cutaneous lymphomas using the polymerase chain reaction. **J. Cutan. Pathol.**, 19:353-356.

Willemze R, CJLM Meijer, E Scheffer, PM Kluin, WA van Vloten, J Toonstra and SC Van Der Putte, 1987a. Diffuse large cell lymphomas of follicular center origin presenting in the skin. A clinicopathologic and immunologic study of 16 patients. **Am. J. Pathol.**, 126:325-333.

Willemze R, CJLM Meijer, HJ Sentis, E Scheffer, WA van Vloten, J Toonstra, and SC Van Der Putte, 1987b. Primary cutaneous large cell lymphomas of follicular center cell origin. **J. Am. Acad. Dermatol.**, 16:518-526.

CHANGING CONCEPTS ON CUTANEOUS PSEUDO-B CELL LYMPHOMAS AND THEIR RELATIONSHIP TO CUTANEOUS B CELL LYMPHOMAS

Udo Rijlaarsdam*†
Victor Bakels*†
Johan W. van Oostveen*†
Marie-Louise Geerts‡
Chris J.L.M. Meijer*†
Rein Willemze*†

* Departments of Dermatology
† Department of Pathology
  Free University Hospital
  Amsterdam, The Netherlands

‡ Department of Dermatology
  University Hospital
  Ghent, Belgium.

Correspondence to: Dr. U. Rijlaarsdam, Department of Dermatology,
University Hospital, Free University, de Boelelaan 1117,
1081 HV Amsterdam, The Netherlands

ABSTRACT

In this chapter the various criteria that are used to differentiate between pseudo-B cell lymphomas and cutaneous B cell lymphomas are reviewed. The changing concepts that have resulted from the introduction of new diagnostic techniques such as immunohistochemistry and immunoglobulin gene rearrangement analysis are emphasized.

Basic Mechanisms of Physiologic and Aberrant Lymphoproliferation in the Skin
Edited by W.C. Lambert *et al.*, Plenum Press, New York, 1994

INTRODUCTION

Pseudo-B cell lymphomas of the skin are characterized by a benign cutaneous hyperplasia of B cells that clinically and histologically may simulate cutaneous B cell lymphoma (Kerl and Ackerman, 1987). Other terms that have been used to designate these conditions are lymphadenosis benigna cutis, lymphocytoma cutis, sarcoid of Spiegler-Fendt and cutaneous lymphoid hyperplasia. The differentiation between pseudo-B cell lymphomas and cutaneous B cell lymphomas (CBCL) may be extremely difficult. For many decades the differential diagnosis was based on clinical and histologic criteria. In the late seventies, when immunohistochemical analysis of tissue sections for expression of intracytoplasmatic or membrane-bound immunoglobulins became widely available, demonstration of monotypic light chain expression became the "gold standard" for differentiation between benign and malignant lymphoproliferative B cell disorders. More recently, immunoglobulin gene rearrangement analysis by Southern blot hybridization has proven to be a more sensitive and objective method to demonstrate clonality and lineage in lymphoproliferative disorders. Here the various criteria that have been used in the past decades to differentiate between benign and malignant cutaneous B cell infiltrates are reviewed and the changing concepts that have resulted from the introduction of new diagnostic methods are discussed.

DIFFERENTIATION BETWEEN PSEUDO-B CELL LYMPHOMAS AND CUTANEOUS B CELL LYMPHOMAS

Clinical and Histologic Criteria

Previously, before the introduction of immunohistochemical analysis, differentiation between benign and malignant cutaneous B cell infiltrates was based on clinical and histologic criteria. In studies attempting to define histologic criteria for the differentiation between these groups, the patients were often selected on the basis of clinical criteria, with lack of systemic involvement five years after the initial skin biopsy as the decisive criterion for the benign character of the initial lesion (Caro and Helwig, 1969; Evans et al., 1979). The clinical and histologic differential diagnostic criteria derived from these studies have been summarized in Table 1. In recent studies and handbooks, many of these criteria are still mentioned as useful for the differentiation between pseudo-B cell lymphomas and primary cutaneous B cell lymphomas (Burg and Braun-Falco, 1983; Kerl and Ackerman, 1987). It must be emphasized, however, that at the time these studies were performed, it was firmly believed that B cell lymphomas found in the skin were always manifestations of systemic disease, and generally associated with a poor prognosis (Evans et al., 1979). Since primary CBCL generally have a very good prognosis, it is conceivable that the group of pseudo-B cell lymphomas in these studies include many cases that would now be considered to be examples of primary CBCL.

Immunohistochemical Analysis

With the introduction of immunohistochemical studies using polyclonal antibodies directed against immunoglobulins (Ig), it was shown that, in nodal B cell lymphomas, the malignant cells exhibited monotypic light chain expression, in contrast to the polytypic light chain expression in reactive B cell populations (Levy et al., 1977). As a result, demonstration of clonality by means of immunohistochemical analysis became the gold standard in the differential diagnosis between benign and malignant B-cell proliferative disorders (Picker et al., 1987). Application of these immunohistochemical techniques to cutaneous B cell infiltrates demonstrated that a proportion of the patients that previously were considered to have a pseudo-B cell lymphoma, on the basis of clinical criteria, showed monotypic Ig light chain expression or lacked detectable immunoglobulin. Because extensive staging procedures did not reveal extracutaneous disease in these cases, the concept of primary cutaneous B cell lymphomas was introduced (Willemze et al., 1987; Garcia et al., 1986; Santucci et al., 1991). The large majority of these primary cutaneous B cell lymphomas are composed of variable numbers of small and large centrocytes (cleaved cells) and centroblasts (large noncleaved cells), cells that are usually found in germinal centers of follicles in lymph nodes. According to data obtained from the registry of the Dutch Cutaneous Lymphoma Working Group these follicular center cell lymphomas comprise up to 25% of primary cutaneous lymphomas. These lymphomas, characterized by localized infiltrated plaques or tumors on the trunk or scalp, have an excellent prognosis after proper treatment with radiotherapy or polychemotherapy (Willemze, et al., 1987). In elderly patients, in whom this type of lymphoma often presents with localized lesions on the lower aspects of the legs, however, the prognosis is less favorable, because systemic spread occurs in a considerable proportion of cases (Rijlaarsdam and Willemze, 1990). In addition, immunocytomas and B immunoblastic lymphomas may be limited to the skin, but these lymphomas constitute no more than 1-2% of the total number of primary cutaneous lymphomas. The rationale for the division between benign and malignant cutaneous B cell infiltrates, based on the presence of clonal B cell populations, is that the former does not have the potential to disseminate to extracutaneous sites, whereas the latter may do so. Therefore, patients with primary CBCL are extensively staged and treated more aggressively, with radiotherapy in the case of localized disease or polychemo-therapy in the case of more widespread disease, whereas cutaneous pseudo-B cell lymphomas are not staged and may be treated with topical or intralesional steroids, or -- if unresponsive -- with low-dose radiotherapy. Using monotypic light chain expression as a decisive criterion to differentiate between pseudo-B cell lymphomas and primary cutaneous B cell lymphomas, many of the clinical and extensively histologic differential diagnostic criteria that are summarized in Table 1 proved to be not valid for the differentiation of these two entities (Rijlaarsdam et al., 1990). Criteria that had been reported to be specific for pseudo-B cell lymphomas in older studies (a polymorphous infiltrate, presence of lymphoid follicles, eosinophils, a top-heavy infiltrate etc., Table 1) were also present in a considerable proportion of primary cutaneous B cell lymphomas (Rijlaarsdam et al., 1990). It was therefore concluded that, although differenti-ation between the two conditions is often possible using a combination of criteria, there is no single clinical or histologic criterion that can reliably do so in all cases.

Table 1. Clinical and histologic criteria for the differentiation between pseudo-B cell lymphoma and primary CBCL from the literature (Caro and Helwig, 1969; Evans et al. 1979).

	Pseudo-BCL	CBCL
Clinical criteria:		
Age	Children/adults	Adults
Etiology	Insect bites/trauma	Unknown
Lesions	Usually solitary	Usually multiple
Prognosis	Good	Progression
Histologic criteria:		
Architecture	"Top heavy"	"Bottom heavy"
Infiltrate	"Polymorphous"	"Monomorphous"
Germinal centers	Often present	Rare
Eosinophils	Often present	Absent
Nuclear debris	Frequently present	Rare

Gene-Rearrangement Analysis

In recent years, Ig-gene rearrangement analysis by Southern blot hybridization has been introduced as a more sensitive and objective method to detect clonality in a B cell population than immunohistochemical analysis. In primary cutaneous B cell lymphomas, gene rearrangement analysis confirmed clonality in the majority of cases (Delia et al., 1989; Rijlaarsdam et al., 1992). Clonality was also demonstrated in some pseudo-B cell lymphomas, however. Wood et al. (1989) investigated 14 cases of pseudo-B cell lymphoma, defined by polyclonal light chain expression detected by immunohistochemistry, and demonstrated clonal B cell populations in five of them. In our own study we demonstrated clonality in four of seven cases of pseudo-B cell lymphoma (Rijlaarsdam et al., 1992). Furthermore, the study of Wood et al., suggests that these clonal pseudolymphomas may have an increased risk to a develop true cutaneous malignant lymphoma. These results may contribute to the view that CBCL and pseudo-B cell lymphomas represent a continuous spectrum of B cell neoplasia, ranging from polyclonal and clonal reactive B cell proliferations to malignant B cell lymphomas.

CUTANEOUS B CELL LYMPHOMAS AND PSEUDO-B-CELL LYMPHOMAS: A CONTINUOUS SPECTRUM OF B CELL NEOPLASIA?

The presence of clonal B cell populations in lymphoproliferative lesions that clinically, histologically and immunophenotypically lack evidence of malignant lymphoma has not only been demonstrated in cutaneous pseudo-B cell lymphomas but also in noncutaneous extranodal lymphoid hyperplasias and in Epstein-Barr Virus (EBV) related lymphoproliferative disorders in immunocompromized patients. Knowles et al. (1989) investigated 16 cases of lymphoid proliferations occuring in the ocular adnexa, salivary glands, breast and thyroid gland satisfying the histopathologic and immunophenotypic criteria of benign lymphoid hyperplasia for the presence of clonal Ig-gene rearrangements, and demonstrated clonal Ig heavy and/or light chain rearrangements in all cases. Two of these cases eventually developed a histopathologically confirmed malignant lymphoma in an anatomically unrelated extranodal site. In three of 16 cases these authors demonstrated rearrangement of the proto-oncogenes, bcl-1 or bcl-2. In contrast to the lymphoid proliferations associated with severe immunosuppression, none of their cases contained Epstein-Barr viral (EBV) DNA sequences. EBV has been demonstrated in hyperplastic lymph nodes of patients with AIDS (Pelicci et al., 1986) and in lymphoid tumors from transplant patients receiving cyclosporine A (Nalesnik et al., 1988; Locker and Nalesnik, 1989). Pelecci et al. (1986) reported clonal immunoglobulin gene rearrangements in hyperplastic lymph nodes of patients with AIDS. Although none of their patients developed overt lymphoma during 18 months of follow-up, they suggested that this finding may be related to the increased incidence of malignant lymphoma in AIDS patients. In the EBV related post-transplant lymphoproliferative disorders, a spectrum from clinically benign lesions to rapidly fatal lymphomas is found. In a proportion of the histologically and immunophenotypically benign lesions, clonal rearrangements of immunoglobulin genes have been demonstrated (Nalesnik et al., 1988; Locker and Nakesnik, 1989). Although reduction of immunosuppression resulted in resolution of the lymphoproliferative lesions in a considerable proportion of these patients, in other cases these lesions were progressive and eventually fatal. The above-mentioned studies have in common that clonal B cell populations are identified in lymphoproliferative lesions that are clinically, histologically and immunophenotypically benign, but that at the same time are associated with an increased incidence of malignant lymphoma. These findings have been explained by the concept that the division between reactive and malignant B-cell lymphoproliferations is not absolute, but rather these lymphoproliferative lesions represent a continuous and progressive spectrum of B cell neoplasia (Knowles et al., 1989; Locker and Nalesnik, 1989). In cutaneous pseudo-B cell lymphomas, the transition to malignant lymphoma has also been frequently described (Shelley et al., 1981; Nakayama et al., 1987; Wood et al., 1989), and not all cases can be explained by the fact that the pseudolymphoma represented an incorrectly diagnosed malignant lymphoma. Wood et al. (1989) described one patient with a clonal pseudo-B cell lymphoma that eventually developed a histologically and immunophenotypically cutaneous B cell lymphoma. Similar to noncutaneous lymphoid hyperplasia and EBV associated lymphoproliferative disorders, the existence of clonal pseudo-B cell lymphomas as well as the transition of cutaneous pseudo-lymphomas to primary CBCL can be explained by the concept that pseudo-B cell lymphomas and primary CBCL are part of a spectrum of B cell neoplasia ranging from reactive polyclonal pseudolymphomas, via oligoclonal and clonal pseudolymphomas, to malignant lymphomas. This concept also explains why it has never been possible to formulate indisputable clinical and/or histological criteria for the differentiation between pseudo-B cell lymphomas and CBCL. In this concept, the clonal B cell populations in histologically and immunophenotypically benign cutaneous B-cell proliferations may result as a consequence of local or general defects in immune surveillance and/or in the mechanisms that normally regulate B cell proliferation (Knowles et al., 1989). Ultimately, these clonal B cell populations may undergo additional genetic alterations that result in malignant transformation. The molecular basis of these additional genetic alterations leading to the development of a primary CBCL is unknown. A relationship with EBV has not been shown and specific translocations, e.g., involvement of the protooncogenes c-myc and bcl-2, have not been reported (Delia et al., 1989). Unraveling the molecular basis of primary CBCL should eventually allow us to distinguish more reliably between the different groups of patients in this spectrum of benign and malignant cutaneous B cell infiltrates.

CLINICAL IMPLICATIONS

The concept that cutaneous pseudo-B cell lymphomas and primary CBCL represent a continuous and progressive spectrum of B cell neoplasia may have consequences for the management of patients with a pseudo-B cell lymphoma. Both cutaneous pseudo-B cell lymphomas and primary CBCL have an excellent prognosis in most cases. Although clonal pseudo-B cell lymphomas may probably progress to CBCL, development of systemic malignant lymphoma has never been reported in such patients. Nevertheless, since only a few cases have been published thus far, the safest therapeutic approach for these patients is to establish that there is no concurrent extracutaneous disease, eradicate the skin lesions, and carefully monitor them for development of malignant lymphoma.

REFERENCES

Burg G and O Braun-Falco, 1983. **Cutaneous lymphomas, pseudolymphomas and related disorders**. Springer, New York.

Caro W and E Helwig, 1969. Cutaneous lymphoid hyperplasia. **Cancer**, 24:48.

Delia D, MG Borello, E Berti, MA Pierotti, D Biassoni, R Gianotti, E Alessi, MG Rizzetti, R Caputo and G Della Porta, 1989. Clonal immunoglobulin gene rearrangements and normal T-cell receptor, bcl-2 and c-myc genes in primary cutaneous B-cell lymphomas. **Cancer Res.**, 49:4901.

Evans H, R Winkelmann and P Banks, 1979. Differential diagnosis of malignant and benign cutaneous infiltrates. **Cancer**, 44:699-717.

Garcia CF, LM Weiss, RA Warnke and GS Wood, 1986. Cutaneous follicular lymphoma. **Am. J. Surg. Pathol.**, 10:454-4631.

Kerl H and A Ackerman, 1987. Cutaneous pseudolymphomas, in: TB Fitzpatrick, AZ Eisen, K Wolff and F Austen, Eds: **Dermatology in General Medicine** 3rd Ed. McGraw-Hill, New York pp. 1118-1130.

Knowles DM, E Athan, A Ubriaco, L Mc Nally, G Inghirami, R Wieczorek, M Finfer and FA Jacobiec, 1989. Extranodal noncutaneous lymphoid hyperplasias represent a continuous spectrum of B-cell neoplasia: Demonstration by molecular genetic analysis. **Blood**, 73:1635-1645.

Locker J and M Nalesnik, 1989. Molecular genetic analysis of lymphoid tumors arising after organ transplantation. **Am. J. Pathol.**, 135:977-987.

Levy R, R Warnke, RF Dorfman and J Haimovich, 1977. The monoclonality of human B-cell lymphomas. **J. Exp. Med.**, 145:1014-1028.

Nakayama H, M Mihara and S Shimao, 1987. Malignant transformation of lymphadenosis benigna cutis: A possibly transformed case and B-cell lymphoma. **Int. J. Dermatol.**, 14:266-269.

Nalesnik MA, R Jaffe, TE Starzl, AJ Demetris, K Porter, JA Burnham, L Mskowka, M Ho and J Locker, 1988. The pathology of post-transplant lymphoproliferative disorders occuring in the setting of cyclosporine A-prednisone immunosuppression. **Am. J. Pathol.**, 133:173-192.

Pelicci PG, DN Knowles, ZA Arlin, RM Wieczorek, P Luciw, D Dina, C Basilico and R Dalla-Favera, 1986. Multiple monoclonal B cell expansions and c-myc oncogene rearrangements in acquired immune deficiency-related lymphoproliferative disorders. **J. Exp. Med.**, 164:2049-76.

Picker LJ, LM Weiss, LI Medeiros, GS Wood and RA Warnke, 1987. Immunophenotypic criteria for the diagnosis of Non-Hodgkin's lymphomas. **Am. J. Dermatol.**, 128:181-201.

Rijlaarsdam JU, CJLM Meijer and R Willemze, 1990. Differentiation between lymphadenosis benigna cutis and primary cutaneous follicular center cell lymphomas. A clinicopathologic study of 57 patients. **Cancer**, 65:2301-2306.

Rijlaarsdam JU and R Willemze, 1990. Primary cutaneous large cell lymphoma of follicular centre cell origen. **Br. J. Dermatol.**, 123:536.

Rijlaarsdam JU, V Bakels, JW Van Oostveen, RJL Gordijn, ML Geerts, CJLM Meijer and R Willemze, 1993. Demonstration of immunoglobulin gene rearrangement in cutaneous B cell lymphomas and pseudo-B cell lymphomas: Differential diagnostic and pathogenetic aspects. **J. Invest. Dermatol.**, 99:749-754.

Santucci N, N Pimpinelli and L Arganini, 1991. Primary cutaneous B-cell lymphoma: A unique type of low-grade lymphoma. **Cancer**, 67:2311-2326.

Shelley WB, M Gray Wood, JF Wilson and R Goodman, 1981. Premalignant lymphoid hyperplasia. **Arch. Dermatol.**, 117:500-503.

Willemze R, CB De Graaff-Reitsma, WA van Vloten and CJLM Meijer, 1983. The cell population of cutaneous B-cell lymphomas. **Br. J. Dermatol.**, 108:395-409.

Willemze R, CJLM Meijer, E Sentis, E Scheffer, WA van Vloten, J Toonstra and SCJ Van der Putte, 1987. Primary cutaneous large cell lymphomas of follicular center cell origin. **J. Am. Acad. Dermatol.**, 16:518-526.

Wood GS, B Ngan, R Tung, TE Hoffman, EA Abel, RT Hoppe, RA Warnke, ML Cleary and J Sklar, 1989. Clonal rearrangement of immunoglobulin genes and progression to B cell lymphoma in cutaneous lymphoid hyperplasia. **Am. J. Pathol.**, 135:13-19.

DIAGNOSTIC AND PROGNOSTIC SIGNIFICANCE OF CLONAL T-CELL RECEPTOR GENE REARRANGEMENTS IN THE PERIPHERAL BLOOD OF PATIENTS WITH CUTANEOUS T-CELL LYMPHOMA

Victor Bakels *
Johan W. van Oostveen *†
Roel L.J. Gordijn *†
Jan M.M. Walboomers †
Chris J.L.M. Meijer †
Rein Willemze *

* Department of Dermatology
† Department of Pathology
Free University Hospital
Amsterdam, The Netherlands

Correspondence to: Prof. Dr. R. Willemze, Department of Dermatology,
University Hospital, de Boelelaan 1117,
1081 HV Amsterdam, The Netherlands

ABSTRACT

The results of recently published T-cell receptor gene rearrangement studies on peripheral blood lymphocytes of patients with mycosis fungoides and Sézary syndrome are reviewed. The significance of detecting clonal T-cell populations in the peripheral blood for the diagnosis and prognosis of these conditions is discussed, along with potential pitfalls in the interpretation of the results of these studies.

INTRODUCTION

Cutaneous T-cell lymphomas (CTCL) represent a heterogeneous group of lymphoproliferative disorders of (primarily helper) T cells, which initially present in the skin. The two main representatives of this group of diseases are mycosis fungoides (MF) and Sézary syndrome (SS). Whether SS is simply a leukemic phase of MF or a distinct entity within the spectrum of CTCL is a matter of controversy.

Basic Mechanisms of Physiologic and Aberrant Lymphoproliferation in the Skin
Edited by W.C. Lambert *et al.*, Plenum Press, New York, 1994

363

Demonstration of peripheral blood involvement in CTCL is important both from a diagnostic and a prognostic point of view. Evaluation of the results of previously reported cytologic studies is difficult, however, because of differences in patient selection, differences in the techniques used to demonstrate peripheral blood involvement, and lack of uniform criteria for the identification of circulating neoplastic T-cells (Bunn et al., 1980; Vonderheid, et al., 1985: Schechter et al., 1987). Cells morphologically similar to the neoplastic cells seen in CTCL have been demonstrated, both by light and electron microscopy, in the peripheral blood of a wide variety of benign dermatoses (van der Loo et al., 1981; Duncan and Winkelmann 1978; Willemze et al., 1983; Duangurai et al., 1988).

Recent studies have shown that T-cell receptor (TCR) gene rearrangement analysis using Southern blot hybridization is a sensitive and objective technique to detect clonal T-cell populations in tissue infiltrates and peripheral blood that may serve as an important adjunct in the diagnosis of CTCL. Results of recent gene rearrangement studies using Southern blot hybridization on peripheral blood mononuclear cells of patients with MF and SS are reviewed here. Attention is focused on the diagnostic and prognostic significance of detecting clonal TCR gene rearrangements in the peripheral blood of patients with MF and SS. The relationship between the results of routine cytologic examination of peripheral blood smears and those of gene rearrangement analysis will be discussed first.

SOUTHERN BLOT ANALYSIS VERSUS CONVENTIONAL LIGHT MICROSCOPY

In two recent studies, results of studies of TCR gene rearrangements on peripheral blood mononuclear cells (PBMC) of patients with CTCL were compared with those of conventional light microscopy (Weiss et al., 1989; Whittaker et al., 1991). Weiss et al. examined peripheral blood of 26 patients with MF/SS. Morphologically atypical circulating lymphocytes were found in 6 patients. Seven of 26 patients had clonal TCR beta gene rearrangements, including the four patients with the greatest percentages of atypical cells, but also including 3 patients without atypical cells by cytologic examination. In two patients with 3% and 4% atypical lymphocytes, respectively, only germline configurations were found. Taken together, there was agreement between the two techniques in 21 of 26 patients. The authors concluded that gene rearrangement analysis is a more sensitive and specific technique than conventional light microscopy. The results of the study of Weiss et al. are roughly similar to those of a recent study by our own group on peripheral blood samples of a large group of patients with erythroderma (Bakels et al., 1991). In 22 of 42 patients both gene rearrangement analyses and quantitative electron microscopic (morphometric) studies were performed. In previous studies we have demonstrated that the presence of more than 20% lymphoid cells with a nuclear contour index (NCI) > 6.5 and/or the presence of lymphoid cells with a NCI > 11.5 is a useful additional criterion for the diagnosis of SS in the peripheral blood (Willemze et al., 1983). Comparison of the morphometric results with those of gene rearrangement analysis revealed agreement between both methods in 16 of 22 blood samples. Four of 11 blood samples classified as malignant by morphometric criteria showed only germline configurations on Southern blot analysis. By contrast, clonal T-cell populations were detected in 2 of 11 cases considered benign on the basis of nuclear contour indexing. The results of this study and those of Weiss et al., indicate an overall agreement between morphologic and gene rearrangement studies in approximately 75% of patients.

In a more recent study, Whittaker et al. (1991) examined peripheral blood samples of 24 patients with MF in various stages of the disease and 14 patients with SS. Clonal T-cell populations were detected in 8 of 24 patients with MF. These included clonal rearrangements of both the beta and gamma TCR chain in 4 patients and of the TCR gamma chain alone in another 4 patients. In two of eight cases, cytologic examination showed abnormal circulating lymphocytes with morphologic features typical of Sézary cells. In the other six patients peripheral blood smears contained 1 to 12% small atypical cells with clefted or folded nuclei; however, these were also identified in blood smears from MF patients without detectable clonal T-cell populations. The poor relationship between conventional cytology and gene rearrangement analysis in this study is underscored by the observation that only 8 of 14 patients considered to have SS had detectable clonal T-cell populations on Southern blot analysis. On the basis of these results, the authors concluded that conventional light microscopy cannot accurately distinguish reactive lymphoid cells from their neoplastic counterparts in CTCL, and that TCR gene analysis is a much more specific technique.

T-CELL RECEPTOR GENE REARRANGEMENT ANALYSIS ON PERIPHERAL BLOOD LYMPHOCYTES IN PATIENTS WITH SÉZARY SYNDROME

SS is characterized by a pruritic exfoliative or infiltrated erythroderma, generalized lymphadenopathy and the presence of circulating atypical cells (Sézary cells). Patients with well established SS show highly increased percentages of $CD3^+/CD4^+$ T cells in the peripheral blood and demonstrate characteristic histologic changes in skin and lymph nodes. In the early stages of the disease, however, clinical and histologic features may be non-diagnostic and do not always allow differentiation from erythroderma caused by benign conditions, such as chronic or atopic dermatitis, psoriasis or drug eruptions. In these early stages differentiation between SS and these benign forms of erythroderma depends heavily on demonstration of Sézary cells in peripheral blood samples. As noted above, however, there are no uniform criteria to differentiate characteristic Sézary cells from morphologically similar cells in benign conditions. As a result, various investigators have used either 10%, 15% or 20% circulating Sézary cells, or an absolute count of 10^3 Sézary cells per millimeter of blood, as a minimum criterion for the diagnosis of SS (Duncan and Winkelmann, 1978; Prunieras, 1978; Willemze et al., 1983; Vonderheid et al., 1985). Recent studies have suggested that demonstration of clonal T-cell populations by Southern blot hybridization on peripheral blood samples of patients with erythroderma is a more objective and more sensitive technique to differentiate between SS and benign forms of erythroderma (Bertness et al., 1985; Waldmann et al., 1985; Ralfkiaer et al., 1987; Weiss et al., 1989; Bakels et al., 1991; Whittaker et al., 1991; Zelickson et al., 1991). In our own study on a large group of patients with erythroderma, including 10 patients with SS and 19 patients with a benign form of erythroderma, clonal TCR beta gene rearrangements were found in the peripheral blood of 8 of 10 patients with SS, and only in one of 19 patients with a benign erythroderma (Bakels et al., 1991). In the two SS patients that initially showed only germline configurations, clonal T-cell populations were detected in blood samples obtained during follow-up. It is of interest that one patient with a lymphomatoid drug eruption, in whom the histologic features in skin and lymph nodes and a highly elevated CD4/CD8 ratio, as well as the results of morphometric analysis, had been highly suggestive of SS, showed only the germline configurations. It was therefore concluded that TCR beta gene rearrangement analysis on peripheral blood of patients with erythroderma is not only a sensitive, but also a highly specific, technique that may contribute significantly to the early diagnosis of SS. However, our results conflict with those of Whittaker et al. (1991). In their study, clonal T-cell populations were detected in the peripheral blood of only 8 of 14 SS patients. It is of interest that their 6 patients without detectable clonal T-cells in the peripheral blood ran a favorable clinical course. Only one of these six patients died (of an unrelated cause), whereas five of the eight patients with clonal disease died during the study. The authors therefore suggested that there is a subset of SS patients with a polyclonal population of circulating atypical lymphoid cells, and that these patients have a better prognosis than patients with clonal disease. Since the authors did not specify which morphologic criteria they used for the diagnosis of SS, however, the possibility cannot be excluded that the difference in sensitivity of TCR gene analysis in the diagnosis of SS between their study and the other studies simply resulted from differences in patient selection.

CLONAL T-CELL POPULATIONS IN THE PERIPHERAL BLOOD OF PATIENTS WITH MYCOSIS FUNGOIDES

Although previous studies have suggested that systemic involvement in CTCL is frequent, generally asymptomatic and develops early via the circulation (Bunn et al., 1980), most investigators agree that peripheral blood involvement is not an early event in MF. Patients with MF generally present with eczematous patches and/or infiltrated plaques that may be the only manifestation of the disease for many years or even decades. With progression of the disease, a proportion of patients may develop tumors or erythroderma, and dissemination to lymph nodes and visceral organs may occur. The frequency of peripheral blood involvement in the various stages of MF is not precisely known. Previous studies have selected primarily patients with CTCL, and often contain a considerable proportion of SS patients (Bunn et al., 1980; Vonderheid et al., 1985; Schechter et al., 1987). Since data on individual patients have generally not been presented, it is not always clear how many patients had MF. In addition, these studies focused mainly on the frequency of peripheral blood involvement in the various skin stages of CTCL, and did not always specify which proportion of patients in these different subgroups had lymph node involvement. Recent studies by our group suggest that peripheral blood involvement in MF is rare (Bakels et al., 1992). Using Southern blot hybridization, clonal T-cell populations were found in only 5 of 46 patients (11%), including 1 of 31 patients (3%) with disease limited to the skin, and 4 of 15 patients (27%) with histologically confirmed lymph node involvement. With respect to skin stage, clonal rearrangements were found in 1 of 23 patients (4%) with plaque stage disease, 2 of 19 patients (10%) with tumor stage disease and 2 of 4 patients (50%) with erythrodermic MF. All five patients with detectable clonal T-cell populations had longstanding MF, varying from 30 to 212 months (median, 104 months), and blood samples had been obtained during progression of the disease in all of them. Roughly similar percentages have been found by Weiss et al. (1989) and Whittaker et al. (1991).

Previous studies have suggested that peripheral blood involvement in CTCL is associated with a poor survival (Bunn et al., 1980; Schechter et al., 1987). However, since there was an almost complete overlap in those studies between groups with peripheral blood involvement and those with lymph node involvement, conclusions as to the relative prognostic importance of peripheral blood involvement cannot be made. In our study, it was found that, in the group of MF patients with histologically proven lymph node involvement, the median survival of patients with detectable clonal TCR beta gene rearrangements was much shorter (3 months; range 1-28 months) than that of patients showing no clonal T-cell populations in the peripheral blood (116 months; range 3-135 months). In conclusion, the results of our study indicate that clonal T-cell populations, as detected by Southern blot analysis, are rare in the peripheral blood of patients with MF, in particular in patients without histologically documented lymph node involvement. They also indicate that the presence of clonal T-cell populations in the peripheral blood of MF patients with lymph node involvement is usually associated with rapidly fatal disease.

CONCLUSIONS

The studies reviewed here suggest that TCR gene rearrangement analysis is a much more sensitive and/or specific technique for the assessment of peripheral blood involvement in patients with MF and SS than other methods now in use. One of the great advantages of gene rearrangement analysis is the lack of the considerable observer variation that is associated with conventional morphologic methods. Additional prospective studies on well-defined groups of patients with MF/SS and control patients are necessary, however, before final conclusions as to the diagnostic and prognostic value of TCR gene analysis can be made. It must be realized that the interpretation and comparison of studies published thus far may be hampered by the fact that various investigators have used different criteria for the selection of patients, in particular in SS. Moreover, it must always be kept in mind that demonstration of a clonal T-cell population does not always imply malignant biologic behavior. The clinical significance of clonal T-cell populations in the peripheral blood of MF patients with early plaque stage disease without concurrent lymph node involvement, as occasionally observed, is as yet unknown. Therefore, the results of gene rearrangement analysis should always be considered in conjunction with all relevant clinical and histologic information.

REFERENCES

Bakels V, JW van Oostveen, RLJ Gordijn, JJM Walboomers, CJLM Meijer and R Willemze, 1991. Diagnostic value of T-cell receptor gene rearrangement analysis on peripheral blood lymphocytes of patients with erythroderma. **J. Invest. Dermatol.**, 97:782.

Bakels V, JW van Oostveen, RLJ Gordijn, JJM Walboomers, CJLM Meijer and R Willemze, 1992. Frequency and prognostic significance of clonal T-cell receptor beta gene rearrangements in the peripheral blood of patients with mycosis fungoides. **Arch. Dermatol.**, 128:1602.

Bertness V, I Kirsch, G Hollis, B Johnson and PA Bunn, 1985. T-cell receptor gene rearrangements as clinical markers of human T-cell lymphomas. **N. Engl. J. Med.**, 313:534.

Bunn PA, MS Huberman, J Whang-Peng, GP Schechter, JG Guccion, MJ Matthews, AF Gazdar, NR Dunnick, AB Fischmann, DC Ihde, MH Cohen, B Fossieck and JD Minna, 1980. Prospective staging evaluation of patients with cutaneous T-cell lymphomas. Demonstration of a high frequency of cutaneous dissemination. **Ann. Intern. Med.**, 93:223.

Duangurai K, T Piamphongsant and T Himmungnan, 1988. Sézary cell count in exfoliative dermatitis. **Int. J. Dermatol.**, 27:248.

Duncan SC and RK Winkelmann, 1978. Circulating Sézary cells in hospitalized dermatology patients. **Br. J. Dermatol.**, 99:171.

Ralfkiaer E, NTJ O'Connor, J Crick, GL Wantzin and DY Mason, 1987. Genotypic analysis of cutaneous T-cell lymphomas. **J. Invest. Dermatol.**, 88:762.

Schechter PG, EA Sausville, AB Fischmann, F Soehlen, J Eddy, M Matthews, A Gazdar, J Guccion, D Munson, R Makuch and PA Bunn, 1987. Evaluation of circulating cells provides prognostic information in cutaneous T cell lymphoma. **Blood**, 69:841.

Van der Loo EM, CJLM Meijer, E Scheffer and WA van Vloten, 1981. The prognostic value of membrane markers and morphometric characteristics of lymphoid cells in blood and lymph nodes from patients with mycosis fungoides. **Cancer**, 48:738.

Vonderheid EC, EL Sobel, PC Nowell, JB Finan, MR Helfrich and DS Whipple, 1985. Diagnostic and prognostic significance of Sézary cells in peripheral blood smears from patients with cutaneous T cell lymphoma. **Blood**, 66:358.

Waldmann TA, MM Davis, KF Bongiovanni and SJ Korsmeyer, 1985. Rearrangements of genes for the antigen receptor on T cells as markers of lineage and clonality in human lymphoid neoplasms. **N. Engl. J. Med.**, 313:776.

Weiss LM, GS Wood, E Hu, EA Abel, RT Hoppe and J Sklar, 1989. Detection of clonal T-cell receptor gene rearrangements in the peripheral blood of patients with mycosis fungoides/Sézary syndrome. **J. Invest. Dermatol.**, 92:601.

Whittaker SJ, NP Smith, R Rusgell, R Jones and L Lazzatto, 1991. Analysis of beta, gamma and delta T-cell receptor genes in mycosis fungoides and Sézary syndrome. **Cancer**, 68:1572.

Willemze R, WA van Vloten, J Hermans, WJM Damsteeg and CJLM Meijer, 1983. Diagnostic criteria in Sézary's syndrome: A multiparameter study of peripheral boood lymphocytes in 32 patients with erythroderma. **J. Invest. Dermatol.**, 81:392.

Zelickson BD, MS Peters, SA Muller, SN Thibodeau, JA Lust, LM Quam and MR Pittelkow, 1991. T-cell receptor gene rearrangement analysis: Cutaneous T cell lymphoma, peripheral T cell lymphoma, and premalignant and benign cutaneous lymphoproliferative disorders. **J. Am. Acad. Dermatol.**, 25:787.

ANALYSIS OF T CELL-RECEPTOR GENE CONFIGURATIONS IN MYCOSIS FUNGOIDES

Lucia Crosti*

Vincenzo Rossi†

Andrea Biondi†

Elena Roscetti*

Emilio Berti*

Ruggero Caputo*

*   First Department of Dermatology

†   Department of Pediatrics

University of Milan

Milan, Italy

Correspondence to: Dr. L. Crosti, Department of Dermatology I, University of Milano, Via Pace 9, 20122 Milano, Italy

ABSTRACT

Histologic and immunophenotypic diagnosis of mycosis fungoides (MF) may be difficult. As an alternative approach to diagnosis, we analyzed DNA from skin biopsies from 21 patients with MF for the configurations of beta, gamma and delta T cell receptor (TCR) genes. Clonal rearrangement of TCR beta genes was detected in 14 of these patients, whereas clonal rearrangement of TCR gamma genes was noted in 16 of them. For the TCR delta chain gene, we detected a mono- or bi-allelic deletion in specimens from all 21 patients. The higher frequency of rearrangement of the TCR gamma gene suggests that this may be a better candidate than the TCR beta gene for detection of monoclonality using the polymerase chain reaction (PCR).

Basic Mechanisms of Physiologic and Aberrant Lymphoproliferation in the Skin
Edited by W.C. Lambert *et al.*, Plenum Press, New York, 1994

INTRODUCTION

Mycosis Fungoides (MF) is a unique cutaneous T-cell malignancy characterized by infiltration of lesional skin by T lymphocytes and by a long clinical course. MF begins as a skin eruption referred to as erythema or patch stage and progresses to tumor stage. The histological picture of fully developed MF is that of a dense lymphocytic infiltrate which occupies the papillary dermis extending into the epidermis. The lymphocytes may invade the epidermis either singly or in groups, forming so-called Pautrier microabscesses. The early stages of MF do not usually have such a characteristic histological pattern, so that the routine histologic diagnosis of early MF is difficult and may require numerous skin biopsies. This is because MF often has a polymorphous infiltrate closely resembling that of other chronic dermatitides. For this reason, many investigators have attempted to develop adjunctive techniques to aid in the evaluation of cutaneous lymphoid infiltrates. Recently, DNA hybridization has been found to be useful in the diagnosis of T-cell malignancy by demonstrating the clonal nature of the disease (Minden et al., 1985; O'Connor et al., 1985; Waldman et al., 1985). Several reports have documented the clonal nature of tumor lesions of MF patients through the demonstration of consistent T cell receptor (TCR) beta chain gene rearrangements (Dosaka et al., 1989; LeBoit and Parslow 1987; Pelicci et al., 1985; Ralfkiaer et al., 1987; Weiss et al., 1985; 1988).

Moreover, in lymph nodes with histologically documented MF involvement, as well as in most lymph nodes of MF patients that histologically showed only dermatopathic lymphadenopathy, clonal TCR beta chain gene rearrangements have been found (Ralfkaier et al., 1987; Weiss et al., 1985; 1989). These data suggest that analysis of TCR genes can be used not only as additional criteria for diagnosing MF, but also for staging of the disease. Skin lesions of early MF (patch or plaque lesions) appear to have the germ-line TCR beta chain gene, however, so that the value of such DNA analysis in the early diagnosis remains unclear (Dosaka et al., 1989; Ralfkaier et al., 1987). Moreover, there is only scattered information about the configuration of the TCR gamma chain gene, and none of the cited studies analyzed the recently characterized TCR delta chain gene. In this study, we have analyzed the configuration of the TCR beta, gamma and delta chain genes in 21 skin biopsies from patients with MF in different stages of the disease in order to clarify when the monoclonality of T cells becames detectable. The results have been correlated with the histologic features and associated immunophenotypes.

MATERIALS AND METHODS

Patients

Biopsy specimens were obtained from 21 patients affected by MF in various stages (Table 1). Each case was evaluated clinically, histologically and immunohistochemically. The clinical evaluation included physical examination, blood count, chest X ray and skin biopsy; patients with enlargement of lymph nodes were further investigated by bone marrow examination and

370

lymph node biopsy. The staging system proposed by the Scandinavian Mycosis Fungoides Cooperative Group was adopted :

Stage I: clinically and histopathologically suspicious lesions of MF

Stage II: plaque lesions of MF , no extracutaneous disease

Stage III: tumor lesions of MF , no extracutaneous disease

Stage IV: MF with enlargement of lymph nodes histologically
                  showing either dermatopathic lymphadenopathy (Stage IVa)
                  or malignant lymphoma (Stage IVb).

A portion of the biopsies were snap frozen in liquid nitrogen and stored at -80° C until used.

Phenotypic analysis

Frozen sections (4μm) of each biopsy specimen were incubated with the following monoclonal antibodies: CD2 (Leu5, Becton Dickinson, Mountain View, CA), CD3 (UCHT1, IV International Workshop on Leukocyte Antigens), CD4 (Leu3a, Becton Dickinson), CD5 (Leu1, Becton Dickinson), CD7 (Leu1, Becton Dickinson), CD8 (Leu2a, Becton Dickinson), CD25 (IL-2R, Becton Dickinson), CD30 (Ber-H2,IV International Workshop on Leukocyte Antigens), BerAct 8 (kindly provided by H. Stein), TCRδ1 (T Cell Science, Cambridge, MA) and BF1 (T Cell Science). A sensitive alkaline phosphatase anti-alkaline phosphatase (APAAP) method was performed (Cordell et al., 1984).

DNA analysis

High molecular weight DNA was extracted from skin, digested to completion with BamHI, EcoRI, Hind III and Bgl II (BRL, Gaithersburg, MD), size fractionated by electrophoresis through a 0.8% agarose gel and transferred to nylon membranes (Genescreen Plus, New England Nuclear, Boston, MA). Prehybridization and hybridization was performed for 16 to 24 hours at 42°C in a solution containing 1 M NaCl, 1% SDS, 10% dextran sulfate and 50% deionized formamide; hybridization solution also contained 100μg/ml salmon sperm DNA. 1×10^6cpm/ml of the labeled probe was added to the hybridization solution. Membranes were washed for 30 minutes successively in 2x SSC/0.1%SDS, followed by a second 30 minute washing in 0.1x SSC/0.1%SDS at 65° C and exposed to XAR-5 film (Eastman Kodak, Rochester, NY) with an intensifying screen at -70°C for one to six days.

DNA probes

The TCR beta chain probe was a 400 base pair(bp) Bgl II cDNA fragment that hybridizes to the constant domains (C) of the TCR beta 1 and beta 2 genes (provided by Dr. T. Mak, Toronto, Canada) (Yoshikai et al., 1984). The TCR gamma chain gene probe was a 0.7 kb Hind III-EcoR I genomic fragment containing the Jγ1 gene (Lefranc et al., 1985).

The TCR delta chain gene probe was a 5 kb EcoR I genomic fragment mapping between Jδ1 and Jδ2 (Hara et al., 1974; Biondi et al., 1989).

Probes were labeled to a high specific activity with ^{32}P using the random primer method (Feinberg and Vogelstein, 1983).

RESULTS AND DISCUSSION

Clinical and immunophenotypic features are summarized in Tables 1 and 2. We examined 21 patients (11 men and 10 women) with MF ranging in age from nine to 80 years. All cases showed typical clinical appearances and satisfied histologic criteria, including epidermotropic lymphoid infiltrates with classical Pautrier microabscesses and several pleomorphic lymphoid cells with medium and large, hyperchromatic and irregular nuclei. With the single exception of case 14, the prevalent immunophenotype of lymphocytes was CD3$^+$, CD2$^+$, CD4$^+$, CD5$^+$, and BF1$^+$ (Table 2). After BamHI, EcoRI and Hind III analysis (Table 3), rearrangements of the TCR beta locus were found in 14 of the patients analyzed (66.6%). In case 13, a rearranged band of 7.9 Kb became apparent after EcoRI digestion, whereas DNA cut by Hind III and BamHI showed a germline configuration. As previously reported, this finding is probably due to an incomplete digestion (van Dongen and Wolvers-Tettero, 1991). The configuration of the TCR gamma locus was determined by probing BamHI, EcoRI and HindIII cut DNA with the Jγ1 probe, which recognizes both Jγ1 and Jγ2 segments. The gamma chain was rearranged in 16 of the patients tested (76.1%). Uniallelic or biallelic deletions of Jδ1 after MH6 hybridization of Bgl II cut DNA were found in all cases. On the basis of the results shown in Tables 2 and 3, no significant difference could be detected in the phenotype with respect to TCR beta and gamma chain rearrangements. Representative patterns of TCR beta and gamma chain gene rearrangements of MF patients are shown in Figures 1 and 2.

Definitive diagnosis of MF, especially in cases of early cutaneous involvement, is still difficult. More recently, Southern blot analysis of antigen receptor gene rearrangements has been helpful in identifyng the clonal nature of some lymphoid tumors (Minden et al., 1985: O'Connor et al., 1985; Waldman et al., 1985), in assigning B or T lineage in cases of unclear phenotype, and in monitoring residual disease. In MF, information about T cell antigen receptor gene rearrangements is scanty and limited to small numbers of cases. In the present study, we analyzed a large panel of cases of MF at different stages of the disease. Over 70% of these were found to have clones of cells rearranged at the TCR beta and gamma loci. Of interest are

Table 1. Clinical and laboratory evaluation of patients with mycosis fungoides.

Case	Age	Sex	Stage	Therapy	Evolution
1	46	M	III er	PUVA + polychemotherapy	Relapse
2	65	M	III	PUVA + Interferon alfa	Remission
3	74	F	III	Radiotherapy + corticosteroid + Interferon alfa	Relapse
4	35	M	II	PUVA	Remission
5	60	F	II + follicular mucinosis	PUVA, retinoids, interferon alfa, corticosteroid	Relapse
6	50	F	II + LP	UVB	Relapse
7	55	M	IVa er	Polychemiotherapy	Relapse
8	55	M	III	PUVA	Remission
9	30	F	III	Polychemiotherapy radiotherapy	Relapse
10	34	F	III	PUVA, electron beam	Remission
11	80	F	III	Inteferon alfa	Exitus
12	20	F	III	Radiotherapy	Remission
13	65	M	III er	Radiotherapy + polychemotherapy	Relapse
14	65	M	III	PWA	Exitus
15	80	F	III + LP	No therapy	Remission
16	70	M	III	PUVA	Remission
17	55	M	III + LP	DDS	Remission
18	70	M	IVa	PUVA	Relapse
19	13	M	I	UVB	Relapse
20	17	F	I	UVB	Remission
21	9	F	I	No therapy	Remission

LP:	Lymphoid papulosis
er:	Erythroderma
PUVA:	Psoralens with ultraviolet A light
DDS:	Diaminodiphenylsulfone (Dapsone)

Table 2. Immunophenotypic analysis of patients with mycosis fungoides.

Case	CD2	CD3	CD4	CD5	CD7	CD8	CD25	CD30	BerAct[s]	Tcrδ1	BF1
1	++	++	++	++	++	-	++	++	-	-	++
2	+·+	++	+	++	++	-	+	-	-	-	++
3	++	++	+	++	-	-	++	++	-	-	++
4	++	++	+	+	+	++	+/-	-	+/-	-	++
5	++	++	++	++	++	-	-	-	-	-	++
6	++	++	++	+	+/-	+/-	-	+/-	-	-	+
7	++	++	++	++	+	+/-	+	-	-	-	+
8	++	++	++	+	++	-	-	+	-	-	+
9	++	++	++	++	+	-	-	-	-	-	+/-
10	++	++	++	+	+/-	+/-	+	-	-	-	++
11	++	++	++	-	-	++	-	-	-	-	++
12	++	++	-	++	-	-	+/-	-	+	-	+
13	++	++	++	++	+/-	+/-	-	-	-	-	-
14	++	++	+	-	+/-	-	-	-	-	+	+/-
15	++	++	++	++	+	-	-	+/-	-	-	++
16	++	++	++	-	-	-	+/-	-	-	-	++
17	++	++	++	++	+	-	-	-	-	-	++
18	++	++	++	++	+	-	-	-	-	-	++
19	++	++	++	+	+	+/-	-	-	-	-	++
20	++	++	++	+	+	+/-	-	-	-	-	++
21	++	++	++	+	+	+/-	-	-	-	-	++

- = 0-10% of positive cells
+/- = 10-30% of positive cells
+ = 30-70% of positive cells
++ = > 70% of positive cells

the results obtained in case 7. The patient showed a clinical enlargement of lymph nodes that histologically were interpreted as dermatopathic lymphadenopathy; DNA analysis revealed the same pattern of rearrangement present in the affected skin, suggesting a secondary localization. No clear correlation between the stage of the disease and the presence of detectable rearranged bands was found. Patients 10 and 17 showed a germ-line configuration at TCR beta and gamma loci even in clinical lesions of tumor stage. Moreover, in other cases (4,5 and 6), we detected clonal rearrangements in patients with plaque lesions of MF. Three cases (19,20 and 21) of suspected MF in a very early stage (unilesional MF) did not show any rearranged bands. Interpretation of these negative results should take into account the sensitivity of the Southern blot analysis, which can

Table 3. Clonal rearrangements of T cell receptor genes in patients with mycosis fungoides.

T CELL RECEPTOR GENES

Case	Stage	Beta			Gamma			Delta
		EcoR I	BamH I	Hind III	EcoR 1	BamH I	Hind III	Bgl II
1	III	R[1]	R	G[2]	R	R	R	D[3]
2	III	R	R	R	R	R	R	D
3	III	RR	R	R	RR	RR	R	D
4	II	RR	R	R	RR	R	R	D
5	II	R	R	R	RR	R	R	D
6	II	R	R	R	R	R	R	D
7 Skin	IVa	R	RR	R	RR	R	RR	D
7 Lymph node		R	R	R	R	R	R	D
8	III	R	R	R	R	R	R	D
9	III	RR	R	G	R	R	R	D
10	III	G	G	G	G	G	G	D
11	III	R	R	G	R	ND[4]	RR	D
12	III	R	R	G	R	ND	RR	D
13	III	R	G	G	R	R	R	D
14	III	R	R	R	R	R	R	D
15	III	G	G	ND	R	ND	R	D
16	III	R	RR	R	R	RR	RR	D
17	III	G	G	G	G	G	G	D
18	IVa	R	ND	R	R	R	R	D
19	I	G	G	G	G	G	G	D
20	I	G	G	G	G	G	G	D
21	I	G	G	G	G	G	G	D

[1]R= rearranged bands (RR, rearrangement of both alleles)
[2]G= germline
[3]D= deleted
[4]ND= not analyzed

detect a clonal lymphoid population comprising 1-5% of the total cells. More recently, the strategy of using polymerase chain reaction (PCR) amplification of the V-D-J junctions has provided a useful tool for monitoring leukemic clones in acute lymphocytic leukemia (ALL) (Macintyre et al., 1990). In this context, due to its limited repertoire of V and J segments and to its extensive junctional diversity, the TCR gamma gene may represent an ideal target for PCR based detection of clonal populations in early stages of MF.

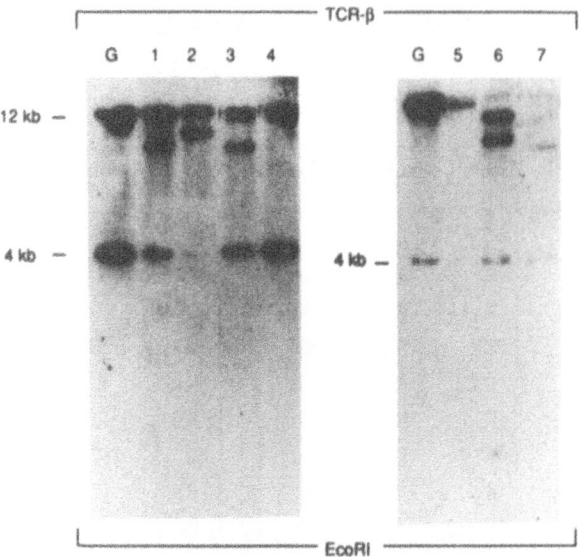

Figure 1. Representative patterns of TCR beta chain gene rearrangements in patients with MF. Lane numbers refer to patients as identified in Table 1. Lane G shows the germline control. DNAs were digested with EcoR I.

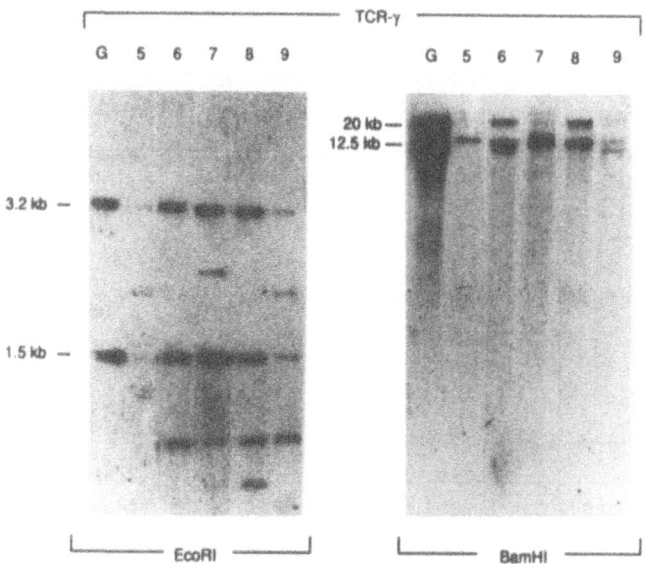

Figure 2. Representative patterns of TCR gamma chain gene rearrangements in patients with MF. Lane number refer to individual patients (See Table 1). Lane G shows the germline control. DNAs were digested with EcoR I and BamH I.

REFERENCES

Biondi A, E Champagne, V Rossi, G Giudici, A Cantu-Rajnoldi, G Masera, A Mantovani, TW Mak and MD Minden, 1989. T Cell receptor delta gene rearrangement in childhood T cell acute lymphoblastic leukemia. **Blood**, 73:2133-2138.

Cordell J, B Falini, WN Erber, A Ghosh, Z Abdulaziz, S MacDonald, K Pulford, H Stein, and DJ Mason: Immunoenzymatic labelling of monoclonal antibodies using immune complexes of alkaline phosphatase and monoclonal anti-alkaline phosphatase (APAAP complexes). **J. Histochem. Cytochem.**, 32:219-229, 1984.

Dosaka N, T Tanaka, M Fujita, Y Miyachi, T Horio, and S Imamura, 1989. Southern blot analysis of clonal rearrangements of T-cell receptor gene in plaque lesion of mycosis fungoides. **J. Invest. Dermatol.**, 93:626-629.

Feinberg AP and B Vogelstein, 1983. A technique for radiolabelling DNA restriction endonuclease fragments to high specific activity. **Anal. Biochem.**, 132:6.

Hara J, SH Benedict, E Champagne, Y Takihara, TW Mak and M Minden, 1988. T cell receptor delta gene rearrangements in acute lymphoblastic leukemia. **J. Clin. Invest.**, 82:1974.

Ho VC, O Baadsgaard, JT Elder, ER Hansen, CA Hanson, GL Vejlsgaard and KD Cooper, 1990. Genotypic analysis of T cell clones derived from cutaneous T cell lymphoma lesions demonstrating selective growth of tumour infiltrating lymphocytes. **J. Invest. Dermatol.** 95:4-8.

Le Boit PE and TG Parslow, 1987. Gene rearrangements in lymphoma: Applications to dermatopathology. **Am. J. Dermatopathol.**, 9:212-218.

Lefranc MP, A Forster and Th Rabbitts, 1985. Two distinct T cell gamma variable region genes rearranged in human DNA. **Nature**, 319:420.

Macintyre EA, L d'Auriol, N Duparc, G Leverger, F Galibert and F Sigaux, 1990. Use of oligonucleotide probes directed against T cell antigen receptor gamma delta variable(diversity) joining junctional sequences as a general method for detecting minimal residual disease in acute lymphoblastic leukemias. **J. Clin. Invest.**, 86:2125-2135.

Minden MD, B Toyonaga, K Ha, Y Yanagi, B Chin, E Gelfand and T Mak, 1985. Somatic rearrangement of T-cell antigen receptor gene in human T-cell malignancies. **Proc. Natl. Acad. Sci. USA**, 82:1224-1227.

O'Connor NTJ, DJ Weatherall, AC Fellen et al., 1985. Rearrangement of the T cell receptor beta chain gene in the diagnosis of lymphoproliferative disorders. **Lancet**, i:1295-1297.

Pelicci PG, DM Knowles and R Dalla Favera, 1985. Lymphoid tumors displaying rearrangements of both immunoglobulin and T cell receptor genes. **J. Exp. Med.**, 162:1015-1024.

Ralfkiaer E, NTJ O'Connor, J Crick, GL Wantzin and DY Mason, 1987. Genotypic analysis of cutaneous T-cell lymphoma. **J. Invest. Dermatol.**, 88:762-765.

Van Dongen JJM and ILM Wolvers-Tettero, 1991. Analysis of immunoglobulin and T cell receptor genes. **Clinica Chimica Acta**, 198:1-174.

Waldmann TA, MM Davis, KF Bongiovanni and SJ Korsmeyer, 1985. Rearrangements of genes for the antigen receptor on T cells as markers of lineage and clonality in human lymphoid neoplasms. **N. Engl. J. Med.**, 313:776-783.

Weiss LM, E Hu, GA Wood GA et al., 1985. Clonal rearrangements of T cell receptor genes in mycosis fungoides and dermatopathic lymphadenopathy. **N. Engl. J. Med.**, 313:539-544.

Weiss LM, GS Wood, BJ Nickoloff and J Sklar, 1988. Gene rearrangement studies in lymphoproliferative disorders of skin. **Adv. Dermatol.**, 3:141-160.

Weiss LM, GS Wood, E Hu, EA Abel, RT Hoppe, J Sklar, 1989. Detection of clonal T cell receptor gene rearrangements in the peripheral blood of patients with mycosis fungoides/Sézary syndrome. **J. Invest. Dermatol.**, 92: 601-604.

Yoshikai Y, D Anatoniou, SP Clark et al., 1984. Sequence and expression of transcripts of the human T cell receptor beta chain genes. **Nature**, 312:521.

THE PATHOGENESIS OF LYMPHOMATOID PAPULOSIS

Sean J. Whittaker

St John's Dermatology Center
St Thomas' Hospital
London, United Kingdom

Correspondence to: Dr. S. J. Whittaker, Department of Dermatology,
St. Thomas' Hospital, Lambeth Palace Road,
London SE1 7H, England, United Kingdon

ABSTRACT

The histogenesis of lymphomatoid papulosis has remained unclear since Macaulay's original studies. Histological and immunohistochemical studies have indicated that the cellular infiltrate is heterogenous and an association with mycosis fungoides, large cell anaplastic lymphoma and Hodgkin disease has been documented. Recent genotypic studies have indicated that the majority of lesions of lymphomatoid papulosis consist of monoclonal T cell populations (Weiss et al., 1986; Kadin et al., 1987). Our studies of eighteen patients, in which we have analyzed immunoglobulin (Ig) and T-cell receptor (TCR) genes, have confirmed these reports and established that recurrent lesions from individuals contain identical T cell clones (Whittaker et al., 1991). In these studies there was no evidence of oligoclonal T cell proliferation, and, in one third of biopsies, no Ig or TCR gene rearrangement was detected. Correlation of our results with the clinicopathologic and immunophenotypic data revealed that T cell clones were limited to patients with "Willemze type B" lymphomatoid papulosis or "mixed type" lymphomatoid papulosis, whereas patients with "type A" lymphomatoid papulosis consistently showed a germline configuration of TCR genes. Therefore, the precise lineage of the atypical CD30 positive cells of "type A" lymphomatoid papulosis has yet to be determined. In addition, recent Southern blot hybridization studies, using a full length HTLV-1 probe (Lambda 23-3) and

Basic Mechanisms of Physiologic and Aberrant Lymphoproliferation in the Skin
Edited by W.C. Lambert *et al.*, Plenum Press, New York, 1994

379

an EBV probe for the large internal repetitive sequence (Bam H1W), have failed to reveal the presence of viral DNA in tissues from these patients with lymphomatoid papulosis.

INTRODUCTION

Lymphomatoid papulosis was originally defined by Macaulay in 1968 as a recurrent, self-healing, cutaneous papulonodular eruption which, although clinically benign, showed histological evidence of malignancy (Macaulay, 1968). While this definition has proved valuable for clinicians, however, the precise histogenesis of lymphomatoid papulosis has been the subject of considerable debate. It is clear from the literature that 10 to 19% of patients with lymphomatoid papulosis may develop an associated malignancy, and development of mycosis fungoides, Hodgkin disease and anaplastic large cell (CD30⁺) lymphomas have all been documented (Sanchez et al., 1983; Weinman et al., 1989; Willemze et al., 1983). At present, however, there are no specific biological markers to delineate this important subgroup of patients. Some authors regard lymphomatoid papulosis and pityriasis lichenoides as part of a clinical and histological spectrum, but this concept has been the subject of intense debate (Black and Wilson Jones, 1972). Clinically, lymphomatoid papulosis is characterised by successive crops of papules, nodules and, occasionally, large ulceronecrotic lesions which undergo necrosis before healing spontaneously to leave varioliform scars. The histological features include a superficial and deep wedge-shaped perivascular infiltrate obscuring the dermoepidermal junction and often associated with epidermal necrosis. The infiltrate usually consists of reactive inflammatory cells, including mononuclear cells, neutrophils and eosinophils, with exocytosis of erythrocytes. The cardinal feature of all biopsies, however, is the presence of medium sized or large atypical mononuclear cells associated with increased numbers of mitoses. By contrast, most authors would agree that the histology of pityriasis lichenoides acuta (PLEVA) is only rarely characterized by a relatively few atypical cells (<10% of the infiltrate) (Black and Wilson Jones, 1972).

Particular controversy surrounds the nature of the cytologically abnormal cells which are characteristic of lymphomatoid papulosis. In 1982, Willemze et al. distinguished two histological subsets of lymphomatoid papulosis: Type A is characterized by predominance of large, atypical cells with abundant cytoplasms, pale vesicular nuclei, and prominent nucleoli with occasional multinucleated cells resembling the Reed-Sternberg cell of Hodgkin disease. Type B is characterized by a population of small or medium-sized mononuclear cells with a hyperchromatic, cerebriform nucleus similar to the Sézary cell of mycosis fungoides (Figure 1). This subdivision is particularly useful because it has served to highlight histological similarities between Type A lymphomatoid papulosis and Hodgkin disease. Indeed, earlier case reports of primary cutaneous Hodgkin disease almost certainly represented lesions of Type A lymphomatoid papulosis (Szur et al., 1970). Unfortunately, this histological distinction has been of less value to clinicians, partly because most lesions of lymphomatoid papulosis consist of a mixed population of atypical cells, and also because both types may be found in different but concurrent lesions from the same patient.

IMMUNOPATHOLOGY

There have been numerous studies attempting to characterize the phenotype of the atypical cells within lesions of lymphomatoid papulosis; various cellular origins have been

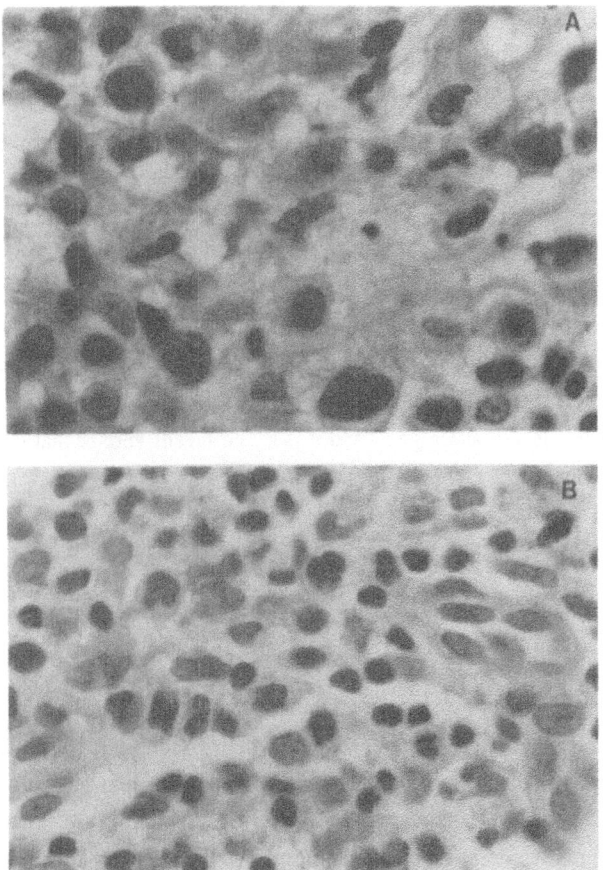

Figure 1. Lymphomatoid papulosis, Willemze's Type A and Type B. (A) Large atypical cells of Willemze Type A lymphomatoid papulosis with abundant cytoplasm, pale vesicular nuclei and prominent nucleoli, with occasional multinucleated forms also present (H&E/oil). (B) Medium sized atypical cells of Willemze Type B lymphomatoid papulosis with hyperchromatic, clefted or cerebriform nuclei (H&E/oil).

suggested, including the monocyte, macrophage, Langerhans cell, interdigitating reticulum cell and activated T lymphocyte (Ralfkiaer et al., 1985). Poppema et al. (1983) suggested that the atypical cells were of monocyte/macrophage origin on the basis of lack of expression of pan T cell markers, enzyme histochemistry and ultrastructural features. Subsequently Willemze et al.

(1983), in their original paper, suggested that the atypical cells in Type A lymphomatoid papulosis had the immunocytochemical and ultrastructural characteristics of Langerhans cells/interdigitating reticulum cells. By contrast, the atypical cells of Type B lymphomatoid papulosis had the immunophenotype of activated T helper lymphocytes. Recent investigations have clearly established that the infiltrates in Type A lesions contain clusters or sheets of large atypical cells which are Ki-1/BerH2 (CD30) positive (Kadin et al., 1985; Kaudewitz et al., 1986; Ralfkiaer et al., 1987). Both these monoclonal antibodies are reactive with Reed-Sternberg and Hodgkin cells and also with some activated T and B lymphocytes (Schwab et al., 1983). Although the large bizarre atypical cells of Type A also express some T cell antigens, specific T cell markers, such as CD3, are frequently lost. Thus the immunological profile of these large atypical cells is similar to that of the Reed-Sternberg cell in Hodgkin disease (Stein et al., 1985). These studies also confirmed earlier impressions that, in Type B lymphomatoid papulosis, the atypical cells represent activated T lymphocytes of the helper subset. Therefore, these phenotypic findings may help to explain the apparent clinical association between lymphomatoid papulosis and both Hodgkin disease and mycosis fungoides, and, indeed, this has prompted Kadin to suggest that these three conditions have a common activated helper T cell origin (Kadin, 1985). However, although this hypothesis is attractive, the origin of the Reed-Sternberg cell of Hodgkin disease is still an enigma, and it is by no means certain that this cell is derived from activated T lymphocytes (Jones, 1987).

LARGE CELL ANAPLASTIC LYMPHOMAS AND REGRESSING ATYPICAL HISTIOCYTOSIS

Over the past few years, it has become apparent that a subgroup of anaplastic lymphomas exists in which the tumor cells express the CD30 antigen. Most of the original cases involved peripheral lymph nodes and were associated with a poor prognosis. It has been established, however, that primary cutaneous large cell anaplastic lymphomas may have a much better prognosis (Feller and Sterry, 1989; Kaudewitz et al., 1989). These CD30+ lymphomas consist, histologically, of a non-epidermotropic monomorphic population of large atypical cells with eccentric oval or reniform shaped nuclei, prominent nucleoli and abundant cytoplasms. Occasionally these cells may resemble immunoblasts or Reed-Sternberg cells. Multinucleated cells are also sometimes present and numerous mitoses are common. Immunohistochemical studies have established that the CD30+ atypical cells have an aberrant T cell phenotype with variable absence of specific T-cell antigens such as CD2, CD3, CD5 and CD7 and expression of the CD4 antigen (Kaudewitz et al., 1989).

In 1982, Flynn et al. described patients with large, self-healing, ulceronecrotic lesions for which he suggested the term, regressing atypical histiocytosis, reflecting the presumed cellular origin. Biopsies show an admixture of reactive inflammatory cells and sheets of large bizarre atypical cells as seen in cutaneous anaplastic lymphomas. An additional striking feature is the presence of pseudoepitheliomatous hyperplasia and occasional erythrophagocytosis. In practice, it can be difficult to distinguish the histological features from lymphomatoid papulosis (Type A) and large cell CD30[+] lymphomas. Furthermore, it has subsequently been established that the atypical cells express the CD30 antigen and have an aberrant T cell phenotype (Headington et al., 1987). Intriguingly, lymphomatoid papulosis has also been described in association with regressing atypical histiocytosis and large cell CD30[+] lymphomas, suggesting that these disorders may have a common histogenesis and that they represent part of a clinical spectrum of CD30[+] cutaneous lymphoproliferative disorders (Cerio and Black, 1990; Murphy et al., 1991).

MOLECULAR GENETICS

Analysis of immunoglobulin and T cell receptor genes has been used extensively to determine the lineage and clonality of lymphoid cell populations (Arnold et al., 1983), and such techniques have now provided considerable insight into the histogenesis of lymphomatoid papulosis. Weiss et al., (1986) reported rearrangements of beta and gamma T cell receptor genes in tissue DNA from five of six patients, while Kadin et al., (1987) found evidence of beta rearrangement in four patients and a polyclonal pattern in a fifth patient. In our studies, we have identified T cell receptor gene rearrangements in tissue DNA from ten of eighteen patients (Whittaker et al., 1991a). Two additional patients had evidence of a polyclonal gamma T cell receptor pattern and six patients consistently had evidence of a germline configuration (Figure 2). Immunoglobulin genes were always present in a germline configuration. These results clearly establish that lymphomatoid papulosis may represent a clonal T cell lymphoproliferative disorder. Weiss et al., (1986) also interpreted the pattern of rearrangement in one patient as being consistent with an oligoclonal T cell proliferation. In our series of thirty one biopsies from eighteen patients, however, we did not find evidence of oligoclonal proliferation, despite analyzing multiple lesions from seven patients. Furthermore, it is also clear from these studies that a significant minority of patients do not have evidence of a clonal T or B-cell population.

TECHNICAL ASPECTS

There are a number of potential explanations for the failure to detect a clonal TCR gene rearrangement; First, with Southern blot analysis, rearranged bands can co-migrate with germline bands, but the use of multiple restriction enzymes and prolonged electrophoresis ensures that this should be a rare occurrence. Second, T cell lymphomas may occasionally have germline configurations for the beta T cell receptor gene while gamma and/or delta T cell receptor genes are rearranged (Foroni et al., 1989; Whittaker et al., 1991b). We did not detect gamma or delta T cell receptor gene rearrangements in biopsies from the six patients with a germline configuration, however. Third, it has been suggested that some lymphomas with a T cell phenotype and a germline configuration may have deleted individual rearranged TCR genes (Weiss et al., 1988), but there is no evidence to support this hypothesis, and, indeed, coincidental deletion of both beta and gamma T cell receptor genes would be extremely unusual, since the genes are located at different chromosomal sites. Finally, a small lymphoid clone could escape detection using conventional Southern blot analysis. Dilution experiments in our laboratory have established that a clone must comprize more than 5% of the total cellular infiltrate before its specific rearrangement can be detected (S. Whittaker and Y. Ng, unpublished data). Of these considerations, the most plausible is that a small T cell clone is present which has escaped detection by Southern blot hybridization. This conclusion may be difficult to accept, however, if the proportion of atypical cells is greater than 10% of the cellular infiltrate, as in our study. In this situation there are two further possible interpretations: Either the atypical cells represent a polyclonal lymphoid population or a proliferation of non-lymphoid cells. (An additional remote possibility is that there is a third, uncharacterized, human TCR molecule, as has been described in other vertebrates). Polyclonal lymphoid populations can be distinguished on Southern blot analysis in two ways: In EcoRI digests, hybridization with a C beta TCR probe produces two germline bands of 12 and 4 kb; absence of the 12 kb band is characteristic of a polyclonal lymphoid population. This pattern was not observed in our studies. In analyzing DNA from skin biopsies, however, this band is invariably detected due to the presence of a significant population of non-lymphoid cells. The gamma TCR gene has only a limited repertoire of V gamma genes, and, therefore, analysis of polyclonal T cell populations produces a series of seven distinct, but faint, rearranged bands of variable intensity after hybridization with a J gamma probe (Le Franc et al., 1986). Such a pattern reflects the proportion of T cells present, and was detected in two of our patients but not in six others with a germline beta TCR gene configuration (Figure 2).

CELLULAR ORIGINS OF CD30 POSITIVE CELLS IN LYMPHOMATOID PAPULOSIS

In our study, a correlation between the abovementioned genotypic studies and histological subtype revealed some interesting observations. Essentially T cell clones were detected in lesions from patients with histological features characteristic either of Willemze Type B lymphomatoid papulosis or of a mixed proliferation of atypical cells. By contrast no evidence of a monoclonal or polyclonal T or B cell proliferation was detected in biopsies with a purely Type A histology. In light of the previous considerations, these observations suggest that the atypical CD30[+] cells may not be of T or B-cell lineage. This interpretation was also supported by the proportions of CD30[+] cells in these six patients (>10%) and results in one patient with a CD3 negative CD4, CD30 positive cutaneous lymphoma in which a germline configuration was detected in both the tumor DNA and a lesion of Type A lymphomatoid papulosis. In Weiss and Kadin's studies, biopsies were classified as either Type A or Type B, and no comment was made regarding lesions with a mixed A/B histology. Both of these patients without evidence of a clonal T cell population had Type A lesions, but, in contrast to our findings, clones were identified in other lesions classified as Type A.

Intriguingly, similar discordant findings have been reported in genotypic studies of patients with both Hodgkin disease and systemic CD30[+] large cell lymphomas (Carbone et al., 1990; Knowles et al., 1986; O'Connor et al., 1987). In Hodgkin disease, immunoglobulin gene rearrangements have been detected in some patients, and T cell receptor gene rearrangements only rarely (Roth et al., 1988). Moreover, in an important study, Knowles et al. (1986) failed to identify either immunoglobulin or T cell receptor gene rearrangements in biopsies containing more than 25% Reed-Sternberg cells. In studies of CD30[+] systemic lymphomas, O'Connor et al., (1987), found evidence of a clonal B or T cell proliferation in some patients and a non-B, non-T cell proliferation in others. These findings suggest that the CD30 antigen may not be lineage-specific and, indeed, embryonic carcinoma cells (Pallesen and Hamilton-Dutiot, 1988)

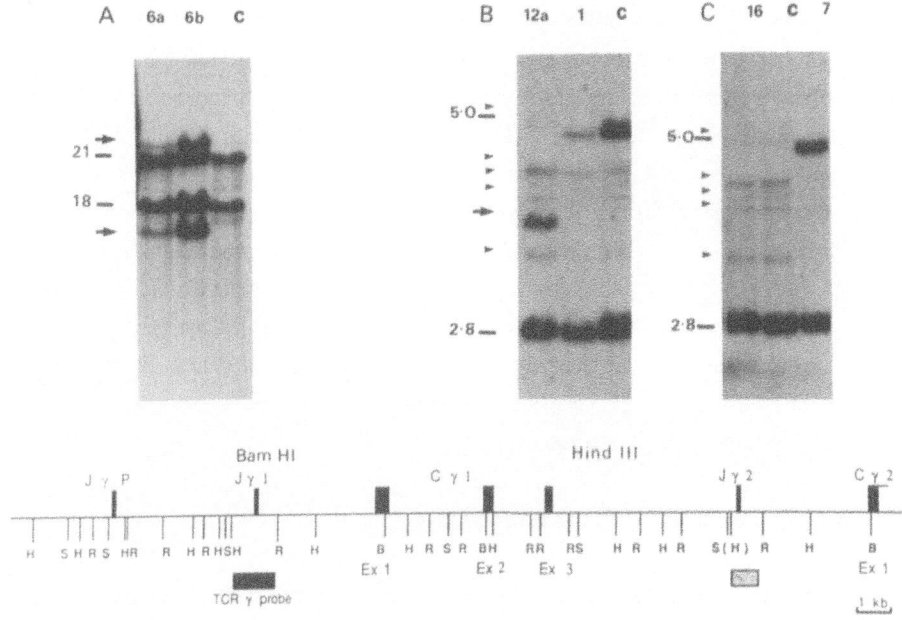

Figure 2. Southern blot analysis of DNA from patients with lymphomatoid papulosis and from peripheral blood mononuclear cells of normal individuals (C) digested with Bam H1 (A) and Hind III (B and C), and hybridized with JY TCR probe (M13H60) indicated by the solid bar. The dotted bar identifies a region of DNA (Jα2) which shows a high degree of homology to this probe. The position and size (kb) of germline fragments are indicated by bars, while discrete rearranged bands are identified by large arrows. Multiple discrete rearranged bands characteristic of polyclonal T cell populations are indicated by small arrows. (A) Identical discrete rearranged bands are present in two different lesions (6a and 6b) from the same patient. (B and C) Analysis of sample 12a shows a discrete rearranged band indicative of a monoclonal T cell population with additional bands of weaker intensity. Multiple additional bands of similar intensity are also present in samples 1, 16 and both controls, consistent with a polyclonal T cell population. By contrast, analysis of tissue from patient 7 only reveals 2 germline fragments. Absence of the 5.0 kb germline band in samples 1, 12a, 16 and one of the controls is due to the presence of a polymorphic Hind III restriction site (H).

and monocytes/macrophages have also been found to express this antigen (Andreesen et al., 1989). Therefore, while the term, CD30[+] lymphoma, is a useful clinicopathological and immunophenotypic designation, it does not necessarily imply that of all these lymphomas share a common histogenesis.

TUMOR PROGRESSION

Unfortunately, there is still insufficient data to accurately predict the biological behavior of lymphomatoid papulosis. Weiss et al., (1987) identified T cell clones in three patients with pityriasis lichenoides acuta, and we have confirmed this result in one patient (S. Whittaker and Y. Ng, unpublished data). This finding strengthens the case of those who have proposed that lymphomatoid papulosis and pityriasis lichenoides are related disorders which are only distinguished by the degree of cellular atypia. It emphasizes, however, that the presence of a T cell clone is not synonymous with malignant progression. We have also had the opportunity to study one patient with coexistent poikiloderma, plaque stage mycosis fungoides and lymphomatoid papulosis in whom we found identical T cell clones in biopsies from lesions of both lymphomatoid papulosis and mycosis fungoides (Whittaker et al., 1991b). This clearly establishes that both conditions can be derived from the same lymphoid clone. By contrast, we failed to identify a T cell clone in one patient with lymphomatoid papulosis (Type A) and a $CD30^+$ cutaneous lymphoma. Intriguingly, in a patient with both lymphomatoid papulosis and "regressing atypical histiocytosis," we found a T cell clone within lesions of lymphomatoid papulosis but not in those of the latter entity (Murphy et al., 1991). These findings require confirmation in larger studies, but clearly establish that clonality is not necessarily a marker of malignant progression in lymphomatoid papulosis.

VIRUSES AND LYMPHOMATOID PAPULOSIS

Despite these advances, the underlying etiology of lymphomatoid papulosis remains unknown. The retrovirus, HTLV-1, is associated with adult T cell leukemia/lymphoma, which frequently involves the skin (Yoshida et al., 1982). This has prompted speculation that mycosis fungoides may also be associated with a retroviral infection, possibly related to HTLV-1. In fact, 11% of patients from a non-endemic area had positive serology for HTLV-1 using an ELISA technique, including three patients with lymphomatoid papulosis (Lange Wantzin et al., 1986). Type C retroviral particles have been identified in tissues from patients with mycosis fungoides using electron microscopy, but no such similar findings have been described in lymphomatoid papulosis (Slater et al., 1985). Weiss et al. (1986) suggested that lymphomatoid papulosis may be associated with a viral infection because of the presence of oligoclonal T cell proliferation in one of their patients. This pattern has been described in EBV associated B-cell lymphomas developing in immunosuppressed patients, particularly after organ transplantation (Cleary and Sklar, 1984). Recently, Anagnostopoulos et al. (1990) detected HTLV-1 proviral sequences in CD30 positive large cell cutaneous lymphomas, and it is known that CD30 antigen expression may be induced on lymphoid cells after viral transformation. As part of a larger study, we have attempted to determine whether there is evidence of HTLV-1, proviral integration within tumor DNA from patients with lymphomatoid papulosis and other forms of CTCL. This has involved the use of Southern blot hybridization with a full length HTLV-1 probe (Lambda 23-3) (Clarke et al., 1983) and in vitro amplification of a specific HTLV-1 polymerase (pol) gene sequence using primers SK 54 and 55 (Kwok et al., 1988). In patients with lymphomatoid papulosis, however, these methods have consistently produced negative results. Epstein-Barr viral (EBV) infection is associated with endemic forms of Burkitt lymphoma and has been occasionally implicated in the etiology of other lymphomas. In particular, recent reports have identified EBV DNA in 19% of patients with Hodgkin disease: In situ hybridization techniques have localized EBV nucleic acid to Reed-Sternberg cells; and Southern blot hybridization studies have suggested that a subset of patients with Hodgkin disease have a clonal proliferation of EBV infected cells (Weiss et al., 1989). In addition, EBV viral DNA has been detected in some peripheral T cell lymphomas, suggesting that the virus may not only infect B-cells, but also T cells (Jones et al., 1988). We have, therefore, analyzed tissue DNA from patients with lymphomatoid papulosis for evidence of EBV genome using Southern blot hybridization with a specific EBV probe for an internal repetitive sequence of the EBV genome (BAM H1W) (Fischer et al., 1981). This probe does not cross-hybridize with human genomic DNA, and so represents a valuable screening method. No evidence of EBV DNA was found in BAM H1 digests from the patients studied, however. The use of PCR techniques would allow the detection of small numbers of EBV infected cells within lesions of lymphomatoid papulosis, but this technique would potentially amplify EBV genome from rare, immortalized B cells, which are present in most adults who have been exposed to Epstein-Barr virus. Obviously, these studies do not exclude a viral etiology, and an association between lymphomatoid papulosis and a retrovirus, which might be closely related to HTLV-1, merits further study.

FUTURE PERSPECTIVES

It has now been clearly established that, in the majority of patients, lymphomatoid papulosis represents a monoclonal T cell lymphoproliferative disorder. This is consistent with the clinical course of the disease in most patients, because clonality is a cardinal feature of neoplasia, whether it be benign or malignant. Indeed, lymphomas are known to show evidence of regression occasionally (Krikorian et al., 1980), and the concept of benign lymphomas has recently been proposed (Slater, 1990). The cellular origin of the large Reed-Sternberg-like cells characteristic of Willemze Type A lymphomatoid papulosis remains elusive, however. In fact, the confusion is reminiscent of that surrounding the origin of the Reed-Sternberg cell in Hodgkin disease itself. Methods of in vitro amplification using PCR are now being employed to detect clonal T cell receptor gene rearrangements in lymphoid neoplasms (McCarthy et al., 1991) and, perhaps, such techniques may help to clarify the cellular origin of the atypical cells in Type A lymphomatoid papulosis. Could it be that these cells are hybrids, formed by somatic fusion of macrophages and lymphocytes, as has been suggested for the Reed-Sternberg cell of Hodgkin disease?

Further clarification of the histogenesis of lymphomatoid papulosis awaits the characterization of specific chromosomal abnormalities. Cytogenetic studies on cells from lesions of lymphomatoid papulosis are technically difficult, and have previously failed to reveal non-random karyotypic abnormalities. A specific chromosomal translocation involving 5q35 has been identified, however, in a large proportion of CD30[+] large cell lymphomas (Mason et al., 1990). The establishment of cell lines from a number of these patients should allow the cloning of the break-point on chromosome 5 in the near future. A full characterization of this cytogenetic abnormality may explain the expression of the CD30 antigen in these lymphomas, and it will be essential to explore the involvement of this translocation in cases of lymphomatoid papulosis.

The relationship of lymphomatoid papulosis to other disorders, such as pityriasis lichenoides acuta, regressing atypical histiocytosis, mycosis fungoides and CD30[+] lymphomas may well reflect the presence of both specific chromosomal abnormalities and the degree of host immune response. As such, lymphomatoid papulosis represents a unique in vivo model of tumorigenesis, because it provides the seeds of its own destruction. An elucidation of the mechanism of regression would be of great potential interest and may well reflect the interaction of the two distinct populations of atypical cells originally delineated by Willemze.

REFERENCES

Anagnostopoulos I, M Hummel, P Kaudewitz, H Hubst, O Braun Falco, and H Stein, 1990. Detection of HTLV-1 proviral sequences in CD30 positive large cell cutaneous T cell lymphomas. **Am. J. Pathol.**, 137:1317.

Andreesen R, W Bruffer, G Lohr and K Bross, 1989. Human macrophages can express the Hodgkin cell-associated antigen Ki-1 (CD30). **Am. J. Pathol.**, 134:187

Arnold A, J Cossman, A Bakhshi, E Jaffe, TA Waldman and SJ Korsmejer, 1983. Immunoglobulin gene rearrangements as unique clonal markers in human lymphoid neoplasms. **N. Engl. J.** Med., 29:1593.

Black M and E Wilson Jones, 1972. Lymphomatoid pityriasis lichenoides; A variant with histological features simulating a lymphoma. **Brit. J. Dermatol.**, 86:329.

Carbone A, A Gloghini, V De Re, P Tamaro, M Boiocchi and R Volpe, 1990. Histopathologic, immunophenotypic and genotypic analysis of Ki-1 anaplastic large cell lymphomas that express histiocyte associated antigens. **Cancer**, 66:2547.

Cerio R and M Black, 1990. Regressing atypical histiocytosis and lymphomatoid papulosis: Variants of the same disorder. **Brit. J. Dermatol.**, 123:515.

Clarke M, E Gelmann and M Reitz, 1983. Homology of human T cell leukaemia virus envelope gene with class 1 HLA gene. **Nature**, 305:60.

Cleary M and J Sklar, 1984. Lymphoproliferative disorders in cardiac transplant recipients are multiclonal lymphomas. **Lancet**, 2:489.

Espinoza C, B Erkman-Balis and N Feuske, 1985. Lymphomatoid papulosis: A pre-malignant T cell disorder. **J. Am. Acad. Dermatol.**, 13:736.

Feller, A. and W. Sterry, 1989. Large cell anaplastic lymphoma of the skin. **Brit. J. Dermatol.**, 121:593.

Fischer D, G Miller, L Gradoville, L Heston, M Weststrate, W Maris, J Wright, J Brandsma and W Summers, 1981. Genome of a mononucleosis Epstein-Barr virus contains DNA fragments previously regarded to be unique to Burkitt's lymphoma isolates. **Cell**, 24:543.

Flynn K, L Dehner, K Gajl-Peczalska, M Dahl, N Ramsey and N Wang, 1982. Regressing atypical histiocytosis. **Cancer**, 49:959.

Foroni L, M Laffan, T Boehm, TH Rabbitts, D Catovsky and L Luzzatto, 1989. Rearrangement of the delta-cell receptor genes in human T cell leukaemias. **Blood**, 73:559.

Headington J, M Roth and B Schnitzer, 1987. Regressing atypical histiocytosis: A review and critical appraisal. **Sem. Diag. Pathol.**, 4:28.

Jones D, 1987. The histogenesis of the Reed-Sternberg cell and its mononuclear counterparts. **J. Pathol.**, 151:191.

Jones J, S Shurin, C Abramowsky, R Tubbs, C Sciotto, R Wahl, J Sands, D Gottman, B Katz and J Sklar, 1988. T cell lymphomas containing Epstein-Barr viral DNA in patients with chronic Epstein-Barr virus infections. **N. Engl. J. Med.**, 318:733.

Kadin M, 1985. Common activated helper-T cell origin for lymphomatoid papulosis, mycosis fungoides and some types of Hodgkin disease. **Lancet**, 864.

Kadin M, K Nasu, D Sako, J Said and E Vonderheid, 1985. Lymphomatoid papulosis: A cutaneous proliferation of activated helper-T cells expressing Hodgkin disease associated antigens. **Am. J. Pathol.**, 119:315.

Kadin M, E Vonderheid, D Sako, L Clayton and S Olbricht, 1987. Clonal composition of T cells in lymphomatoid papulosis. **Am. J. Pathol.**, 126:13.

Kaudewitz P, H Stein, G Burg, D Mason and O Braun-Falco, 1986. Atypical cells in lymphomatoid papulosis express the Hodgkin cell-associated antigen Ki-1. **J. Invest. Dermatol.**, 86:350.

Kaudewitz P, H Stern, F Dallenbach, F Eckert, K Bleber, G Burg and O Braun-Falco, 1989. Primary and secondary cutaneous Ki-1 (CD30+ve) anaplastic large cell lymphomas. **Am. J. Pathol.**, 135:359.

Knowles D, A Neri, P Pelicci, J Burke, A Wu, C Winberg, K Sheiban and R Dalla-Favera, 1986. Immunoglobulin and TCR chain gene rearrangement analysis of Hodgkin disease: Implications for lineage determination and differential diagnosis. **Proc. Natl. Acad. Sci. USA.**, 83:7942.

Krikorian J, C Portlock, D Cooney and S Rosenberg, 1980. Spontaneous regression of non-Hodgkin lymphoma: A report of nine cases. **Cancer**, 46:2093.

Kwok S, G Ehrlich, B Poiesz, R Kalish and J Sninsky, 1988. Enzymatic amplication of HTLV-1 viral sequences from peripheral blood mononuclear cells and infected tissues. **Blood**, 72:1117.

Lange Wantzin G, K Thamsen, N Nissen, C Saxinger and R Gallo, 1986. Occurrence of human T cell lymphotropic virus (type 1) antibodies in cutaneous T cell lymphoma. **J. Am. Acad. Dermatol.** 15:598.

Le Franc M, A Forster, R Baer, M Stinson and TH Rabbitts, 1986. Diversity and rearrangement of the human T cell rearranging genes: Nine germline gamma variable genes belonging to two subgroups. **Cell**, 45:237.

Macaulay WL, 1968. Lymphomatoid papulosis: A continuing self healing eruption, clinically benign-histologically malignant. **Arch. Dermatol.**, 97:23.

Mason D, C Bastard, R Rimokh, N Dastugue, JL Huret, U Kristoffersson, JP Magaud, C Nezelof, H Tilly, JP Vanner, J Hemet and R Warnke, 1990. CD30 positive large cell lymphomas (Ki-1 lymphoma) are associated with a chromosomal translocation involving 5q35. **Brit. J. Haematol.**, 74:161.

McCarthy K, J Sloane, J Kabarowski, E Matutes and L Wiedemann, 1991. The rapid detection of clonal T cell proliferations in patients with lymphoid disorders. **Am. J. Pathol.**, 138:821.

Murphy G, R Cerio, S Whittaker, E Wilson Jones and W Griffiths, 1991. Regressing atypical histiocytosis - like lesions in association with lymphomatoid papulosis. **Proc. 1st Congress. E.A.D.V.**, 573.

O'Connor N, H Stein, K Gatter, J Wainscoat, J Crick, T Saati, B Fallini, G Delsol and D Mason, 1987. Genotypic analysis of large cell lymphomas which express the Ki-1 antigen. **Histopathology**, 11:733.

Pallesen G and S Hamilton-Dutiot, 1988. Ki-1 (CD30) antigen is regularly expressed by tumor cells of embryonal carcinoma. **Am. J. Pathol.**, 133:446.

Poppema S, P Voorst Vader, T Rozeboom-Uiterwijk and J Dijkstra, 1983. Lymphomatoid papulosis. **Cancer**, 52:1178.

Ralfkiaer E, J Bosce, K Gatter, R Schwarting, J Gerdes, H Stein and D Mason, 1987. Expression of a Hodgkin and Reed-Sternberg cell-associated antigen (Ki-1) in cutaneous lymphoid infiltrates. **Arch. Dermatol. Res.**, 279:285.

Ralfkiaer E, H Stein, G Lange Wantzin, K Thomsen, N Ralfkiaer and D Mason, 1985. Lymphomatoid papulosis: Characterisation of skin infiltrates by monoclonal antibodies. **Am. J. Clin. Pathol.**, 84:587.

Roth M, B Sghnitler, E Bingham, C Harnden, D Hyder and D Ginsburg, 1988. Rearrangement of immunoglobulin and TCR genes in Hodgkin disease. **Am. J. Pathol.**, 131:331.

Sanchez N, M Pittelkow, S Muller, P Banks and R Winkelmann, 1983. The clinicopathological spectrum of lymphomatoid papulosis: Study of 31 cases. **J. Am. Acad. Dermatol.**, 8:81.

Schwab U, H Stein, J Gerdes, H Lemke, H Kirchner, M Schaadt and V Diehl, 1983. Production of a monoclonal antibody specific for Hodgkin and Sternberg-Reed cells of Hodgkin disease and a subset of normal lymphoid cells. **Nature**, 299:65.

Slater D, 1990. Clonal dermatoses: A conceptual and diagnostic dilemma. **J. Pathol.**, 162:1.

Slater D, N Rooney, S Bleehen and A Hamed, 1985. The lymph node in mycosis fungoides: A light and electron microscopy and immunohistological study supporting the Langerhans cell retrovirus hypothesis. **Histopathology**, 9:587.

Stein H, D Mason, J Gerdes, N O'Connor, J Wainscoat, G Pallesen, K Gatter, B Falini, G Delsol, K Lemke, R Schwarting and K Lennert, 1985. The expression of the Hodgkin's disease associated antigen Ki-1 in reactive and neoplastic lymphoid tissue: Evidence that Reed-Sternberg cells and histiocytic malignancies are derived from activated lymphoid cells. **Blood**, 66:848.

Szur L, C Harrison, G Levene and P Samman, 1970. Primary cutaneous Hodgkin disease. **Lancet**, 1:1016.

Weinman VF and AB Ackerman, 1981. Lymphomatoid papulosis: A critical review and new findings. **Am. J. Dermatopathol.**, 3:129.

Weiss L, L Movahed, R Warne and J Sklar, 1989. Detection of Epstein-Barr viral genomes in Reed-Sternberg cells of Hodgkin disease. **N. Engl. J. Med.**, 320:520.

Weiss L, L Picker, T Grogan, R Warnke and J Sklar, 1988. Absence of clonal beta and gamma T cell receptor gene rearrangements in a subset of peripheral T cell lymphomas. **Am. J. Pathol.**, 130:436.

Weiss L, F Wood, L Ellisen, T Reynolds and J Sklar, 1987. Clonal T cell populations in pityriasis lichenoides et varioliformis acuta (Mucha-Habermann disease). **Am. J. Pathol.**, 126:417.

Weiss L, G Wood, M Trela, R Warnke and J Sklar, 1986. Clonal T cell populations in lymphomatoid papulosis. **N. Engl. J. Med.**, 315:475.

Whittaker S, N Smith, R Russell Jones and L Luzzatto, 1991a. Analysis of beta, gamma and delta TCR genes in lymphomatoid papulosis: Cellular basis of two distinct histologic subsets. **J. Invest. Dermatol.**, 96:786.

Whittaker S, N Smith, R Russell Jones and L Luzzatto, 1991b. Analysis of beta, gamma and delta TCR genes in mycosis fungoides and Sézary syndrome. **Cancer.** 68:1572.

Willemze R, CM Meijer, W Van Vloten and E Scheffer, 1982. The clinical and histological spectrum of lymphomatoid papulosis. **Br. J. Dermatol.**, 107:131.

Willemze R, E Scheffer, DJ Ruiter, W Van Vloten and CM Meijer, 1983. Immunological, cytochemical and ultrastructural studies in lymphomatoid papulosis. **Br. J. Dermatol.**, 108:381.

Willemze R, E Scheffer, W Van Vloten and CM Meijer, 1983. Lymphomatoid papulosis and Hodgkin disease: Are they related? **Arch. Dermatol. Res.**, 275:159.

Yoshida M, I Miyoshi and Y Hinuma, 1982. Isolation and characterisation of retrovirus from cell lines of human adult T cell leukaemia and its implication in the disease. **Proc. Natl. Acad. Sci. USA**, 79:2031.

T CELL RECEPTOR VARIABLE REGION GENE EXPRESSION IN CUTANEOUS T-CELL LYMPHOMA

Martine Bagot
Janine Wechsler
Marie-Claude Lescs
Jean Revuz
Philippe Gaulard

Department of Dermatology
Department of Pathology
Henri Mondor Hospital
Creteil, France

Correspondence to: Dr. M. Bagot, Department of Dermatology, Hosp. Henri Mondor, 51 Av. du M. de Lattre de Tass, 94010 Creteil, France

ABSTRACT

T lymphocytes interact with antigen and major histocompatibility complex via a specific T-cell receptor (TCR). Monoclonal antibodies to the variable region of TCR gene products have been produced that identify minor populations of normal peripheral blood T lymphocytes. These antibodies may detect clonal T-cell proliferations which express the same $V\beta$ gene. An initial report using two anti-V region antibodies suggested that cutaneous T-cell lymphomas preferentially express the $V\beta8$ gene. However, several other studies with a larger panel of seven antibodies have not confirmed the restricted use of some $V\beta$ segments. Indeed, we and others have found that, using this antibody panel, only a minority of cutaneous T-cell lymphomas was stained by one of these anti-V region antibodies, although, in two cases, it allowed us to demonstrate the strictly epidermotropic localization of clonal proliferation in plaque stage mycosis fungoides. Therefore, at the present time, immunohistological staining with these antibodies

Basic Mechanisms of Physiologic and Aberrant Lymphoproliferation in the Skin
Edited by W.C. Lambert *et al.*, Plenum Press, New York, 1994

393

cannot replace molecular biological methods, either for the demonstration of clonality in T-cell lymphoma, or for distinguishing between benign lymphoid infiltrates and malignant lymphoma. Their usefulness as potentially virtually clonotypic markers in T-cell lymphoma needs to be reevaluated when a larger panel of antibodies becomes available.

INTRODUCTION

Specific immune recognition by T lymphocytes resides within the T cell receptor (TCR), a heterodimeric glycoprotein non-covalently linked to the T cell surface antigen, CD3 (Acuto et al., 1985). This molecule is responsible for recognition of antigen associated with the major histocompatibility complex (MHC). The majority of mature T lymphocytes bears an $\alpha\beta$ TCR, composed of a 50 kD α-chain and a 43 kD β-chain. The variable regions of the α and β chains create a V domain that binds antigen and MHC molecules (Marrack et al., 1987). α and β chains have variable (V), junctional (J), and constant (C) region genes coding for the corresponding regions of the T cell receptor, and the β chain has an additional diversity (D) region (Wilson et al., 1988). The great diversity of T cell specificities is induced by rearrangements of these germline segment genes. These rearrangements occur in the thymus during T cell ontogeny and lead to the T cell antigen receptor repertoire. In humans, the pool of $V\gamma$ gene segments is estimated to contain a hundred members grouped into at least 19 families based on percent homology at the nucleic acid level (Klein et al., 1987; Toyonaga et al., 1987). The pool of $V\beta$ gene segments contains approximately 70 members grouped into at least 18 families (Acuto et al., 1989; Concannon et al., 1986; Kimura et al., 1986). Each family is composed of 1 to 10 homologous members. Monoclonal antibodies to V region TCR gene products have been produced by immunizing mice with human T cell tumor lines (Bigler et al., 1983; Boylston et al., 1984). Some of them identify minor populations of normal peripheral blood T lymphocytes (Boylston et al., 1986; Carrel et al., 1986). They recognize either all members of a V region family, a subset of the V region within a family or a particular V region only. The exact epitope, however, is not always precisely defined.

$V\beta$ GENE EXPRESSION IN NORMAL AND PATHOLOGIC TISSUES

In spite of the broad diversity of V genes, it has been shown that the T cell receptor uses only a limited repertoire of expressed $V\beta$ segments, and that somatic mutations are extremely rare (Barth et al., 1985). Moreover, preferential use of TCR V genes by T cells responsive to defined antigens has been demonstrated in several studies (Hochgeschwender et al., 1987; Kappler et al., 1989; Morel et al., 1987; Sorger et al., 1987). TCR $V\beta$ genes may be linked to certain diseases (Seboun et al., 1989). Anti-V region antibodies therefore appear to be useful tools to study T cell mediated immune responses and T cell mediated human diseases. Stimulation of lymphoid cells with staphylococcal toxins leads to proliferation of T lymphocytes expressing a restricted range of $V\beta$ families (Kappler et al., 1989). Preferential usage of particular V genes has also been found in autoimmune diseases (Wraith et al., 1989). Murine experimental encephalomyelitis is characterized by the expansion of $V\beta8$-expressing T-lymphocytes, and can be reversed by the injection of anti-Vβ8 antibodies (Acha-Orbea et al., 1988; Urban et al., 1988). Patients with active pulmonary sarcoidosis have expanded proportions of T cells expressing the Vβ8 idiotope in lung and blood (Moller et al., 1988). Such a preferential use of Vβ8 genes has also been demonstrated in lymphocytes from patients with Crohn disease (Posnett et al., 1990).

ANTI-V REGION ANTIBODIES IN LYMPHOMA AND LEUKEMIA

The diagnosis of T-cell lymphoma relies on histological examination and immunohisto-chemistry. In B-cell lymphoma, clonality is easily demonstrated by the presence of light chain restriction. By contrast, no adequate immunohistological technique is currently available for the demonstration of T-cell monoclonality. Molecular biological methods are necessary to detect clonality, using TCR gene probes. Immunohistological staining with anti-V region antibodies may have potential as a simple method useful in routine pathology, able to detect clonal proliferations of T-cells expressing the same Vβ gene. This might also be useful for evaluation of response to therapy, and for detection of an early relapse. Each anti V region antibody reacts with a minor population of normal peripheral blood lymphocytes (0-5%). Staining of normal lymph nodes shows only scattered lymphocytes, with no evidence of clustering (Clark et al., 1989; O'Grady et al., 1990).

Only a few studies using these antibodies for evaluation of lymphomas have been reported so far. Clark et al., have studied twenty T-cell lymphomas and four T-cell leukemias with two monoclonal antibodies specific for Vβ5 and Vβ8. Three cases of T-cell lymphoma were positive (two with anti-Vβ8 and one with anti-Vβ5; Clark et al., 1986).

A larger panel of seven antibodies to TCR V-region products was used by O'Grady et al., (1990) to stain three reactive lymph nodes, 10 B-cell lymphomas, and 35 T-cell lymphomas, including four cases of mycosis fungoides and two of Sézary syndrome. Five cases (three of mycosis fungoides, one of immunoblastic lymphoma and one of lymphoblastic lymphoma) were stained by one of these antibodies (one with Vβ5a, three with Vβ8a and one with Vβ6), whereas other antibodies stained less than 1% of cells. One case of mycosis fungoides showed reactivity with both anti-Vβ5a and anti-Vβ8a. All positive cases also expressed CD3 and reacted with βF1, an antibody to a nonpolymorphic determinant on the intracytoplasmic portion of the TCR-β chain. None of the cases showing loss of expression of the TCR β-chain or of CD3 was stained by the anti-clonotypes (O'Grady et al., 1990).

Poppema and Hepperle (1991) studied a series of 44 T-cell lymphomas (8 lymphoblastic lymphomas, 8 lymphocytic lymphomas including 3 cases of Sézary syndrome, 16 mixed small and large cell lymphomas and 12 large cell lymphomas) with a panel of seven reagents reactive with four different TCR β-chain variable region families. Nine cases (20%) showed clonal staining with one of the antibodies (four with Vβ5.1, one with Vβ5.2, one with Vβ6.7, two with Vβ8 and one with Vβ12). These cases represented 29% of TCR positive lymphomas. Most large cell T-cell lymphomas did not express TCR despite the presence of cytoplasmic CD3. No preferential use of specific families could be demonstrated (Poppema, and Hepperle, 1991).

ANTI-V REGION ANTIBODIES IN CUTANEOUS T-CELL LYMPHOMA

Some other studies have focused on cutaneous T-cell lymphomas. Charley et al., tested three Sézary patients and found, in one, that anti-Vβ5 antibody stained the majority of peripheral blood and nodal lymphocytes and induced proliferation of leukemic cells in vitro (Charley et al., 1990).

Using two anti-V region antibodies (Vβ5 and Vβ8), Jack et al., studied the skin infiltrates of 16 cases of mycosis fungoides. They found that 10 of them were stained by the monoclonal antibody specific for the Vβ8 family, one of them reacting with both anti-Vβ5 and Vβ8 antibodies (Jack et al., 1990). All cases of plaque or tumor stage cutaneous T-cell lymphoma were positive, whereas the 6 negative cases were reported as eczematoid stage. These exciting results suggested that cutaneous T-cell lymphoma might derive from defined lymphocyte subpopulations, possibly selected by some specific antigenic contacts.

These results have not been confirmed by more recent studies using a wider range of seven commercially available antibodies, however. The expression of TCR V genes in the skin was studied by Ho et al., in eight cutaneous T cell lymphomas and a T-cell line derived from a patient with Sézary syndrome. They could find no reactivity with any of the anti-V region antibodies (Ho et al., 1991). Hunt et al., studied the V region expression of ten cases of cutaneous T cell lymphoma (6 with plaque/tumor stage mycosis fungoides, three with Sézary syndrome and one with follicular mucinosis). Only one patient with Sézary syndrome had significant anti-Vβ5 staining (Hunt et al., 1991).

Using the immunoalkaline phosphatase (APAAP) technique, we have studied the expression of seven TCR variable region genes in 18 cutaneous T cell lymphomas (14 mycosis fungoides, 1 Sézary syndrome, 1 pleomorphic lymphoma, 1 anaplastic large cell lymphoma, and 1 HTLV-1-related pleomorphic lymphoma). All cases showed strong staining with anti-CD3 and βF1. In all cases, except two patients with mycosis fungoides, the anti-V region antibodies stained only scattered cells, representing 1 to 5% of the infiltrate. In one patient, the majority of cells of the infiltrate in both the epidermis and the dermis stained with anti-Vγ2 antibody. These cells expressed all pan-T antigens and were CD4$^+$, CD8$^-$. In another patient with plaque stage mycosis fungoides, lymphoid cells were CD2$^+$, CD3$^+$, CD4$^+$, CD7$^-$, CD8$^-$. Loss of the CD5 antigen and staining with anti-V$\alpha\beta$ antibody were restricted to intraepidermal cells.

Similar results have been reported by Boehncke et al., who were unable to demonstrate clonality in most of 30 cases of mycosis fungoides. However, a strictly epidermotropic clone, with 26% of proliferating cells staining with anti-Vβ8, was found in two early lesions in one patient (Boehncke et al., 1991).

ANTI-V REGION ANTIBODIES IN BENIGN CUTANEOUS LYMPHOID INFILTRATES

Benign lymphoid reactions of the skin may develop T-cell predominant lymphoid infiltrates. Clinical and histological differentiation from malignant lymphoma is often very difficult. In these conditions, it is interesting to evaluate whether immunohistological staining with anticlonotypic antibodies can help to detect early clonal proliferations or demonstrate preferential use of some TCR Vβ genes.

In a limited study of eight cutaneous T-cell lymphoid infiltrates (two of parapsoriasis en plaques, one of lymphomatoid papulosis, one of drug-induced pseudolymphoma, and four of chronic contact dermatitis), we found no evidence of clonality, and only random use of TCR Vβ genes, since the anti-V region antibodies stained only a few scattered cells.

CONCLUSIONS

Anti-TCR V region antibodies are new tools to study cutaneous T-cell lymphomas and lymphoid infiltrates. These antibodies can help to identify the malignant clone in TCR-positive T-cell lymphomas, and may show the strictly epidermotropic localization of clonal proliferation in some cases of plaque stage mycosis fungoides. They may help us to better understand the pathophysiology of lymphoproliferative disorders and to study the repertoire of T lymphocytes in the skin. However, the panel of antibodies currently available does not identify all variable region epitopes, and only a minority of cutaneous T-cell lymphomas are stained. Thus, several recent studies have not confirmed the preferential usage of Vβ8 initially reported in cutaneous T cell lymphoma. Positivity may also be hampered by loss of TCR expression by neoplastic cells. Therefore, as of now, immunostaining with these antibodies cannot replace genotypic studies, either for demonstration of clonality in T-cell lymphomas, or for distinguishing benign lymphoid infiltrates from malignant lymphoma. The usefulness of V region expression as a virtually clonotypic marker in T-cell lymphoma needs to be reevaluated when a larger panel of antibodies covering nearly all V-region specificities becomes available.

REFERENCES

Acha-Orbea H, DJ Mitchell, L Timmermann, DC Wraith, GS Tausch, MK Waldor, SS Zamvil, HO McDevitt and L Steinman, 1988. Limited heterogeneity of T cell receptors from lymphocytes mediating autoimmune encephalomyelitis allows specific immune intervention. **Cell**, 54:263.

Acuto O and E L Reinherz, 1985. The human T cell receptor: Structure and function. **N. Engl. J. Med.**, 312:1100.

Acuto O and T Meo, 1989. TCR Vβ genes in man and mouse and the factors that shape the linkage pattern of immune receptor genes. **Immunol. Today**, 10:14.

Barth RK, BS Kim, NC Lan, T Hunkapiller, N Sobieck, A Winoto, H Gershenfeld, C Okada, D Hansburg, IL Weissman and L Hood, 1985. The murine T cell receptor uses a limited repertoire of expressed Vβ segments. **Nature**, 316:517.

Bigler RD, DE Fisher, CY Wang, EA Rinnooy Kan and H Kunkel, 1983. Idiotype like molecules on cells of a human T cell leukemia. **J. Exp. Med.**, 158:1000.

Boehncke WH, S Krettek and W Sterry, 1991. Mycosis fungoides does not show preferential usage of T-cell receptor variable region genes. **J. Invest. Dermatol.**, 96:1017A.

Boylston AW, J Borst, H Yssel, D Blanchard, H Spits and JE de Vries, 1986. Properties of a panel of monoclonal antibodies which react with the human T cell antigen receptor on the leukemic line HPB-ALL and a subset of normal peripheral blood T lymphocytes. **J. Immunol.**, 137:741.

Boylston AW, RD Goldin and CS Moore, 1984. A human T cell tumour which expresses the putative T cell antigen receptor. **Eur. J. Immunol.**, 14:273.

Carrel S, P Isler, M Schreyer, A Vacca, S Salvi, L Giuffre and JP Mach, 1986. Expression on human thymocytes of the idiotypic structures (Ti) from two leukaemic T cell lines, Jurkatt and HPB-ALL. **Eur. J. Immunol.**, 16:649.

Charley M, JP McCoy, JS Deng and B Jegasothy, 1990. Anti-V region antibodies as "almost clonotypic" reagents for the study of cutaneous T cell lymphomas and leukemias. **J. Invest. Dermatol.**, 95:614.

Clark DM and AW Boylston, 1989. T-cell antigen receptor beta-chain variable region families: A study of their distribution in normal and reactive tissues. **J. Pathol.**, 158:9.

Clark DM, AW Boylston, PA Hall and S Carrel, 1986. Antibodies to T cell antigen receptor beta chain families detect monoclonal T cell proliferation. **Lancet**, 2:835.

Concannon P, L Pickering, P Kung and L Hood, 1986. Diversity and structure of human T cell receptor β chain variable region genes. **Proc. Natl. Acad. Sci. USA**, 83:6598.

Ho VC, CB Gilks, RD Gascoyne, DJ Ellison and DT McLean, 1991. T-cell receptor variable region gene expression in cutaneous T-cell lymphoma. **J. Invest. Dermatol.**, 96:604A.

Hochgeschwender U, HG Simon, HU Weltzien, F Bartels, A Becker and JT Epplen, 1987. Dominance of one T-cell receptor in the H-2Kb/TNP response. **Nature**, 326:307.

Hunt SJ, MR Charley and BV Jegasothy, 1991. Immunohistochemical staining of cutaneous T-cell lymphoma by antibodies to the variable regions of the human T-cell antigen receptor. **J. Invest. Dermatol.**, 96:602A.

Jack AS, AW Boylston, S Carrel and I Grigor, 1990. Cutaneous T cell lymphoma cells employ a restricted range of T-cell antigen receptor variable region genes. **Am. J. Pathol.**, 136:17.

Kappler J, B Kotzin, L Herron, EW Gelfand, R Bigler, AW Boylston, S Carrel, DN Posnett, Y Choi and P Marrack, 1989. Vβ-specific stimulation of human T cells by staphylococcal toxins. **Science**, 244:811.

Kimura N, B Toyonaga, Y Yoshikai, MD Minden and TW Mak, 1986. Sequence and diversity of human T cell receptor beta chain genes. **J. Exp. Med.**, 164:739.

Klein MH, P Concannon, TM Evert, LD Kim, T Hunkapiller and L Hood, 1987. Diversity and structure of human T-cell receptor α-chain variable region genes. **Proc. Natl. Acad. Sci. USA**, 84:6884.

Marrack P, J Kappler, 1987. The T-cell receptor. **Science**, 238:1073.

Moller DR, K Konishi, M Kirby, B Balbi and RG Crystal, 1988. Bias towards use of a specific T-cell receptor β-chain variable region in a subgroup of individuals with sarcoidosis. **J. Clin. Invest.**, 82:1183.

Morel PA, AM Livingstone and CG Fathman, 1987. Correlation of T cell receptor Vβ family with MHC restriction. **J. Exp. Med.**, 166:583.

O'Grady J, AS Krajewski and EF Ramage, 1990. Demonstration of clonality in T-cell lymphoma using an anti-T-cell receptor variable region antibody panel. **Histopathology.**, 17:553.

Poppema S and B Hepperle, 1991. Restricted V gene usage in T-cell lymphomas as detected by anti-T-cell receptor variable region reagents. **Am. J. Pathol.**, 138:1479.

Posnett DN, I Schmelkin, DA Burton, A August, H McGrath and LF Mayer, 1990. T cell antigen receptor V gene usage: Increases in V$\beta8^+$ T cells in Crohn's disease. **J. Clin. Invest.**, 85:1770.

Seboun E, MA Robinson, TH Doolittle, TA Ciulla, TJ Kindt and SL Hauser, 1989. A susceptibility locus for multiple sclerosis is linked to the T cell receptor β chain complex. **Cell**, 57:1095.

Sorger SB, SM Hendrick, PL Fink, MA Bookman and LA Matin, 1987. Generation of diversity in T cell receptor repertoire specific for pigeon cytochrome C. **J. Exp. Med.**, 165:279.

Toyonaga B and TW Mak, 1987. Genes of the T cell antigen receptor in normal and malignant T cells. **Ann. Rev. Immunol.**, 5:585.

Urban JL, V Kumar, DH Kono, C Gomez, SJ Horwath, J Clayton, DG Ando, EE Sercaz and L Hood, 1988. Restricted use of T-cell receptor V genes in murine autoimmune encephalomyelitis raises possibilities for antibody therapy. **Cell**, 54:577.

Wilson RK, E Lai, P Concannon, RK Barth and LE Hood, 1988. Structure, organization and polymorphism of murine and human T-cell receptor α and β chain gene families. **Immunol. Rev.**, 101:149.

Wraith DC, HO McDevitt, L Steinmann, H Acha-Orbea, 1989. T cell recognition as the target for immune intervention in autoimmune disease. **Cell**, 57:709.

SÉZARY SYNDROME IS CHARACTERIZED BY GENOTRAUMATIC T CELLS

Keld Kaltoft*
Susanne Bisballe*
Wolfram Sterry†
Helmer Søgaard#
Kristian Thestrup-Pedersen‡

* Institute of Human Genetics
  The Bartholin Building
‡ Department of Dermatology
  Aarhus University
  DK-8000 Aarhus C
  Denmark

Aarhus Municipal Hospital
  Denmark

† Department of Dermatology
  University of Ulm
  Germany

Correspondence to: Dr. K. Kaltoft, Instutite of Human Genetics
University of Aarhus, Bartholin Building
DK-8000 Aarhus C, Denmark

ABSTRACT

Karyotyping of peripheral blood leucocytes of patients with Sézary syndrome often reveals cells with multiple chromosome changes primarily characterized by the existence of several structurally abnormal chromosomes (marker chromosomes). Here we show that these cells represent malignant T cells. Malignant T cells with multiple and complex chromosomal aberrations belong to a family of T cells for which we suggest the name "genotraumatic T cells".

Basic Mechanisms of Physiologic and Aberrant Lymphoproliferation in the Skin
Edited by W.C. Lambert *et al.*, Plenum Press, New York, 1994

A genotraumatic T cell, unlike a normal T lymphocyte, is characterized by its ability to develop clonal chromsomal aberrations. We propose that a genotraumatic T cell generates by successive cell divisions multiple and complex chromosome aberrations. Surprisingly, several different genotraumatic T cell clones may exist in a given patient. Genotraumatic T cells are also detected in patients with mycosis fungoides.

INTRODUCTION

The definition of cutaneous T cell lymphoma relies on an often troublesome clinicohistological investigation (Edelson, 1980; Sterry, 1985). Over the years a single, cellular parameter, which can be used to define the syndrome, has been the goal of many research projects. Candidates for a single, cellular characteristic include the morphology of the Sézary cell nucleus (Lutzner et al., 1968), antigens on leukemic cells detected by monoclonal antibodies (Berger et al., 1982), and, in recent years, T cell receptor gene rearrangement (Weiss et al., 1985). The latter investigations are based on the assumption that demonstration of a T cell clone reflects the presence of a malignant rather than a reactive T cell clone (Lee, 1991). None of these parameters, however, is specific for cutaneous T cell lymphoma (Flaxman et al.,1971; Ralfkiaer et al., 1986; Weiss et al., 1986; Wechsler et al., 1990).

Mycosis fungoides and Sézary syndrome are considered to be low and intermediate malignancies, respectively. Several papers have reported that karyotyping of cells in affected tissues often reveals clones with multiple chromosome changes, and such clones are believed to identify the malignant cells (Whang-Peng et al., 1982; Berger et al., 1987; Shapiro et al., 1987; Kaltoft et al., 1991). In recent years, T cell receptor gene rearrangement studies have shown that clonal T cells appear in peripheral blood of patients with Sézary syndrome (Bertness et al., 1985). It is reasonable to suppose that the karyotypically abnormal clone and the clone detected by T cell receptor analysis are identical.

In this paper, we show that a combination of cell culture, phenotyping, genotyping and karyotyping can define the malignant cell in four patients with Sézary syndrome. This malignant T cell is primarily characterized by multiple chromosome aberrations, often represented by many morphologically abnormal chromosomes (marker chromosomes). It is generally assumed that only malignant cells show clonal chromosome aberrations. Besides the malignant genotraumatic T cell clone, non-malignant, genotraumtic T cell clones can be detected by cell culture. This suggests that Sézary syndrome is characterized by genotraumatic T cells and that one of these T cell clones eventually becomes malignant.

We report here that the malignant cell, in all four of the Sézary patients we investigated, is represented by a genotraumatic T cell clone. Furthermore, we illustrate by two examples that genotraumatic T cell clones also exist in patients with mycosis fungoides.

MATERIALS AND METHODS

Patients and cell lines

Four cell lines (Se-Ax, Se-La, Se-Le, and Se-Se) were established from peripheral blood of patients with a diagnosis of Sézary syndrome (Sterry, 1985). Mononuclear cells were cultured at an initial density of 10^6/ml in medium consisting of RPMI 1640 80%, human AB serum 20%, 100 pM IL-2, 500 pM IL-4, 100 u/ml penicillin G and 25 μg/ml streptomycin. When proliferation was evident, cells were subcultured at a 1:2 ratio.

From a 42-year old male patient with mycosis fungoides, stage IV, a cell line, My-Ta, was obtained from a lymph node showing malignant lymphoma. The My-Ta cell line was cultured and derives from the patient called MF3 described in an earlier publication (Kaltoft et al., 1984).

The establishment of the so-called My-La cell lines from a patient with mycosis fungoides stage II has been described in detail (Kaltoft et al., 1991). In short, a plaque was taken from an 82-year old man who had been suffering from the disease for 10 years. The skin biopsy was divided into two parts. One part was used for confirmatory diagnosis; the other part was placed in culture medium with IL-2 and IL-4 and cells were allowed to proliferate. Two cell lines could be identified: i) a primary clonal CD4[+] cell line with normal karyotype and with an immunophenotype that represented the majority of the T cells in the skin biopsy; and ii) a second clonal cell line, detected after extensive cell culturing, with CD8[+] phenotype and multiple chromosome aberrations. CD8[+] cells represented less than 10% of the T cells in the plaque.

T cell receptor gene expression was analyzed as previously described (Kaltoft et al., 1991), and was kindly performed at the Department of Molecular Genetics, Novo-Nordisk, Denmark, by Drs. E. Boel, P.B. Rasmussen, and T. Dyrberg. Immunophenotyping on living cells was done according to standard procedures (Kaltoft et al., 1987).

Karyotyping was performed on all primary cultures with phytohemagglutinin M at 10 μg/ml in the medium described above. If the mitotic index was low, other mitogens, like con A (10 μg/ml) or pokeweed mitogen (10 μg/ml), were tried in order to increase mitotic activity. Karyotyping was also performed at regular intervals to follow the development of the cell lines. The nomenclature of the Paris Conference ISCN (1985) was used.

RESULTS

The Sézary syndrome is characterized by a family of genotraumatic T cell clones

The Se-Ax patient demonstrated, on 3 separate occasions, leucocytosis and typical Sézary cells with a CD3[+], CD4[+], TCR phenotype (Kaltoft et al., 1987). When mononuclear cells were cultured with recombinant IL-2 and IL-4, the same immunophenotype was detected in the continuous cell strain.

T cell receptor gene expression demonstrated that the continuous cell line was a clone

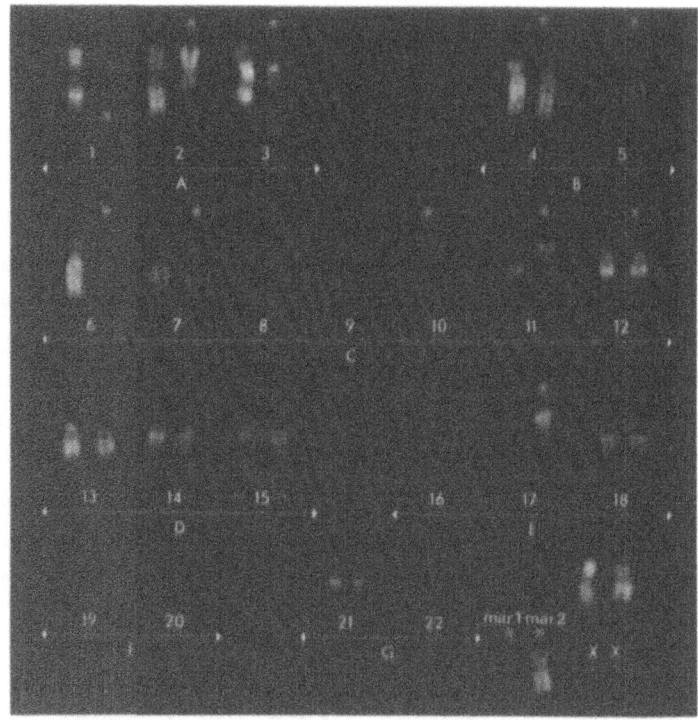

Figure 1. Shows the representative karyotype of the near diploid subclone in peripheral blood of the Se-Ax patient. Se-Ax, 2n-: 44, XX, -8, -8, -9, -10, +mar1, +mar2, inv(1)(p36;q21), del(2)(q21), t(3;?)(q21;?), t(4;?)(p16;?), del(5)(p13), del(6)(q21), del(7)(p11;p15), t(10;?)(p14;?), del(11)(q23), del(12)(p13), t(17;?)(p11;?).

with Vβ3 expression. Karyotyping of peripheral blood leucocytes from the Se-Ax patient demonstrated the presence of a clonal cell population. Mitotic activity in PHA stimulated leucocytes was good, with a mitotic index of 2% to 5% in 3 separate blood samplings. Numerous metaphases were thus available for identification of the malignant cell. Two very aberrant chromosomal subclones could be detected, a near diploid clone and a near tetraploid

404

clone. The two subclones clearly originated from the same clone and represented approximately 40% of the metaphases. Although minor chromosome changes were recognized from metaphase to metaphase, a representative karyotype of the near diploid and the near tetraploid cell could be obtained and are shown in Figure 1 and Figure 2, respectively. By inspection of the near diploid karyotype it can be seen that 13 marker chromosomes appear. Furthermore, other numerical aberrations are also evident. In the near tetraploid karyotype, several of the same marker chromosomes as seen in the near diploid cell are present. However, some are missing and additional ones can be recognized (like mar 3 and mar 4).

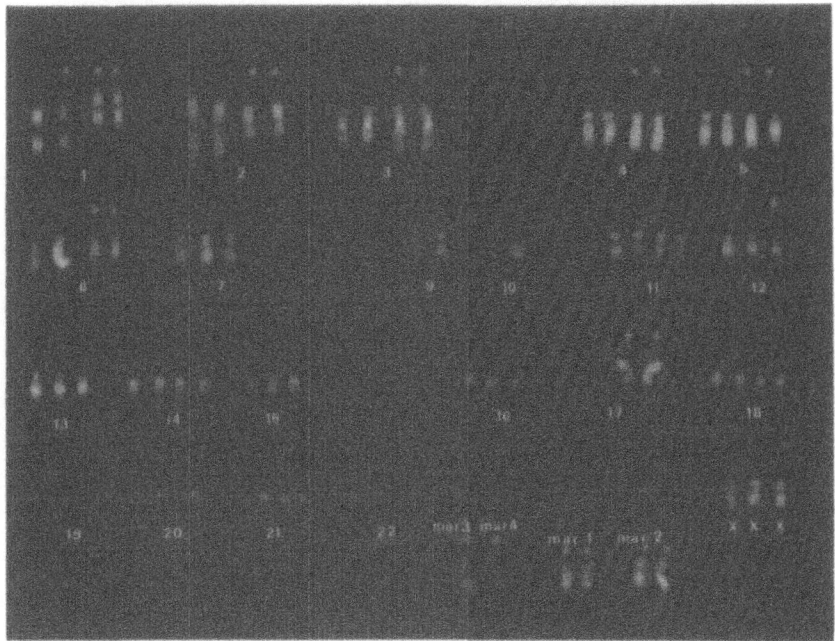

Figure 2. Shows the representative karyotype of the near tetraploid subclone in peripheral blood of the Se-Ax patient. Se-Ax, 4n-: 85, XXX, -7, -8, -8, -8, -8,-9, -9, -10, -10, -12, -13, -15, +2mar1, +2mar2, +mar3, +mar4, i(1q), (inv(1)(p36;q21), inv(1)(p36;q21), del(2)(q21), del(2)(q21), t(3;?)(q21;?), t(3;?)(q21;?), t(4;?)(p16;?), t(4;?)(p16;?), del(5)(p13), del(5)(p13), del(6), (q21), del(6)(q21), del(12)(p13), t(17;?)(p11;?), t(17;?)(p11;?).

In the continuous (immortal) Se-Ax T cell line only metaphases similar to the representative metaphases shown in Figure 1 and Figure 2 can be detected. By continuous culture novel chromosome aberrations occur, demonstrating genetic instability of the Se-Ax cell strain.

In summary, the malignant cell demonstrated on 3 separate occasions in the Se-Ax patient is a CD3$^+$, CD4$^+$, TCR-2, Vβ3 clonal T cell. By karyotyping, this cell could be shown to consist of two subclones, with 44 and 85 chromosomes, respectively. Of the 44 chromosomes in the near diploid cell, 13 are marker chromosomes. Generation of a single marker chromosome involves rearrangement or loss of genetic material of several million base pairs. The chromosomes in the malignant cell were thus far from the normal human chromosome

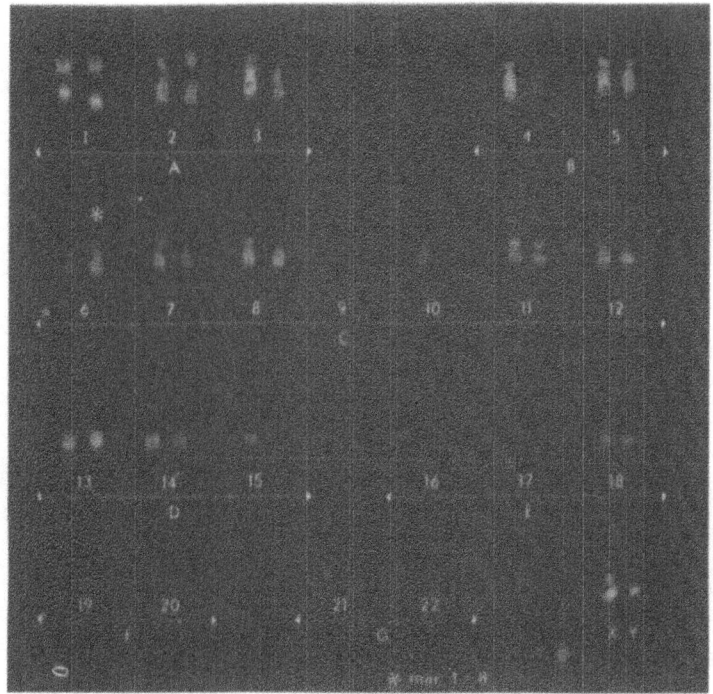

Figure 3. Shows the representative karyotype 46, XY, -9, -10, -15, -17, -17, -19, -20, -22, +mar1-8, t(6;?) (p25;?) of the Se-La cell line which also dominates the karyotypes in peripheral blood lymphocytes (1984).

complement. We consider that this reflects a genetic trauma, and hence we propose that the Se-Ax cell strain belongs to a family of T cells which we classify as "genotraumatic" T cells.

The malignant T cells from the blood of another Sézary patient, were investigated over a 3-year period. During this time phenotyping and karyotyping showed, on all occasions, that the malignant T cell was basically the same genotraumatic T cell. A typical analysis of

406

peripheral blood leucocytes revealed that more than 90% of the lymphocytes were CD3$^+$, CD4$^+$, TCR-2 positive. A karyotype as shown in Figure 4 could be identified in more than 90% of metaphases. Again, minor chromosomal variations occurred from metaphase to metaphase. Larger variations could be detected when karyotypes obtained 3 years apart were compared (Figure 3 is the representative karyotype from 1984 and Figure 4 the karyotype from 1987). However, since several of the same marker chromosomes and most of the numerical aberrations are present in both karyotypes, the malignant cell clearly originated from the same clone. From the blood of the patient (in 1987) a finite cell line (Se-La) with a life span of approximately 20

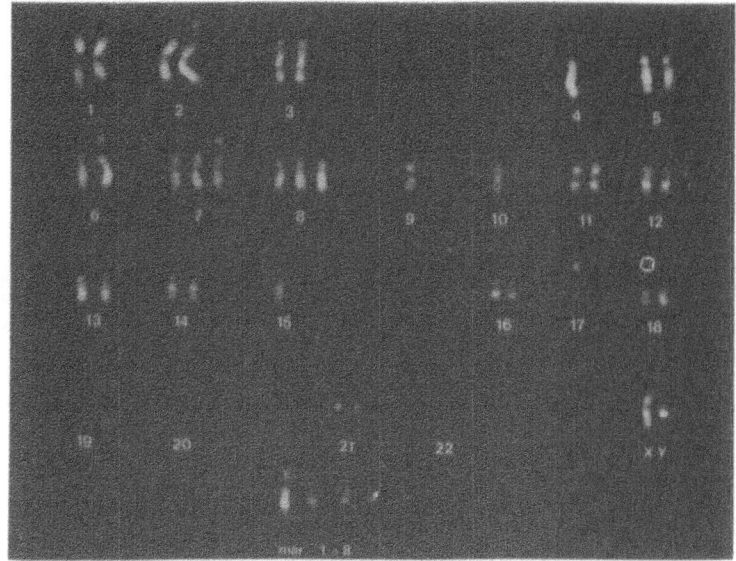

Figure 4. Shows the representative karyotype 46, XY, -4, -9, -10, -15, -17, -19, -20, -20, -22, -22, +del(7)(p15), +8, +marl-8, t(2;?)(q37;?), inv(6)(p25q25), t(17;?)(p13;?) in 1987 of the clonal Se-La cell line. A similar karyotype dominates in peripheral blood.

cell population doublings was established. This cell line has a CD3$^+$, CD4$^+$, TCR-2$^+$ phenotype and only the representative karyotype as shown in Figure 4 appeared after the first cell population doubling. This clonal cell line thus represents the malignant T cells. Here the malignant cell is characterized by 12 marker chromosomes and several numerical chromosome aberrations. The data from the Se-La patient demonstrate again that the malignant T cell can primarily be described as a genotraumatic T cell, and that a genotraumatic T cell in vivo also shows genetic instability.

The phenotype and DNA content of uncultured lymphocytes of the Sézary patient, Se-Le, was determined by flow cytometry. Approximately 95% of mononuclear cells had the CD3$^+$, CD4$^+$ phenotype, and 90% of the cells had a near-tetraploid DNA content. A representative karyotype, present in 87% of the metaphases analyzed is shown in Figure 5. The near-tetraploid lymphocyte clone could be detected for approximately 5 cell population doublings and was then overgrown by lymphocytes with a CD3$^+$, CD4$^+$ phenotype and a 45,XY,-14,-21, +t(14;21) karyotype. In the last of the four Sézary patients investigated, (Se-Se), a genotraumtic T cell clone could easily be identified in peripheral blood. A representative karyotype is shown in Figure 6 (a near diploid cell with 15 marker chromosomes). Besides the near diploid karyotype, a near tetraploid karyotype could also be recognized originating from the same clone. By culturing mononuclear cells, a clonal cell line with the same karyotype (in all metaphases) as in Figure 6 could be established. This clonal cell line has a CD3$^+$, CD4$^+$ phenotype and this again demonstrates that the malignant cell detected by karyotyping in peripheral blood is a T cell. The Se-Se cell line stopped proliferating after approximately 10 cell population doublings.

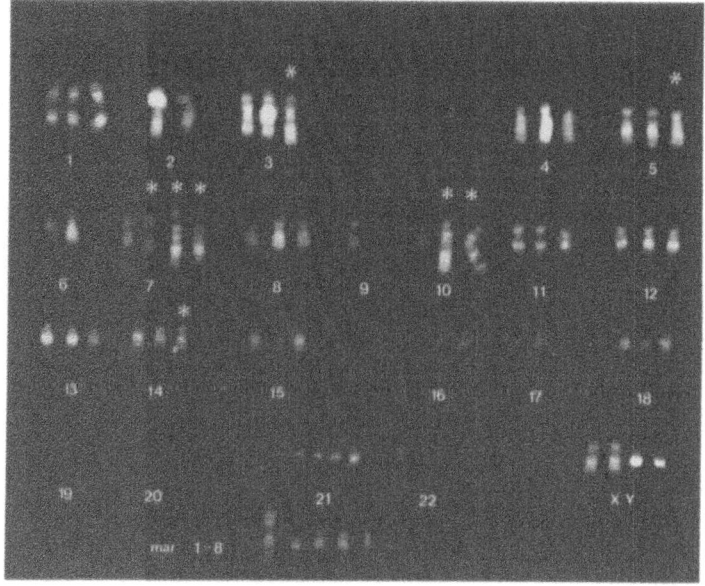

Figure 5. Shows the representative karyotype in peripheral blood and in cultured lymphocytes of the Se-Le patient. 77, XXYY, -1, -2, -2, -3, -4, -5, -6, -6, -8, -9, -9, -10, -11, -12, -13, -14, -15, -16, -17, -18, -19, -20, -20, +mar1-8, t(3;?)(q28;?), del(5)(p13p15,1), (i(7q), t(7;?)(p11;?)t(7;?) (q32;?), t(7;?)-(p11;?)t(7;?)(q32;?), t(10;?)(q26;?), t(10;?)(q26;?), t(14;?)(p11;?).

By comparing a primary blood culture with cultured, clonal cell lines, the following conclusion can be made: The malignant cell in peripheral blood leucocytes is clearly a T cell with the expected phenotype. Furthermore, the malignant T cell in all four Sézary patients is a genotraumatic T cell, which we define as a T cell with the ability to develop clonal chromosomal aberrations. In the four Sézary patients reported here the malignant clones have multiple and complex chromosome aberrations.

Genotraumatic T cells can also be detected in mycosis fungoides

The malignant cell in Sézary syndrome can often be recognized by karyotyping of peripheral blood. Since mycosis fungoides and Sézary syndrome are related by similar clinical appearance and histology, the genotraumatic T cell is also expected to be the malignant cell in mycosis fungoides. Several examples confirm the existence of such a cell in mycosis fungoides, particularly in advanced stages (Whang-Peng et al., 1982; Shapiro et al., 1987). We illustrate here that a genotraumatic T cell is the malignant cell in a patient with mycosis fungoides, stage IV. Figure 7 shows the karyotype of the My-Ta CD3$^+$, CD4$^+$ cell line derived from a biopsy of a lymph node. The karyotype represents approximately 70% of the metaphases in the

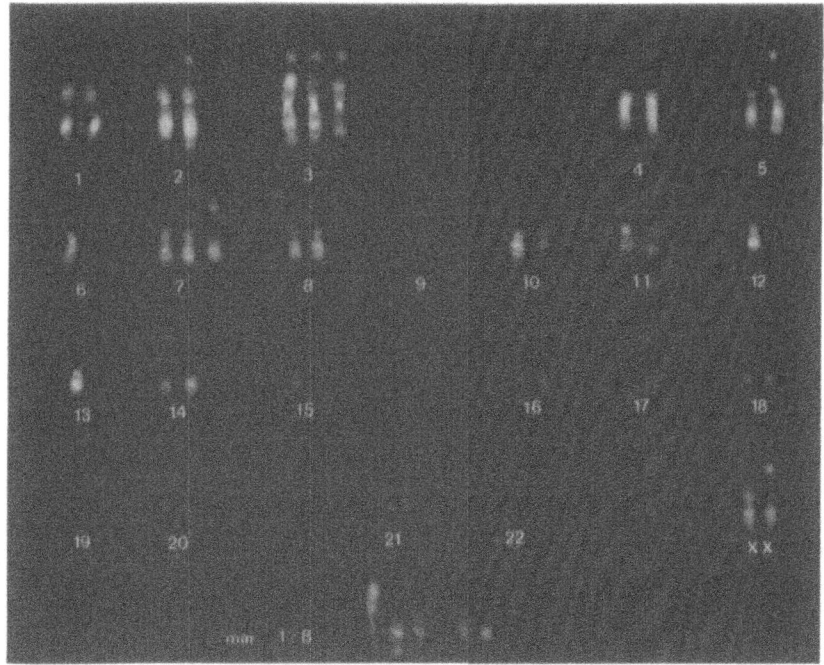

Figure 6. Shows the representative karyotype of the clonal Se-Se cell line which also dominates in PHA-stimulated leucocytes: 47, X, del(X)(p11p21), -6, -9, -9, -12, -13, -15, -17, -21, -22, +3, +7, +marl-8, t(2;?)(q36;?), t(3;?)(p25;?)t(3;?)(q29;?), t(3;?)(q29;?), t(3;?)(q29;?), t(5;?)(q35;?), del(7)(p12).with the expected phenotype. Furthermore, the malignant T cell in all four Sézary patients is a genotraumatic T cell which we define as a T cell with the ability to develop clonal chromosomal aberrations. In the four Sézary patients reported here the malignant clones have multiple and complex chromosome aberrations.

primary culture and, with its 22 marker chromosomes and other chromosome aberrations, it has the same complexity of chromosomal aberrations as the malignant T cells reported here for Sézary syndrome. We were not able to detect this clone in the peripheral blood.

In early stage mycosis fungoides, genotraumatic T cells may be difficult to detect. The My-La patient illustrates this problem. The clinico-histological picture is diagnostic for mycosis fungoides, stage II, with a predominant CD4$^+$ cell infiltrate in the skin (Kaltoft et al., 1991). A primary cell line from this biopsy had a CD4$^+$ phenotype representing a clone with Vβ18 T cell receptor expression and normal 46,XY karyotype. When the Hayftick limit was reached (after approximately 40 cell population doublings) (Effros et al., 1984), the cell culture entered a crisis. The CD4$^+$ cell line was occasionally overgrown by an abnormal CD8$^+$ cell clone with Vβ13 T cell receptor expression and a karyotype as shown in Figure 8 (Kaltoft et al., 1991). Extensive analysis clearly demonstrates that both the CD4$^+$ and the CD8$^+$ clonal cell lines derive from the My-La patient (Kaltoft et al., 1991).

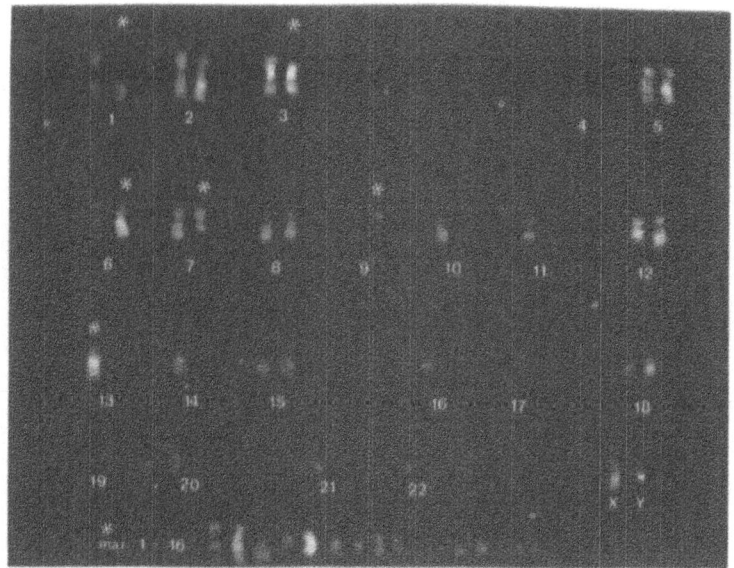

Figure 7. Demonstrates the representative karyotype 49, XY, -4, -4, -10, -11, -13, -14, -16, -17, -17, -19, -20, -21, -22, +marl-16, del(1)(p13), del(3)(p14), del(6)(q25), del(7)(q22), del(9)(q21), t(13;?)(q34;?) of the My-Ta cell line from a lymph node of a patient with mycosis fungoides, stage IV.

The My-La CD8$^+$ cell clone, with its 13 marker chromosomes and other chromosome aberrations, resembles the malignant, genotraumatic T cells described here in patients with Sézary syndrome. It is reasonable to assume that it represents the malignant cell in the skin infiltrate. Immunophenotyping of the plaque from which the My-La, CD8$^+$ cell line derives shows that it probably represents a minor fraction of the lymphocytes in affected skin. This implies that the percentage of truly malignant cells in the plaque is rather low.

DISCUSSION

We have shown, in four patients with Sézary syndrome, that the malignant T cell belongs to a family of genotraumatic T cell clones. This conclusion is based on a combination of methods, including cell culture, phenotyping, genotyping, and karyotyping. In cancer cytogenetics it is generally accepted that a malignant clone can be defined if two or more metaphases with identical structural anomalies are present. We want to stress that our analysis

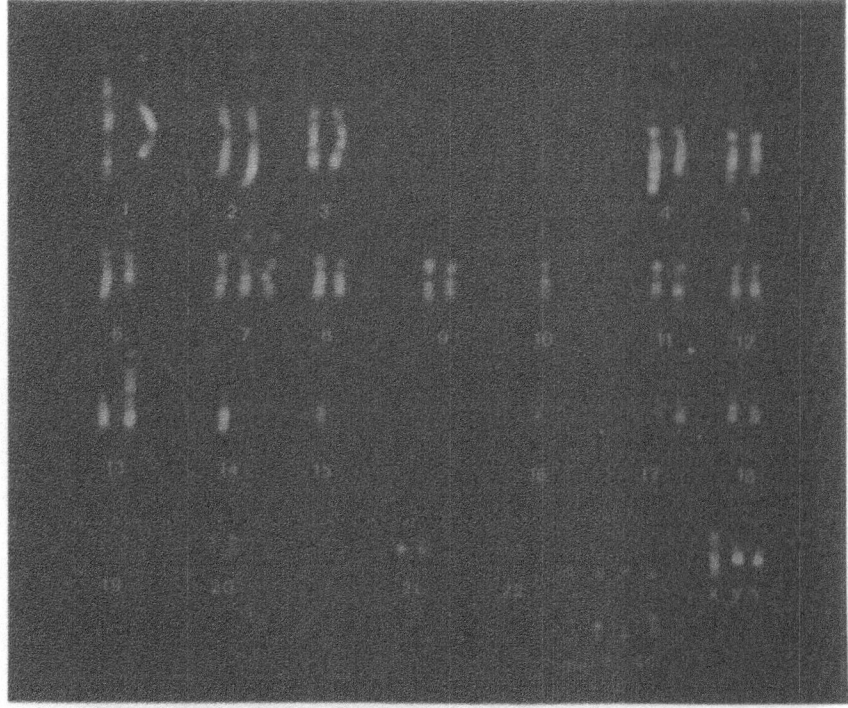

Figure 8. Shows the representative karyotype 49, XYY, -10, -14, -15, -16, +del(7)(p15.2), +17, +marl-4, t(1;?)(p36.2;?), del(1)(q32.2), t(2;?)(q37.2;?), del(4)(q31.2), del(5)(q21q23.1), del(6)(q23.2), del(7)(p15.2), t(10q13q) of the CD8$^+$ clonal cell line appearing after extensive culture of lymphocytes of a skin biopsy from a patient with mycosis fungoides, stage II.

is based on detecting the abnormal clone in a substantial fraction of the metaphases in a primary culture. Often more than 100 karyotypically abnormal metaphases could be seen in a single investigation. This makes us confident that karyotyping shows the malignant clone. We have subsequently used cell culture phenotyping, genotyping, and karyotyping in order to characterize the malignant cell. Not surprisingly, this approach shows that the malignant cell is a T cell with the expected phenotype. Our results demonstrate that the clonal T cell which others have detected by T cell receptor gene rearrangement studies, can be identified in some Sézary patients by karyotyping.

In principle, T cell receptor analysis only demonstrates the presence of a clone but not whether this clone is malignant. In our hands, karyotyping may give information additional to that obtained by T cell receptor gene rearrangement studies. For instance, whereas T cell receptor analysis of the Se-Ax cell line only demonstrates one clone with Vβ3 T cell receptor expression, karyotyping shows that there are two subclones, a near diploid and a near tetraploid clone. Karyotyping also shows that variations exist in the chromosome complement within a given subclone. Furthermore, the presence of a very abnormal karyotype in a substantial fraction of the metaphases in a primary culture leaves little doubt that this clone represents the leukemic cells.

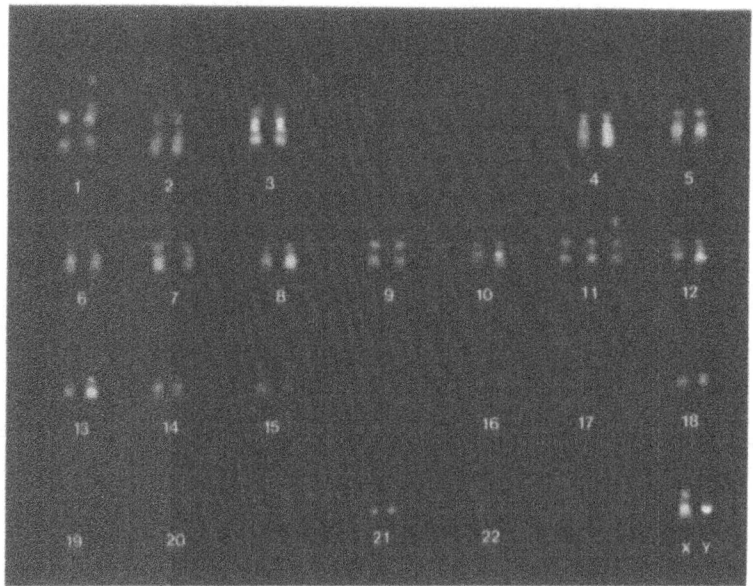

Figure 9. Shows the karyotype 47, XY, +del(11)(q11q13), t(1;?)(q32;?) of a non-B, non-T cell line established from the Se-La patient.

Several reports, in addition to our work confirm the existence of very aberrant chromosomal clones in Sézary syndrome (Johnson et al., 1985; Gamperl, 1986; Berger et al., 1987; Shapiro et al., 1987; Solé et al., 1990; D'Allesandro et al., 1990; Santos et al., 1990; Todd Abrams et al., 1991a; Todd Abrams et al., 1991b). The presence of genotraumatic T cells in Sézary syndrome may be greatly underestimated. We and others (Kaltoft et al., 1984;

Goldstein et al., 1986; Kaltoft et al., 1987; Ho et al., 1990; Rheinhold et al., 1990; Todd Abrams et al., 1991b) have noticed that malignant T cells often do not proliferate well in vitro. Thus, their existence may be missed by karyotyping. Stimulation of peripheral blood lymphocytes with a single mitogen (like PHA) may not allow the clonal leukemic cells to proliferate. In such a case other mitogens, such as phorbol ester or monoclonal antibodies, can be tried in order to make the malignant clone proliferate. Certain growth factors and cytokines also seem to promote proliferation of Sézary cells (Todd Abrams et al., 1991a; 1991b; Dalloul et al., 1992).

By comparing the individual karyotypes shown here, it can be seen that each genotraumatic T cell clone is unique in the sense that the pattern of chromosome changes differs from patient to patient. The karyotyping has been based on routine Q-banding of chromosomes. The resolution of banded chromosomes by this technique is not high and only major chromosomal aberrations are detected. With the limitation of this banding technique, apparently no single chromosome aberration appears to be common to all 8 karyotypes shown here. This does not imply that the chromosome changes are completely random (Berger et al., 1987). For instance, we (this paper) and others (Berger et al., 1987; Shapiro et al., 1987) have frequently found monosomy for chromosome 10 or a translocation involving chromosome 10 (the Se-Se patient being the only exception).

In contrast to the classical Philadephia chromosome (Ph[1]-chromosome), which is one of the two specific marker chromosomes in most cases of chronic myelocytic leukemia, the karyotypes described here for Sézary syndrome and mycosis fungoides are characterized by multiple chromosome aberrations ("chromosome jam") rather than by specific marker chromosomes. This does not exclude the possibility that a single (specific) chromosome mutation or single gene mutation(s) could be present in all genotraumatic T cells and that this mutation could be implicated in generation of the many chromosome aberrations. If this is the case, the chromosomal aberrations are secondary to a primary mutational event. This implies that karyotyping with Q-banding is unlikely to reveal the primary genetic defect in the genotraumatic T-lymphocytes.

At present, we have no clue as to how a genotraumatic T cell with multiple and complex chromosome changes is generated. Lymphocytes are unique among somatic cells, however, in that they express their paratopes by recombination and mutation. A karyotypically complex genotraumatic T cell could have arisen through a series of timely spaced chromosome changes and could be an ongoing process. This would explain the additional chromosome changes of the Se-La 1987 compared to the Se-La 1984 karyotype and the generation of novel chromosome aberrations in the continuous Se-Ax cell strain.

Cells that we define as genotraumatic T cells have, besides Sézary syndrome and mycosis fungoides, also been described in non-Hodgkin's lymphoma of T cell origin (Fischer et al.,

1988; Ohno et al., 1988; Kubonishi et al., 1990; Morikawa et al., 1991). The definition of a genotraumtic T-lymphocyte can, of course, be extended by analogy to a genotraumatic lymphocyte. Apparently, Hodgkin's disease often demonstrates the presence of genotraumatic lymphocytes (Tilly et al., 1991). It has been suggested that cutaneous T cell lymphoma and Hodgkin disease may develop from a common T cell clone (Kadin, 1990; Davis et al., 1992). We suggest that genotraumatic lymphocytes are a common denominator for both diseases.

A genetic predisposition for mycosis fungoides has been suggested (Dick et al., 1977). We have previously shown that in Epstein-Barr virus harbouring B cells of patients with mycosis fungoides and Sézary syndrome, several chromosome aberrations develop rapidly during culture (Kaltoft et al., 1985). The fact that some B and T cells show chromosome aberrations may point to a genetic defect making lymphocytes of patients with cutaneous T cell lymphoma prone to develop chromosome aberrations. The apparent genetic instability in lymphocytes of patients with cutaneous T cell lymphoma means that karyotyping sometimes reveals a clone that is not the malignant cell. Use of karyotyping, demonstrating a chromosomally aberrant clone, as the only method for depicting the malignant cell should thus be met with caution. In the blood of the Se-Le patient a non-malignant CD3$^+$, CD4$^+$ T cell with a 45,XY,-14,-21,+t(14;21) karyotype was observed. Figure 9 further illustrates this problem. The karyotype shown here was seen in CD4 depleted mononuclear cells of the Se-La patient (depletion obtained with dynal CD4 beads as described by the manufacturer). This clone required IL-2 and IL-4 for growth. Another minor, clonal T cell population with a 47,XX,+2 karyotype could also be demonstrated in the blood of the Se-La patient. However, the karyotype of the malignant T cell in the Se-La patient is, as shown in Figure 4, based on a combination of phenotyping, karyotyping, and cell culture.

In lymphocytes of the Se-Ax patient a non-malignant CD8$^+$ T cell clone with a chromosomal aberration could be detected (Kaltoft et al., 1987), and in the My-La CD4$^+$ cell line also a clonal chromosomal aberration developed during culture (Kaltoft et al., 1991). These cell lines are, by definition, genotraumatic, emphasizing that some lymphocytes of patients with cutaneous T cell lymphoma, unlike normal T-lymphocytes, are able to develop clonal chromosomal aberrations. Although these genotraumatic cell lines do not represent the malignant cell, they could be cancer prone clones. The results of the cell culture experiments also suggest that several genotraumatic T cell clones may exist in a given patient, which is an exceptional property of cutaneous T cell lymphoma.

In addition to a genetic element, other hypotheses concerning the etiology of mycosis fungoides and Sézary syndrome have also been suggested. A chronic antigen stimulation by contact allergens has been hypothesized (Fischmann et al., 1979), but recent investigations have failed to support the idea that environmental factors are etiologically important in cutaneous T cell lymphoma (Whittemore et al., 1989). Also, a retrovial hypothesis for mycosis fungoides has been intensively investigated, ever since it was first proposed by MacKie (1981), but the assumption is not supported by experimental data (Capesius et al., 1991). In none of the patients, nor in the cell lines reported here, have we found evidence for human T-lymphotropic viruses. We prefer the hypothesis that a hallmark for cutaneous T cell lymphoma is genotraumatic T cells.

Fibroblasts of the Li-Fraumeni syndrome express during continuous culture only mutant p53 (Yin et al., 1992) and develop chromosome aberrations (Bischoff et al., 1990). A mutant tumor suppressor gene may thus be involved in converting a T cell with a normal karyotype into a clonal, chromosomal aberrant clone. It should be noticed that p53 is located on chromosome 17 and that most of the malignant T cells reported here have aberrations for chromosome 17. We believe that the molecular mechanisms generating the (malignant) genotraumatic T cell will be a central issue in future research of cutaneous T cell lymphoma.

ACKNOWLEDGEMENT

This work was supported by grant number 93-026 from the Danish Cancer Society.

REFERENCES

Berger, CL, S Morrison, A Chu, J Patterson, A Estabrook, S Takezaki, J Sharon, D Warburton, O Irigoyen and RL Edelson, 1982. Diagnosis of cutaneous T cell lymphoma by use of monoclonal antibodies reactive with tumor-associated antigens. **J. Clin. Invest.**, 70:1205.

Berger, R and A Bernheim, 1987. Cygogenetic studies of Sézary cells. **Cancer Genet. Cytogenet.**, 27:79.

Bertness, V, I Kirsch, G Hollis, B Johnson and PA Bunn Jr., 1985. T cell receptor gene rearrangement as clinical markers of human T cell lymphomas. **N. Engl. J. Med.**, 313:534.

Bischoff, FZ, SO Yim, S Pathak, G Grant, MJ Siciliano, BC Giovanella, LC Strong and MA Tainsky, 1990. Spontaneous abnormalities in normal fibroblasts from patients with Li-Fraumeni cancer syndrome: Aneuploidy and immortalization. **Cancer Res.**, 50:7979.

Capesius, C, F Saal, E Maero, A Bazarbachi, J Lasneret, L Laroche, A Gesain, F Hojman and J Peries, 1991. No evidence for HTLV-I infection in 24 cases of French and Portuguese mycosis fungoides and Sézary syndrome (as seen in France). **Leukemia**, 5:164.

D'Allesandro, E, P Paterlini, ML Lo Re, M Di Cola, C Ligas, D Quaglino and G. Del Porto, 1990. Cytogenetic Follow-up in a case of Sézary syndrome. **Cancer Genet. Cytogenet.**, 45:231.

Dalloul, A, L Laroche, M Bagot, MD Mossalayi, C Fourcade, DJ Thacker, DE Hogge, H Merie-Béral, P Debré and C Schmitt, 1992. Interleukin-7 is a growth factor for Sézary lymphoma cells. **J. Clin. Invest.**, 90:1054.

Davis, TH, CC Morton, R Miller-Cassman, SP Balk and E Kadin, 1992. Hodgkin's disease, lymphomatoid papulosis, and cutaneous T cell lymphoma derived from a common T cell clone. **N. Engl. J. Med.**, 326:1115.

Dick, HM and R Mackie, 1977. Distribution of HLA antigens in patients with mycosis fungoides. **Dermatol.**, 155:275.

Edelson, RL, 1980. Cutaneous T cell lymphoma: mycosis fungoides, Sézary syndrome, and other variants. **J. Am. Acad. Dermatol.**, 2:89.

Effros, RB and RL Walford, 1984. T cell cultures and the Hayflick limit. **Human Immunol.**, 9:49.

Fischer, P, E Nacheva, DY Mason, PD Sherrington, C Hoyle, FGJ. Hayhoe and A Karpas, 1988. A Ki-1 (CD30)-positive human cell line (Karpas 299) established from a high-grade non-Hodgkin's lymphoma, showing a 2;5 translocation and rearrangement of the T cell receptor β-chain gene. **Blood**, 72:234.

Fischmann, AB, PA Bunn Jr. and JG Guccion et al., 1979. Exposure to chemicals, physical agents, and biologic agents in mycosis fungoides and the Sézary syndrome. **Cancer Treat. Rep.**, 63:591.

Flaxman BA, G Zelazny and EJ van Scott, 1971. Nonspecificity of characteristic cells in mycosis fungoides. **Arch. Dermatol.**, 104:141.

Gamperl R, 1986. Clonal chromosome aberrations in a case of cutaneous T cell lymphoma. **Cancer Genet. Cytogenet.**, 19:341.

Golstein, MM, C Farnarier-Seidel, P Daubney and S Kaplanski, 1986. An OKT4$^+$ T cell population in Sézary syndrome: Attempts to elucidate its lack of proliferative capacity and its suppressive effect. **Scand. J. Immunol.**, 23:53.

Ho, VC, O Baadsgaard, JT Elder, ER Hansen, CA Hanson, GL Vejlsgaard and KD Cooper, 1990. Genotypic analysis of T cell clones derived from cutaneous T cell lymphoma lesions demonstrates selective growth of tumor-infiltrating lymphocytes. **J. Invest. Dermatol.**, 95:4.

Johnson, GA, GW Dewald, WR Strand and RK Winkelmann, 1985. Chromosome studies in 17 patients with the Sézary syndrome. **Cancer**, 55:2426.

Kadin, ME, 1990. Spectrum of cutaneous T cell lymphomas. **Curr. Probl. Dermatol.**, Basel, Karger, 19:132.

Kaltoft, K, K Thestrup-Pedersen, JR Jensen, S Bisballe and H Zachariae, 1984. Establishment of T and B cell lines from patients with mycosis fungoides. **Br. J. Dermatol.**, 111:303.

Kaltoft, K, S Bisballe and K Rasmussen, 1985. Balanced terminal chromosome translocations develop in EBV-derived, but non-immortal cell lines from patients with mycosis fungoides. **Acta Dermatovener. Suppl.**, 120:60.

Kaltoft, K, S Bisballe, HF Rasmussen, K Thestrup-Pedersen, K Thomsen and W. Sterry, 1987. A continuous T cell line from a patient with Sézary syndrome. **Arch. Dermatol. Res.**, 279:293.

Kaltoft, K, S Bisballe, T Dyrberg, E Boel, PB Rasmussen and K Thestrup-Pedersen. Establishment of two continuous cell strains from a single plaque of a patient with mycosis fungoides. **In Vitro Cell Dev.**, 28A:161.

Kubonishi, I, H Sonobe, T Miyagi, Y Iwahara, JH Ohyashiki, K Ohyashiki, K Toyama, Y Ohtsuki and I Miyoshi, 1990. A Ki-1 (CD3[+])-positive T (E[+], CD4[+], Ia[+])-cell line, DL-40, established from aggressive large cell lymphoma. **Cancer Res.**, 50:7685.

Lee, LA, 1991. A patient-specific probe for cutaneous T cell lymphoma. **J. Invest. Dermatol.**, 96:297.

Lutzner, MA and H.W. Jordan, 1968. Ultrastructure of an abnormal cell in Sézary's syndrome. **Blood**, 31:719.

MacKie, RM, 1981. Initial event in mycosis fungoides is viral infection of epidermal Langerhans cells. **Lancet** ii,1:283.

Morikawa, S, K Morikawa, J Hara, M Nagasaki, A Nakano and F Oseko, 1991. Establishment of a novel cell line with T-lineage phenotype(HPB-MLp-W) from a non-Hodgkin's lymphoma patient. **Leukemia Res.**, 15:381.

Ohno, T, S Fukuhara, Y Arita, S Doi, R Takahashi, H Fuji, T Honjo, T Sugiyama and H Uchino, 1988. Establishment of a peripheral T cell lymphoma cell line showing amplification of the c-myc oncogene. **Cancer Res.**, 48:4959.

Ralfkiaer, E, KC Gatter, GL Wantzin, K Thomsen and DY Mason, 1986. Immunohistological reactivity pattern of the anti-cutaneous T-lymphoma antibody BE$_2$. **Br. J. Dermatol.**, 114:677.

Rheinhold, U, G Pawelec, A Fratila, S Leippold, R Bauer and H-W Kreysel, 1990. Phenotypic and functional characterization of tumor infiltrating lymphocytes in mycosis fungoides: Continuous growth of CD4[+] CD45R[+] T cell clones with suppressor-inducer activity. **J. Invest. Dermatol.**, 94:304.

Santos, M, I Benitez and C Rivas, 1990. Possible correlation between a specific alteration t(7;14) and the rearrangement of TCR observed in a Sézary's syndrome. **Cancer Genet. Cytogenet.**, 46:261.

Shapiro, PE, D Warburton, CL Berger and RL Edelson, 1987. Clonal chromosomal abnormalities in cutaneous T cell lymphoma. **Cancer Genet. Cytogenet.**, 28:267.

Solé, F, N Tarrida, MD Coll, MR Caballin, A De Miguel, S Woessner and J Egozcue, 1990. Cytogenetic study of a patient with the Sézary syndrome. **Cancer Genet. Cytogenet.**, 44:193.

Sterry, W, 1985. Mycosis fungoides. **Curr. Top. Pathol.**, 74:167.

Tilly, BH, C Bastard, T Delastre, C Duval, M Bizet, B Lenormand, J-P Daucé, M. Monconduit and H. Piguet, 1991. Cytogenetic studies in untreated Hodgkin's disease. **Blood**, 77:1298.

Todd Abrams, J, S Lessin, SK Ghosh, W Ju, EC Vonderheid, P Nowell, G Murphy, B Elfenbein and E DeFreitas, 1991a. A clonal CD4-positive T cell line established from the blood of a patient with Sézary syndrome. **J. Invest. Dermatol.**, 96:31.

Todd Abrams, J, SR Lessin, SK Ghosh, PC Nowell, W Ju, EC Vonderheid, AH Rook and E. DeFreitas, 1991b. Malignant and nonmalignant T cell lines from human T cell lymphotropic virus type I-negative patients with Sézary syndrome. **J. Immunol.**, 146:1455.

Wechsler, J, M Bagot, T Henni and P Gaulard, 1990. Cutaneous pseudolymphomas: Immunotypical and immunogenotypical studies. In: WA van Vloten, R Willemze, GL Vejlsgaard K. Thomsen EdS: **Cutaneous lymphoma. Curr. Probl. Dermatol.**, 19:183.

Weiss, LM, GS Wood, M Trela, RA Warnke and J Sklar, 1986. Clonal T cell populations in lymphomatoid papulosis. Evidence of a lymphoproliferative origin for a clinically benign disease. **N. Engl. J. Med.**, 315:475.

Weiss LM, E Hu, GS Wood, C Moulds, ML Cleary, E. Warnke and J. Sklar, 1985. Clonal rearrangements for the T cell receptor genes in mycosis fungoides and dermatopathic lymphadenopathy. **N. Engl. J. Med.**, 313:539.

Whang-Peng, J, PA Bunn, T Knutsen, MJ Matthews, T Schechter and JD Minna, 1982. Clinical implications of cytogenetic studies in cutaneous T cell lymphoma (CTCL). **Cancer**, 50:1539.

Whittemore, AS, EA Holly, I-M Lee, EA Abel, RM Adams, BJ Nickoloff, L Bley, JM Peters and C Gibney, 1989. Mycosis fungoides in relation to environmental exposures and immune response: A case-control study. **J. Natl. Cancer Inst.**, 81:1560.

Yin, Y, MA Tainsky, FZ bischoff, LC Strong and GM Wahl, 1992. Wild-type p53 restores cell cycle control and inhibits gene amplification in cells with mutant p53 alleles. **Cell**, 70:937.

CHROMOSOME ABNORMALITIES IN CUTANEOUS B-CELL LYMPHOMAS

Anne Marie Busschots *
Marie-Louise Geerts †
Cristina Mecucci ‡
Michel Stul *
Jean-Jacques Cassiman *
Herman Van den Berghe *

* Center for Human Genetics
  University of Leuven
  Leuven, Belgium

† Department of Dermatology
  University of Gent
  Gent, Belgium

‡ Institute of Hematology
  University of Perugia
  Perugia, Italy

Correspondence to: Dr. A. M. Busschots, Center for Human Genetics,
UZ Gasthuisberg, Herestraat 49,
B-3,000, Leuven, Belgium

ABSTRACT

A case of cutaneous B-cell lymphoma (CBCL) is described in which a specific translocation, t(8;14)(q24;q32), was found. As far as we are aware, this is the first report of a cytogenetic abnormality in CBCL.

Basic Mechanisms of Physiologic and Aberrant Lymphoproliferation in the Skin
Edited by W.C. Lambert *et al.*, Plenum Press, New York, 1994

INTRODUCTION

Cytogenetic investigations have demonstrated that a variety of human malignancies are characterized by a specific chromosome abnormality (Mitelman, 1991). The fact that these karyotypic changes are consistently shared by a neoplastic entity from unrelated patients indicates that the characteristic chromosomal event may play a key role in the malignant transformation of the cell. Non-random breakpoints have been shown to be the sites of cancer related genes, namely oncogenes and growth factor genes. Several mechanisms potentially accounting for how a chromosomal abnormality could relate to malignant disease have been identified. These include: a translocation producing juxtaposition of an oncogene with a very active gene (such as an immunoglobulin gene), thereby resulting in elevated production of a cellular protein; formation of a new gene, also by juxtaposition, with an abnormal gene product being created as a consequence; and a deletion resulting in the loss or alteration of a gene encoding one or more important regulatory proteins, such as a tumor suppressor gene (for review see Sandberg, 1990).

To date, little is known about the pathogenic mechanisms responsible for cutaneous lymphomas. Only a limited number of reports have dealt with cytogenetic analysis of cutaneous T-cell lymphomas (CTCL). The karyotypic changes that have been found are complex, characterization has often been incomplete and no consistent change has been found. We describe a specific translocation, t(8;14)(q24;q32), in a cutaneous B cell lymphoma (CBCL). As far as we know, this is the first report of a cytogenetic abnormality in CBCL.

CASE REPORT

A 62-year-old man presented with multiple facial tumors and two enlarged cervical lymph nodes. Skin lesions had been noticed six months prior to lymph node involvement.

Pathologic examination revealed a follicular and diffuse centroblastic-centrocytic or large cell lymphoma, according to the Kiel classification and Working Formulation, respectively (Gerard-Marchant et al., 1974; Non Hodgkin's lymphoma pathologic classification project, 1982).

Immunohistochemically, the malignant cells were $\delta\mu\lambda^+$HLA-DR$^+$ CD20$^+$CD22$^+$ MB1$^+$MB2$^+$CD5$^-$CD10$^-$.

There was no involvement of blood or bone marrow.

Cytogenetic analysis performed on both involved skin and lymph node revealed the following karyotype: 47,XY,inv dup(1) (q11→q32),+3,t(8;14)(q24;q32) (Figure 1).

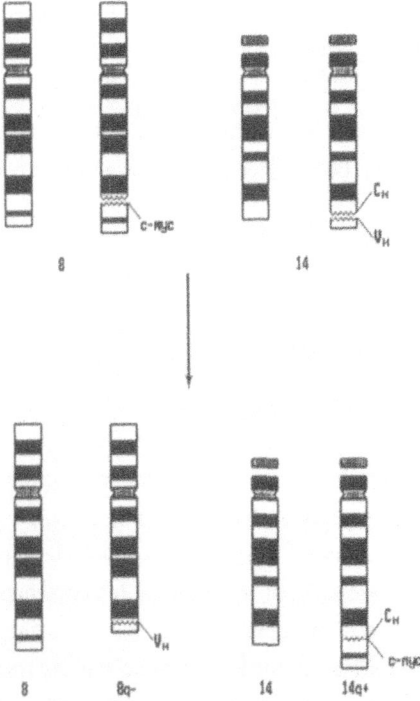

Figure 1. Diagram of the (8;14)(q24;q32) chromosome translocation

Southern blot analysis, performed on Bam HI, Eco RI and Hind III digested lymph node DNA, revealed a rearrangement of immunoglobulin heavy and lambda light chain genes, indicative of a monoclonal B-cell proliferation. A germline configuration was found with TCR, bcl-1 and bcl-2 probes as well as a first exon probe of the c-myc oncogene.

More details have been presented elsewhere (Busschots et al., 1993).

DISCUSSION

Within the group of lymphoproliferative disorders, different cytogenetic and molecular abnormalities have been found to be consistently associated not only with histologically distinct B- and T-cell neoplasms, but even with distinct subgroups of those neoplasms. Among the B cell malignancies, a 14q+ chromosome is the most frequent chromosomal abnormality. The t(8;14)(q24;q32) of Burkitt's lymphoma, the t(11;14)(q13;q32) of intermediately differentiated lymphocytic lymphoma, the t(14;18)(q32;q21) of follicular lymphoma and the t(14;19)(q32;q13) of an aggressive subtype of B-chronic lymphocytic leukemia are well-known chromosomal changes (Yunis et al, 1982; Yunis, 1983; Vandenberghe et al, 1991; Busschots et al, 1991).

They are associated with rearrangement of the (putative) oncogenes, c-myc, bcl-1, bcl-2 and bcl-3, located at 8q24, 11q13, 18q21 and 19q13, respectively (Dalla-Favera et al, 1982; Tsujimoto et al, 1984a;b; McKeithan et al., 1987).

In our case of CBCL there was a classical t(8;14)(q24;q32). The primary site of tumor involvement, however, could have been either the skin or a lymph node.

A translocation of the distal end (q24→qter) of the long arm of chromosome 8 to chromosome 14q32 (Figure 1) is the chromosome anomaly in 75 % of Burkitt lymphoma (BL) (Zech et al., 1976). Other types of non-Hodgkin lymphoma, however, may show the same translocation, especially large cell lymphoma (Mitelman, 1991). The c-myc oncogene and the immunoglobulin heavy chain gene have been mapped in or near the breakpoints involved in BL (8;14) (Taub et al., 1982). It has been demonstrated that the c-myc gene (8q24) comes under the influence of enhancers in or adjacent to the immunoglobulin heavy chain locus (14q32), resulting in a deregulation of its expression (Hayday et al., 1984; Nishikura et al., 1983). The c-myc oncogene comprises three exons. The first exon contains termination codons on all three reading frames and therefore represents an untranslated leader sequence. The breakpoints on chromosome 8 are always 5' (i.e., "upstream") of the c-myc coding exons (II and III) in the (8;14) translocations. The breaks may occur at variable distances from the 5' end of the gene or they may involve either the first exon or the first intron (Croce and Nowell, 1985; Shiramizu and Magrath, 1990; Boehm and Rabbitts, 1989; Figure 2).

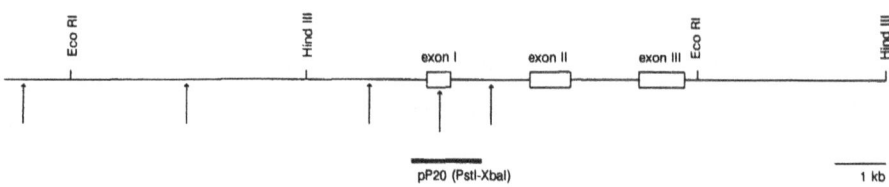

Figure 2. Restriction map of the human c-myc locus at chromosome 8 showing the location of the first exon probe and restriction endonuclease sites. Possible sites for a chromosomal break in t(8;14) lymphomas are indicated by arrows.

As no rearrangement of the c-myc oncogene was detected with an exon I probe on Eco RI and Hind III digested DNA, we cannot exclude the possibility that in the present case the breakpoint was far 5' of the first c-myc exon.

In our review of the literature on CBCL, we found no description of rearrangement of the c-myc oncogene, including c-myc (Delia et al., 1989). Moreover, cytogenetic data on CBCL are not available.

Indeed, while molecular genetics provides a set of techniques theoretically capable of isolating any gene from the genome, potentially leading to a detailed understanding of genotypic changes, those techniques are sometimes insufficient for identifying the altered DNA sequences in neoplasia. Clues from other information sources, such as a karyotype, must therefore be used to direct molecular studies to the correct region of the genome. Cytogenetic changes reflect events which pertain to certain molecular mechanisms which may be key events in the genesis of neoplasia. Therefore, in order to clarify the pathogenic mechanisms responsible for CBCL, and for cutaneous lymphomas in general, more cytogenetic analyses should be performed on skin and/or on metastatic tissue.

ACKNOWLEDGEMENT: This research was supported by the Inter-University Network for Fundamental Research sponsored by the Belgian Government (1991-1995).

REFERENCES

Boehm T and TH Rabbitts, 1989. A chromosomal basis of lymphoid malignancy in man. **Eur. J. Biochem.**, 185:1-17.

Busschots AM, ML Geerts, C Mecucci, M Stul, JJ Cassiman and H. Van den Berghe, 1993. A translocation (8;14) in a cutaneous large B-cell lymphoma. **Am. J. Clin. Pathol.**, in press.

Busschots AM, C Mecucci, M Stul, E Vandenberghe, JL Michaux, H Noel, JJ Cassiman and H Van den Berghe, 1991. Translocation (14;19)(q32;q13.1) in a young patient who developed a large cell lymphoma after an initial diagnosis of CLL. **Leukemia and Lymphoma**, 5:281-286.

Croce CM and PC Nowell, 1985. Molecular basis of human B cell neoplasia. **Blood**, 65:I-VII.

Dalla-Favera R, M Bregni, J Erikson, D Patterson, RC Gallo and CM Croce, 1982. Human c-myc oncgene is located on the region of chromosome 8 that is translocated in Burkitt lymphoma cells. **Proc. Natl. Acad. Sci. USA**, 79:7824-7827.

Delia D, MG Borrello, E Berti, MA Pierotti, D Biassoni, R Gianotti, E Alessi, MG Rizzetti, R Caputo and G Della Porta, 1989. Clonal immunoglobulin gene rearrangements and normal T-cell receptor, bcl-2 and c-myc genes in primary cutaneous B-cell lymphomas. **Cancer Res.**, 49:4901-4905.

Gerard-Marchant R, I Hamlin, K Lennert, F Rilke, AG Stansfeld and JAM Van Unnik, 1974. Classification of non-Hodgkin's lymphomas. **Lancet**, 2:406-408.

Hayday AC, SD Gillies, H Saito, C Wood, K Wiman, WS Hayward and S Tonegawa, 1984. Activation of a translocated human c-myc gene by an enhancer in the immunoglobulin heavy-chain locus. **Nature**, 307:334-340.

McKeithan TW, JD Rowley, TB Shows and MO Diaz, 1987. Cloning of the chromosome translocation breakpoint junction of the t(14;19) in chronic lymphocytic leukemia. **Proc. Natl. Acad Sci U.S.A.**, 84:9257-9260.

Mitelman F, 1991. **Catalog of Chromosome Aberrations in Cancer**, 4th ed. New York, Wiley-Liss, Editor.

Nishikura K, A Ar-Rushdi, J Erikson, R Watt, G Rovera and CM Croce, 1983. Differential expression of the normal and of the translocated human c-myc oncogenes in B cells. **Proc. Natl. Acad. Sci. USA**, 80:4822-4826.

(The) Non-Hodgkin's lymphoma pathologic classification project, 1982. National Cancer Institute Sponsored Study of Classification of Non-Hodgkin's lymphomas. Summary and Description of a Working Formulation for Clinical Usage. **Cancer** (Phila.), 49:2112-2135.

Sandberg AA, 1990. **The Chromosomes in Human Cancer and Leukemia**, 2nd ed. New York, Elsevier North-Holland, Inc.

Shiramizu B and I Magrath, 1990. Localization of breakpoints by polymerase chain reactions in Burkitt's lymphoma with 8;14 translocations. **Blood**, 75:1848-1852.

Taub R, I Kirsch, C Morton, G Lenoir, D Swan, S Tronick, S Aaronson and P Leder, 1982. Translocation of the c-myc gene into the immunoglobulin heavy chain locus in human Burkitt lymphoma and murine plasmacytoma cells. **Proc. Natl. Acad. Sci. USA**, 79:7837-7841.

Tsujimoto Y, LR Finger, J Yunis, PC Nowell and CM Croce, 1984a. Cloning of the chromosome breakpoint of neoplastic B cells with the t(14;18) chromosome translocation. **Science**, 226:1097-1099.

Tsujimoto Y, J Yunis, L Onorato-Showe, J Erikson, PC Nowell and CM Croce, 1984b. Molecular cloning of the chromosomal breakpoint of B-cell lymphomas and leukemias with the t(ll;14) chromosome translocation. **Science**, 224:1403-1406.

Vandenberghe E, C De Wolf-Peeters, J Van Den Oord, I Wlodarska, J Delabie, M Stul, J Thomas, JL Michaux, C Mecucci, JJ Cassiman and H Van den Berghe, 1991. Translocation (11;14): A cytogenetic anomaly associated with B-cell lymphomas of nonfollicle centre cell lineage. **J. Pathol.**, 163:13-18.

Yunis JJ, MM Oken, ME Kaplan, KM Ensrud, RR Howe and A Theologides, 1982. Distinctive chromosomal abnormalities in histologic subtypes of non-Hodgkin's lymphoma. **New Engl. J. Med.**, 307:1231-1236.

Yunis JJ, 1983. The chromosomal basis of human neoplasia. **Science**, 221:227-236.

Zech L, U Haglund, K Nilsson and G Klein, 1976. Characteristic chromosomal abnormalities in biopsies and lymphoid cell lines from patients with Burkitt and non-Burkitt lymphomas. **Int. J. Cancer**, 17:47-56.

MECHANISM FOR TUMOR PROGRESSION IN LYMPHOMATOID PAPULOSIS: HYPOTHESIS BASED ON STUDIES OF TUMOR CELL LINES CLONALLY DERIVED FROM LYMPHOMATOID PAPULOSIS

Marshall E. Kadin*
Thomas H Davis†
Steven P Balk‡
Samuel R Newcom‡
Sela Cheifitz#
Joan Massague#

* Department of Pathology
† Department of Medicine
  Beth Israel Hospital
  Harvard Medical School
  Boston, MA

‡ Department of Medicine
  Emory University
  Atlanta, GA

Cell Biology and Genetics Program
  Memorial Sloan-Kettering Cancer Center
  New York, NY, U.S.A.

Correspondence to: Dr. M. E. Kadin, Department of Hematopathology,
Beth Israel Hospital, 330 Brookline Avenue,
Boston, MA 02215, U.S.A.

Basic Mechanisms of Physiologic and Aberrant Lymphoproliferation in the Skin
Edited by W.C. Lambert *et al.*, Plenum Press, New York, 1994

425

INTRODUCTION

Lymphomatoid papulosis (LyP) is a recurrent, multifocal cutaneous eruption characterized pathologically as an infiltration of large atypical cells surrounded by inflammatory cells (Macaulay, 1968). The large atypical cells resemble Reed Sternberg (RS) cells of Hodgkin disease (HD) (type A LyP cells), or Sézary cells of cutaneous T cell lymphoma (CTCL) (type B LyP cells) (Willemze et al., 1982). In most cases the large atypical cells have an activated helper T cell phenotype (CD30+, CD4+) (Kadin et al., 1985). Approximately 10-20% of LyP cases are associated with a malignant lymphoma, usually CTCL, HD, or a CD30+ large cell anaplastic lymphoma (ALCL), (Weinman and Ackerman, 1981; Willemze et al., 1982; Sanchez et al., 1983; Wantzin et al., 1985; Harrington et al., 1989; Kaudewitz et al., 1990). The skin lesions of LyP can precede, coexist with, or follow the associated lymphoma (Ibid).

The high frequency of malignant lymphomas in LyP patients and their similar morphologic and immunophenotypic characteristics to the large atypical cells comprising LyP lesions have led to the hypothesis that these lymphomas represent tumor evolution from common T cell clones present in LyP (Kadin, 1985). Thus we suggest that LyP can be used to understand the biology of lymphoma development and progression, as well as host interactions, early in the pathogenesis of a significant proportion of human lymphoid malignancies.

DEVELOPMENT AND CHARACTERIZATION OF LyP-RELATED CELL LINES

We had the opportunity to test this hypothesis in a patient who presented with LyP (in 1971) and later developed HD (in 1975) and a CD30+ CTCL (in 1983). Three clonally related tumor cell lines were developed from clinically indolent (Mac-1) and advanced tumor-forming stages (Mac-2A and Mac-2B) of this patient's CTCL. Cell line Mac-1 was developed from circulating Sézary-like cells in the blood in 1983 and two cell lines (Mac-2A and Mac-2B) were developed from separate skin tumor nodules in 1985. Cell line Mac-1 was initiated with interleukin-2 (IL-2), but subsequently it became evident that this cell line was not IL-2 dependent. Cell lines Mac-2A and Mac-2B were started without IL-2. All cell lines are maintained in RPMI 1640 medium supplemented with 15% fetal calf serum.

Morphology

The lymphoma cell lines grow in suspension as clusters of tumor cells. Cell line Mac-1 contains mostly small and intermediate size lymphocytes with approximately 5% multinucleated RS-like cells. Cell lines Mac-2A and Mac-2B contain a higher percentage of large cells and more frequent RS-like cells (Figure 1).

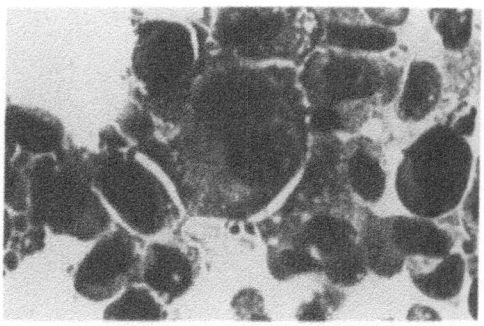

Figure 1. CD30⁺ CTCL line Mac 2B containing Reed-Sternberg-like cells.

Cytogenetics

All cell lines have a balanced translocation, t(8;9)(p22;p24), also identified in a "dermatopathic" lymph node in 1983. Cell lines Mac-2A and Mac-2B have additional chromosomal abnormalities, consistent with clonal evolution and tumor progression (Davis et al., 1992).

Immunophenotyping

Cell line Mac-1 has an activated helper T cell phenotype with expression of leukocyte common antigen (CD45), T cell antigens CD2 and CD4, and activation antigens CD30 and CD25, but not CD15. Cell lines Mac-2A and Mac-2B have a less well differentiated phenotype, lacking CD45, CD2 and CD4, but expressing both CD15 and CD30 (ibid). The immunophenotype of cell lines 2A and 2B is similar to that of RS-cells in most cases of mixed cellularity and nodular sclerosing HD.

Evidence that CTCL cell lines are clonally related to LyP

The T cell receptor (TCR) alpha chain gene was cloned and sequenced from cell line Mac-2B. From these alpha chain sequences, it was possible to construct V and J region primers to amplify, and a tumor specific N region probe to detect, identical TCR alpha chain sequences in other tissues of this patient. DNA amplified by the polymerase chain reaction (PCR) from a 1971 LyP skin lesion and a 1975 HD lymph node hybridized specifically with the TCR N region probe derived from the patient's CTCL (Figure 2). A DNA densitometry study comparing rearranged alpha chain DNA versus total DNA was consistent with derivation of specifically amplified product from atypical cells in the LyP lesions and RS-cells in the HD lymph node.

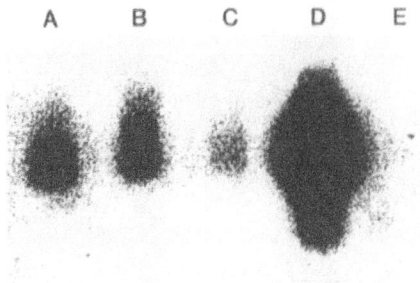

Figure 2. Southern blot showing hybridization of DNA amplified from 1971 LyP lesion (A and B), 1975 HD lymph node (C), and autopsy lymph node (D) with N region probe derived from TCR alpha chain of CTCL line Mac-2B. No hybridization is seen in lane E containing DNA from another patient with HD. Reproduced from Figure 6, Davis et al., 1992.

Cloning and sequencing of the amplified DNA confirmed that the identical TCR alpha chain was present in the patient's CTCL, HD and LyP. These results indicate that the patient's CTCL and HD were derived from a single T cell clone present in the earlier LyP (Davis et al., 1992).

Growth inhibition by transforming growth factor-beta (TGF-β1)

IL-2 dependent DNA synthesis of nonmalignant activated T lymphocytes is suppressed 60-80% by TGF-β1 (Kerhl et al., 1986). To determine whether Mac-1 cells from clinically indolent CTCL are also inhibited by TGF-β1, Mac-1 cells were cultured in serum-free medium with low concentrations of TGF-β1 and IL-2 (Newcom et al., 1988). Addition of 2 ng/ml TGF-β suppressed IL-2 dependent DNA synthesis of Mac-1 cells by 40-45%, or about one-half the suppression obtained with nonmalignant activated T- lymphocytes. This suppression correlated with a 40-65 % reduction in the number of IL-2 receptors measured by immunofluoresence. By contrast, no suppression of DNA synthesis by cell line L428 from advanced HD was observed. L428 cells have no detectable receptors for IL-2 or TGF-β.

TGF-β1 inhibits colony formation of cell line Mac-1 from clinically indolent CTCL but not cell lines Mac-2A and Mac-2B from advanced CTCL

Colony formation in methylcellulose of Mac-1 cells was significantly inhibited (70-80%) by low concentrations (1.0-10.0 ng/ml) of TGF-β1 (Kadin et al., 1990). By contrast, the same concentrations of TGF-β1 did not inhibit colony formation of cell lines Mac-2A and 2B from advanced disease. These results demonstrate that disease progression in this LyP-related CTCL is correlated with loss of response to growth inhibition by TGF-β1.

Fluorescence measurement of TGF-β1 membrane binding in cell lines

To investigate the mechanism of TGF-β resistance in advanced disease, binding of fluorescein labelled TGF-β to membrane receptors of cell lines was evaluated. Fluorescein labelled TGF-β was incubated with cell lines Mac-1, Mac-2A and Mac-2B in the presence of excess unlabelled TGF-β1. Binding of fluorokine TGF-β is shown in Figure 3. Unexpectedly, cell lines Mac-2A and Mac-2B, which are resistant to TGF-β growth inhibition, demonstrated slightly greater fluorescence, or more binding of TGF-β, than line Mac-1.

Loss of TGF-ß receptors type I and II in advanced disease (cell lines MAC-2A and 2B)

Cell lines were affinity labeled with iodinated TGF-β as previously described (Massague

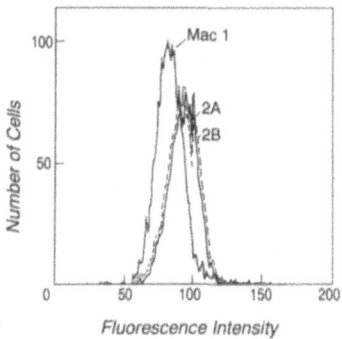

Figure 3. Fluorescence histogram showing greater binding of fluorokine TGF-β-biotin to cell lines Mac-2A and Mac-2B than to Mac-1 (FACS analysis).

and Like, 1985). Following removal of unbound ligand, bound TGF-β was chemically cross-linked to cells and affinity labeled protein extracts analyzed by SDS-PAGE on 5-8% linear polyacrylamide gels and visualized by autoradiography. Under these conditions, normal cells express three types of TGF-β receptors, type I, type II and type III, a ß-glycan. Affinity labeling of Mac-1 cells revealed that they express beta glycan, the TGF-β binding proteoglycan, and receptors type I and II (Figure 4). By contrast, no type I or II receptors were detected on cell lines Mac-2A or Mac-2B. These cells did express ß-glycan at a higher relative intensity than Mac-1 cells, presumably accounting for the increased fluoresence observed with the fluorokine, TGF-β. Type I and type II receptors appear to mediate the growth inhibitory functions of TGF-β1 as shown by experiments with receptor-deficient mutants of mink lung epithelial cells commonly used to assay the inhibitory effects of TGF-β1 (Cheifitz, et al.). Thus, disease progression in this LyP related CTCL appears to be associated with loss or markedly decreased expression of type I and type II receptors for growth inhibition by TGF-β1.

Correlation with in vivo observations, a: TGF-β activity detected immunohistochemically in advanced disease

To determine whether these in vitro observations on cell lines correlate with disease

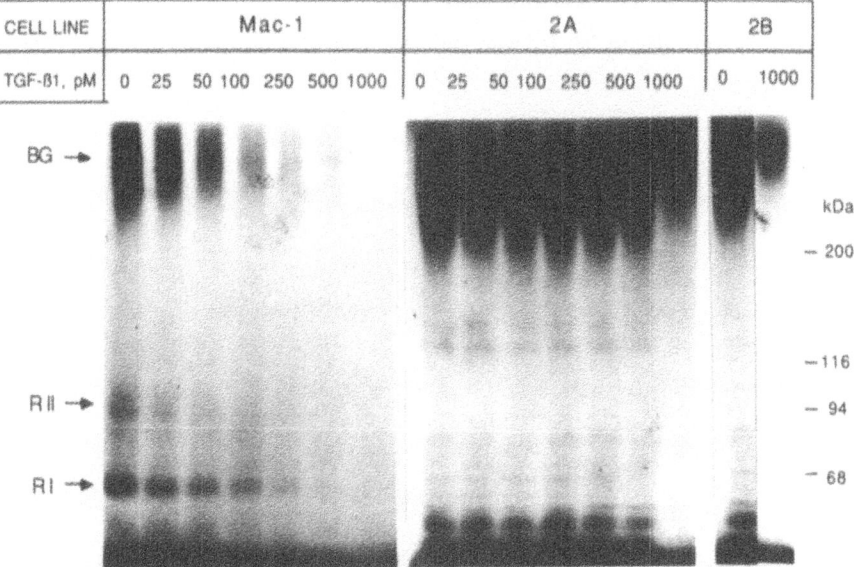

Figure 4. Affinity labeling of cell lines Mac-1, Mac-2A and Mac-2B with ¹²⁵I-TGF-β1. Radiolabeled products corresponding to beta glycan (BG), and receptor (R) types I and II are indicated by arrows. Cell lines Mac-2A and Mac-2B lack detectable receptors type I and II shown in cell line Mac-1. There is 2.5 x greater density of ß-glycan in cell lines Mac-2A and Mac-2B.

progression in vivo, immunohistochemistry was performed with antibody CC (1-30), which detects activated TGF-β (Ellingsworth, et al., 1986). TGF-β activity was detected in a skin tumor from the advanced stage of CTCL from which cell line Mac-2B was derived. Apparently, failure of this lesion to regress was not due to absence of active TGF-β, but more likely was due to absence of TGF-β receptors on tumor cells as demonstrated in vitro. Unfortunately, antibodies to detect TGF-β receptors in fixed tissue sections of the tumor are not available at the time of this writing.

Correlation with in vivo observations, b: TGF-ß activity detected in regressing LyP lesions but not in LyP associated persistent patch lesions of CTCL

In two other patients who had coexistent LyP and CTCL, TGF-β activity was detected immunohistochemically in the regressing LyP type A lesions but not the persistent patch lesions of CTCL (Figure 5). The LyP lesions had numerous inflammatory cells and large atypical cells whereas coexistant CTCL lesions contained mainly cerebriform lymphocytes and few inflammatory cells. TGF-β is normally secreted in latent form and requires, for biological

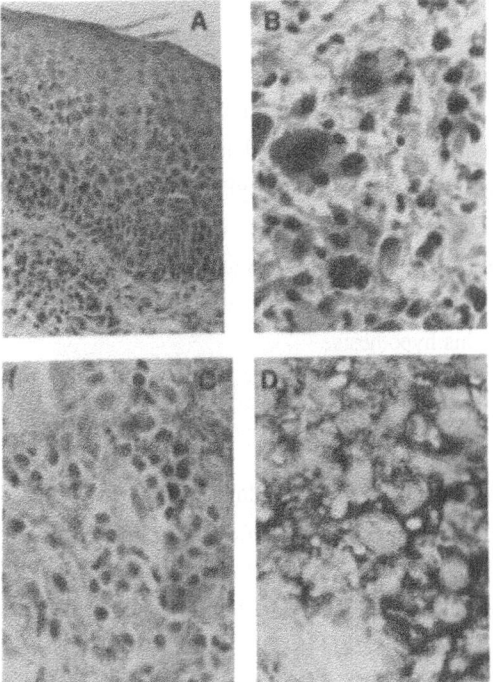

Figure 5. Biopsies of coexistent patch stage MF (left) and LyP type A (right). TGF-β1 activity is detected immunohistochemically as dark precipitate on cell surface and extracellular matrix in LyP lesion (lower right) but not in MF (lower left).

activation, certain conditions such as environmental acidification (Jullien et al., 1989), heparin dissociation of the TGF-β/α-2 macroglobulin inactive complex (Mc Caffrey et al., 1989) and cleavage by plasmin (Lyons et al., 1990). One or more of the appropriate conditions for TGF-β activation may be provided by inflammatory cells which infiltrate regressing LyP type A lesions but are less numerous or are infrequent in chronic LyP type B or CTCL lesions. Thus it is possible that incomplete local activation of TGF-β may contribute to tumor progression in LyP-associated lymphomas.

Correlation with in vivo observations, c: Eosinophils are a major source of TGF-ß1 in Hodgkin disease

Another possibility is that the TGF-β is actually secreted by inflammatory cells infiltrating regressing LyP lesions. Recently, we demonstrated TGF-β mRNA in eosinophils of nodular sclerosing HD (Kadin et al., 1993) suggesting that eosinophils can be a major source of TGF-β in human lymphoproliferative disorders.

Model for tumor progression in LyP

In this model, tumor progression can occur when atypical/tumor cells lose receptors for growth inhibition by TGF-β as demonstrated in cell lines Mac-2A and Mac-2B from advanced CTCL and in cell line L428 from advanced HD. Alternatively, a deficient host immune response could result in inadequate local production or activation of TGF-β. TGF-β activity was detected immunohistochemically in regressing LyP lesions but not in coexistent patch lesions of CTCL in two patients. The two mechanisms are not exclusive and may be operative at different clinical stages (early and late) of tumor progression from LyP. Further studies on fresh tissues and cell lines derived from different stages in the progression of LyP to malignant lymphoma should permit testing of this hypothesis.

REFERENCES

Cheifitz, S, B Like and J Massague, 1986. Cellular distribution of type I and type II receptors for transforming growth factor-ß. **J. Biol. Chem.**, 261:9972-78.

Davis, TH, CC Morton, R. Miller-Cassman, SP Balk and ME Kadin, 1992. Hodgkin's disease, lymphoblastoid papulosis, and cutaneous T cell lymphoma derived from a common T cell clone. **N. Engl. J. Med.**, 326:1115-22.

Ellingsworth, LR, JE Brennan, X Fok, DM Rosen, H Bentz, KA Piez and SM Seyedin, 1986. Antibodies to the N-terminal portion of cartilage-inducing factor A and transforming growth factor B. **J. Biol. Chem.**, 261:12362-12367.

Harrington, DS, SW Braddock, KS Blochr, DD Weisenburger, W Sanger and JO Armitage, 1989. Lymphomatoid papulosis and progression to T cell lymphoma: An immunophenotypic and genotypic analysis. **J. Am. Acad. Dermatol.**, 21:951-957.

Jullien, P, TM Berg and DA Lawrence, 1989. Acidic cellular environments: Activation of latent TGF-beta and sensitization of cellular responses to TGF-ß and EGF. **Int. J. Cancer**, 43:886-891.

Kadin, ME, 1985. Common activated helper T cell origin for lymphomatoid papulosis, mycosis fungoides and some types of Hodgkin's disease. **Lancet** ii: 864-865.

Kadin, ME, K Nasu, D Sako, J Said and EC Vonderheid, 1985, Lymphomatoid papulosis. A cutaneous proliferation of activated helper T cells expressing Hodgkin's disease associated antigens. **Am. J. Pathol.**, 119:315-325.

Kadin, ME, MW Cavaille-Coll and CC Morton, 1990. Tumor progression in Ki-1[+] cutaneous lymphomas is related to escape from inhibition by transforming growth factor-ß. **Blood**, 76, Suppl 1, 354a.

Kadin, ME, J Butmarc, A Elovic and D Wong, 1993. Eosinophils are a major source of transforming growth factor-beta (TGF-β) in nodular sclerosing Hodgkin's disease. **Am. J. Pathol.**, 142:11-16.

Kaudewitz, P, H Stein, G Plewig et al, 1990. Hodgkin's disease followed by lymphomatoid papulosis: Immunophenotypical evidence for a close relationship between lymphomatoid papulosis and Hodgkin's disease. **J. Am. Acad. Dermatol.**, 22:999-1006.

Kehrl, JH, AB Roberts, LM Wakefield, S Jakeloew, MB Sporn and AS Fauci, 1986. Production of transforming growth factor beta by human T lymphocytes and its potential role in the regulation of T cell growth. **J. Exp. Med.**, 163: 1037-1050.

Lyons, RM, LE Gentry, AF Purchio and HL Moses, 1990. Mechanism of activation of latent recombinant TGFβ1 by plasmin. **J. Cell Biol.**, 110:1361-1367.

Massague, J and B Like, 1985. Cellular receptors for type B transforming growth factor. Ligand binding and affinity labeling in human and rodent cell lines. **J. Biol. Chem.**, 260:1626-1645.

McCaffrey, TA, DJ Falcone, CT Brayton, LA Agarwal, FGP Welt and BB Weksler, 1989. Transforming growth factor-ß activity is potentiated by heparin via dissociation of the transforming growth factor-α/ß-2-macroglobulin complex. **J. Cell Biol.**, 109:441-448.

Macaulay, WL, 1968. Lymphomatoid papulosis: A continuing self healing eruption, clinically benign histologically malignant. **Arch. Dermatol.**, 97:23-30.

Newcom, SR, ME Kadin and AA Ansari, 1988. Production of transforming growth factor-ß activity by Ki-1 positive lymphoma cells and analysis of its role in the regulation of Ki-1 positive lymphoma growth. **Am. J. Pathol.**, 131:569-577.

Sanchez, NP, MR Pittelkow, SA Muller, PM Banks and RK Winkelmann, 1983. The clinicopathologic spectrum of lymphomatoid papulosis: Study of 31 cases. **J. Am. Acad. Dermatol.**, 8:81-94.

Wantzin, GL, K Thomsen, F Brandup and JK Larsen, 1985. Lymphomatoid papulosis. Development into cutaneous T cell lymphoma. **Arch. Dermatol.**, 121:792-794.

Weinman, VF and AB Ackerman, 1981. Lymphomatoid papulosis. A critical review and new findings. **Am. J. Dermatopathol.**, 3:129-163.

Willemze, R, CJ Meyer, WA van Vloten and E Scheffer, 1982. The clinical and histological spectrum of lymphomatoid papulosis. **Br. J. Dermatol.**, 107:131-44.

SHEDDING OF INTERLEUKIN-2 RECEPTOR IN CUTANEOUS LYMPHOMAS: AN EFFECTIVE MECHANISM TO CIRCUMVENT IMMUNOSURVEILLANCE?

Reinhard Dummer*
Frank Nestle*
Gerhard Posseckert†
Jurgen C Becker‡
Günter Burg*

* Department of Dermatology
University of Zurich
Zurich, Switzerland

† Department of Biochemistry
‡ Department of Dermatology
University of Würzburg
Würzburg, Germany

Correspondence to: Dr. R. Dummer, Department of Dermatology,
University Hospital, Gloriastrasse 31,
CH-8091 Zurich, Switzerland

ABSTRACT

Serum levels of soluble interleukin-2 receptor (sIL-2R) were determined by an ELISA technique and cytotoxic activity of peripheral mononuclear cells (PMC) measured by a four hour ^{51}Cr release assay in patients with cutaneous T cell lymphoma (CTCL). In addition, the clinical course of these patients was followed. A significant negative correlation between serum sIL-2R and NK-activity was found ($p < 0.05$, $n = 19$). Both parameters seem to be prognostic factors for disease progression. After a four day IL-2 stimulation, the increase in cytotoxicity of CTCL PMC resembled the increase observed in control PMC. In CTCL serum, however, IL-2 dependent augmentation of cytotoxicity was reduced. IL-2 affinity chromatography of serum from one CTCL patient produced an enrichment of sIL-2R which was able to inhibit IL-2 effects.

Basic Mechanisms of Physiologic and Aberrant Lymphoproliferation in the Skin
Edited by W.C. Lambert *et al.*, Plenum Press, New York, 1994

435

Western blotting characterized this IL-2 inhibitor as multimeric TAC-protein (sIL-2R α-chain).

Transfection of NIH 3T3 fibroblasts resulted in production of a recombinant TAC-protein present in monomeric (45 kDa) and dimeric (90 kDa) forms.

In vitro studies revealed a dose-dependent inhibition of IL-2 induced lymphokine-activated killer cell activity and of phytohemagglutinin (PHA) blast proliferation by recombinant sIL-2R.

Our data demonstrate that sIL-2R is capable of inhibiting IL-2 dependent cell proliferation and induction of cytotoxicity. We conclude that the negative correlation between sIL-2R and NK-activity in CTCL patients may be caused by neutralization of IL-2 by sIL-2R. This could be an important mechanism for escape from immunosurveillance in lymphoma patients.

INTRODUCTION

Immunosuppression in CTCL patients

The progression of neoplastic diseases depends on the proliferative capacity of the tumor cells as well as on immunologic functions of the host. Cutaneous T-cell lymphomas are mainly monoclonal neoplasms of T helper memory lymphocytes (Sterry et al., 1989) which play a central role in the regulation of the immune defense (Sanders et al., 1988).

There are hints that the malignant clones in these lymphoproliferative disorders retain some immunoregulatory capabilities. Mono- or oligo-clonal enhancement of immunoglobulins occurs regularly in these patients, which might be due to stimulation of the corresponding B lymphocytes by the malignant clones. In one patient suffering from a T cell gamma/delta receptor bearing cutaneous lymphoma, tumor cells isolated from a biopsy produced large amounts of interferon gamma, which was found to be increased in the serum of this patient and might account for the augmented natural killer cell (NK) activity exerted by his peripheral blood cells (Burg et al., 1991). The malignant cells might also have an impact on host defense mechanisms, however. The high risk in CTCL patients of developing secondary neoplasms (Kantor et al., 1989) is one clue to impaired immunofunction in these patients. Another well known point is the stage-related decrease in natural killer cell activity (Levy et al., 1984, Laroche et al., 1983), which appears in non-leukemic CTCL patients.

Various clinical observations suggest that the defense mechanisms of the host determine the outcome of these lymphoproliferative disorders. Reports of rapidly progressing CTCL after cyclosporine A therapy (Moreland et al., 1985, Thomsen et al., 1987), which blocks interleukin-2 transcription and selectively inhibits lymphocytic immune responses without reducing granulocyte or macrophage-mediated immune responses, and the relative inability of aggressive chemotherapy to improve the prognosis of CTCL patients (Kaye et al., 1989) support this notion.

Receptor shedding: Immunological implications

Shedding of plasma membrane materials has been demonstrated for all membrane compounds, including the heterogeneous populations of lipids, glycolipids, proteoglycans and glycoproteins (van Blitterswijk et al., 1979). The general concept of antigen shedding as an immunosuppressive mechanism was proposed as early as the early seventies (Alexander, 1974).

The stepwise promotion and final transformation of a normal lymphocyte into a malignant lymphocyte may be accompanied by the expression of antigens normally associated with early maturation stages or fetal tissues, or, in the case of viral transformation, with virus-associated antigens. Immunocompetent hosts have an effective arsenal of elimination pathways for mounting an immune response against the tumor. Antigens associated with MHC class I and class II molecules allow a specific T-cell dependent cytotoxic reaction to take place. The antigenic epitopes for natural killer cells (NK) are still only operationally defined. Since NK cells, as well as macrophages, possess receptors for immunoglobulins, antibodies could support NK-dependent or macrophage-mediated tumor elimination. Shed antigen fragments might provide protection for the tumor by competing for tumor recognition in humoral mechanisms, such as specific antibodies or the nonspecific complement system, or by blocking cell-bound receptors. In this way, the effector processes of the immune system may be substantially inhibited (Raz et al., 1978).

Within the last several years, it has become obvious that receptor molecules are involved in the shedding process under physiologic as well as pathophysiologic conditions (Weber et al., 1984). Since cytokines, such as IL-1, IL-2, IL-4, and interferons, are key molecules of immune responsiveness, escape from immunosurveillance might imply an interruption of the cytokine cascade. Membrane-bound cytokine receptors provide high affinity binding, which renders them candidates for cytokine neutralization after detachment from their respective cell surfaces.

A broad spectrum of other molecules might interact with effector mechanisms for immunosurveillance as well, however. These include T-cell antigens such as CD8 (Fujimoto et al., 1983), CD4 (Symons et al., 1991), adhesion molecules such as intercellular adhesion molecule-1 (Becker et al., 1991) or leukocyte-function antigen-1 (Meuer and Schirren, personal communication). This repertoire of specific proteins could be the basis for a general mechanism for regulation of biological functions.

Soluble receptor molecules in CTCL patients

On the basis of these concepts regarding immunosuppression in CTCL patients and potential relevance of shed cytokine receptors, we chose to analyze the interactions of NK activity, soluble interleukin-2 receptor (sIL-2R) and clinical outcome, since interleukin-2 is a potent stimulatory factor for NK activity (Yamada et al., 1987) and sIL-2R is able to bind IL-2 efficiently (Rubin et al., 1986). In addition, serum levels of soluble CD8 (sCD8) and soluble

CD4 (sCD4) in CTCL patients were studied and compared with the corresponding serum levels in inflammatory skin diseases. In order to define the role of the soluble TAC protein (sIL-2R α-chain) in IL-2 dependent proliferation and generation of cytotoxicity, sIL-2R was concentrated from the serum of a CTCL patient and a recombinant molecule was produced. Their impact on interleukin-2 effects in vitro was then studied.

PATIENTS AND METHODS

Patients

24 patients with histologically proven CTCL in different stages were investigated. Before entering the study, systemic treatment had been stopped for at least two weeks. A physical examination was done on day 0 and repeated six months later. Peripheral blood mononuclear cells were obtained for ^{51}Cr release assay on day 0 in 17 patients. Serum samples for sIL-2R assessment were collected in 23 patients. sCD8 and sCD4 serum levels were determined in CTCL patients and in patients with inflammatory skin disease (eczema) as well as in healthy donors.

Clinical course

In order to estimate the cutaneous tumor mass in a semiquantitative manner, a tumor burden index (TBI) was introduced. Physical examination of all subjects was done by only one investigator. The percentage of involved skin was documented using the rule of the nines (i.e., The head and neck region was assigned 9%, the arms 9%, each, the anterior and posterior torso 18%, each, the legs 18%, each, and the perineum 1% of total body surface area). Specific skin lesions were differentiated into patches (flat lesions, diameter larger than 1 cm), plaques (flat or slightly elevated lesions with increased consistency) and tumors (large nodular lesions, diameter larger than 1 cm) (Kerl et al., 1987). The surface area covered by tumors, patches and plaques was estimated and the tumor burden index (TBI) calculated as:

$$TBI = 4 \times (\% \text{ skin surface covered by tumor}) + 2 \times (\% \text{ skin surface covered by plaque}) + 1 \times (\% \text{ skin surface covered by patch})$$

Under these conditions the maximal achievable TBI was 400. In our patients the TBI was 41 ± 59 (mean $\pm$ standard deviation, minimum 2, maximum 280). The clinical course of the patients was determined as the difference between the tumor burden index (∂ TBI) at day 0 and six month later. It was calculated as:

$$\partial \text{ TBI} = \text{TBI after six months} - \text{TBI on day 0}$$

Patients with stable disease or regressing lesions were defined as ∂ TBI = 0 for the sake of statistical calculations.

Quantification of soluble interleukin-2 receptors

Soluble CD8 protein (sCD8), soluble CD4 protein (sCD4) and sIL-2R in the serum or in culture medium were determined by commercially available sandwich ELISAs (T Cell Sciences Inc., Cambridge, MA, USA). After development of the color, the ELISA plates were read at 490 nm, using a Dynatech MR 700 microplate reader. Units of sIL-2R, sCD8 and sCD4 were calculated from a standard curve constructed on the basis of a supernatant fluid from phytohemagglutinin-stimulated peripheral blood mononuclear cells (T Cell Sciences). Interassay variation was 5%.

Preparation of peripheral mononuclear cells (PMC)

Human PMC were obtained from healthy age-matched volunteers and from CTCL patients, after informed consent, and separated by Ficoll-Hypaque gradient centrifugation. After separation the cells were washed twice and immediately resuspended in complete medium (CM) consisting of RPMI 1640 (Gibco/BRL, Eggenstein, FRG) supplemented with 5% fetal calf serum (Gibco/BRL) or human serum as indicated, 2 mM L-glutamine (Seromed, Berlin, FRG), 10 mM sodium pyruvate (Seromed), 100 U/ml penicillin (Seromed), 100 μg/ml streptomycin (Seromed), and 50 μg/ml gentamycin (Seromed). For determination of NK activity, cells were used immediately after preparation in the ^{51}Cr release assay.

Induction of cytotoxicity

PMC were incubated for four days in CM supplemented with different concentrations of recombinant IL-2, kindly provided by Eurocetus, Frankfurt, FRG. As indicated in the results, in some experiments CM contained 25% allogeneic serum from healthy volunteers or CTCL patients. In the stimulation experiments using recombinant or natural TAC protein, PMC were taken from healthy donors and incubated in CM supplemented with 5% autologous serum.

sIL-2R release after phytohemagglutinin stimulation

PMC from healthy donors (n=10) and from patients with CTCL (n=10) were stimulated with phytohemagglutinin (PHA) for two days. The supernatant fluid was harvested and the released sIL-2R were determined by ELISA.

^{51}Cr release assay

Cytotoxic activity was determined in a four hour ^{51}Cr release assay using "NK-sensitive" erythroblastoma cell line K562 as target cells and the specific lysis (SL) was calculated as we have described (Dummer et al., 1991).

Proliferation assays

In order to study the influence of CTCL serum or TAC-protein on IL-2 dependent proliferation, PMC of healthy donors were stimulated with phytohemagglutinin for two days. After washing, they were incubated with various concentration of recombinant IL-2 for three days. Proliferation was quantified by ^{3}H-thymidine uptake in triplicate or by a colorimetric assay which uses hexosaminidase as the indicator substrate.

Expression system for sIL-2R

The gene coding for a soluble TAC species, consisting of 223 amino acids and lacking the 28 C-terminal residues (i.e., most of the membrane anchor and the whole intracytoplasmatic domain (Rusk et al., 1988)), was prepared by Bcn I digestion and BamH I conversion from a human cDNA clone. It originated from peripheral blood lymphocytes and was modified by inserting the stop-signal bearing oligonucleotide, TGACTGCAGTCA, into the Nae I site within the terminal region of the TAC gene sequence (Nikaido et al., 1984). The isolated modified gene was cloned into the Xho I site of the BMGneo expression vector (kindly provided by F. Melchers, Basel (Karasuyama and Melchers, 1988)) by filling with Klenow polymerase and blunt-end ligation (enzymes from Boehringer Mannheim, FRG).

Cultivation of fibroblast cells used for IL-2R expression

NIH3T3 fibroblasts were cultivated in Dulbecco's modified Eagle medium (DMEM) supplemented with 10% fetal calf serum, 2 x 10 M L-glutamine, 100 U/ml penicillin and 100 μg/ml streptomycin (Biochrom KG, Berlin, FRG) at 10% CO_2, 37˚C and 100% humidity. For selection, isolation and maintenance of transfected cells, 700 μg/ml G 418 (Geneticin , Gibco/-BRL) were added to the complete medium.

Transfection

Stable transfection of NIH 3T3 cells was performed using the calcium phosphate precipitation method (Chen and Okayama, 1987).

Purification of soluble TAC from fibroblast supernatant or CTCL serum

The purification of sIL-2R was performed using IL-2 affinity chromatography. About 80 mg of recombinant IL-2 U 94/T125 (Weigel et al., 1989) were coupled to 4.2 g (dry weight) CNBr preactivated sepharose 4B (Pharmacia) according to the manufacturer's protocol. A small syringe column was filled with about 1.5 ml swollen affinity matrix and equilibrated with phosphate buffered saline (PBS) buffer, pH 7,4. For purification of recombinant sIL-2R, about 250 ml of conditioned fibroblast medium was pumped continuously through the column for 14 hours at a low flow rate of about 0.5 ml/min. After loading, the column was washed with PBS until the extinction at 280 nm returned to starting levels. Elution was performed with 0.2 M acetic acid/0.2 M NaCl (Weber et al., 1988). 1 ml fractions of eluate were collected, neutralized with 0.3 volumes of 1 M Tris/Cl, pH 8, to a final pH of 7, and stored frozen. TAC-free control buffer was treated in the same way. The analogous procedure was performed using twenty ml of 1:1 PBS diluted CTCL serum.

Western blot analysis

Western blots were performed according to standard procedures under reducing and nonreducing conditions using 7G7/B6 (kindly provided by D.L. Nelson, NIH, Bethesda, USA) and R23g (kindly provided by R.J. Robb, Glenoden, Pennsylvania, USA) as primary antibodies and an alkaline phosphatase coupled secondary antibody (Sigma, Taufkirchen, FRG).

RESULTS

Statistical analysis of clinical course, NK activity and sIL-2R

sIL-2R was found to be significantly ($p < 0.01$, Student's one tailed t-test) higher in CTCL patients than in age-matched control patients. NK activity of fresh PMC was significantly lower in CTCL patients compared to healthy controls ($p < 0.01$, t-test). Statistical analysis of the in vivo immunological findings revealed a negative correlation between NK activity and sIL-2R in CTCL patients (Spearman's rank correlation coefficient $= -0.5423$, $p < 0.03$, $n = 17$) as well as in CTCL patients plus ten control patients, whose sIL-2R and NK activity had been determined simultaneously (Spearman's rank correlation coefficient $= -0.4568$, $p < 0.02$, $n = 27$).

In addition, statistical analysis of our data revealed correlations between NK activity, sIL-2R and disease progression, which was described by the ∂ TBI. There was a negative correlation between NK activity and ∂ TBI ($p \leq 0.05$). A strong positive correlation was found between sIL2R and ∂ TBI ($p < 0.005$). No correlation between staging and sIL-2R or staging and NK activity was observed.

Analyzing the reliability of sIL-2R as a prognostic factor, we suggest that a ∂ TBI of 10 or greater should be considered a significant change. Moreover, to be significant, sIL-2R should exceed the upper range of normal by a factor of 2 (> 1000 U/ml). Under these conditions the specificity of sIL-2R for tumor progression was 90.9% ($n = 11$). There was no false-positive value, indicating a high degree of specificity.

sCD4 and sCD8 SERUM LEVELS

Both serum sCD4 and sCD8 were found to be elevated in CTCL patients, as well as in patients with inflammatory skin diseases, compared to normal controls (Figure 1). sCD4 and sCD8 levels did not correlate with the clinical outcome, however.

Stimulation experiments using CTCL and normal donor PMC

The average increase in cytotoxic activity in a four day stimulation of PMC (1000 IU IL-2/ml) from CTCL patients (n = 12) showed no significant difference compared with the increase in controls (n = 10).

sIL-2R release after PHA-stimulation

After PHA stimulation there was no significant difference in the soluble sIL-2R levels in the supernatant fluids of CTCL patients' PMC (n=10) compared to controls (n=10).

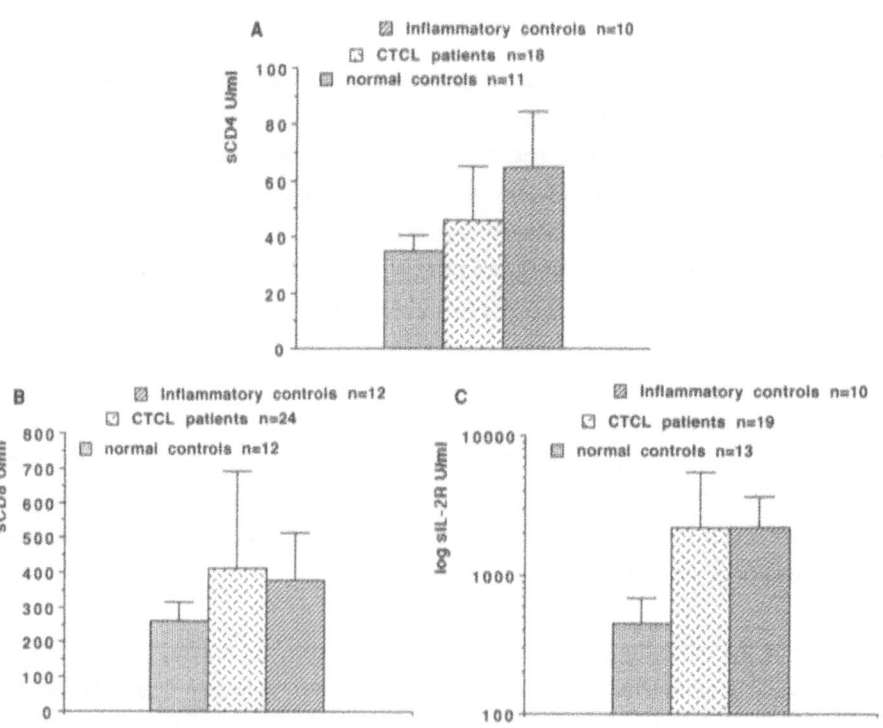

Figure 1. Serum levels of soluble CD4 (A) and CD8 (B) protein and soluble interleukin-2 receptor (C) in cutaneous T-cell lymphoma patients, healthy donors and patients with inflammatory skin diseases.

Stimulation experiments using CTCL and normal donor serum

PMC from healthy donors were stimulated in the serum of three CTCL patients (sIL-2R 3,000, 7,330, and 10,700 U/ml, respectively) and in control serum (sIL-2R 320, 400, and 420 U/ml, respectively). A four-day stimulation of a normal donor's PMC with 50 IU or 5 IU IL-2 in 25% CTCL serum resulted in reduced induction of cytotoxic activity compared to control serum. In a similar manner, IL-2 dependent PHA-blast proliferation was 60% lower (with 50 IU IL-2/ml) or 50% lower (with 5 IU IL-2/ml) in CTCL serum (sIL-2R = 3,000 U/ml) compared to control serum (sIL-2R = 400 U/ml).

TAC production by transfected fibroblasts

Soluble TAC concentrations (determined by ELISA) in the supernatant fluids of transfected fibroblasts reached up to 30,000 U/ml during four days of incubation, i.e., about 6,000 U/24 hr/10^6 cells. 1,000,000 U were determined to represent about 3 mg TAC protein.

Purification of sIL-2R

Using fibroblast supernatant fluids, peak fractions of IL-2 affinity chromatography exhibited soluble TAC concentrations of up to about 1,000,000 U/ml. Thus, a single purification step was able to concentrate the protein more than 30-fold. TAC peak fractions were highly pure, and proteins derived from the culture medium, such as albumin, were removed efficiently (data not shown).

Using 20 ml of one CTCL patient's serum (patient ST, sIL-2R = 3000 U/ml), a single affinity chromatography purification step resulted in a maximal concentration of 8,000 U/ml sIL-2R.

Western blotting of purified recombinant TAC proteins

Western blots were performed using 7C7/B6 (non-reducing conditions) and R23g (reducing and non-reducing conditions) as primary antibodies. Large amounts of recombinant sIL-2R (180,000 u/ml) completely blocked enhancement of cytotoxicity induced by IL-2 (5 IU/ml). The main band, seen at about 45 kD, corresponds to the soluble TAC monomer, while the band seen at about 100 kD -- present only under non-reducing conditions -- is ostensibly due to dimer formation (Smart et al., 1990). Extra bands below and above the main bands probably correspond to glycosylation modifications.

Inhibition of IL-2 induced generation of cytotoxicity and proliferation by natural and recombinant TAC protein

In the presence of a control fraction, 5 IU IL-2/ml induced a specific lysis (SL) of 56.7%

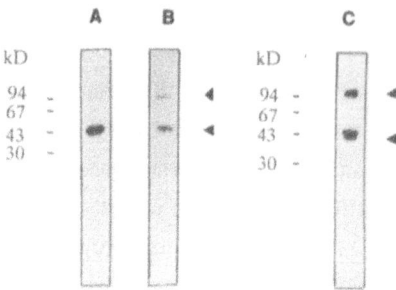

Figure 2. Western blots of IL-2 affinity purified recombinant sIL-2R. Lanes A,B: R23g as primary antibody. Lane C: 7G7/B6 as primary antibody. Lane A: reducing conditions. Lanes B,C: Non-reducing conditions.

in healthy donors' PMC. Addition of the TAC-enriched fraction resulted in a SL of 32.3%, representing a 57% inhibition. Proliferation of PHA blasts was reduced by 78.5% in the presence of the control fraction compared to the TAC-enriched fraction. Healthy donors' PMC developed reduced enhancement of cytotoxic activity in the presence of recombinant TAC protein in a dose-dependent manner. Large amounts of recombinant sIL-2R (180,000 U/ml) completely blocked enhancement of cytotoxicity induced by IL-2 (5 IU/ml). IL-2 dependent proliferation of PHA blasts was inhibited in a dose-dependent manner. A 50% inhibition was achieved by a sIL-2R concentration of 18,000 U/ml (50 IU IL-2).

DISCUSSION

CTCL patients demonstrate an obvious state of immunosuppression which is poorly understood. To obtain more insight into this phenomenon, we have analyzed the clinical course of CTCL patients in conjunction with their serological as well as functional immune markers.

Statistical evaluation revealed a correlation between decrease in NK-activity and progression of the disease, which suggests that NK-activity may be a prognostic factor for CTCL patients. We are well aware that NK-activity is a complex immunological factor. In the peripheral blood, no phenotypically defined cell type fulfills this activity exclusively. NK-cells (CD16$^+$, CD56$^+$) as well as MHC restricted and non-restricted T-lymphocytes (CD4$^+$ or CD8$^+$) contribute to this parameter of cytotoxicity. Our patients had a normal CD4/CD8 ratio and excessive numbers of cells with malignant morphology were not found by electron microscopy. Therefore, we can rule out a displacement of CD8 positive cytotoxic T lymphocytes by malignant T cells which do not exert cytotoxic activity. We do not know, however, whether the circulating CD4$^+$ lymphocytes express a T helper/inducer or T suppressor/inducer phenotype or whether a shift to an increased percentage of T helper/inducer cells is associated with diminished NK-activity. There seems to be a functional difference between CTCL patients' PMC and healthy donors' PMC. Phenotypic changes in T helper subsets in the peripheral blood of CTCL patients have been reported (Gilmore et al., 1991) which may explain some of our observations.

We and others (Kaudewitz et al., 1988; Dummer et al., 1991) have reported elevated levels of soluble IL-2 receptor proteins (TAC-proteins) in the serum of CTCL patients, a phenomenon which has also been observed in patients with inflammatory skin diseases (Kapp et al., 1988).

Regarding the strong correlation between tumor progression in CTCL patients and presence of sIL-2R, we suggest that this protein may be of great prognostic value. It shows promise as a guide for planning treatment modalities in these patients. By contrast, sCD8 protein does not correlate with the clinical stage or with the clinical outcome, whereas sCD4 seems to be a marker for the tumor burden in CTCL, but has no prognostic value for the clinical course. In comparison to inflammatory diseases associated with benign lymphoproliferation, serum levels of these soluble proteins do not differ significantly, a fact which underscores the similarities between aberrant and physiologic lymphoproliferation in the skin.

Elevated sIL-2R serum levels seem to be predictors of an unfavorable prognosis in patients with other immunoproliferative disorders, such as Hodgkin disease (Gause et al., 1990) or lymphoblastic lymphoma (Wagner et al., 1987). They might also reflect tumor burden in lymphoblastoid lymphomas or CTCL. Immunoprecipitation of tumor cell lysates with an antibody against the TAC-protein demonstrated not only bands at 55 kD, as was expected, but also at 30 kD (Wagner et al., 1987). Since the TAC-protein is coded on eight exons on chromosome 10 (Leonhard et al., 1985), it would appear possible that during physiologic and aberrant lymphoproliferation mRNA splicing produces different TAC proteins. Lack of exon 8 would cause a defect in the anchor mechanism in the cell membrane and result in an easily releasable protein which is still able to bind, and thus to neutralize IL-2, but which is unable to function as cell-bound high-affinity IL-2R and to transmit signals into the cell. In this regard, it is interesting that chromosomal aberrations on precisely this chromosome (i.e., 10) have been previously reported in CTCL patients (Shapiro et al., 1987)

Under physiologic conditions, membrane-bound and soluble forms of the TAC protein are observed after T-cell stimulation, for example by antigen presenting cells and interleukin-1. As a consequence, the stimulated T lymphocytes produce interleukin-2.

It remains to be determined whether these regulatory cascades remain intact when aberrant lymphoproliferation is taking place in cases of CTCL. An increased expression of interleukin-1 in CTCL lesions has been reported (Tron at al, 1988). The suppressed NK-activity in CTCL patients' peripheral blood, however, could be interpreted as indirect evidence for decreased or neutralized interleukin-2 activity.

We provide evidence that sIL-2R may account for the diminished NK activity in CTCL patients' peripheral blood. Stimulation experiments with IL-2 demonstrated that the reponse of PMC from CTCL patients to the IL-2 signal resembles that of normal donor PMC. This supports the notion that serum factors might have an impact on cytotoxic functions in the patients' peripheral blood. Proliferation and cytotoxicity experiments indicated an IL-2 inhibitory activity in the serum of these patients associated with high sIL-2R serum levels. sIL-2R from one CTCL patient's serum was concentrated by IL-2 affinity chromatography. This sIL-2R enriched fraction inhibited IL-2 dependent proliferation more efficiently than the native serum. Therefore, the IL-2 inhibitor in CTCL serum seems to be able to bind to IL-2. Since large volumes of CTCL serum were not available, and since the presence of other IL-2 binding proteins such as antibodies to IL-2 or shed fragments of the beta-chain of the high-affinity IL-2 receptor (Honda et al., 1990) in the purified serum fraction cannot be excluded, transfection experiments were performed to clarify the specific role of the TAC protein on IL-2 dependent effects.

Transfection of a modified TAC gene using a BMCneo expression vector system resulted in the production of a recombinant TAC protein. In order to rule out obfuscating factors in the supernatant fluids of the transfected fibroblasts, the recombinant protein was purified using an IL-2 affinity column. These purified TAC proteins were characterized by Western blotting. As previously described, the protein was found in monomeric and dimeric forms (Weber et al, 1988; Smart et al., 1990). The free sulfhydral (SH)-residue at position Cys 192 could explain the dimer formation of the recombinant soluble TAC species used in our experiments (Rusk et al., 1988; Miedel et al., 1988). Using this recombinant protein we found a dose-dependent inhibition of IL-2 mediated proliferation and induction of cytotoxicity. These results correspond well to the observation that the released IL-2 receptor is able to bind IL-2 efficiently.(Rubin et al., 1986). Comparing the neutralizing capacity of recombinant and native sIL-2R, however, the natural protein seems to be more effective than the recombinant sIL-2R. Possible explanations for this phenomenon include unequal affinities for their ligands due to different degrees of dimer formation or changes in protein structure due to glycosylation. Another hypothesis could be a simultaneous release of the IL-2R alpha and beta chains, resulting in a soluble high-affinity receptor.

Therefore, sIL-2R seems to be a physiological inhibitor of IL-2. This has also been suggested by the observation that, in the synovial fluid of rheumatoid arthritis, IL-2 inhibitory activity correlates with sIL-2R (Symons et al., 1988). Since this cytokine is able to stimulate its own production by a positive feed-back mechanism (Yamada et al., 1987), release of the surface receptor neutralizing the corresponding cytokine might be an elegant mechanism for limiting its biological effects.

Recently, proteins isolated from human urine have been shown to be structurally related to the tumor necrosis factor alpha receptor. These proteins were able to bind tumor necrosis factor alpha, and provided protection against cytotoxic effects of its ligand in vitro (Engelmann et al., 1990). From the serum of cancer patients, a soluble tumor necrosis factor-alpha receptor was purified (Gatanga et al., 1990) which has a high affinity for tumor necrosis factor alpha, but not for lymphotoxin. This finding offers an interesting perspective concerning the regulation of tumor necrosis factor and the interaction between the tumor and the immune system in cancer patients. As an example of molecular mimicry, the Shope fibroma virus DNA encodes for a soluble protein with a striking homology to the tumor necrosis factor-alpha receptor (Smith et al., 1991). Since this cytokine seems to be involved in the elimination processes for virus infected cells, a large amount of released "tumor necrosis factor-alpha receptor-like" molecule in the immediate surroundings of the cell might allow its survival in a deadly microenvironment.

In addition, the soluble extracellular portion of the interleukin-1 receptor seems to be a regulator of allograft rejection, probably due to its biological efficacy for neutralizing interleukin-1 (Fanslow et al., 1990). At the present time, soluble receptors are also known to exist for cytokines such as interleukin-1 (Fanslow et al., 1990), interleukin-2 (Rubin et al., 1985), interleukin-4 (Mosley et al., 1989), tumor necrosis factor-alpha (Engelmann et al., 1990) and a broad spectrum of other molecules. Therefore, we suggest that receptor shedding might be a general mechanism for regulating biological functions under physiologic conditions. Based on our in vitro findings on the interaction of sIL-2R and its ligand, we suggest that elevated levels of this soluble cytokine receptor chain have an impact on IL-2 dependent immunosurveillance during aberrant lymphoproliferation in CTCL, and possibly also in other lymphomas such as Hodgkin disease.

REFERENCES

Alexander P, 1974. Escape from immune destruction by the host through shedding of surface antigens: Is this a characteristic shared by malignant and embryonic cells? **Cancer Res.**, 34: 2077-2082.

Becker JC, R Dummer, G Burg and RE Schmidt, 1991. Shedding of ICAM-1 from human melanoma cell lines induced by IFN-gamma and TNF-alpha: Functional consequences on cell mediated cytotoxicity. **J. Immunol.**, 147:4398-4401.

Blitterswijk WJ van, P Emmelot, HA Hilkmann, J Hilgers and CA Feltkamp, 1979. Rigid plasma-membrane derived vesicles, enriched in tumour-associated surface antigens (MLr) occuring in the ascites fluid of a murine leukemia (GRSL). **Int. J. Cancer**, 23:62-70.

Bunn PA and SI Lamberg, 1979. Report of the committee on staging and classification of cutaneous T-cell lymphomas. **Cancer Treat Rep.**, 63:725-728. In: G Burg, O Braun-Falco, Eds: **Cutaneous Lymphomas, Pseudolymphomas and Related Disorders**. Springer, Berlin, Heidelberg, New York, Tokyo, 1983.

Burg G, R Dummer, M Wilhelm, F Nestle, MM Ott, A Feller, H Hefner, U Lanz, A Schwinn and J Wiede, 1991. Primary subcutaneous ("lipotropic") lymphoma of T-cell receptor delta-positive, interferon-gamma producing T-cells. **N. Engl. J. Med.** 325:1078-1081.

Dummer R, F Nestle, J Wiede, E Schafer, J Roger, JC Becker, T Vogt and G Burg, 1991. Coincidence of increased interleukin-2 receptors, diminished natural killer cell activity and progressive disease in cutaneous T-cell lymphomas. **Eur. J. Dermatol.** 1:135-138.

Dummer R, G Posseckert, F Nestle, M Burger, R Witzgall, JC Becker, E Schafer, J Wiede, W Sebald and G Burg, 1992. Soluble interleukin-2 receptors inhibit interleukin-2 dependent proliferation and cytotoxicity: Explanation for diminished NK activity in cutaneous lymphomas in vivo? **J. Invest. Dermatol.**, 98:50-54.

Engelmann H, D Novick and D Wallach, 1990. Two tumor necrosis factor-binding proteins purified from human urine. Evidence for immunological cross-reactivity with cell surface tumor necrosis factor receptors. **J. Biol. Chem.**, 265:1531-1536.

Fanslow WC, JE Sims, H Sassenfeld, PJ Morrissey, S Gillis, SK Dower and MB Widmer, 1990. Regulation of alloreactivity in vivo by a soluble form of the interleukin-1 receptor. **Science**, 248:739-742.

Fujimoto J, S Levy and R Levy, 1983. Spontaneous release of the Leu-2 (T8) molecule from human T cells. **J. Exp. Med.**, 159: 752-766.

Gilmore SJ, EM Benson and JWI Kelly, 1991. T-cell subsets with a naive phenotype are selectively decreased in the peripheral blood of patients with mycosis fungoides. **J. Invest. Dermatol.**, 96:50-56.

Gatanga T, C Hwang, W Kohr, F Cappuccini, JA Lucci, EWB Jeffes, R Lentz, J Tomich, RS Yamamoto and GA Granger, 1990. Purification and characterization of an inhibitor (soluble tumor necrosis factor receptor) for tumor necrosis factor and lymphotoxin obtained from the serum ultrafiltrates of human cancer patients. **Proc. Natl. Acad. Sci. USA**, 87:8781-8784.

Gause A, V Roschansky, A Tschiersch, R Schmits, V Diehl and M Pfreundschuh, 1990. The prognostic value of low pretreatment serum interleukin-2 receptor (sIL-2R) in patients with Hodgkin's disease (HD). **J. Cancer Res. Clin. Oncol.**, 116:320.S

Honda M, K Kitamura, T Takeshita, K Sugamura and T Tokunaga, 1990. Identification of a soluble IL-2 receptor β-chain from human lymphoid cell line cells. **J. Immunol.**, 145:4131-4135.

Kantor AF, EC Rochelle, EC Vonderheid, EJ Van Scott and JFF Fraumeni, 1989. Risk of second malignancy after cutaneous T-cell lymphoma. **Cancer**, 63:1612-1615.

Kapp A, A Piskorski and E Schop, 1988. Elevated levels of interleukin-2 receptors in sera with atopic dermatitis and psoriasis. **Br. J. Dermatol.**, 119:707-710.

Karasuyama H and F Melchers F, 1988. Establishment of mouse cell lines which constitutively secrete large quantities of interleukin 2, 3, 4, 5 using modified cDNA expression vectors. **Eur. J. Immunol.**, 18:97-104.

Kaudewitz P, O Josimovic-Alasevic, T Diamantstein, F Eckert, K Klepzig and G Burg, 1988. Soluble IL-2 receptor serum levels in cutaneous T-cell lymphoma: Correlation with clinical stage and IL-2 receptor status in cutaneous infiltrates. **J. Invest. Dermatol.**, 91:386-387.

Kaye FJ, PA Bunn, SM Steinberg, DC Ihde, AB Fischmann, EJ Glatstein, GP Schechter, RM Phelbs, FM Foss, HL Parlette, MJ Anderson and EA Sausville, 1989. A randomized trial comparing combination electron-beam radiation and chemotherapy with topical therapy in the initial treatment of mycosis fungoides. **N. Engl. J. Med.**, 321:1784-1790.

Kerl K and W Sterry, 1987. Classification and staging. In: G Burg, W Sterry, Eds: **EORTC/BMFT Cutaneous Lymphoma Project Group: Recommendations for staging and therapy of cutaneous lymphomas.** EORTC, Brussels, pp 1-10.

Laroche L and D Kaiserlian, 1983. Decreased natural killer cell activity in cutaneous T-cell lymphomas. **New Engl. J. Med.,** 306:101-102.

Leonard WJ, JM Depper, M Kanehisa, M Krönke, NJ Peffer, PB Svetlik, M Sullivan and WC Greene, 1985. Structure of the human interleukin-2 receptor gene. **Science,** 230:633-639.

Levy S, JL Tempe, P Caussade, A Aleksijevic, E Grosshans, S Mayer and JM Lang, 1984. Stage related decrease in natural killer cell activity in untreated patients with mycosis fungoides. **Cancer Immunol. Immunother.,** 18:138-140.

Miedel MC, JD Hulmes, DV Weber, P Bailon and YCE Pan, 1988. Structural analysis of recombinant soluble human interleukin 2 receptor. **Biochem. Biophys. Res. Commun.,** 54:372-379.

Moreland AA, DB Robertson and LT Heffner, 1985. Treatment of cutaneous T-cell lymphoma with cyclosporin A. **J. Am. Acad. Dermatol.,** 12:886-887.

Mosley B, MP Beckmann, CJ March, RL Idzerda, SD Gimpel, T VandenBos, D Friend, A Alpert, D Anderson, J Jackson, JM Wignall, C Smith, B Gallis, JE Sims, D Urdal, MB Widmer, D Cosman and LS Park, 1989. The murine interleukin-4 receptor: Molecular cloning and characterization of secreted and membrane bound forms. **Cell** 59:335-348.

Nikaido T, A Shimizu, N Ishida, H Sabe, K Teshigawara, M Maeda, T Uchiyama, J Yodoi and T Honjo, 1984. Molecular cloning of cDNA encoding human IL-2 receptor. **Nature,** 311:631-635.

Raz A, R Goldmann, I Yuli and M Inbar, 1978. Isolation of plasma membrane fragments and vesicles from ascites fluids of lymphoma bearing mice and their possible role in the escape mechanism of tumours from host immune rejection. **Cancer Immunol. Immunother.,** 4:53-59..

Robb RJ, A Munck and KA Smith, 1981. T cell growth factor receptors: Quantification, specifity and biological relevance. **J. Exp. Med.,** 154:1455-1472.

Rubin LA, G Jay and DI Nelson, 1986. The released interleukin-2 receptor binds interleukin-2 efficiently. **J. Immunol.,** 137: 3841-3844.

Rubin LA, CC Kurman, ME Fritz, WE Biddison, R Boutin, R Yarchoan and DL Nelson, 1985. Soluble interleukin-2 receptors are released from activated human lymphoid cells in vitro. **J. Immunol.,** 135:3172-3177.

Rusk CM, MP Neeper, L-M Kuo, RM Kutny and RJ Robb, 1988. Structure-activity analysis of modified and truncated forms of the TAC receptor protein: Site specific mutagenesis of cysteine residues. **J. Immunol.,** 140:2249-2259.

Sanders ME, MW Makgoba and S Shaw, 1988. Human naive and memory cells: Reinterpretion of helper-inducer and suppressor-inducer subsets. **Immunol. Today,** 9:195-198.

Shapiro PE, D Warburton, CL Berger and RL Edelson, 1987. Clonal chromosomal abnormalities in cutaneous T-cell lymphoma. **Cancer Genet Cytogenet,** 28:267-276.

Smart JE, PC Familletti, DV Weber, RF Keeney and P Bailon, 1990. Purification of the IL-2 receptor (TAC) by ligand-affinity chromatography and utilization of the immobilized receptor for receptor-affinity chromatography (RAC) purification of IL-2, mutant IL-2, and IL-2 fusion proteins. **J. Invest. Dermatol.**, 94:158-163.

Smith CA, T Davis, JM Wignall, WS Din, T Farrah, C Upton, G McFadden and RG Goodwin, 1991. T2 open reading frame from the Shope fibroma virus encodes a soluble form of the TNF receptor. **Biochem. Biophys. Res. Commun.**, 176:335-342.

Sterry W and V Mielke, 1989. CD 4$^+$ cutaneous T-cell lymphomas show the phenotype of helper/inducer T cells. **J. Invest. Dermatol.**, 93:413-416.

Symons JA, NC Wood, FS DiGiovine and GW Duff, 1988. Soluble IL-2 receptor in rheumatoid arthritis: Correlation with disease activity, IL-1 and IL-2 inhibition. **J. Immunol.**, 141:2612-2618.

Symons JA, JF McCulloch, NC Wood and GW Duff, 1991. Soluble CD4 in patients with rheumatoid arthritis and osteoarthritis. **Clin. Immunol. Immunopathol.**, 60:72-82.

Thomsen X and GL Wantzin, 1987. Extracutaneous spreading with fatal outcome of mycosis ·fungoides in a patient treated with cyclosporin A: A word of caution. **Dermatologica**, 174:236-238.

Tron VA, DR Rosenthal and DN Sauder, 1988. Epidermal interleukin-1 is increased in cutaneous T-cell lymphoma. **J. Invest. Dermatol.**, 90:378-381.

Wagner DK, J Kiwanuka, BK Edwards, LA Rubin, DL Nelson and IT Magrath, 1987. Soluble interleukin-2 receptor levels in patients with undifferentiated and lymphoblastic lymphomas: Correlation with survival. **J. Clin. Oncol.**, 5:1262-1274.

Weber DV, RF Keeney, PC Familletti and P Bailon, 1988. Medium scale ligand-affinity purification of two soluble forms of human IL-2 receptor. **J. Chromatogr.**, 431:55-63.

Weber W, G Gill and J Spiess, 1984. Production of an epidermal growth factor receptor-related protein. **Science**, 224:294-297.

Weigel U, M Meyer and W Sebald, 1989. Mutant proteins of human interleukin-2. **Eur. J. Biochem.**, 180:295-300.

Yamada S, FW Ruscetti, WA Overton, RB Herbermann, MC Birchenall Sparks and JR Ortaldo, 1987. Regulation of human large granular lymphocyte and T cell growth by recombinant interleukin 2: Induction of interleukin 2 receptor and promotion of growth of cells with enhanced cytotoxicity. **J. Leuk. Biol.**, 41:505-517.

THE SKIN AS A TARGET ORGAN DURING IL-2 ADMINISTRATION

Günter Burg*
Reinhard Dummer*
Jurgen C. Becker†

* Department of Dermatology
University of Zurich
Zurich, Switzerland

† Department of Dermatology
University of Würzburg
Würzburg, Germany

Correspondence to: Prof. Dr. G. Burg, Department of Dermatology,
University Hospital, Gloriastrasse 31,
CH 8091, Zurich, Switzerland

ABSTRACT

During treatment of patients with metastatic malignant melanoma with high dose interleukin-2 (IL-2), eczematous rashes appeared in all patients within the first few days of treatment. In other patients adjuvant treatment with IL-2 subcutaneously lead to panniculitis-like infiltrates. The purpose of this study was to investigate, using both routine histology and immunohistochemistry, the skin changes following either high dose intraveneous application of IL-2 or low dose subcutaneous application of IL-2 during adjuvant treatment. IL-2 in both treatment modalities lead to marked accumulation of (activated) T-cells in the dermis or in the subcutaneous tissue.

These histologic and immunohistochemical findings indicate that the skin serves as a target organ during IL-2 administration.

Basic Mechanisms of Physiologic and Aberrant Lymphoproliferation in the Skin
Edited by W.C. Lambert *et al.*, Plenum Press, New York, 1994

INTRODUCTION

The active role played by the skin in the immune system is now well recognized (Bos, 1990). The permament or transient cellular constituents represent the structural background for a broad pathophysiological scenario of immunological skin diseases in the different cutaneous compartments (Table 1).

Table 1. Compartmental manifestations of immune reactions in the skin.

Compartment	Major cellular constituents	Examples of nosologic manifestations of immune reactions
Epidermis	Keratinocytes	Contact dermatitis
	Langerhans cells	Atopic eczema
	"Thy-1-cells"	Acantholysis
	Melanocytes	Lupus erythematosus
	Merkel cells	Erythema multiforme
		Vitiligo
Dermo-epidermal Grenz zone	Basal layer	Subepidermal blister
	Basement membrane and subunits	formation (Bullous pemphigoid, Dermatitis
	Anchoring fibrils	herpetiformis, Epider-
		molysis bullosa)
		Lichen planus (?)
Dermis	Vessels	Vasculitis
	Fibroblasts	Graft-versus-host reaction
	Elastic fibers	Scleroderma
	Mast cells	Urticaria
	Adnexal structures	Granulomas
		Alopecia areata

Cytokines are polypeptide hormone-like substances which regulate growth, differentiation and proliferation of cells and play an important role in inflammatory as well as in neoplastic processes. They form a mutually interacting (suppression or stimulation) network. Interleukin-2 (IL-2) is produced mainly by activated T-cells and promotes T-cell division (T-cell growth factor) and cytokine release, which again activates T-cells and constituent cells of the skin to release interferon-gamma. IL-2 is being used in various clinical trials in patients with metastatic cancer or in adjuvant treatment regimens. It can be given alone or in combination with other cytokines, with lymphokine-activated killer (LAK) cells (Rosenberg et al., 1987), with tumor infiltrating lymphocytes (TIL) or with chemotherapy.

Malignant melanoma, renal cell carcinoma and colonic carcinoma appear to be responsive to this therapy. IL-2 treatment is associated with severe side effects, however, such as pyrexia (fever), chills, hematologic abnormalities (thrombocytopenia, eosinophilia and anemia), hepatic and renal toxicity, hypotension and fluid retention (Rosenberg et al., 1987). In addition, patients treated with IL-2 develop dermatological changes such as macular lesions, exfoliative generalized dermatitis, erythema nodosum, dyshidrosiform eruptions and acantholytic bulla formation, as well as triggering of polymyositis, dermatomyositis and psoriatic eruptions (Gaspari et al., 1987; Ramseur et al., 1989, and our own observations).

In order to study the pathophysiology of these eruptions, skin biopsies and serum levels of cytokines from patients undergoing immunotherapy with systemic or subcutaneous application of IL-2 were analyzed.

MATERIALS AND METHODS

Patients and treatment

Six patients with metastatic malignant melanoma underwent 12 treatment cycles consisting of dacarbazine ($250mg/m^2$) on days 1 through 5 and recombinant interleukin-2 (18 million I.U., equivalent to 3 million Cetus $U/m^2/24$ hours) intraveneously by continous infusion on days 21 through 24 and 27 through 30. After a rest of 7 to 14 days the treatment was restarted. All patients were treated with 500mg paracetamol six times per day, ranitidine, 150mg every 12 hours, and furosemide, 40 to 140mg per day to prevent fever, gastric ulcer and fluid retention, respectively.

Seven patients with high risk malignant melanoma (tumor thickness > 1.5mm) in complete remission received interleukin-2 subcutaneously (9 million I.U., equivalent to 1.5 million Cetus U/m^2) for 4 consecutive days every 5 weeks for up to two years. During weeks 2-5, interferon-alpha-2b (3 million units) was administered subcutaneously 3 times per week.

Biopsy specimens

Six biopsies were taken from the skin on day 29 during IL-2 administration in five patients receiving IL-2 intraveneously and in six patients receiving IL-2 subcutaneously. Each biopsy specimen was divided into two parts. Half of each biopsy specimen was snap-frozen, the other half was fixed with buffered formalin, embedded in paraffin and sections stained with hematoxylin and eosin (H&E).

Immunostaining of frozen tissues

Snap-frozen biopsy specimens were stored at -70° C until use. They were stained by an alkaline phosphatase-anti-alkaline phosphatase monoclonal antibody (APAAP) technique as previously described (Cordell et al., 1984), using a panel of monoclonal antibodies (Table 2). Evaluation of the mononuclear cell infiltrate was performed semiquantitatively.

Table 2. Monoclonal antibodies used for phenotyping of the mononuclear cell infiltrate in skin reactions following intraveneous or subcutaneous application of IL-2.

CD[*]	Antibody	Predominant reactivity	Mononuclear cell infiltrate	
			Intravenous application[a]	Subcutaneous application[b]
CD1	T6	Langerhans cells	0/+	+/++
CD3	Leu4	Pan T-cell marker	++++	++++
CD4	Leu3a	T helper/inducer cells	++++	++++
CD8	Leu2a	T suppresor/cytotoxic cells	+/++	+/++
CD19	B4Pan	B-cells	0	0
CD20	L26	B-cells	0	0
CD25	anti-TAC	α-chain of IL-2 receptor	+/++	+/++
CD30	Ki-1/BerH2	proliferating cells	0	+/++
-	TCR-δ1	T-cell receptor δ-chain	+	0/+
-	TCR-α	T-cell receptor α-chain	+++	+++/++++
-	HLA-DR	activated cells	++/+++[c]	+/++[c]
CD11a	IOT-16	leukocytes	++/+++	++/+++
CD54	ICAM-1	intercellular adhesion molecule-1	++/+++[c]	+/++[c]
-	MAC 387	monocytes/macrophages	+/++	+/++

Percentage of mononuclear cells stained: 0, none; +, less than 10%; ++, 10-25%; +++, 25-50%; ++++, more than 50%. * CD: cluster designation

[a] Scattered mononuclear cell infiltrate in the upper and mid dermis

[b] Dense nodular infiltrate in subcutaneous fat tissue

[c] Also endothelial cells and keratinocytes

RESULTS

Skin changes

All patients receiving IL-2 intraveneously developed a persistent, macular, erythematous rash with scaling. Lesions in different patients differed in intensity and extent. Erythema started on the face 24 to 72 hours following IL-2 infusion and subsequently spread to the lower parts of the body. The patients noted that the skin was warm and "itchy". These sensations were also present in the mucosa of the upper respiratory tract. About 24-48 hours after cessation of interleukin-2 administration, the erythema resolved with a desquamation starting on the face and scalp and extending to the trunk. Fine adherent scales were observed on the face, palms and soles, and large, confluent desquamative sheets on the trunk. The total duration of this inflammatory desquamation was 14-20 days. The cutaneous changes regressed spontaneously, but reappeared during the following treatment cycles. No correlation between the intensity of cutaneous changes and IL-2 dosage was observed.

Patients receiving IL-2 subcutaneously developed a localized plaque-like inflammatory reaction within 2-3 days. It persisted for 1 to 2 weeks.

Histological analysis

Histologtic examination of the skin rash related to intraveneous application of IL-2 showed a few necrotic keratinocytes, spongiotic foci in the epidermis and edema in the upper and mid dermis. In areas of single-cell epidermotropism of mononuclear cells, there was focal basal cell degeneration and papillary edema. In addition, a perivascular infiltrate consisting mainly of mononuclear cells and a few eosinophils was observed. No sign of vasculitis was present, with the exception of inconspicuous swelling of endothelial cells.

Subcutaneous injection of IL-2 lead to a dense inflammatory mononuclear cell infiltrate resembling lobular panniculitis, containing scattered large blast cells.

Immunohistochemistry of skin biopsy specimens (Table 2)

In all biopsies, endothelial cells and, less intensively, keratinocytes stained positive for intercellular adhesion molecule-1 (ICAM-1). The mononuclear infiltrate was mainly CD3$^+$/CD4$^+$ (Figure 1a,b)/ CD8$^-$, suggesting a T-helper phenotype. In one patient receiving IL-2 intraveneously, lymphocytes accumulated around nests of nerve cells. Only a few CD8$^+$ T-lymphocytes were seen. Some of the mononuclear cells stained for HLA-DR and CD25 (TAC) expression, reflecting an activated, functional state. In the subcutaneous infiltrates seen following local application of IL-2, scattered blast cells showed CD30 (Ki-1) positivity (Figure 1c).

No influence on the normal distribution of T-cell receptor delta chain bearing T lymphocytes, Langerhans cells (CD1) or natural killer cells (CD57) was observed. The number of B-lymphocytes (CD19, CD20), macrophages and granulocytes (MAC 387) was low. Differences between intraveneous and subcutaneous IL-2 application were quantitative rather than qualitative.

DISCUSSION

Scarlatiniform skin reactions followed by desquamation occurred regularly during long-term, high-dose, intraveneous IL-2 administration. Although some patients showed only minor dermatological changes, skin reactions were observed in each treatment cycle. The histological features included spongotic foci and mononuclear infiltrations of varying intensity. The infiltrates were localized, mainly perivascularly, but also involved the epidermis. They consisted of activated T helper lymphocytes (CD3$^+$/CD4$^+$/CD8$^-$/CD25$^+$/HLADR$^+$) (Gaspari et al., 1987). However, this phenotypic pattern is not specific, and can also be seen in other types of "interface dermatitis" (Shiohara et al., 1988).

Subcutaneous application of IL-2 lead to panniculitis-like lymphoid infiltrates consisting of activated T-helper cells (CD3$^+$/CD4$^+$/CD8$^-$/CD25$^+$/HLA-DR$^+$/ scattered CD30$^+$ cells). Activated lymphocytes are probably the source for elevated serum levels of interferon-gamma (Dummer et al., 1991; Lotze et al., 1985); Pearlstein et al., 1983). Interferon-gamma may

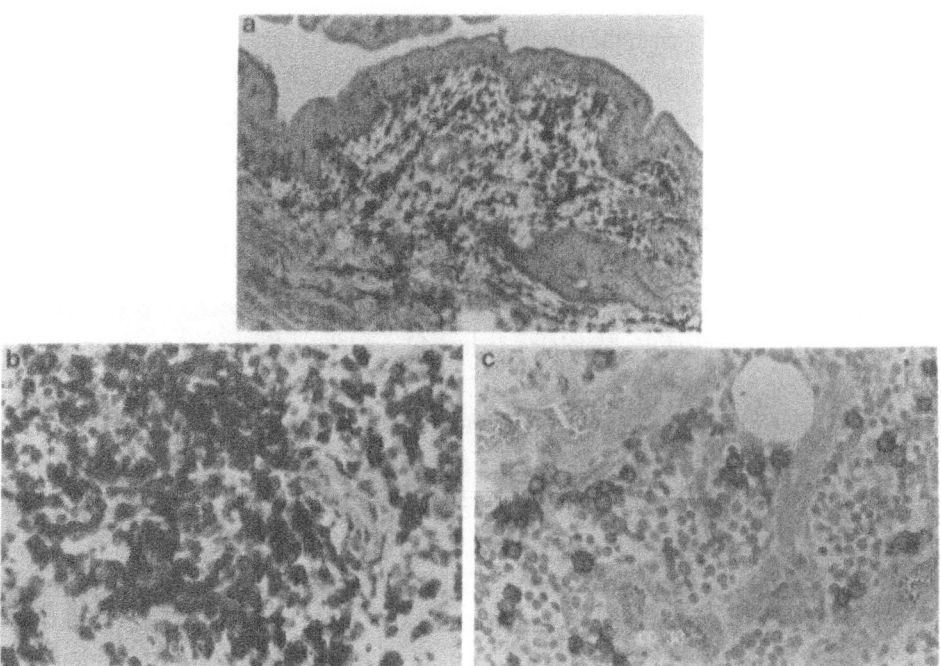

Figure 1. Mononuclear cell infiltrate in the skin following IL-2 administration.
    A,   Intraveneously: CD4$^+$ cells are observed in the upper and mid-dermis. (x 100);
    B,   Subcutaneously: CD3$^+$ cells are observed in the subcutis. (x 400);
    C,   Subcutaneously: Scattered CD30$^+$ blast cells are observed. (x 400).

cause upregulation of ICAM-1 on endothelial cells and keratinocytes (Cotran et al., 1987; Nickoloff et al., 1989). Stimulation of macrophages, endothelial cells or keratinocytes by interferon-gamma results in the production of various cytokines, such as TNF-alpha, granulocyte-macrophage colony-stimulating factor and interleukin-6 (Kupper, 1988; Luger et al.,

1988; Nedwin et al., 1985). Increase of TNF-alpha serum levels; causing a febrile reaction in cancer patients receiving IL-2, has indeed been demonstrated by immunoradiometric assay (Mier et al., 1988). The expression of adhesion molecules, like ICAM-1, a ligand for the lymphocyte function-associated antigen-1 (LFA-1), on leukocytes and production of various cytokines may provide a suitable micronviroenment for activated lymphocytes. Consequently, dermatological changes during immunotherapy with IL-2 are likely to be the result of a complicated network of cellular intractions involving various cytokines, rendering the skin an "immunoreactive" target organ during IL-2 administration.

In allergic contact dermatitis, antigens are presented by Langerhans cells; consequently interleukin-1 is released, inducing activation of T-lymphocytes with production of gamma-interferon. In patients treated with IL-2, activated T-lymphocytes produce interferon-gamma, which stimulates antigen expression in endothelial cells and keratinocytes. These cells may be the source of other cytokines, such as interleukin-1 or interleukin-6, which are able to initate a dermal inflammatory reaction.

Thus, IL-2 is responsible for an inflammatory lymphoid reaction which must be differentiated from an allergic drug eruption.

REFERENCES

Bos JD, 1990. Ed: **Skin Immune System (SIS)**. CRC Press, Inc. Boca Raton, Florida.

Cordell JL, G Falini, WN Erber, AK Ghosh, Z Abdulaziz, S Macdonald, KAF Pulford, H Stein and DY Mason, 1984. Immunoenzymatic labeling of monoclonal antibodies using immune complexes of alkine phosphatase and monoclonal anti-alkaline phosphatase antibodies (APAAP complexes). **J. Histochem. Cytochem.**, 32:219.

Cotran RS, JS Pober, MA Gimbrone, TA Springer, EA Wiebke, AA Gaspari, SA Rosenberg and MT Lotze, 1987. Endothelial activation during interleukin 2 immunotherapy. A possible mechanism for the vascular leak syndrome. **J. Immunol.**, 139:1883.

Dummer R, K Miller, C Eilles and G Burg, 1991. The skin: An immunoreactive target organ during interleukin-2 administration? **Dermatologica**, 183:95.

Gaspari AA, MT Lotze, SA Rosenberg, JB Stern and SI Katz, 1987. Dermatologic changes associated with interleukin-2 administration. **JAMA**, 258:1 624.

Kupper TS, 1989. Mechanism of cutaneous inflammation. **Arch. Dermatol.**, 125:1406.

Lotze MT, YL Matory, SE Ettinghausen, AA Rayner, SO Sharrow, CAY Seipp, MC Custer and SA Rosenberg, 1985. In vivo administration of purified human interleukin-2. II. Half life, immunologic effects, and expansion of peripheral lymphoid cells in vivo with recombinant IL 2. **J. Immunol.**, 135:2865.

Luger TA, T Schwarz, 1988. Epidermal cell derived cytokines, In: JD Bos, Ed: **Skin Immune System**, (SIS), CRC Press, Boca Raton, Florida, p 257.

Mier JW, G Vachino, JW van der Meer, RP Numerof, S Adams, JG Cannon, HA Berheim, MB Atkins, DR Parkinson and CA Dinarello, 1988. Induction of circulating tumor necrosis factor (TNF alpha) as the mechanism for the febrile response to interleukin-2 (IL-2) in cancer patients. **J. Clin. Immunol.**, 8:426.

Nickoloff BJ and CE Griffiths, 1989. T lymphocytes and monocytes bind to keratinocytes in frozen sections of biopsy specimens of normal skin treated with gamma interferon. **J. Am. Acad. Dermatol.**, 20:736.

Nedwin GE, LP Svedfesky, TS Bringman, MA Palladino and DV Goeddel, 1985. Effect of interleukin-2, interferon-gamma and mitogens on the production of tumor necrosis factor-alpha and beta. **J. Immunol.**, 135:2492.

Pearlstein KT, MA Palladino, K Welte and J Vilcek, 1983. Purified interleukin-2 enhanced induction of immune interferon. **Cell Immunol.**, 80:1.

Ramseur WL, F Richards and DB Duggan, 1989. A case of fatal pemphigus vulgaris in association with beta interferon and interleukin-2 therapy. **Cancer**, 63:2005.

Rosenberg SA, MT Lotze, LM Muul, AE Chang, FP Avis, S Leitman, WM Lineham, CN Robertson, RE Lee, JT Rubin, CA Simpson and DE White, 1987. A progress report on the treatment of 157 patients with advanced cancer using lymphokine activated killer cells and interleukin-2 or high dose interleukin-2 alone. **N. Engl. J. Med.**, 316:889.

Shiohara T, N Moriya and M Nagashima, 1988. The lichenoid tissue reaction. **Int. J. Dermatol.**, 27:365.

SPECIFIC IMMUNE RESPONSE AGAINST MELANOMA: ANALYSIS AT A CLONAL LEVEL

Jurgen C. Becker*
C. Bormann*
R. Dummer†
A. Schwinn*
G. Burg†

* Department of Dermatology
University of Würzburg
Würzburg, Germany

† Department of Dermatology
University of Zurich
Zurich, Switzerland

Correspondence to: Prof. Dr. G. Burg, Department of Dermatology,
University Hospital, Gloriastrasse 31,
CH 8091 Zurich, Switzerland

ABSTRACT

The means by which tumor-infiltrating lymphocytes (TIL) exert their antitumor effects in vivo are unknown. Our study was designed to characterize the phenotype and functional capacity of TILs in early primary melanoma and in the corresponding metastases. Therefore, melanoma cell lines and cloned TIL lines were established from primary and secondary melanomas from the same patients. TIL clones were analyzed using flow cytometry and proliferation and cytotoxicity assays. Phenotypic analysis revealed that all clones expressed CD2, CD3, CD11, and CD25. About 28% of clones reacted with CD4 monoclonal antibodies (mAb) and 72% with CD8 mAb. Proliferation of TIL clones were tested in response to irradiated (50

Basic Mechanisms of Physiologic and Aberrant Lymphoproliferation in the Skin
Edited by W.C. Lambert *et al.*, Plenum Press, New York, 1994

459

Gray) melanoma cell lines and low concentrations of recombinant interleukin-2 (rIL-2) (30 I.U./ml). Co-culture of TIL clones with autologous, lesion-specific tumor lines and rIL-2 induced up to a 460% greater proliferative response than that with rIL-2 alone. If TIL clones were co-cultured with autologous, but not lesion-specific tumor lines, melanoma (MM) lines from primary tumors induced a strong proliferative response in TIL clones from secondary melanomas. By contrast, MM lines obtained from metastatic tumors did not induce a greater proliferative response than that induced by rIL-2 alone. 57% of TIL clones were able to mediate cytotoxicity against the corresponding tumor cell lines with up to 35% specific lysis in a four hour ^{51}Cr release assay. Two TIL clones generated from from metastatic tumors were able to lyse MM lines from primary tumors, whereas none of the clones from primary tumors was able to kill tumor lines from metastatic tumors.

INTRODUCTION

The idea that the tumor environment is intrinsically immunogenic and, therefore, contains lymphocytes with the potential to induce tumor regression, has led to the use of tumor-infiltrating lymphocytes (TIL) in clinical trials (Muul et al., 1987; Tefany et al., 1991; Takagi et al., 1989). In this procedure, lymphocytes are grown ex vivo directly from tumors in the presence of the lymphokine, IL-2 (Topalian et al. 1987). Although 60% of metastatic melanoma patients who had not previously received any immunotherapy showed objective responses in the largest clinical TIL trial performed to date (Rosenberg et al., 1988), the characteristics of the tumor environment that produce TILs in vivo remains unclear. Two classes of stimuli -- one derived from cell-cell contact between tumor cells and immunocytes and the other from soluble factors -- may influence T-cell homing and proliferation (Gromo et al., 1987). The induction of the high affinity p55/p75 IL-2 receptor (IL-2R) on T-cells by antigen via the T-cell receptor reflects the cooperation of these two stimuli (Caliguri et al., 1990; Wang et al., 1987). Furthermore, it has been demonstrated that secreted factors from tumor cell lines provide mitogenic activation of TILs (Packard et al., 1990).

Recent studies have demonstrated that cell lines cultured from lesions early in the pathway of melanocytic tumor progression stimulate autologous T-cell proliferation in vitro, whereas cell lines derived from late melanocytic lesions do not (Alexander et al., 1989). This was confirmed by in situ studies demonstrating that certain precursors and early lesions of primary melanoma are characterized by an activated T-cell infiltrate, which is attenuated or absent in advanced metastatic lesions (Tefany et al., 1991; Alexander et al., 1989). Our study was designed to characterize the phenotype and the functional capacity of TILs in primary melanoma and in the corresponding metastases and their interaction with the specific tumors. Therefore, melanoma cell lines and cloned TIL lines were established from primary and secondary melanomas from the same patients.

MATERIALS AND METHODS

Melanoma cell lines

Dispersed cells were obtained by grating tumor fragments from freshly resected melanomas against a 0.3 x 0.3 mm metalic mesh immersed in RPMI 1640 medium supplemented with 10% fetal calf serum (FCS), 1% penicillin, 1% streptomycin, 1% glutamine, and 1% sodium pyruvate (CM). A portion of these cells was frozen for later use in T-cell stimulation and cytotoxicity assays. The other cells were plated into 12-well collagen-coated culture plates at 2,000 cells per well in CM and grown in humidified incubators at 37°C with 5% CO_2. Fibroblast contamination was suppressed by adding geneticin (250 μg/ml). During the initial 3 weeks of growth, a volume no greater than one-fourth of the spent medium was removed and replaced three times per week. Tumor lines were maintained in monolayer and passaged by trypsinization with 0.0625% trypsin plus EDTA as required. Melanoma lines were designated pM, if derived from a primary tumor, and sM, if derived from a secondary tumor.

Preparation of tumor infiltrating lymphocytes (TIL)

Tumor cell suspensions were prepared by mincing freshly resected tumors into small pieces, digesting them for 12 hours in CM containing 0.1% collagenase type IV (200 U/g) and 0.005% deoxyribonuclease type I (100 U/mg; Sigma, St. Louis, MO), and passing them through a steel sieve. After washing twice with Hank's balanced salt solution (HBSS), viable cells were separated on a Ficoll/Hypaque gradient at 600 x g for 20 minutes, washed twice, counted, and placed into 6-well tissue culture plates in CM at a concentration of 5 x 10^5 cells per ml. CM was supplemented with 30 I.U. IL-2 per ml (Eurocetus, Amsterdam, Netherlands).

Immunomagnetic isolation of CD25$^+$ cells

The indirect immunomagnetic isolation of CD25$^+$ cells has been described in detail (Naume et al., 1991). The TILs were diluted in CM to a concentration of 1 x 10^8 cells/ml. Thereafter, 0.1 mg CD25 mAb/10^6 TILs was added and the cells were incubated for one hour at 4°C. The cells were washed twice in HBSS, diluted in CM and incubated with sheep anti-mouse IgG Ab coated Dynabeads M-450 (DYNAL, Oslo, Norway; 7.5 x 10^5 beads/10^6 PBMC) for 30 minutes with gentle rotation. Cells attached to Dynabeads were recovered with a MPC-6 magnet (DYNAL) and washed thrice in CM. The cell/bead suspension was incubated for 24 hours at 37°C, resulting in detachment of most beads from the cells. Thereafter, the cells were separated from the beads using a MPC-6 magnet. The efficiency of cell separation was confirmed by flow cytometry (< 5% contaminating cells).

Generation of cloned human TIL lines

TIL clones were obtained using a limiting dilution technique by plating 0.5 cells per well onto a feeder layer of 5×10^3 autologous irradiated (50 Gray) melanoma cells -- obtained from the same tumor specimen -- per well and 5×10^3 irradiated (50 Gray) LAZ 509 cells per well. Only CD25$^+$ TILs were used for cloning (Becker et al., 1990; Anichini et al., 1989). Colonies were expanded by addition of culture medium containing rIL-2 (30 U/ml) every 3 days. The culture medium was RPMI 1640 medium supplemented with 20% human AB serum, 1% penicillin streptomycin, 1% glutamine, and 1% sodium pyruvate. All cell lines used in this study had been subcloned at least three times at 10^3/cells per well. TIL lines were designated pT, if derived from a primary tumor and sT, if derived from a secondary tumor.

Monoclonal antibodies

Monoclonal antibodies (mAbs) utilized in this study have been previously described in detail. All mAbs are commercially available (Becton Dickinson, San Jose, CA)

Phenotypic analysis by flow cytometry (FCM)

Cε''s were washed twice with PBS and then incubated with purified human IgG for 10 minutes to inhibit subsequent mAb binding (to Fc receptor (FcR)). 10^6 cells were incubated for 30 minutes with a first step mAb. After two washes with HBSS containing 0.2% sodium azide, cells were stained for 30 minutes with Fab'2 goat anti-mouse IgG FITC conjugate. After two washes, the cells were incubated 20 minutes with excess mouse IgG to block free goat anti-mouse IgG-binding sites. The goat anti-mouse IgG and blocking steps were omitted for samples stained with directly FITC-conjugated mAbs. After the blocking step, directly PE-conjugated mAb was added for 30 minutes, followed by two washes. All incubations and washes were performed at 4°C. Cells were analyzed with a FACScan (Becton Dickenson, San Jose, CA; 488nm or 590nm, respectively). The noise threshold was set to exclude volume signals below those of lymphocytes. All analyses were performed using photomultiplier voltages and gain settings that were standardized using fluorescent calibration beads, and all signals were processed using logarithmic amplification. FITC-conjugated mouse IgG2a mAb controls were used to assess the degree of nonspecific antibody binding to each cell preparation and to allow for the establishment of markers for distinguishing positive and negative cell populations.

Proliferation assay

The proliferative response was measured by culturing 5×10^4 cells per well for 6 hours in flat-bottom microtiter plates. Tritiated thymidine was added 18 hours before harvesting.

Cytotoxicity assay

Cell-mediated lysis was measured in a standard four hour ^{51}Cr release assay as described. U-bottom plates were utilized. The medium for the cytotoxicity assay was RPMI 1640 supplemented with 10% FCS. Assays were performed at various effector cell/target cell (E/T) ratios using 5 x 10^3 ^{51}Cr labeled target cells per well. Plates were incubated for four hours, a 70 μl aliquot was removed from each well, and specific ^{51}Cr release measured.

Statistical analysis

Student's paired t test was used to determine the significance of differences between two groups. A result was considererd significant if the p value was less than 0.01.

RESULTS and DISCUSSION

TIL clones were generated using a limiting dilution technique with low concentrations of IL-2 (30 I.U.). Selection of TILs expressing the p55 α-chain of the IL-2R for cloning increased the cloning efficiency from 0.4 clones/96 wells to 3.2 clones/96 wells (Poisson corrected, from 0.4% to 3.4% cloning efficiency).

The TIL clones were tested for cell surface marker expression using monoclonal antibodies against T cell subsets. The results for the clones used in this study are summarized in Table 1.

Table 1. Characterization of TIL clones.

Clone Origin	Phenotype[1]						Cytotoxic against autologous tumor[2]
	CD2	CD3	CD4	CD8	CD11	CD25	
pTB1 primary	+	+	−	+	+	+	+
pTB3 primary	+	+	+	−	+	+	−
pTB5 primary	+	+	−	+	+	+	+
sTB2 secondary	+	+	−	+	+	+	−
sTB3 secondary	+	+	−	+	+	+	+
sTB5 secondary	+	+	+	−	+	+	−
sTB6 secondary	+	+	−	+	+	+	+

[1] Phenotype of clones determined by FACS analysis.

[2] Cytotoxicity was tested against autologous, lesion specific, fresh tumor cells in a standard four hour ^{51}Cr-release assay.

All clones expressed CD2, CD3, CD11, and CD25. About 28% of clones reacted with CD4 mAb and 72% with CD8 mAb. No correlation of CD4 or CD8 expression with the origin of the TIL clones from a primary versus metastatic (secondary) tumor could be found. In addition, testing was done for reactivity with mAb directed against antigens mainly expressed on NK cells. As expected, a number of clones showed a low reactivity with CD56 mAb (40%), whereas none of the clones showed a high reactivity against this mAb (data not shown). Since CD56 is not a specific marker for NK cells in long-term cultures, we also used CD16 mAb, which is thought to be more specific. None of the clones showed CD16 expression.

Proliferation of TIL clones was tested in response to irradiated (50 Gray) melanoma cell lines and low concentrations of rIL-2 (30 I.U./ml) (Figure 1) after 48 hour culture in CM without any further stimuli. Under these conditions rIL-2 alone was not sufficient to induce a good proliferative response. Co-culture of TIL clones with autologous, lesion-specific tumor lines and rIL-2 induced up to a 460% greater proliferative response as compared to rIL-2 alone. If TIL clones were cocultured with autologous, but not lesion-specific tumor lines, MM lines from primary tumors induced a strong proliferative response in TIL clones from secondary melanomas. By contrast, MM lines obtained from metastatic tumors did not induce a greater proliferative response than that induced by Il-2 alone (Figure 1).

The TIL clones obtained under the conditions described above showed no or almost no NK activity as measured by killing of K562 cells (less than 10% lysis in a E/T ratio of 40:1, data not shown). LAK cell activity, as determined by the killing of Daudi cells, ranged from 17% to 25% in an E/T ratio of 40:1 in a four hour-^{51}Cr release assay for the following clones: pTB1, pTB5, sTB3, and sTB6 (data not shown).

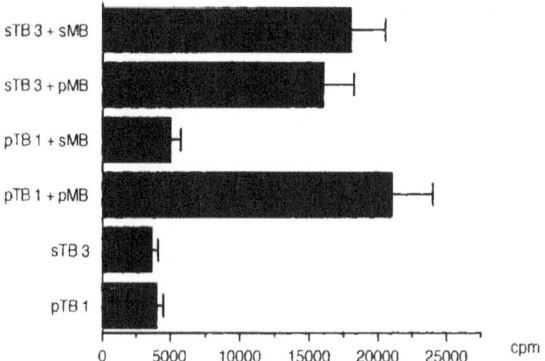

Figure 1. Proliferation of TIL clones. TIL clones were cultured without any stimuli in CM for 48 hours. Subsequently, 10^5 cells per well of pTB1 and sTB3 were stimulated with IL-2 (30 I.U./ml) or IL-2 in combination with the MM lines pMB and sMB for six hours. Proliferation was assessed by ^{3}H-thymidine incorporation over 18 hours. Results are given as mean ± SEM of four experiments.

Table 1 documents the lytic activity of TIL clones against the autologous, lesion-specific tumor cell line. 57% of TIL clones were able to mediate cytotoxicty against the corresponding tumor cell lines with up to 35% specific lysis in a four hour-^{51}Cr release assay. sTB3 and sTB6 generated from metastatic tumors were able to lyse MM lines from primary tumors, whereas none of the clones from primary tumors were able to kill tumor lines from metastatic tumors (Figure 2).

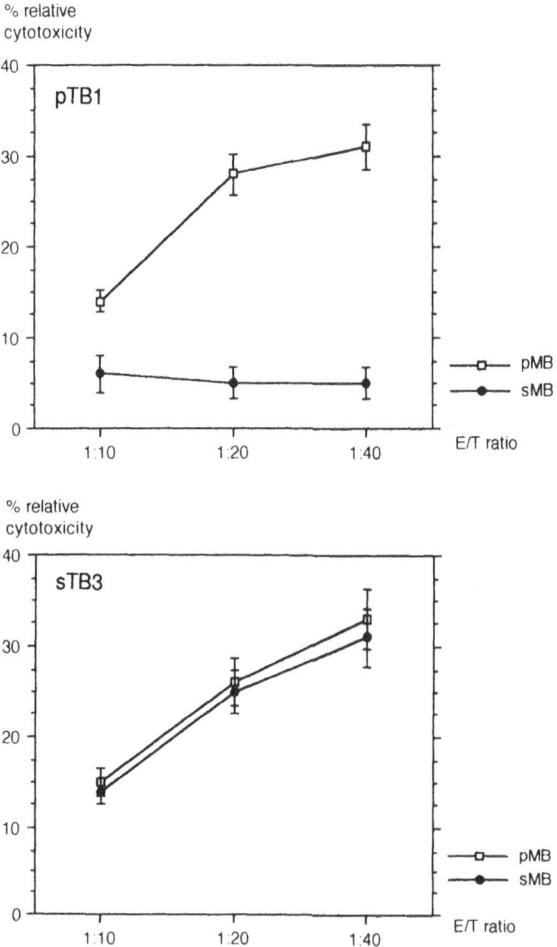

Figure 2. Killing of autologous tumor lines by TIL clones. TIL clones pTB1 and sTB3 were tested for their ability to lyse ^{51}Cr-labeled autologous MM lines pMB and sMB in a four hour assay. ^{51}Cr release was measured as described in Materials and Methods. Results are given as mean ± SEM of three experiments.

In this study we have demonstrated a specific immune response against melanoma. Specific effector cell-target cell interaction not only triggers cytotoxicty against the tumor, but also stimulates the proliferative response of the effector cells to low concentrations of IL-2. The different behavior of TIL clones obtained from primary and secondary tumors towards tumor cell lines from primary and secondary melanomas indicates that the tumor loses some of the target structures recognized by specific TIL clones during progression of the disease (Degiovanni et al., 1988; Natali et al., 1990; Pandolfi et al., 1991; Topalian et al., 1990).

REFERENCES

Alexander MA, J Bennicelli and D Guerry, IV, 1989. Defective antigen presentation by human melanoma cell lines cultured from advanced, but not biologically early disease. **J. Immunol.**, 142:4070.

Anchini A, A Mazzocchi, G Fossati, and G Parmiani, 1989. Cytotoxic T lymphocyte clones from peripheral blood and from tumor site detect intratumor heterogeneity of melanoma cells. **J. Immunol.**, 142:3692.

Becker JC, W Kolanus, C Lonnemann and RE Schmidt, 1990. Human natural killer clones enhance in vitro antibody production by tumor necrosis factor alpha and gamma interferon. **Scand. J. Immunol.**, 32:153.

Caliguri MA, A Zmuiddzinas, TJ Manley, H Levine, K A Smith and J Ritz, 1990. Functional consequences of interleukin 2 receptor expression on resting human lymphocytes: Identification of a novel natural killer subset with high affinity receptors. **J. Exp. Med.**, 171:1509.

Degiovanni G, T Lahaye, M Herin, P Hainaut, and T Boon, 1988. Antigenic heterogeneity of a human melanoma tumor detected by autologous CTL clones. **Eur. J. Immunol.**, 18:671.

Gromo G, RL Geller, L Inveradi and FH Bach, 1987. Signal requirement in the step-wise functional maturation of cytotoxic T lymphocytes. **Nature**, 327:424.

Natali P, MR Nicotra, R Cavaliere, A Bigotti, G Romano, M Temponi and S Ferrone, 1990. Differential expression of intercellular adhesion molecule 1 in primary and metastatic melanoma lesions. **Cancer Res.**, 50:1271.

Naume B, U Nonstad, B Steinkjer, S Funderud, E Smeland and T Espevik, 1991. Immunomagnetic isolation of NK and LAK cells. **J. Immunol. Methods**, 136:1.

Markey AC, LJ Churchill, MH Allen and DM MacDonald, 1990. Activation and inducer subset phenotype of the lymphocytic infiltrate around epidermally derived tumors. **J. Am. Acad. Dermatol.**, 23:214.

Muul LM, PJ Spiess, EP Director and SA Rosenberg, 1987. Identification of specific cytolytic immune responses against autologous tumor in humans bearing malignant melanoma. **J. Immunol.**, 138:989.

Packard BS, 1990. Mitogenic stimulation of human tumor-infiltrating lymphocytes by factor(s) from human tumor cell lines. **Proc. Natl. Acad. Sci. USA**, 87:4058.

Pandolfi F, LA Boyle, L Trentin, JT Kurnick, KJ Isselbacher and S Gattoni-Celli, 1991. Expression of HLA-A2 antigen in human melanoma cell lines and its role in T-cell recognition. **Cancer Res.**, 51:3164.

Rosenberg SA, BS Packard, PM Aebersold, D Solomon, SL Topalian, ST Toy, P Simon, MT Lotze, LV Yang, CA Seipp, C Simpson, C Carter, S Bock, D Schwartzenruber, JP Wei and

DE White, 1988. Use of tumor-infiltrating lymphocytes and interleukin-2 in the immunotherapy of patients with metastatic melanoma. **N. Eng. J. Med.**, 319:1976.

Takagi S, K Chen, R Schwarz, S Iwatsuki, RB Herberman and TL Whiteside, 1989. Functional and phenotypic analysis of tumor infiltrating lymphocytes isolated from human primary and metastatic liver tumors and cultured in recombinant IL-2. **Cancer**, 63:102.

Tefany FJ, RS Barnetson, GM Halliday, SW McCarthy and WH MacCarthy, 1991. Immunocytochemical analysis of the cellular infiltrate in primary regressing and non-regressing malignant melanoma. **J. Invest. Dermatol.**, 7:197.

Topalian SL, LM Muul, D Solomon and SA Rosenberg, 1987. Expansion of human tumor infiltrating lymphocytes for use in immunotherapy trials. **J. Immunol. Methods**, 102:127.

Topalian SL, A Kasid and SA Rosenberg, 1990. Immunoselection of a human melanoma resistant to specific lysis by autologous TILs: Possible mechanisms for immunotherapeutic failures. **J. Immunol.**, 144:4487.

Wang HM and KA Smith, 1987. The interleukin 2 receptor:Functional consequences of its bimolecular structure. **J. Exp. Med.**, 166:1055.

RESPONSE OF EARLY STAGE CUTANEOUS T-CELL LYMPHOMA TO ULTRAVIOLET B PHOTOTHERAPY

David L. Ramsay
Karen M. Lish
Cynthia B. Yalowitz
Nicholas A. Soter

Perelman Department of Dermatology and Photomedicine Section
New York University School of Medicine
New York, New York, U.S.A.

Correspondence to: Dr. D. Ramsay, Perelman Department of Dermatology,
New York University Medical Center, 550 First Avenue,
New York, New York, 10016, U.S.A.

ABSTRACT

Twenty-five (71%) of 35 patients with cutaneous T-cell lymphoma (CTCL) treated with ultraviolet B (UVB) phototherapy achieved a total remission. Median time to remission was 5 months, and median duration of the remission was 22 months. Twenty-five (83%) of patients with disease limited to patches (Stage I) achieved remission, whereas none of the patients with plaque level disease (Stage II) achieved remission. Of the 25 patients who achieved complete remission, five (20%) had a recurrence of CTCL. These results suggest that UVB phototherapy is an effective treatment for patients with early stage I disease.

INTRODUCTION

Cutaneous T-cell lymphoma (CTCL) initially presents in the skin and slowly progresses to

Basic Mechanisms of Physiologic and Aberrant Lymphoproliferation in the Skin
Edited by W.C. Lambert *et al.*, Plenum Press, New York, 1994

469

involve the lymph nodes and viscera. The cutaneous involvement begins with erythematous patches and may advance to indurated plaques and eventually ulcers and tumors.

CTCL most often presents on non-sunlight-exposed regions of the body, which suggests a possible protective role for ultraviolet B (UVB) radiation. UVB phototherapy may be beneficial because of its effects on Langerhans cells (Rowden et al., 1979; Tron et al., 1988). UVB has been shown to produce suppression of the antigen-presenting function of Langerhans cells, which results in suppression of both antigen and mitogen-induced lymphocyte proliferation as well as a decrease in Langerhans cells surface markers (Aberer et al., 1981; Austad et al., 1985; Sauder et al., 1983; Stingl et al., 1981). UVB irradiation has produced a delayed increase of interleukin-1 (IL-1) production in human epidermal cells (Ansel et al., 1983; Kupper et al., 1987; Oxholm et al., 1988; Rasanen et al., 1989), and has induced an increased release of interleukin-6 (IL-6) by human keratinocytes into the circulation (Urbanski et al., 1990). In addition, increased amounts of tumor necrosis factor (TNF) in human epidermis (Oxholm et al., 1988) and an increased tumor cell immunogenicity have been detected after UVB irradiation (Hostetler et al., 1986). UVB has also been found to produce an immediate inhibition of expression of intercellular adhesion molecule 1 (ICAM-1) at 24 hours, and a delayed induction at 48, 72, and 96 hours in human keratinocytes (Norris et al., 1990). These observations suggest that the UVB induced alterations in cell function and cytokine release may serve an immunotherapeutic role in controlling the progression of CTCL.

Currently, the three most widely used therapeutic modalities for CTCL are topical mechlorethamine hydrochloride (nitrogen mustard) (Hoppe et al., 1987; Price et al., 1983; Volden and Larsen, 1978; Vonderheid et al., 1979; 1989; Zachariae et al., 1985), electron beam (Hamminga et al., 1982; Hoppe et al., 1979; Le Bourgeois et al., 1987; Nisce et al., 1979; Slevin et al., 1987; Tadros et al., 1983; van Vloten et al., 1985), and oral psoralen with ultraviolet A (PUVA) photochemotherapy (Abel et al., 1981; Gilchrist, 1979; Lowe et al., 1979; Powell et al., 1984; Roenigk et al., 1990; Rosenbaum et al., 1985). Systemic chemotherapy is generally used only in patients unresponsive to other therapeutic modalities and in those who demonstrate internal involvement (Bunn et al., 1979; Gronzea et al., 1979; Hamminga et al., 1982b; Kaye et al., 1989; Maddox et al., 1985; Mc Donald and Bertino, 1978; Merlo et al., 1987; Molin et al., 1987; Moreland et al., 1985; Tirelli et al., 1982; Zachariae et al., 1982; Zakem et al., 1986). In addition, a therapeutic role for interferons and monoclonal antibodies has recently been demonstrated (Bunn and Norris, 1990; Kaplan et al., 1990; Knox et al., 1991; Kuzel et al., 1990; Olsen et al., 1989; Roenigk et al., 1990; Vegna et al., 1990). While extracorporeal photochemotherapy has been successful in treating patients with the erythrodermic form of CTCL (Edelson et al., 1987), no studies have been reported as to its appropriateness in non-erythrodermic disease. Limited data are available regarding use of UVB phototherapy in treating CTCL (Milstein et al., 1982).

At the New York University (NYU) Medical Center, the majority of patients are treated with topical mechlorethamine hydrochloride (Hostetler et al., 1986). UVB phototherapy, however, has been utilized in younger individuals in their procreative years in whom there is a reluctance to use chemotherapeutic agents. UVB phototherapy also has been used in patients who developed an immediate hypersensitivity urticarial reaction to topical mechlorethamine hydrochloride, and in whom continuation might have provoked an anaphylactoid response, as well as in patients manifesting a delayed-type hypersensitivity reaction to topical mechlorethamine that could not be overcome by further reduction of its concentration. Patients who objected to topical mechlorethamine hydrochloride or more aggressive forms of therapy were also treated with UVB phototherapy. We report on the effective use of UVB phototherapy in early CTCL.

PATIENTS AND METHODS

After giving informed consent, 37 patients were treated with UVB phototherapy by our

Table 1. Staging classifications of cutaneous T-cell lymphoma.

Stage*	Clinical characteristics of skin lesions	Lymph node involvement	Organ involvement
I	Erythematous patches	No	No
II	Infiltrated plaques	No	No
III	Tumors or ulcers	No	No
IV	Any of above	Yes	No
V	Any of above	Yes	Yes

* Stages are further divided into substages A and B. A indicates lesions that involve $\leq 10\%$ of the body; B indicates lesions that involve $> 10\%$ of the body.

clinical investigative group at the NYU Medical Center between April, 1984, and April, 1991. Thirty-two patients had histologically proven CTCL and five had parapsoriasis en plaques, considered to be the first stage of CTCL (Sanchez and Ackerman, 1979). The patients were staged according to the criteria set forth by Vonderheid et al. (1979) (Table 1), with the additional designation of A, indicating cutaneous involvement of less than or equal to 10%, and

B, indicating greater than 10% cutaneous involvement. Of the 37 patients who used UVB phototherapy, 31 (84%) had stage I disease, 5 (13%) had stage II disease, and one began UVB phototherapy after achieving remission with mechlorethamine hydrochloride (Table 2). Eleven patients had previously been treated with topical mechlorethamine hydrochloride, and two of these also had received other therapies including electron beam or localized irradiation.

Table 2. Stage of patients at initiation of UVB phototherapy.

Stage/Substage	No. of Patients (%)	
0	1	(3%)
1A	25	(68%)
1B	6	(16%)
2A	3	(8%)
2B	2	(5%)
Total Patients: 37		

A profile of the patient population shows an almost equal number of women and men (51% F, 49% M) (Table 3). The median age of the patients was 43 years with a range of 17 to 86 years.

Seventeen (49%) of the patients were started on home UVB phototherapy, 10 (29%) began treatment in an outpatient setting and subsequently switched to home UVB therapy, and 8 (23%) received UVB phototherapy exclusively in an outpatient hospital setting.

Patients on home UVB phototherapy were exposed to four Westinghouse 40 watt FS 40 fluorescent lamps, each 1.2 meters in length, on a daily basis. They were instructed to stand approximately 0.5 meters from the bulbs and to expose the anterior and posterior aspects of their body on one day alternating with exposure of the lateral aspects of their body on the subsequent day. The dose was slowly increased in increments of 15 seconds on alternate days. Upon clearing, patients were maintained at that dose of UVB exposure. The mean exposure was 4 minutes.

For those patients who began UVB phototherapy in the Photomedicine Section using a walk-in irradiation chamber, a minimal erythema dose (MED) was determined using a high output UVB lamp (FS 72T12). Phototherapy was administered starting at 50-60% of the MED with subsequent increases by increments of 50, 40, 30 and 20%, respectively, of the previous dose, at each of the next four treatments. After the fifth treatment, increases in UVB were determined by the individual patient's tolerance. In all cases, the end point of increase was a generalized faint erythema 24 hours after exposure. Most patients initially received irradiation three times per week. The subsequent treatments varied with individual patient improvement, usually decreasing to twice and then once a week upon achieving remission, and then to every other week upon achieving a maintained remission of several months' duration.

RESULTS

Patients received UVB phototherapy for a median duration of 22 months, with a range of one to 79 months (Table 5).

Table 3. Sex and age of patients with cutaneous T-cell lymphoma at initiation of UVB phototherapy.

Age (year)	Sex M	F	Total	(%)
≤20	2	0	2	(5%)
20-29	4	4	8	(22%)
30-39	4	3	7	(19%)
40-49	1	6	7	(19%)
50-59	3	2	5	(14%)
60-69	2	3	5	(14%)
70-79	1	0	1	(3%)
>80	1	1	2	(5%)
Totals	18(49%)	19(51%)	37	

The median interval between the onset of symptoms and initiation of UVB phototherapy was 6.0 years (mean 8.6), with a range of 0.25 to 49 years (Table 4).

Table 4. Duration of symptoms prior to UVB phototherapy.

Years Prior to Treatment	No. of Patients (%)	
<1	4	(11%)
1-4	10	(27%)
5-9	10	(27%)
10-14	5	(14%)
15-19	6	(16%)
≥20	2	(5%)

Table 5. Duration of UVB phototherapy.

Months	No. of Patients
≤4	5
5-12	6
13-24	7
25-36	8
37-48	3
49-60	3
61-72	1
73-84	2

Twenty-five (71%) of the 35 patients available for analysis (two were lost to follow-up) achieved a complete clinical remission, defined as the clearance of all cutaneous lesions for greater than three consecutive months (Table 6). In addition, one (3%) achieved clinical improvement with a decreased number of cutaneous lesions and a subsequent reduction within a stage, from stage 1B to 1A. The patient who began UVB phototherapy at stage 0 remained in remission. Twenty-five (83%) of the 30 patients with Stage I disease achieved total remission, and one showed clinical improvement. Thus 26 (87%) Stage I patients demonstrated complete remission or considerable clinical improvement, defined as a reduction in stage or substage. By contrast, none of the four patients beginning therapy in stage II disease were responsive to UVB treatment.

Table 6. Outcome of patients treated with UVB phototherapy.

Stage at onset	No. of patients	No.(%)of Patients Achieving Remission	No.(%)of Patients Improved	No.(%)of Patients Unchanged	No.(%)of Patients Progressed
0	1	-	-	1	-
1A	24	20	-	4	-
1B	6	5	1	-	-
2A	2	-	-	1	1
2B	2	-	-	-	2
Totals	35	25 (71)	1 (3)	6 (17)	3 (9)

Of the 25 patients who achieved remission, the median time to remission was 5 months with a range from one month to 33 months. The median duration of the complete response was 22 months with a range of three to 74 months. Upon achieving remission, 18 patients (72%) continued on maintenance UVB phototherapy. Five patients (20%) had a recurrence of CTCL. In three of these patients, relapse occurred, 24, 18, and 12 months after discontinuing therapy, respectively. The other two patients relapsed while using UVB phototherapy after 32 and 22 months, respectively.

Patients receiving therapy in each of the three different treatment settings achieved remissions (Table 7). Three of 8 (38%) patients treated in the outpatient clinic and 12 of 17 patients (71%) treated with home light therapy achieved remissions. In addition, all 10 patients treated initially in the outpatient section and then converted to home UV light achieved remission, four while receiving outpatient therapy, and six while using home light therapy. In total, eighteen (72%) achieved remission while using home light, and 7 (28%) achieved remission while receiving outpatient therapy. The small number of remissions in the outpatient clinic setting reflects a patient population with more advanced stage II disease.

Table 7. Outcome of patients treated with UVB phototherapy

	Clinic Outpatient (OP) (N=8)	Home Light (HL) (N=17)	Clinic Outpatient + Home light (N=10)
Remission	3	12	10
Improved	0	1	0
Unchanged	2	4	0
Progressed	3	0	0
Totals	8	17	10

UVB phototherapy was found to be well tolerated by the majority of patients, with no evidence of associated cutaneous malignancies. After achieving remission, however, two patients were found to have biopsy-proven dysplastic nevi and maintenance therapy was discontinued, even though these lesions had been of longstanding duration. One patient, however, did continue on maintenance UVB after a dysplastic nevus was diagnosed. Another patient, in whom UVB phototherapy was not proving to be successful, discontinued UVB phototherapy because she experienced pruritus.

DISCUSSION

Our data suggest that UVB phototherapy is an effective treatment for early stage CTCL. Of the 35 patients available for analysis, 71% achieved a total remission, lasting a median duration of 22 months. Total remission occurred in 83% of patients with patch stage disease, while 87% of patients with stage I disease demonstrated complete clearing or considerable improvement. These observations confirm and extend those of Milstein et al. (1982), who demonstrated a 61% remission rate, for a median duration of 18 months, in patients with premycotic disease, parapsoriasis en plaques, or CTCL treated with home UVB phototherapy.

Our study demonstrates that it is important to make a clinical distinction between patch and plaque disease, since UVB phototherapy has proven to be effective only in patch stage disease. The tumor-node-metastasis (TNM) classification system (Bunn and Lamberg, 1979), which groups both patch and plaque disease together, and separates T1 from T2 by percentage of body area with disease involvement (T1 with < 10% and T2 > 10% body area involvement), camouflages the clinical distinction necessary for effective UVB irradiation. Since the only patients in our study to achieve remission or clinical improvement were those with patch stage disease (stage IA and IB), it is not possible to express remission rates in terms of the TNM classification system.

Also of interest, patients who began therapy in either stage IA or IB had equal remission rates, both 83%. Median duration of remission for patients with stage IA disease was 25.5 months, compared to 20 months for patients with stage IB disease.

The results of this study, with 71% overall remission, and 83% remission in patients with stage I disease, suggest that UVB phototherapy may be as effective as other topical modalities in the treatment of early stage I CTCL. Since other studies use the TNM classification system, in which early stage CTCL is a combination of both patch and plaque stage disease, comparison of efficacies is difficult. In our report of the use of topical mechlorethamine in which we used the Vonderheid classification (Vonderheid et al., 1979) of stage I disease, defined as those patients with disease limited to patch level lesions, the remission rate with topical mechlorethamine was 75.8% compared to the UVB remission rate of 83%. In addition, the median time to achieve complete remission was 5 months in patients treated with UVB, compared to 6.5 months in stage I patients treated with topical mechlorethamine hydrochloride (Ramsay et al., 1988).

This non-randomized study suggests that both outpatient and home UVB phototherapy are effective in achieving remission in patch stage disease. While dosage in Joules could not be determined for home UVB phototherapy, such precise quantification does not appear to be necessary, since 18 of 25 patients (72%) achieved remission while using home light therapy. Larger patient populations, however, are necessary to accurately assess the differences among treatment groups with regard to efficacy of treatment, time to remission, and duration of remission.

This preliminary study suggests that UVB phototherapy is an effective therapy for patients in early stage I CTCL. Further prospective studies are necessary to evaluate the duration of remission and the potential side effects of UVB phototherapy.

REFERENCES

Abel EA, DG Deneau, EM Farber et al., 1981. PUVA treatment of erythrodermic and plaque type mycosis fungoides. **J. Am. Acad. Dermatol.**, 4:423-429.

Aberer W, G Schuler, G Stingl et al., 1981. UV light depletes surface markers of Langerhans cells. **J. Invest. Dermatol.**, 76:202-210.

Ansel JC, TA Luger and I Green, 1983. The effect of in vitro and in vivo UV irradiation on the production of ETAF activity by human and murine keratinocytes. **J. Invest. Dermatol.**, 81:519-523.

Austad J and LR Braathen, 1985. Effect of UVB on alloactivating and antigen-presenting capacity of human epidermal Langerhans cells. **Scand. J. Immunol.**, 21:417-423.

Bunn PA, AB Fischmann, GP Schechter et al., 1979. Combined modality therapy with electron-beam irradiation and systemic chemotherapy for cutaneous T-cell lymphomas. **Cancer Treat. Rep.**, 63:713-717.

Bunn PA Jr and SI Lamberg, 1979. Report of the committee on staging and classification of cutaneous T-cell lymphomas. **Cancer Treat. Rep.**, 63:725-728.

Bunn PA and DA Norris, 1990. The therapeutic role of interferons and monoclonal antibodies in cutaneous T-cell lymphomas. **J. Invest. Dermatol.**, 95:209S-212S.

Edelson R, C Berger, F Gasparro et al., 1987. Treatment of cutaneous T-cell lymphoma by extracorporeal photochemotherapy. **N. Engl. J. Med.**, 316:297-303.

Gilchrest BA, 1979. Methoxsalen photochemotherapy for mycosis fungoides. **Cancer Treat. Rep.**, 63:663-667.

Grozea PN, SE Jones, EM McKelvey et al., 1979. Combination chemotherapy for mycosis fungoides: A Southwest oncology group study. **Cancer Treat. Rep.**, 63:647-653.

Hamminga L, J Hermans, EM Noordijk et al., 1982. Cutaneous T-cell lymphoma: Clinocopathological relationships, therapy and survival in ninety-two patients. **Br. J. Dermatol.**, 107:145-156.

Hamminga B, EM Noordijk and WA van Vloten, 1982b. Treatment of mycosis fungoides: Total skin electron beam irradiation vs. topical mechlorethamine therapy. **Arch. Dermatol.**, 118:150-153.

Hoppe RT, EA Abel, DG Deneau et al., 1987. Mycosis fungoides: Management with topical nitrogen mustard. **J. Clin. Oncol.**, 5:1796-1803.

Hoppe RT, RS Cox, Z Fuks et al., 1979. Electron-beam therapy for mycosis fungoides: The Stanford University experience. **Cancer Treat. Rep.**, 63:691-700.

Hostetler LW, HN Ananthaswamy and ML Kripke, 1986. Generation of tumor-specific transplantation antigens by UV radiation can occur independently of neoplastic transformation. **J. Immunol.**, 137:2721-2725.

Kaplan EH, ST Rosen, DB Norris et al., 1990. Phase II study of recombinant human interferon gamma for treatment of cutaneous T-cell lymphoma. **J. Natl. Cancer Inst.**, 82:208-212.

Knox SJ, R Levy, S Hodgkinson et al., 1991. Observations on the effect of chimeric anti-CD4 monoclonal antibody in patients with mycosis fungoides. **Blood**, 77:20-30.

Kaye FJ, PA Bunn, Jr, SM Steinberg et al., 1989. A randomized trial comparing combination electron-beam radiation and chemotherapy with topical therapy in the initial treatment of mycosis fungoides. **N. Engl. J. Med.**, 321:1784-1790.

Kupper TS, AO Chua, P Flood et al., 1987. Interleukin 1 gene expression in cultured human keratinocytes is augmented by ultraviolet irradiation. **J. Clin. Invest.**, 80: 430-436.

Kuzel TM, R Gilyon R, E Springer et al., 1990. Interferon alfa-2a combined with photo-therapy in the treatment of cutaneous T-cell lymphoma. **J. Natl. Cancer Inst.**, 82:203-207.

Le Bourgeois JP, E Haddad, G Marinello et al., 1987. The indications for total cutaneous electron beam radiation therapy of mycosis fungoides. **Int. J. Radiat. Oncol. Biol. Phys.**, 13:189-193.

Lowe NJ, DJ Cripps, PA Dutton PA et al., 1979. Photochemotherapy for mycosis fungoi-des: A clinical and histologic study. **Dermatol.**, 115:50-53.

Maddox AM, BD Kahan, S Tuker, et al., 1985. Remission in skin infiltrate of a patient with mycosis fungoides treated with cyclosporin. **J. Am. Acad. Dermatol.**, 12:952-956.

McDonald CJ and JR Bertino, 1978. Treatment of mycosis fungoides lymphoma: Effectiveness of infusions of methotrexate followed by oral citrovorum factor. **Cancer Treat. Rep.**, 62:1009-1014.

Merlo CJ, RT Hoppe, E Abel et al., 1987. Extracutaneous mycosis fungoides. **Cancer**, 60:397-402.

Milstein HJ, EC Vonderheid, EJ Van Scott et al., 1982. Home ultraviolet phototherapy of early mycosis fungoides: Preliminary observations. **J. Amer. Acad. Dermatol.**, 6:355-362.

Molin L, K Thomsen, G Volden et al., 1987. Retinoids and systemic chemotherapy in cases of advanced mycosis fungoides. A report from the Scandinavian Mycosis Fungoides Group. **Acta Derm. Venereol. (Stockh)**, 67:179-182.

Moreland AA, DB Robertson and LT Heffner, 1985. Treatment of cutaneous T cell lymphoma with cyclosporin A. **J. Am. Acad. Dermatol.**, 12:886-887.

Nisce LZ and B Safai, 1979. Once weekly total skin electron beam therapy for mycosis fungoides. **Cancer Treat. Rep.**, 63:633-638.

Norris DA, MB Lyons, MH Middleton et al., 1990. Ultraviolet radiation can either suppress or induce expression of intercellular adhesion molecule 1 (ICAM-1) on the surface of cultured human keratinocytes. **J. Invest. Dermatol.**, 95:132-138.

Olsen EA, ST Rosen, RT Vollmer et al., 1989. Interferon alfa-2a in the treatment of cutaneous T cell lymphoma. **J. Am. Acad. Dermatol.**, 20:395-407.

Oxholm A, P Oxholm, B Staberg et al., 1988. Immunohistological detection of interleukin I-like molecules and tumour necrosis factor in human epidermis before and after UVB-irra-diation in vivo. **Br. J. Dermatol.**, 118:369-376.

Price NM, RT Hoppe and DG Deneau DG, 1983. Ointment-based mechlorethamine treatment for mycosis fungoides. **Cancer**, 52:2214-2219.

Powell FC, GT Siegel and SA Muller, 1984. Treatment of parapsoriasis and mycosis fungoides: The role of psoralen and long-wave ultraviolet A (PUVA). **Mayo Clin. Proc.**, 59:538-546.

Ramsay DL, PS Halperin and A Zeleniuch-Jacquotte, 1988. Topical mechlorethamine therapy for early stage mycosis fungoides. **J. Am. Acad. Dermatol.**, 19:684-691.

Rasanen L, T Reunala, M Lehto et al., 1989. Immediate decrease in antigen-presenting function and delayed enhancement of interleukin-I production in human epidermal cells after in vivo UVB irradiation. **Br. J. Dermatol.**, 120:589-596.

Roenigk HH, TM Kuzel, AP Skoutelis et al., 1990. Photochemotherapy alone or combined with interferon alpha-2a in the treatment of cutaneous T-cell lymphoma. **J. Invest. Dermatol.**, 95:198S-205S.

Rosenbaum MM, HH Roenigk, WA Caro et al., 1985. Photochemotherapy in cutaneous T cell lymphoma and parapsoriasis en plaques. **J. Am. Acad. Dermatol.**, 13:613-622.

Rowden G, TM Phillips, MG Lewis et al., 1979. Target role of Langerhans cells in mycosis fungoides: Transmission and immuno-electron microscope studies. **J. Cut. Pathol.**, 6:364-382.

Sanchez JL and AB Ackerman, 1979. The patch stage of mycosis fungoides: Criteria for histologic diagnosis. **Am. J. Dermatopathol.**, 1:5-26.

Sauder DN, FP Noonan, EC DeFabo et al., 1983. Ultraviolet radiation inhibits alloantigen presentation by epidermal cells: Partial reversal by the soluble epidermal cell product, epidermal cell-derived thymocyte-activating factor (ETAF). **J. Invest. Dermatol.**, 80:485-489.

Slevin NJ, VBlair and ID Todd, 1987. Mycosis fungoides - Response to therapy and survival patterns in 85 cases. **Br. J. Dermatol.**, 116:47-53.

Stingl G, LA Gazze-Stingl, W Aberer et al., 1981. Antigen presentation by murine epidermal Langerhans cell and its alteration by ultraviolet B light. **J. Immunol.**, 127:1707-1713.

Tadros AAM, BS Tepperman, WM Hryniuk et al., 1983. Total skin electron irradiation of mycosis fungoides: Failure analysis and prognostic factors. **Int. J. Radiat. Oncol. Biol. Phys.**, 9:1279-1287.

Tirelli U, A Carbone, A Veronesi et al., 1982. Combination chemotherapy with cyclophosphamide, vincristine, and prednisone (CVP) in TNM - classified stage IV mycosis fungoides. **Cancer Treat. Rep.**, 66:167-169.

Tron VA, D Rosenthal and DN Sauder, 1988. Epidermal interleukin-1 is increased in cutaneous T-cell lymphoma. **J. Invest. Dermatol.**, 90: 378-381.

Urbanski A, T Schwarz, P Neuner et al., 1990. Ultraviolet light induces increased circulating interleukin-6 in humans. **J. Invest. Dermatol.**, 94:808-811.

Van Vloten WA, H DeVroome and EM Noordijk, 1985. Total skin electron beam irradiation for cutaneous T-cell lymphoma (mycosis fungoides). **Br. J. Dermatol.**, 112:697-702.

Vegna ML, G Papa, D Defazio et al., 1990. Interferon alpha-2a in cutaneous T-cell lymphoma. **Eur. J. Haematol.**, 45:Suppl. 52: 32-35.

Volden G and TE Larsen, 1978. Remissions of mycosis fungoides induced by nitrogen mustard (HN2). **Dermatologica**, 156: 129-141.

Vonderheid EC, ET Tan, AF Kantor et al., 1989. Long-term efficacy, curative potential, and carcinogenicity of topical mechlorethamine chemotherapy in cutaneous T cell lymphoma. **J. Am. Acad. Dermatol.**, 20:416-428.

Vonderheid EC, EJ Van Scott, PE Wallner et al., 1979. A 10 year experience with topical mechlorethamine for mycosis fungoides: Comparison with patients treated by total-skin electron beam radiation therapy. **Cancer Treat. Rep.**, 63:681-689.

Zachariae H, E Grunnet, K Thestrup-Pedersen et al., 1982. Oral retinoid in combination with bleomycin, cyclophosphamide, prednisone, and transfer factor in mycosis fungoides. **Acta Derm. Venereol.**, 62:162-164.

Zachariae H, K Thestrup-Pedersen and H Sogaard, 1985. Topical nitrogen mustard in early mycosis fungoides. **Acta Dermatol. Venereol. (Stockh).**, 65:53-58.

Zakem MH, BR David, DJ Adelstein et al., 1986. Treatment of advanced stage mycosis fungoides with bleomycin, doxorubicin and methotrexate with topical nitrogen mustard (BAM-M). **Cancer**, 58:2611-2616.

A MURINE T-CELL LYMPHOMA MODEL SHOWING PROTECTION AGAINST TUMOR DEVELOPMENT AND TREATMENT OF ESTABLISHED DISEASE

Maritza I. Perez
Richard L. Edelson
Yasuhiro Yamane
Francis M. Lobo

Department of Dermatology
Yale University School of Medicine
New Haven, Connecticut, U.S.A.

Correspondence to: Dr. R. L. Edelson, Department of Dermatology,
Yale University School of Medicine, 333 Cedar Street,
New Haven, CT 06510, U.S.A.

ABSTRACT

Patients suffering from leukemic and erythrodermic cutaneous T-cell lymphoma (CTCL) treated with photopheresis demonstrate a profound and prolonged clinical response that appears to be mediated immunologically. Photopheresis involves exposure of the peripheral blood lymphocytes from a patient to 8-methoxypsoralen (8-MOP) photoactivated with ultraviolet A light (UVA), with subsequent reinfusion of the treated cells.

We have evaluated the capacity of mice pretreated with chemically or photochemically altered tumor cells to induce protection against tumor development in a murine lymphoma model using a T-cell hybridoma. When injected subcutaneously into genetically compatible hybrid mice, a T-cell hybridoma leads to the development of a rapidly progressive lymphoma that metastasizes to internal organs, causing death of all the mice within four to six weeks. For the induction of protection against this murine T-cell lymphoma, mice were immunized with altered

Basic Mechanisms of Physiologic and Aberrant Lymphoproliferation in the Skin
Edited by W.C. Lambert *et al.*, Plenum Press, New York, 1994

483

tumorogenic cells. Our data indicate that the most effective method to induce protection against tumor development in 66% of treated mice involved predamaging tumor cells with 8-methoxypsoralen photoactivated with ultraviolet A light. We have demonstrated that this protection is T-cell mediated by treating nude mice in a similar fashion without inducing protection against tumor development. We have demonstrated that there is cross-protection to another T-cell hybridoma differing in T-cell receptor specificity and to the parental thymoma. We have also demonstrated successful treatment of 64% of mice with established disease. Adoptive transfer experiments have demonstrated that this protection against tumor development is transferable by spleen cells from immune-protected mice. Adoptive transfer experiments with specific-cell-subtype depletion and isolation of immunogenic peptides will help to clarify the conditions most conducive to an anti-T-cell tumor response, and to identify its target molecules and the cells involved.

INTRODUCTION

Cutaneous T-cell lymphoma (CTCL) is a clonal malignancy (Berger et al., 1979) of phenotypic and functional helper/inducer T lymphocytes (Edelson, 1980 a;b), manifested as generalized or localized erythroderma with or without exfoliation, edema, fissures, or tumor formation. The disease progresses to involve the blood and other organs. The incidence of CTCL in the general population was formerly underestimated; in fact, it is comparable to that of Hodgkin disease (Edelson, 1980 a;b). Unfortunately, there is no animal model for CTCL. Development of an animal model is necessary if we are to determine whether cellular vaccination and development of immunity against tumor can explain the clinical responses observed in patients treated by photopheresis. Photopheresis involves the exposure of peripheral blood lymphocytes from the patient to photoactivated 8-methoxypsoralen (8-MOP) with subsequent reinfusion of the treated cells into the same patient. We have reported that patients with CTCL who are treated by photopheresis demonstrate a profound and prolonged clinical response that appears to be mediated immunologically (Edelson et al., 1987). These results occur in the absence of any other systemic therapy and result exclusively from the extracorporeal treatment and return to the patients of approximately only ten percent of their total body burden of malignant T-cells. Therefore, we hypothesized that an immunologic attack on the remaining untreated malignant T-cells had been induced (Edelson et al., 1987).

MATERIALS AND METHODS

We have used T hybridoma cells in genetically compatible mice as an animal model for human T-cell lymphomas. T-cell hybridomas are tetraploid cells produced by polyethylene glycol-mediated fusion of antigen-specific T lymphoblasts with the immortal AKR-derived malignant thymoma, BW5147 (Kappler et al., 1981). Hybridoma 2B4 was raised in B10.A mice and has a membrane T-cell receptor (TCR) with specificity for pigeon cytochrome c presented on Class II molecule I-E^k (Ashwell et al.,1987 a;b). The advantages of utilizing this hybridoma cell are: in vitro immortality, the known specificity of its TCR, and the availability of an anticlonotypic antibody, A2B4, against its TCR (Samelson et al., 1983). In vivo, antigen-specific T hybridoma cells injected subcutaneously (s.c.) into F1 mice produce a progressive lymphoma that metastasizes and kills the inoculated animals (Ashwell et al., 1987a). We have established an experimental murine model for T cell lymphomas using these cells. Varying numbers of viable, antigen-specific T hybridoma cells have been injected s.c. into F1 hybrid mice to determine the minimal number of tumor cells that cause fatal lymphoma in almost all recipient mice. Our preliminary studies show that the minimal number of 2B4 tumor cells capable of killing 100% of the recipient mice is approximately 5×10^6 cells (Table 1).

Table 1. Development of malignant lymphoma in F1 (B10.A x AKR) hybrid mice.

s.c. Injection of 2B4.11 cells	Tumor Development	Death (30-35 Days
1×10^6	2/3	1/3
2.5×10^6	6/7	5/7
5×10^6	8/8	8/8
s.c. Injection of C10.9 cells		
10×10^6	5/5	5/5
10×10^6	5/5	5/5
s.c. Injection of 2B4.11.21.2.2 cells		
10×10^6	0/6	0/6

We have used several approaches to treat these tumor cells in vitro in an attempt to simultaneously enhance their immunogenicity and render them unable to form progressively growing lethal tumors. For this purpose we have tested different methods of cellular inactivation, including treatment with 8-MOP with photoactivation by UVA light, glutaraldehyde, mitomycin C (MMC), and X-irradiation. The rationale for the manipulation in vitro of these tumor cells is as follows: In other systems, attempts have been made to selectively suppress populations of pathogenic T cells. A murine model of autoreactive disease has been developed in which T cell clones specific for myelin basic protein (MBP) induce experimental autoimmune encephalomyelitis if passively transferred into susceptible syngeneic strains of rodents (Holoshitz et al., 1985a). If the same disease-inducing, cloned T cells are first attenuated extracorporeally by X-irradiation, mitomycin C, or glutaraldehyde, and then intravenously reinfused, however, they can immunoprotect syngeneic animals in a clonotypic manner against the same autoreactive disease (Holshitz et al., 1983a;b). We have developed animal models in which potent and defined immunologic responses, such as skin allograft rejection, are expressed in vivo, and for which laboratory correlates, such as the mixed leukocyte culture (MLC) and the delayed-type hypersensitivity (DTh) response, exist. In such a system, which involves transplantation of skin across both major and minor (Perez, 1989) and exclusively major (Perez et al., 1991) mouse histocompatibility barriers, we have reported that the responses in vivo and in vitro to alloantigen are attenuated in a donor-specific fashion. Splenocytes that included expanded populations of effector T cells mediating the relevant allograft rejection were first treated with 8-MOP and UVA and then were infused into naïve syngeneic recipients, which subsequently showed markedly enhanced survival of relevant skin allografts, in parallel with specific inhibition of the MLC response, cytotoxic T cell (CTL) response, and DTH response to alloantigens. We have demonstrated, in adoptive transfer experiments, that CD8$^+$ T-cells are critically involved in these inhibitory responses (Perez et al., 1991b; 1992). In collaboration with Dr. Carole Berger at Columbia University, we have also demonstrated that prophylactic treatment of mice suffering from an autoimmune disease similar to systemic lupus erythematosus with 8-MOP/UVA-damaged autoimmune splenocytes improves the survival and inhibits both the fulminant hyperproliferation of abnormal T-cells and the production of high-titer DNA-specific antibodies found in untreated mice (Berger et al., 1990).

In other systems, the stimulation in vitro of these spontaneously dividing murine T-cell hybridomas by their specific antigen results in an irreversible block in the cell cycle at the G_1/S interphase associated with increased secretion of IL-1 (Ashwell, 1987b) followed by cell lysis (Mercep et al., 1989). A report by Ashwell and coworkers (Mercep et al., 1988; Sussman et al., 1988) indicates that potentially activating these tumor cells via their TCR (using CD3-specific antibodies) or via the use of monoclonal antibodies (mAb) against other surface molecules (such as Thy-1 and Ly-6) induces similar inhibition of growth of these T hybridoma cells. This raises the possibility that activation of neoplastic T-cells by specific and non-specific stimulation might inhibit progression of their malignant growth and induce the development of specific tumor immunity.

RESULTS AND DISCUSSION

8-MOP is a naturally occurring, biologically inert furocoumarin which is transiently transformed by UVA to a state in which it is capable of forming covalent bonds with pyrimidine bases of DNA which, in turn, leads to cross-links between complementary strands of DNA (Scott et al., 1976). The effect on DNA induced by 8-MOP is analogous to the chemical effect of a bifunctional alkylating agent, such as mitomycin C (MMC). However, 8-MOP, unlike MMC, is used in the treatment of patients. In our system, we have used chemical and photochemical cross-linkers in an attempt to abolish the ability of hybridoma cells to form rapidly growing lethal tumors while simultaneously becoming more immunogenic when inoculated into susceptible mice. The efficacy of each attempted inactivation has been determined in terms of inhibition of incorporation of thymidine (Tdr). In preliminary studies, we have determined the optimal conditions for inactivation of tumor cells for all of the previously mentioned modalities of cellular inactivation (Table 2). For example, 2B4 T hybri-

Table 2. Effects of pretreatment with various modalities of cellular inactivation in the inhibition of incorporation of [^{3}H]-thymidine by 2B4 cells (x $\pm$ SD, CPM x 10^{-3}; N =3).

	Day 0	Day 1	Day 3	Day 5	Day 7
No treatment					
Exp. #1	41.5 $\pm$ 3.0	106.7 $\pm$ 10.0	ND	ND	ND
Exp. #2	5.7 $\pm$ 3.4	225.6 $\pm$ 12.3	72.1 $\pm$ 15.5	75.3 $\pm$ 4.5	4.1 $\pm$ 0.1
8-MOP (100 ng/ml)					
UVA (2 J/cm^2)					
Exp. #1	4.9 $\pm$ 0.4	1.3 $\pm$ 0.2	0.3 $\pm$ 0.1	0.5 $\pm$ 0.1	0.4 $\pm$ 0.1
Exp. #2	0.9 $\pm$ 0.2	0.3 $\pm$ 0.0	0.3 $\pm$ 0.2	ND	ND
X-irradiation					
3200 rads	6.5 $\pm$ 0.5	11.0 $\pm$ 0.6	6.3 $\pm$ 0.4	12.0 $\pm$ 1.6	0.9 $\pm$ 0.1
5000 rads					
Exp. #1	7.4 $\pm$ 0.3	1.5 $\pm$ 0.1	.7 $\pm$ 0.1	0.4 $\pm$ 0.2	0.3 $\pm$ 0.1
Exp. #2	6.2 $\pm$ 0.8	3.5 $\pm$ 1.1	3.8 $\pm$ 0.0	6.1 $\pm$ 0.5	0.3 $\pm$ 0.1
7000 rads	5.1 $\pm$ 0.1	1.9 $\pm$ 0.6	3.7 $\pm$ 0.4	13.2 $\pm$ 3.0	0.3 $\pm$ 0.0
10,000 rads	4.2 $\pm$ 0.2	1.6 $\pm$ 0.5	3.2 $\pm$ 0.2	10.0 $\pm$ 0.9	0.3 $\pm$ 0.0
Mitomycin C (MMC)					
25 ug/ml Exp. #1	8.2 $\pm$ 0.6	2.0 $\pm$ 0.1	7.8 $\pm$ 0.7	114.3 $\pm$ 13.0	121.0 $\pm$ 6.4
Exp. #2	2.5 $\pm$ 0.0	4.1 $\pm$ 0.3	1.8 $\pm$ 0.1	8.5 $\pm$ 2.2	0.9 $\pm$ 0.1
50 ug/ml Exp. #1	8.8 $\pm$ 0.5	0.3 $\pm$ 0.1	0.4 $\pm$ 0.2	0.3 $\pm$ 0.1	0.3 $\pm$ 0.1
Exp. #2	1.4 $\pm$ 0.1	5.8 $\pm$ 0.4	2.0 $\pm$ 0.3	9.7 $\pm$ 0.8	0.4 $\pm$ 0.1
75 ug/ml	0.9 $\pm$ 0.0	5.7 $\pm$ 0.4	2.5 $\pm$ 0.6	1.4 $\pm$ 0.3	0.2 $\pm$ 0.0
Glutaraldehyde (0.5%, w/v)	0.4 $\pm$ 0.1	0.4 $\pm$ 0.1	0.4 $\pm$ 0.0	0.2 $\pm$ 0.0	0.3 $\pm$ 0.0

doma cells have been incubated in vitro with 8-MOP at different concentrations and exposed to increasing numbers of Joules of UVA. The dose of the 8-MOP/UVA combination that maximally inhibits the spontaneous proliferation of T hybridoma cells is 200 ng/ml 8-MOP and 2 J/cm^2 UVA light. Further preliminary studies show that the minimal inhibitory dose of glutaraldehyde for inactivation of tumor cells is a 0.5% (w/v) solution of glutaraldehyde in PBS (Table 2). Using the standard procedure for incubation with MMC, we found that the minimum dose of MMC capable of obtaining the same result in vitro was 75 mg/ml (Table 2). The optimal dose of X-irradiation capable of preventing spontaneous growth of tumors was determined to be 5,000 rads (Table 2).

In our clinical experience, erythrodermic CTCL patients presenting with disease realcitrant to conventional therapy responded to photopheresis therapy with an average 64% decrease in cutaneous involvement after a mean of 22 weeks of treatment, without significant systemic toxicity (Edelson et al., 1987). Moreover, erythrodermic CTCL patients treated by photopheresis have demonstrated prolonged survival when compared with historical controls (Heald et al., 1991; 1992). With this clinical correlate in mind, we have conducted preliminary studies to determine the most efficacious tested method of inducing protection against tumor development. Tumor cells, having been damaged by treatment with the optimal combination of 8-MOP (200 ng/ml) and UVA (2 J/cm^2), X-irradiation (5,000 rads), glutaraldehyde (0.5%), or MMC (75 mg/ml), were injected intraperitoneally (i.p.) weekly, for four weeks, into F1 hybrid mice. One week after the fourth injection, mice treated in this manner were challenged with s.c. injection of viable tumor cells of the same specificity. The extent of subsequent development of tumor in treated mice was compared to that in non-treated syngeneic control mice challenged in the same fashion. Preliminary studies have suggested that the most efficacious of these methods of cellular inactivation for inducing protection against tumor development is 8-MOP and UVA (Tables 2 and 3). Tumor growth in the first ten days after challenge was significantly impeded only in mice pretreated with cells inactivated by 8-MOP/UVA; treatments with cells inactivated by mitomycin C, by glutaraldehyde, and by X-irradiation impeded tumor growth to a lesser degree. The incidence of tumor formation was lower in all groups of pretreated mice, especially in the recipients of 8-MOP/UVA and mitomycin C-inactivated tumor cells; tumors were observed to disappear over the first ten days in a small fraction of all experimental groups. Significant regression was noted in the 8-MOP/UVA and mitomycin C treatment groups. No such regression took place in the untreated control group. However, tumors that had not regressed in experimental mice by day ten were neither significantly smaller nor less lethal than those in control mice.

Pretreatment with cells inactivated by 8-MOP/UVA, by mitomycin C, and by X-irradiation led to a significant improvement in 40-day survival compared with untreated control mice; by 80 days, enhancement of survival was significant only for the 8-MOP/UVA (28/42 survivors, Table 3) and mitomycin C (4/10 survivors) groups compared with the control group (37/37 dead). Mice pretreated with cells inactivated by glutaraldehyde also demonstrated enhanced 40-day and 80-day survival, but this protection was not statistically significant with the sample size

Table 3. Short term immunity[a] against tumor by pretreatment[b] with variously inactivated 2B4.11 cells.

Method of inactivation	Tumor Area[c], Days After Challenge (mm² ± SEM) (Number with tumors/Number challenged)			Dead at 40 days	Dead at 80 days
	Day 4	Day 7	Day 10		
None (control) n=37	36 ± 6 (36/37)	123 ± 38 (37/37)	157 ± 23 (37/37)	35/37	37/37
8-MOP/UVA n=42	24 ± 3[d] (12/42)	53 ± 28 (10/42)	141 ± 29 (14/42)[e]	14/42	14/42[f]
Mitomycin C n=10	31 ± 6 (8/10)	72± 17 (6/10)	129 ± 56 (5/10)[e]	4/10[f]	6/10[f]
Glutaraldehyde n=11	36 ±4 (10/11)	76 ± 9 (11/11)	84 ± 29 (7/11)	6/11	9/11
X-irradiation n=12	28 ± 4 (10/12)	58 ± 9 (9/12)	145 ± 35 (8/12)	5/12[f]	10/12

a - Challenged six days after last treatment by s.c.injection of 5×10^6 viable 2B4.11 cells.

b - Pretreatment by four weekly i.p. injections of 5×10^6 inactivated 2B4.11 cells.

c - Mean of tumor areas on tumor-bearing mice only.

d - Significant suppression of tumor growth versus control ($p \leq 0.01$).

e - Significant suppression of tumor incidence versus control ($p \leq 0.04$).

f - Significant increase in survival versus control ($p \leq 0.05$).

in this experiment. Deaths both in the experimental groups and in the control group occurred predominantly within forty days of challenge. The data suggest that 8-MOP/UVA is the most effective form of cellular inactivation for inducing this immunity.

In order to determine the longevity of the observed immunity against tumor, mice were treated with 8-MOP/UVA-damaged tumor cells as above, but were not challenged until thirty days after the last treatment. As detailed in Table 4, these mice demonstrated both a significant decrease in tumor incidence and a significant inhibition of tumor growth. The 80-day survival of treated mice (7/8 survivors) was significantly higher than that of untreated controls (6/6 dead). Indeed, the enhancement of survival was significantly greater than that observed in the recipients of 8-MOP/UVA damaged cells with challenge at day six after the last treatment. Once again, the majority of deaths in the control group occurred within forty days of challenge, while no such rapid death was observed in the experimental group. These data indicate that the immunity against tumor induced by treatments with 8-MOP/UVA-damaged cells is more potent

Table 4. Long term immunity[a] against tumor by pretreatment[b] with 2B4.11 cells inactivated by 8-MOP/UVA.

Method of inactivation	Tumor Area[c], Days After Challenge (mm² ± SEM) (Number with tumors/Number challenged)			Dead at 40 days	Dead at 80 days
	Day 4	Day 7	Day 10		
None (control, not pretreated) n=6	46 ± 9 (5/6)	164 ± 72 (5/6)	175 ± 10	4/6	6/6
8-MOP/UVA n=8	25 ± 5 (5/8)	63 ± 16 (3/8)	118 ± 8[d] (2/8)	0/8[e]	1/8[f]

a - Challenged one month after last treatment by s.c. injection of 5 X 10⁶ viable 2B4.11 cells.

b - Pretreatment by four weekly i.p. injections of 5 X 10⁶ inactivated 2B4.11 cells.

c - Mean of tumor areas on tumor-bearing mice only.

d - Significant suppression of tumor growth versus control ($p \leq 0.02$).

e - Significant increase in survival versus control ($p \leq 0.01$).

f - Very significant increase in survival versus control ($p \leq 0.005$).

at thirty days following the treatment protocol than at six days, suggesting an internal evolution of the mechanism of the observed immunity against tumor.

To determine whether the immune system is involved in the protection against tumor development, BALB/c nude mice had received treatments similar to those previously described and had been tested for tumor development and survival after s.c. challenge with tumor cells of the same specificity (Table 5). Nude BALB/c mice, in general, demonstrated significantly increased tumor growth, earlier death, and decreased survival as compared to immune-competent mice (Table 3), as well as no demonstrable protection against tumor formation by any form of pretreatment. These data demonstrate that this protection against tumor development is immune-mediated.

To determine the specificity of the protection against tumor development, C10.9, a T-cell hybridoma whose TCR is specific for hen-egg lysozyme (HEL) presented on a Class I I-A^k molecule (Ashwell et al., 1987a) and the parental thymoma BW5147 were used. Our preliminary studies have shown that 10 X 10⁶ is the minimal number of C10.9 hybridoma cells capable of killing 100% of the animals. Furthermore, extended preliminary studies suggest that there is cross-protection against a hybridoma of a different TCR specificity than the one used for immunizations as well as for the parental thymoma (Table 6). Mice pretreated with 8-MOP/UVA-damaged 2B4 cells were challenged either with viable 2B4 or with C10.9 hybridoma

Table 5. Immunity[a] against tumor by pretreatment[b] of nude BALB/c mice with variously inactivated 2B4.11 cells.

Method of inactivation	Tumor Area[c], Days After Challenge (mm² ± SEM) (Number with tumors/Number challenged)			Dead at 40 days	Dead at 80 days
	Day 4	Day 7	Day 10		
None (control) n=11	45 ± 6 (10/11)	109 ± 14 (11/11)	238 ±18 (11/11)	11/11	11/11
8-MOP/UVA n=11	32 ± 9 (5/11)	82 ± 14 (9/11)	200 ± 23 (10/11)	10/11	10/11
Mitomycin C n=11	29 ± 7 (6/11)	115 ± 11 (9/11)	253 ± 20 (11/11)	6/11	11/11
Glutaraldehyde n=11	28 ± 8 (4/11)	137 ± 18 (8/11)	208 ± 38 (11/11)	10/11	11/11
X-irradiation n=7	33 ± 4 (6/7)	105 ± 9 (6/7)	ND (7/7)	6/7	7/7

a - Challenged six days after last treatment by s.c. injection of 5 X 10^6 viable 2B4.11 cells.

b - Pretreatment by four weekly i.p. injections of 5 X 10^6 inactivated 2B4.11 cells.

c - Mean of tumor areas on tumor-bearing mice only.

cells and followed for tumor development and survival. In the group of mice pretreated with 8-MOP/UVA-damaged 2B4 cells and challenged with viable cells of the same specificity, 8/12 developed tumors compared with 10/10 of the control mice during the first seven days of tumor growth. These tumors were significantly smaller than those which developed in control mice. However, by the tenth day, significant regression of tumors was noted in this experimental group of mice, leaving statistically smaller tumors in 6/12 mice as compared with tumors in 10/10 control mice. Among those mice that were pretreated with damaged 2B4 tumor cells and challenged with viable C10.9 tumor cells, 9/11 mice developed tumors of sizes similar to those of control mice during the first ten days of evaluation. However, by the tenth day, significant regression of tumors was noticed in this group of experimental mice, leaving growing tumors in 6/11 mice as compared to 10/10 control mice. Among those mice immunized with the parental thymoma BW5147 and challenged with viable 2B4 tumor cells, only 2/12 developed very small tumors that ultimately totally regressed.

Pretreatment of mice with 8-MOP/UVA-damaged tumor cells led to a significant improvement in 40-day and 80-day survival as compared to untreated control mice. However, C10.9 hybridoma cells induce smaller tumors that metastasize slower than 2B4 hybridoma cells,

Table 6. Specificity of tumor immunity in mice pretreated with tumor cells inactivated by 8-MOP/UVA and challenged with viable 2B4.11 or C10.9 or BW5147 cells.

Pretreatment[a]	Challenge[b]	Tumor Area[c], Days After Challenge (mm² ± SEM) (Number with tumors/Number challenged)			Dead at 40 days	Dead at 80 days
		Day 4	Day 7	Day 10		
None (control) n=10	2B4.11	38 ± 3	86 ± 5 (10/10)	143 ± 9 (10/10)	9/10 (10/10)	10/10
None (control) n=15	C10.9	57 ± 10	109 ± 9 (8/10)	120 ± 10 (10/10)	10/15 (10/10)	15/15
None (control) n=11	BW5147	37 ± 6	69 ± 5 (5/11)	85 ± 10 (10/11)	6/11 (10/110	11/11
2B4.11 n=12	2B4.11	27 ± 5	54 ± 6[d] (8/12)	75 ± 17[d] (8/12)	3/12 (6/12)	3/1
2B4.11 n=11	C10.9	20 ± 2	58 ± 8 (9/11)	59 ± 8[e] (8/11)	3/11 (6/11)	4/11
C10.9 n=5	C10.9	21 ± 8[f]	38 ± 8[f] (5/5)	31 ± 0[f] (3/5)	0/5 (1/5)	0/5
C10.9 n=6	2B4.11	33 ± 3	55 ± 8[g] (6/6)	27 ± 8[g] (4/6)	0/6 (3/6)	0/6
BW5147 n=12	2B4.11	36 ± 3	16[h] (2/12)	0 ± 0[h] (1/12)	0/12 (0/12)	1/12
BW5147 n=5	C10.9	35 ± 13[i]	80 ± 29[i] (2/5)	67 ± 16[i] (2/5)	4/5 (3/5)	4/5
BW5147 n=5	BW5147	37 ± 1	63 ± 4 (3/5)	89 ± 15 (5/5)	4/5 (5/5)	4/5

a - Pretreatment by four weekly i.p. injections of 5 X 10⁶ damaged 2B4 or 10 X 10⁶ C10.9 or 15 X 10⁶ BW5147 cells as indicated.

b - Challenged six days after the last treatment by s.c. injection of 5 X 10⁶ viable 2B4 cells or 10 X 10⁶ viable C10.9 cells or 15 X 10⁶ viable BW5147 cells.

c - Mean tumor area on tumor bearing mice only.

d - Significant supression of tumor incidence ($p \leq 0.02$ and growth versus control ($p \leq 0.001$).

e - Significant suppression of tumor incidence and growth versus control ($p \leq 0.04$).

f - Significant suppression of tumor incidence ($p \leq 0.01$) and growth ($p \leq 0.05$) versus control.

g - Significant suppression of tumor growth ($p \leq 0.03$) and ($p \leq 0.002$).

h - Very significant suppression of tumor incidence and growth ($p \leq 0.0001$).

i - Significant suppression of tumor growth ($p \leq 0.01$) versus control.

killing the animals in approximately seventy days. All animals pretreated with either C10.9 or BW5147 damaged tumor cells demonstrated close to 100% survival after challenge with either viable 2B4 or C10.9 tumor cells (Table 6). These results demonstrate cross-protection against the development of tumor induced by pretreatment with a T-cell hybridoma of different TCR specificity as well as the parental thymoma. These data indicate that the tumor associated antigen capable of inducing the protection against tumor development is predominantly presented by a Class I^k MHC molecule.

Table 7. Induction of tumor regression by pretreatment[b] with 2B4.11 cells inactivated by 8-MOP/UVA.

Method of inactivation day of tx[a]	Tumor Area[c], Days After Challenge (mm² ± SEM) (Number with tumors/Number challenged)			Dead at 40 days	Dead at 80 days
	Day 7	Day 11	Day 26		
None (control, not pretreated) n=5	99 ± 21 (5/5)	146 ± 37 (5/5)	508 ± 91 (5/5)	5/5	5/5
8 MOP/UVA Day 1, n=10	54 ± 0 (1/10)	170 ± 48 (6/10)	433 ± 94 (6/10)	3/10[d]	6/10[e]
8 MOP/UVA Day 7, n=8	60 ± 15 (4/8)	149 ± 43 (3/8)	588 ± 90 (3/8)	1/8[d]	3/8[e]

a - Treatment was started either one day or seven days after s.c. injection of 5 X 10⁶ viable 2B4.11 cells. All animals in the group treated seven days after tumor inoculation had palpable tumors. However, the tumors in four mice were diffuse and difficult to measure.

b - Treatment by six weekly i.p. injections of 5 X 10⁶ inactivated 2B4.11 cells.

c - Mean of tumor areas on tumor-bearing mice only.

d - Very significant increase in survival versus control ($p \leq 0.005$).

e - Significant increase in survival versus control ($p \leq 0.02.$).

To determine whether regression of established tumors can be induced, mice that had received viable tumor cells and have established lymphomas received i.p. injections of tumor cells of the same specificity after the cells were damaged with 8-MOP and UVA. These animals have been followed for tumor regression and survival. Although it is difficult to demonstrate tumor regression in the mice which were treated one day after tumor inoculation, the data shown on the mice treated seven days after tumor inoculation demonstrate tumor regression in 5/8 mice. Also, these data demonstrate increases in survival in a significant percentage (40% for day-one-treated mice and 63% for day-seven-treated mice) of all mice with established disease that were treated with 8-MOP/UVA inactivated tumor cells (Table 7).

Adoptive transfer experiments show adoptively transferable protection by spleen cells from immune-protected donors into syngeneic recipients (Table 8). Identification of the phenotype of the cells mediating this adoptively transferable immunity against tumor will be obtained by weekly pretreating the immunized mice with anti-CD-8 mAbs before each immuni-

Table 8. Tumor growth and survival in naive syngeneic recipients of adoptive transfer spleen cells[a] from tumor-immunized mice.

Donor Spleen[b]	Tumor Area[c], Days After Challenge (mm² ± SEM) (Number with tumors/Number challenged)			Dead at 40 days	Dead at 80 days
	Day 4	Day 7	Day 10		
Naïve control n=4	85 ± 30 (2/4)	134 ± 8 (4/4)	168 ± 15 (4/4)	2/4[d]	4/4[d]
Immune-protected n=5	84 ± 10[e] (2/5)	154 ± 0[e] (1/5)	254 ± 0[e] (1/5)	2/5[f]	5/5[f]

a - Adoptive transfer of 2 X 10⁸ spleen cells was performed six days after the last immunization of C10.9-immune-protected donor mice. Immune-recipients were tumor inoculated with 10 X 10⁶ viable C10.9 tumor cells immediately after cell transfer and followed for tumor growth and survival.

b - C10.9-immune-protected donor mice were immunized by four weekly i.p. injections of 5 X 10⁶ 8-MOP/UVA-inactivated C10.9 cells before adoptive transfer. Naïve control mice are donors of 2 X 10⁸ syngeneic naïve spleen cells.

c - Mean of tumor areas on tumor-bearing mice only.

d - All mice dead of tumor metastasis.

e - Significant suppression of tumor incidence versus control ($p \leq 0.02$).

f - Mice dead within three days of each other of dehydration; suspicious of viral infection.

---

zation with 8-MOP/UVA damaged tumor cells followed by tumor inoculation and, in other experiments, by depleting the CD8⁺ T cells from the adoptive transfer inoculum obtained from immune-protected mice.

These cumulative studies have helped to clarify the conditions most conducive to an anti-T-cell subset depletion. Isolation of immunogenic peptides will help to identify the cells involved in the anti-T-cell tumor response and its target molecules.

REFERENCES

Ashwell JD, DL Longo and SH Bridges, 1987a. T-cell tumor elimination as a result of T-cell receptor-mediated activation. **Science**, 237:61.

Ashwell JD, RE Cunningham, PD Noguchi, D Hernandez, 1987b. Cell growth cycle block of T cell hybridomas upon activation with antigen. **J. Exp. Med.**, 165:173.

Beryer CL, D Warburton, J Raafat, P Logerfo and RL Edelson, 1979. Cutaneous T cell lymphoma, neoplasm of T cell with helper activity. **Blood**, 53: 642.

Cohen IR, 1984. Autoimmunity: Physiologic and pernicious. **Adv. Intern. Med.**, 29:147.

Edelson RL, 1980a. Cutaneous T cell lymphoma. **J. Dermatol. Surg. Oncol.**, 6:358.

Edelson RL, 1980b. Cutaneous T cell lymphoma (mycosis fungoides, Sézary syndrome and other variants). **J. Amer. Acad. Dermatol.**, 2:89.

Edelson RL, CL Berger, F Gasparro, B Jegasothy et al., 1987. Treatment of cutaneous T cell lymphoma by extracorporeal photochemotherapy. Preliminary results. **N. Engl. J. Med.**, 316:297.

Heald P, 1991. Photopheresis for cutaneous T-cell lymphoma In: J. Ashwell, R. Edelson, Eds. **"Antigen- and Clone-specific Immunoregulation"**. **Ann. NY Acad. Sci.**

Heald P, A Rook, MI Perez, B Wintroub, R Knobler, R Mescheg, B Jegasothy, F Gasparro, C Berger and RE Edelson, 1992. Treatment of erythrodermic cutaneous T cell lymphoma with extracorporeal photochemotherapy. **J. Am. Acad. Dermatol.**, 27:427.

Holoshitz J, A Frenkel, A Ben-Nun and IR Cohen, 1983a. Autoimmune encephalomyelitis (EAE) mediated or prevented by T lymphocyte lines directed against diverse antigenic determinants of myelin basic protein. Vaccination is determinant-specific. **J. Immunol.**, 131:2810.

Holoshitz J, Y Naparstek, A Ben-Nun and IR Cohen, 1983b. Lines of T lymphocytes induce or vaccinate against autoimmune arthritis. **Science**, 219:56.

Kappler JW, JW Skidmore and P Marrack, 1981. The development of T cell hybridomas. **J. Exp. Med.**, 153:1198.

Mercep M, PD Noguchi and JD Ashwell, 1989. The cell cycle block and lysis of an activated T cell hybridoma are distinct processes with different Ca^{2+} requirements and sensitivity to cyclosporine A. **J. Immunol.**, 142:4085.

Mercep M, JA Bluestone, PD Noguchi and JD Ashwell, 1988. Inhibition of transformed cell growth in vitro by monoclonal antibodies directed against distinct activating molecules. **J. Immunol.**, 140 (1):324.

Perez MI, RL Edelson, LL Lanoche and CL Berger, 1989. Inhibition of anti-skin allograft immunity by infusions with syngeneic photoinactivated effector lymphocytes. **J. Invest. Derm.**, 92:669.

Perez MI, CL Berger, Y Yamane, L John, L LaRoche and RL Edelson, 1991a. Inhibition of anti-skin allograft immunity induced by infusions with photoactivated effector T lymphocytes (PET cells). The Congenic Model. **Transplantation**, 51:1283.

Perez MI, F Lobo, Y Yamane, L John, CL Berger and RL Edelson, 1991b. Inhibition of anti-skin allograft immunity induced by infusions with photoactivated effector T cells (PET cells) is in vivo cell transferable. In: J. Ashwell and R. Edelson, Eds. **"Antigen- and Clone-specific Immunoregulation"**. **Ann. NY Acad. Sci.**, 112.

Perez MI, M Lobo, L John, Y Yamane and RL Edelson, 1992. Induction of a cell-transferable suppression of alloreactivity by photodamaged lymphocytes. **Transplantation**, 54:896.

Samelson LE, RN Germain and RH Schwartz, 1983. Monoclonal antibodies against antigen receptor on a cloned T cell hybrid. **Proc. Natl. Acad. Sci. USA**, 80, 66972.

Scott ER, MA Patak and GR Mohn, 1976. Molecular and genetic basis of furocoumarin reactions. **Mutat. Res.**, 39:29.

Sussman JJ, T Saito, EM Shevach, RN Germain and JD Ashwell, 1988. Thy-1 and Ly-6-mediated lymphokine production and growth inhibition of a T cell hybridoma require co-expression of the T cell antigen receptor complex. **J. Immunol.**, 104:2520.

MOLECULAR MECHANISMS RESPONSIBLE FOR REPAIR OF ADDUCTS INDUCED IN HUMAN CELLULAR DNA BY PUVA

Muriel W. Lambert
David D. Parrish
W. Clark Lambert

Department of Laboratory Medicine and Pathology
UMDNJ-New Jersey Medical School
Newark, NJ U.S.A.

Correspondence to: Dr. M. W. Lambert, Department of Laboratory Medicine
and Pathology, Room C572, Medical Science Bldg.,
UMDNJ-New Jersey Medical School, 185 South Orange Avenue,
Newark, NJ 07103-2714, U.S.A.

ABSTRACT

Psoralen plus UVA (long wavelength ultraviolet radiation) (PUVA) produces three types of adducts in DNA: (i) intercalation of the psoralen molecule between flat, stacked base-pairs, (ii) formation of a monoadduct by UVA radiation-dependent covalent bonding of the psoralen molecule to a base, primarily via a cyclobutane ring to a thymine, on one strand of the DNA, and (iii) formation of a DNA interstrand cross-link by a second UVA radiation-dependent covalent bonding of the psoralen molecule to a base on the opposite strand of the DNA molecule. The latter adduct (iii) is thought to be the most important biologically.

We have isolated two DNA endonuclease complexes from the chromatin of normal human lymphoblastoid cells. One complex, pI 4.6, recognizes and selectively cleaves DNA containing the psoralen intercalation adduct and also the psoralen interstrand DNA cross-link, against which it has the greater activity. The other complex, pI 7.6, recognizes and cleaves the cyclobutane ring psoralen-DNA monoadduct. It also recognizes and cleaves the ultraviolet radiation (254nm;

Basic Mechanisms of Physiologic and Aberrant Lymphoproliferation in the Skin
Edited by W.C. Lambert *et al.*, Plenum Press, New York, 1994

497

UVC) induced pyrimidine dimer, which has a similar cyclobutane ring structure. Kinetic analysis of activities of the endonuclease complexes on DNA treated with PUVA so as to favor cross-link production reveals a reduced K_m, with little or no change in K_{cat} or V_{max}, indicating an increased affinity, or rate of association, of these enzyme complexes for the damaged DNA.

Both complexes contain at least two proteins, one of which is necessary for interaction of the complex with DNA in the form of chromatin, the other(s) of which recognizes the adduct and also cleaves the phosphodiester bond of the DNA molecule. The former protein is defective in cells derived from patients with xeroderma pigmentosum, complementation group A, whereas the latter is defective in the complex, pI 4.6, in cells derived from patients with Fanconi anemia (FA), complementation group A, and in the complex, pI 7.6, in cells derived from patients with FA, complementation group B. Kinetic analysis reveals that all of these deficiencies are due to reduced selective affinity, or rate of association, of the enzyme complexes for their respective damaged nucleosomal or non-nucleosomal DNA substrates. The deficiencies in the mutant cell repair systems correlate with increased sensitivities of these cells to DNA damaging agents in culture, and these hypersensitivities can be corrected by introduction, via electroporation, of the corresponding normal DNA endonuclease complexes into these cultured cells.

INTRODUCTION

Psoralen plus long-wavelength light (UVA) produces clearly beneficial clinical and histologic changes in lesions of CTCL and is now in wide use, but the molecular mechanisms by which cells respond to psoralen plus UVA damage in cellular DNA are poorly understood. We have isolated two DNA endonuclease complexes from the chromatin of normal human lymphoblastoid cells, with pI 4.6 and pI 7.6, which are selectively active on DNA treated with psoralen plus long wavelength (365 nm) ultraviolet radiation (UVA) (Lambert et al., 1988). Our isolation system utilizes a number of special techniques, such as carrying out some procedures at -20°C in liquid phase in ethylene glycol, which maintain these complexes in active form. Our results indicate that the endonuclease complex, pI 4.6, recognizes the psoralen intercalation and, in addition, the psoralen interstrand cross-link, whereas the endonuclease complex, pI 7.6, recognizes the psoralen monoadduct (Lambert et al., 1988; Parrish and Lambert, 1990). We have also shown that the activity of these normal chromatin-associated endonuclease complexes on psoralen-damaged DNA increases approximately two to three fold when the damaged DNA is reconstituted into nucleosomes containing core histones (i.e., histones H2A, H2B, H3 and H4) (Parrish and Lambert, 1990). Addition of histone H1 to the nucleosomes reduces, but does not eliminate, this increase in activity on damaged nucleosomal DNA compared to activity on damaged naked DNA (Parrish and Lambert, 1990). This is consistent with the proposed role of histone H1 in DNA and chromatin packaging (see below).

We now summarize our further characterization of these chromatin-associated DNA repair endonuclease complexes, as well as our analysis of several mutant forms of these complexes obtained from lymphoblastoid cells derived from patients with the DNA repair-deficient genodermatoses, Fanconi anemia and xeroderma pigmentosum. These results serve to further characterize what appears to represent the principal molecular mechanisms by which both normal and neoplastic human cells respond to DNA damage induced by psoralen plus UVA.

Fanconi Anemia Mutant Cell Lines

Fanconi anemia (FA) is a rare, recessively transmitted genetic disorder characterized by specific congenital abnormalities, progressive hypoplastic anemia, an increased frequency of chromosomal aberrations and a predisposition to develop cancer (Fanconi, 1967; German, 1982; Schroeder, 1982; Glanz and Fraser, 1982). Studies have shown that cells derived from patients with FA have a hypersensitivity to DNA interstrand cross-linking agents (Sasaki and Tonomura, 1973; Auerbach and Wolman, 1976; Fujiwara et al., 1977; Weksberg et al., 1979; Ishida and Buchwald, 1982; Papadopoulo et al., 1987; Digweed et al., 1988; Auerbach et al., 1989). They display reduced cell survival and increased chromosome damage when treated with such agents as mitomycin C and nitrogen mustard, as well as psoralen plus UVA (Sasaki and Tonomura, 1973; Lalt et al., 1975; Auerbach and Wolman, 1976; Fujiwara et al., 1977; Weksberg et al., 1979; Kano and Fujiwara, 1982; Wunder and Fleischer-Reischman, 1983; Papadopoulo et al., 1987; Digweed et al., 1988). They are thought to have a defect in repair of lesions in their DNA produced by these cross-linking agents (Fujiwara, 1982; Gruenert and Cleaver, 1985; Plooy et al., 1985; Papadopoulo et al., 1987; Averbeck, et al., 1988; Moustacchi et al., 1989). Patients with FA have been grouped into at least four complementation groups, labeled A, B (i.e., FA-A and FA-B) etc., based on their cellular responses to DNA interstrand cross-linking agents (Duckworth-Rysiecki et al., 1985; Moustacchi et al., 1987; Strathdee et al., 1992). FA-A cells show greater growth inhibition by mitomycin C (Duckworth-Rysiecki et al., 1985), and much greater reduction in rate of semi-conservative DNA synthesis after 8-methoxypsoralen (8-MOP) plus UVA treatment than do FA-B cells (Moustacchi et al., 1987). Although both FA-A and FA-B cells display reduced capacity to incise DNA interstrand cross-links and monoadducts produced by selected cross-linking agents (Papadopoulo et al., 1987; Averbeck et al., 1988; Moustacchi et al., 1989), FA-A cells show a greater reduction in ability to incise DNA containing interstrand cross-links (Papadopoulo et al., 1987; Moustacchi et al., 1989), whereas FA-B cells are more sensitive to psoralen monoadducts (Averbeck et al., 1988; Moustacchi et al., 1989).

Xeroderma Pigmentosum Mutant Cell Lines

Xeroderma pigmentosum (XP) is a rare, recessively transmitted genetic disease characterized by more or less extreme sun sensitivity and development of advanced epidermal changes associated with photoaging, including development of melanomas and non-melanoma skin cancers, at a very early age (Kraemer et al., 1987; Lambert and Lambert, 1987). A subset of patients also have a progressive neurological deficiency which is unrelated to sun exposure

(Kraemer et al., 1987; Lambert and Lambert, 1987). The disease is genetically heterogeneous, with seven complementation groups (formerly nine, with two now withdrawn), labeled A, B (i.e., XPA, XPB), etc., in which there is a well documented deficiency in an endonuclease-mediated step in repair of ultraviolet-light-induced adducts in cellular DNA, as well as at least one additional complementation group, known as the variant group (i.e., XPV), in which a defect in an endonuclease-mediated step has not been documented. There are numerous unanswered questions, as well as considerable controversy, regarding the biochemical genetics of XP: although one DNA repair gene defective in cells from patients with XPA has been cloned (Satokata et al., 1990; Tanaka et al., 1990), it now appears that there may also be a second DNA repair gene defective in XPA cells (Rinaldy et al., 1990) as well as a gene controlling a catalase activity (Vuillaume et al., 1992). We, and subsequently others, have proposed that some or all complementation groups of XP are associated with homozygosity or hemizygosity for defective alleles at more than one locus, a hypothesis known as "Co-Recessive Inheritance," which provides an explanation for these and other findings, as well as a number of epidemiologic data, that are incompatible with a mendelian inheritance mechanism for XP as well as for several other rare genetic disorders, such as ataxia-telangiectasia (Lambert and Lambert, 1985; 1989; 1992).

Modulation of DNA Repair Mechanisms by Nucleosome Structure

Chromatin structure has been shown to play an important role in determining the distribution of repair sites on DNA as well as the accessibility of damaged DNA to enzymatic attack (Lan and Smerdon, 1985; Bohr et al., 1987, Smerdon, 1989). Depending upon the type of damage, a particular lesion may be nonrandomly located and repaired in the core or linker regions of the nucleosome (Cerutti et al., 1980; Smerdon, 1989). Preferential repair of DNA has been demonstrated to occur in transcriptionally active DNA sequences, in which chromatin is in a more open configuration, compared with transcriptionally inactive DNA sequences (Mellon et al., 1986; Bohr et al., 1987; Leadon and Snowden, 1988; Hanawalt et al., 1989). Chromatin configuration has also been shown to play a role in repair processes occurring in higher order chromatin loops in the nuclear matrix (Mullenders et al., 1986, 1989).

Our laboratory has focused on the influence of nucleosome structure on the activity and binding affinity of isolated specific DNA repair enzymes and enzyme complexes on damaged DNA. The results obtained have shown that, whereas the major deficiencies in the FA-A and FA-B DNA endonuclease complexes, pI 4.6 and pI 7.6, lie in a defect in their ability to recognize and incise damaged naked DNA, the XPA complexes show a major defect in ability to interact with damaged DNA when present in the form of nucleosomes.

MATERIALS AND METHODS

Cell Lines and Culture Conditions

Normal human (GM 1989 and GM 3299) and xeroderma pigmentosum, complementation group A (XPA), (GM 2345 and GM 2250A) lymphoblastoid cell lines (all transformed with Epstein-Barr Virus) were obtained from the Coriell Institute for Medical Research, Camden, NJ. Lymphoblastoid cell lines (transformed with Epstein-Barr Virus), obtained from FA patients, complementation group A (HSC 72) and complementation group B (HSC 62), were a gift from Dr. Manuel Buchwald (Hospital for Sick Children, Toronto). The cells were grown in suspension culture in RPMI 1640 medium, supplemented with 12.5% fetal calf serum (Grand Island Biological Co.) and harvested under conditions of maximal proliferation, as previously described (Okorodudu et al., 1982). Cell cultures were routinely tested for mycoplasma (Okorodudu et al., 1982).

Measurement of Unscheduled DNA Synthesis

Cells in culture were treated with 1 μg/ml 8-methoxypsoralen (8-MOP) (Sigma Chemical Company) in phosphate-buffered saline (PBS) (0.15 M) for 20 minutes at room temperature in the dark. They were then irradiated with UVA (principally 366 nm) (10 W/m^2 for 10 minutes). The cells were washed with PBS and exposed to a second dose of UVA (10 W/m^2 for 10 minutes). Alternatively, the cells exposed to angelicin (Elder Company) in PBS for 20 minutes followed by irradiation with UVA light (10 W/m^2 for 5 minutes). The cells were then resuspended in media containing 10 μCi/ml [^{3}H] methylthymidine (specific activity 61 Ci/mmole) (ICN Radiochemicals) and incubated for 2 hours at 37°C (Tsongalis et al., 1990). Unincorporated thymidine was removed by several washes with cold PBS. Cells were smeared onto glass slides and the slides were dipped in Kodak NTB3 nuclear emulsion and exposed for 7 days at 4°C (Tsongalis et al., 1990). The slides were then treated with Kodak Dl9 developer and stained with Giemsa. Grains per nucleus were counted in random fields. Cells with 40-100 grains per nucleus were classified as undergoing UDS. For each individual experiment 300-500 cells were counted.

Electroporation

The normal, FA or XPA endonuclease complexes, pI 4.6 or pI 7.6, or albumin (control), (0.4-1.8 μg in 0.1 ml) were added to a suspension of 0.9 ml cells containing 3 x 10^6 cells and a high voltage electric pulse was applied using a BTX Transfector 300 System (Biotechnologies, Inc.). The cells were exposed to a field strength of 1.7 kV/cm over a distance of 3.5 mm for 4.0 milliseconds. The cells were then kept on ice for 1 minute and resuspended into 2 ml RPMI 1640 medium buffered with HEPES buffer, supplemented with 7.5% fetal calf serum and 7.5% horse serum, prewarmed to 37°C (Tsongalis et al., 1990a; 1990b).

Extraction and Isolation of DNA Endonuclease Complexes

Cell nuclei were isolated and the chromatin-associated proteins separated from the nucleoplasmic proteins in a series of steps, some carried out at -20°C in purified ethylene glycol, passed through a CM sephadex column and electrophoresed on an isoelectric focusing column as previously described (Lambert et al., 1982, 1988). Fractions collected from the column were assayed for DNA endonuclease and exonuclease activity (Lambert et al., 1982). Peaks of endonuclease activity were pooled, dialyzed against 50 mM potassium phosphate (pH 7.1), 1 mM ß-mercaptoethanol, 1 mM EDTA, 0.25 mM phenylmethylsulfonylfluoride (PMSF), and 40% ethylene glycol and stored unfrozen at -20°C (Lambert et al., 1982, 1988). Protein concentrations were determined by the BioRad protein assay (BioRad Laboratories).

Plasmid Growth and Purification

Escherichia coli strain HB101, containing plasmid pWT830/pBR322 (a clone of the entire SV40 and pBR322 genomes), was grown, harvested and lysed as previously described (Kaysen et al., 1986; Lambert et al., 1988). DNA was extracted with phenol, treated with ribonuclease I and electrophoresed on 0.9% agarose gels. The uncleaved, circular, Form I DNA band was cut from the gel, electroeluted and recovered by ethanol precipitation (Parrish and Lambert, 1990). The DNA was further purified on a NACS 37 (Bethesda Research Laboratory) column (Parrish and Lambert, 1990). DNA eluting from the column, consisting of greater than 95% Form I DNA, was recovered by ethanol precipitation and resuspended in 10 mM Tris-HCl, pH 8.0, 1 mM EDTA.

Histone Isolation

Nuclei were isolated from normal and from XPA lymphoblastoid cell lines and histones were extracted and separated as previously described (Kaysen et al., 1986). Histone H1 was removed from total histones by precipitation with 5% perchloric acid (Kaysen et al., 1986). The purity of core (H2A, H2B, H3 and H4) and total (core plus H1) histones was monitored by gel electrophoresis (Kaysen et al., 1986). Protein concentrations were determined by the BioRad protein assay (BioRad Laboratories) using total calf-thymus histones as a standard.

Nucleosome Reconstitution

Plasmid DNA was mixed with histones (with or without histone H1) from normal or XPA cells at a histone:DNA weight ratio of 1.0 in a buffer containing 2 M NaCl, 50 mM Tris-HCl pH 8.0), 0.1 M EDTA and 0.24 mM PMSF (Kaysen et al., 1986, 1987). The NaCl concentration was progressively decreased by stepwise dialysis at 4°C over a 28 hour period to 50 mM NaCl (Kaysen et al., 1986; Parrish and Lambert, 1990).

Reaction of Psoralen with DNA

8-Methoxypsoralen (8-MOP) (Sigma Chemical Co.) was recrystallized and purity checked by thin-layer chromatography (Lambert et al., 1988). Photoreaction of 8-MOP with non-nucleosomal and nucleosomal DNA was carried out utilizing a treatment protocol which involved exposing 8-MOP (7-15 μg/ml) treated DNA to two doses of UVA radiation, an initial dose (10 W/m^2 for 10 minutes) after the 8-MOP intercalated into the DNA and a second dose (again 10 W/m^2 for 10 minutes) after the unbound 8-MOP had been removed by dialysis (Lambert et al., 1988). This procedure has been shown to increase the number of DNA interstrand cross-links (Ben-Hur and Elkind, 1973; Bredberg, 1982) and produced cross-links in 99% of the non-nucleosomal DNA molecules (Lambert et al., 1988). Angelicin (Elder Co.) (25 μg/ml) was reacted with non-nucleosomal and nucleosomal DNA for 20 minutes and then exposed to UVA (10 W/m^2) for 5 minutes (Lambert et al., 1988). Control DNA for the psoralen-treated DNAs was exposed to UVA irradiation only. Cross-linking of psoralen to non-nucleosomal and nucleosomal DNA was determined by alkaline gel electrophoresis (Lambert et al., 1988).

DNA Endonuclease Assay

Endonuclease activity on nucleosomal and non-nucleosomal DNA was measured using a gel electrophoretic assay which measures the conversion of circular, supercoiled Form I DNA to nicked, relaxed circular Form II DNA (Lambert et al., 1988; Parrish and Lambert, 1990). Briefly, 0.10 μg of DNA substrate was reacted with each DNA endonuclease complex from either normal or XPA cells in 10 mM MgCl$_2$, 10 mM Tris-maleate (pH 7.5) at 37°C for 3 hours. The concentration of each DNA endonuclease complex was adjusted, at similar levels of protein, to produce 0.05 $\pm$ 0.01 breaks per DNA molecule on non-damaged non-nucleosomal DNA in these assays. The enzymatic reaction was terminated with 0.1 M EDTA and the DNA samples were treated with 0.4% sarkosyl (Ciba-Geigy) and 50 μg/ml proteinase K (Sigma Chemical Co.) for 1 hour at 37°C (Kaysen et al., 1986; Parrish and Lambert, 1990). Samples were electrophoresed on 1.0% agarose gels which were subsequently stained with 0.5 μg/ml ethidium bromide and photographed. The negatives of the gels were scanned and endonuclease activity, expressed as the number of enzyme induced breaks per DNA molecule, determined as previously described (Lambert and Lambert, 1986; Lambert et al., 1988; Parrish and Lambert, 1990). At the low concentration used here, the binding of ethidium bromide to superhelical versus non-superhelical forms of DNA was completely equivalent and did not influence the calculations of the different forms of DNA. In addition, in the exposure ranges used, the response of the film used in photographing the gels was linear.

Kinetic Analysis

For analysis of the kinetics of these endonuclease-mediated reactions, assays were performed on undamaged and damaged, non-nucleosomal and nucleosomal (with and without histone H1) DNA as described above, but with graduated reductions in substrate concentration (0.1-0.025 μg). Each assay was carried out over a range encompassing at least a four-fold decrease in substrate concentration. Over this range all components of the assay system, described above, remained linear. Results were plotted as $[S]^{-1}$ versus v^{-1} according to Lineweaver and Burke and also as v versus v/[S] according to Eadie and Hofstee, where [S] and v represent initial molar substrate concentration and velocity of the enzymatic reaction, respectively. We have recently reconfirmed the accuracy of these graphic representations within these reagent concentrations using a more accurate system of graphic data representation,

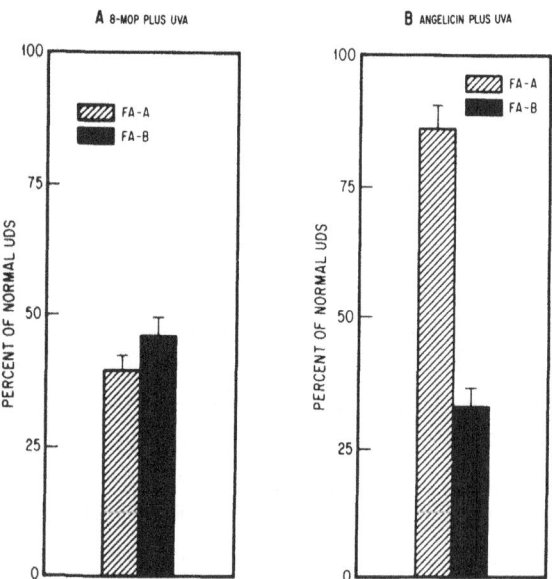

Figure 1. UDS in FA cells, complementation groups A and B, treated with (A) 8-MOP (1 μg/ml) plus two doses of UVA irradiation and (B) angelicin (5 μg/ml) plus UVA irradiation. Results are expressed as percent of normal UDS (100%) ± Standard Error of the Mean (S.E.M.) for 8-10 separate experiments with a total of 2.4×10^3-5.0×10^3 cells counted. (Lambert et al., 1992).

developed by us, based on a more rigorous mathematical formulation where slope = V_{max} and [S] intercept = $-K_m$; (i.e., [S] versus $-t\{\ln(1-[P]/[S])\}^{-1}$, with t = duration of the reaction and [P] = concentration of product produced -- substrate molecules cleaved once or more than once; Lambert et al., 1993). In the classical systems, velocity of the reaction was computed based on cleavages produced per substrate molecule and on the number of substrate molecules present in the assay solution. Values of V_{max} (maximum velocity) and K_m (Michaelis constant) were determined from linear extrapolations on these graphic representations using standard methods based on the Michaelis-Menten equation as well as using the more accurate system we have developed. Values of turnover number, K_{cat}, were computed from these values for V_{max}.

RESULTS

UDS in FA Cells Treated with Psoralen Plus UVA

Non S-phase unscheduled DNA Synthesis (UDS), detected by autoradiography, was observed in both FA-A and FA-B cells in culture exposed to 8-MOP plus two doses of UVA light. The levels were lower, however, than those found in normal cells (Figure 1A). UDS in FA-A cells was approximately 40% of that found in normal cells, whereas in FA-B cells it was approximately 46% of normal levels. UDS was also examined in these cells exposed to angelicin plus UVA. Angelicin plus UVA produces psoralen monoadducts, rather than cross-links, due to the angular structure of angelicin, which prevents cross-link formation. In FA-A and FA-B cells UDS was 87% and 33% of normal levels, respectively (Figure 1B). The effect of these psoralens on UDS was concentration-dependent.

Endonuclease Activity on 8-MOP Plus UVA-Treated Non-Nucleosomal DNA

Nine chromatin-associated DNA endonuclease complexes were isolated from the nuclei of normal human, FA, complementation groups A and B, and XP, complementation group A, cells and examined on DNA treated with 8-MOP plus UVA in separate experiments. As we have previously reported, selective activity against 8-MOP plus UVA-treated DNA was present in two normal endonuclease activities, pIs 4.6 and 7.6, which showed similar levels of activity on this substrate (Figures 2 and 3) (Lambert et al., 1988). Selective activity against 8-MOP plus UVA treated DNA was also found in these same two endonuclease activities from FA-A and FA-B cells (Figure 2, also Figures 5 and 6). However, the levels of activity of both FA-A endonucleases and of the FA-B endonuclease, pI 7.6, were decreased, compared to those of the corresponding normal endonucleases (Figure 2). A relative decrease was observed in activity of the FA-A endonuclease, pI 4.6, compared with activity of the FA-A endonuclease, pI 7.6, as well as in activity of the FA-B endonuclease, pI 7.6, compared with activity of the FA-B endonuclease, pI 4.6 (Figure 2). The FA-A endonuclease, pI 4.6, was approximately 25% and 30% as active on 8-MOP plus UVA-treated DNA as the corresponding normal and FA-B endonucleases, respectively ($p < 0.001$), and 35% as active on this substrate as the FA-A endonuclease, pI 7.6 ($p < 0.001$). The FA-A endonuclease, pI 7.6, was approximately 75% as active as the corresponding normal endonuclease on this substrate ($p < 0.001$). The FA-B endonuclease, pI 7.6, was approximately 50% as active on this substrate as the corresponding normal endonuclease and 55% as active as the FA-B endonuclease, pI 4.6 ($p < 0.001$). The activity of the FA-B endonuclease, pI 4.6, on this substrate was also slightly reduced compared to the activity of the corresponding normal endonuclease, but this reduction was not statistically significant (Figure 2).

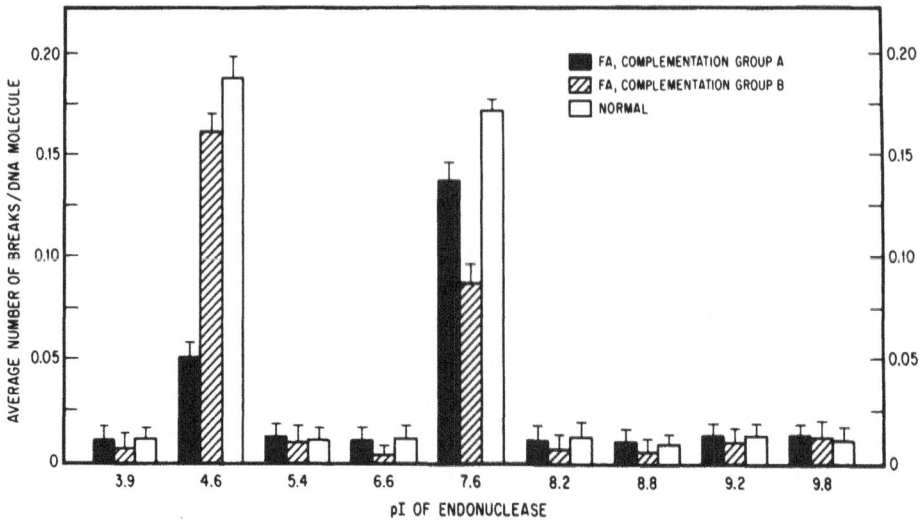

Figure 2. Action of chromatin-associated DNA endonuclease activities from FA cells on DNA treated with 8-MOP plus UVA light. DNA endonuclease activities from normal human cells and FA cells, complementation groups A and B, were examined for activity on plasmid DNA treated with 8-MOP (7 μg/ml) plus two doses of UVA. These values have had subtracted from them the enzyme activity on undamaged DNA (0.05 $\pm$ 0.01 breaks). Vertical lines represent $\pm$ S.E.M. (Lambert et al., 1992).

These same two endonuclease complexes were present in XPA cells and had levels of activity on 8-MOP and angelicin plus UVA treated DNA which were similar to those of the normal complexes (Figure 3A and 3B) (Lambert et al., 1988).

Activity of the Normal and XPA Endonuclease Complexes on Psoralen Plus UVA Irradiated Nucleosomal DNA

The activity of the normal and XPA complexes was examined on damaged nucleosomal DNA. The reconstituted nucleosomal system, which utilizes a plasmid containing the SV40 genome and normal or XPA histones, gave standard patterns of digestion with micrococcal nuclease and DNAase I and showed positioning of nucleosomes in a region near the SV40 origin of replication (Kaysen et al, 1986; Amari et al., 1986; Kaysen et al., 1987). The activity of the two normal endonuclease complexes, pIs 4.6 and 7.6, on core (minus histone H1) nucleosomal DNA treated with 8-MOP plus UVA was increased approximately 2.5-fold compared to their activity on damaged non-nucleosomal DNA (Figure 4) (Parrish and Lambert, 1990). This increase was reduced, but not eliminated, when histone H1 was added to the system, remaining approximately 1.5-fold greater than the activity on damaged naked DNA (Figure 4) (Parrish and Lambert, 1990). These increases in activity, which were not observed on undamaged nucleosomal DNA, were also present on angelicin plus UVA treated DNA (Parrish and Lambert,

1990). In marked contrast, these same two endonuclease complexes from XPA cells did not show any increase in activity on either 8-MOP or angelicin plus UVA treated core nucleosomal DNA and showed a significant decrease in activity when histone H1 was added (Figure 4; Parrish and Lambert, 1990). These difference were not due to the source of the histones, since using either normal or XPA histones in the system made no difference. In addition, we have

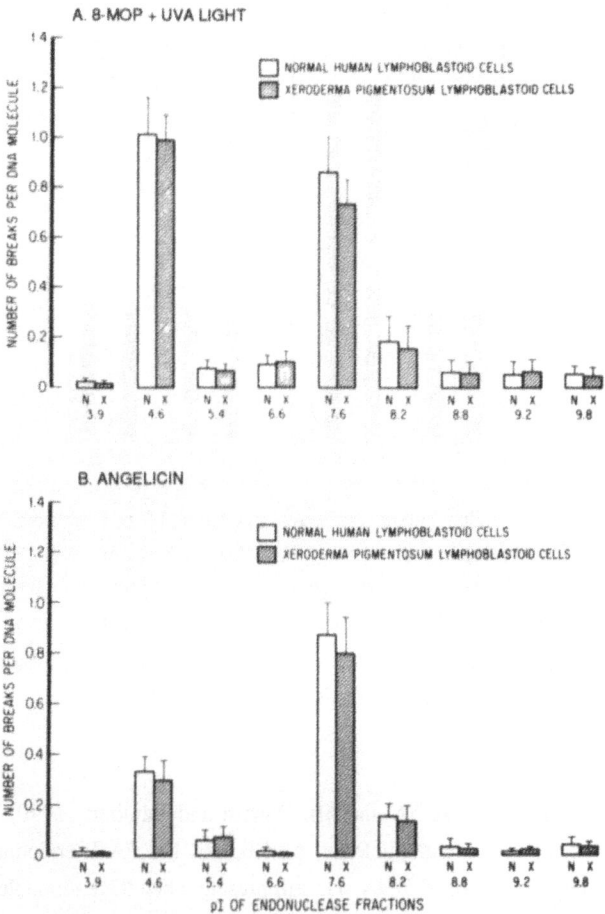

Figure 3. Activity of chromatin-associated DNA endonuclease complexes from normal human and XPA lymphoblastoid cells on non-nucleosomal DNA treated with (A) 15 μg/ml 8-MOP plus two doses of UVA and (B) 25 μg/ml angelicin plus UVA. These values have had subtracted from them the enzyme activity on undamaged DNA. Vertical lines represent ± S.E.M. (Lambert et al., 1988).

previously examined normal and XPA histones and have found no differences quantitatively, qualitatively or in DNA binding affinity (Amari et al., 1986).

The activity of the two endonucleases, pIs 4.6 and 7.6, from both FA-A and FA-B cells on reconstituted core (minus histone H1) nucleosomal DNA treated with 8-MOP plus UVA was increased approximately 2.5-fold compared to their activity on damaged non-nucleosomal DNA. This increase was not observed on undamaged nucleosomal DNA. When histone H1 was added to the reconstituted system, this increase in activity of all of these enzymes was reduced approximately 36% (Figure 5A and 5B). As above, results similar to these were also seen with

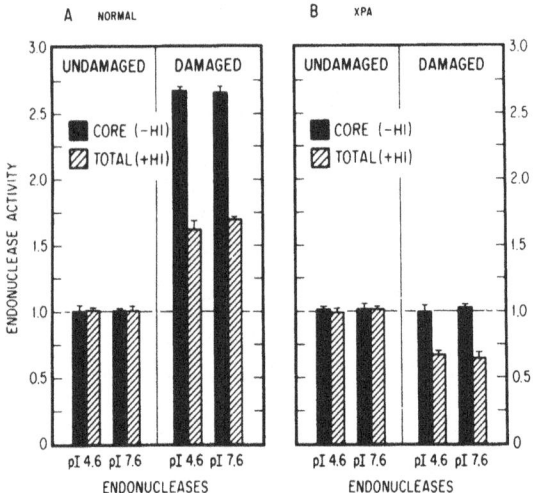

Figure 4. Activity of DNA endonuclease complexes, pIs 4.6 and 7.6, from normal and XPA cells on nucleosomal plasmid DNA treated with 8-MOP plus UVA. (A) Normal and (B) XPA endonuclease complexes (0.41 $\pm$ 0.05 µg) were incubated with undamaged or 8-MOP (15 µg/ml) plus UVA treated DNA reconstituted with total or core histones. Endonuclease activity is expressed as multiples of activity on non-nucleosomal DNA. The solid horizontal line represents enzyme activity on non-nucleosomal DNA. Vertical lines represent $\pm$ S.E.M. (Parrish and Lambert, 1990).

the normal endonucleases (Figure 5A and 5B; Parrish and Lambert, 1990). The decrease in activity observed in the FA-A endonuclease, pI 4.6, and the FA-B endonuclease, pI 7.6, on 8-MOP plus UVA non-nucleosomal DNA was still present when the endonucleases were assayed on nucleosomal DNA (with or without histone H1; Figure 5A and 5B). Thus, the relative activities of both of the normal and of both of the FA endonucleases on nucleosomal DNA remained similar to those on non-nucleosomal DNA.

Endonuclease Activity on Angelicin Plus UVA-Damaged Non-Nucleosomal and Nucleosomal DNA

These two endonuclease activities from normal and FA cells were also examined for ability to incise DNA treated with angelicin plus UVA radiation, which produced monoadducts rather than cross-links in DNA. In both normal and FA cells, the endonuclease activity, pI 7.6, had the greater activity on angelicin-treated DNA (Figure 6). In FA-A and FA-B cells the activity of this endonuclease on damaged non-nucleosomal DNA was 72% and 55%, respectively, of that of the normal endonuclease, pI 7.6. Both in normal and in FA-A and FA-B cells the activity of the endonuclease, pI 4.6, was present but markedly reduced (Figure 6A), compared with its activity on 8-MOP plus UVA-treated DNA (Figure 5A) or with the activity of the endonuclease, pI 7.6, on angelicin plus UVA-treated DNA (Figure 6B). In normal cells the activity of the endonuclease, pI 4.6, was 23% of the activity of the normal endonuclease, pI 7.6, on this substrate (Figures 6A and 6B). The FA-A and FA-B endonucleases, pI 7.6, had 10% and 60%, respectively, of the activity of the corresponding FA-A and FA-B endonucleases, pI 7.6, and 30% and 120%, respectively, of the activity of the normal endonuclease, pI 4.6, on angelicin

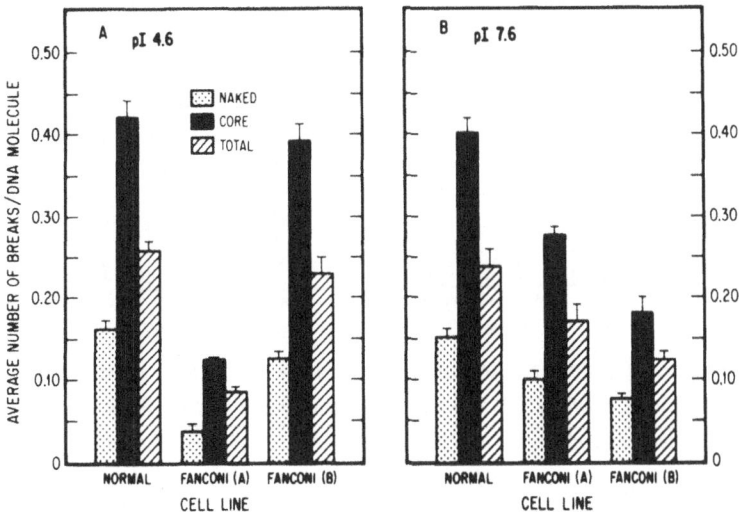

Figure 5. Influence of nucleosome structure on FA endonuclease activity on 8-MOP plus UVA light damaged DNA. The action of the DNA endonuclease activities, pIs 4.6 and 7.6, from normal human, FA-A and FA-B cells was examined on 8-MOP plus UVA treated naked, core (histones H2A, H2B, H3, H4) and total (core + histone H1) nucleosomal DNA. Endonuclease activities (A) pI 4.6 and (B) pI 7.6 (0.34 ± 0.04 μg) were incubated with non-nucleosomal and nucleosomal plasmid DNA (0.1 μg) which had been treated with 8-MOP (7 μg/ml) plus UVA. These values have had subtracted from them the enzyme activity on undamaged DNA. Vertical lines represent ± S.E.M. of 4-6 experiments. (Lambert et al., 1992)

plus UVA-treated DNA. Again, the activity of both of the normal and of both of the FA-A and of the FA-B endonucleases increased approximately 2.5-fold when angelicin plus UVA-treated nucleosomal DNA (minus histone H1) was used as substrate (Figures 6A and 6B), and this increase was reduced, but not eliminated, when histone H1 was added to the system. The same differences in endonuclease activity that were seen on the damaged non-nucleosomal DNA were observed on angelicin plus UVA-damaged nucleosomal DNA (+ histone H1).

Complementation of the XPA Repair Defect by the Normal Human Endonuclease Complexes

We have introduced each of these normal endonuclease complexes, via electroporation, into XPA cells in culture treated with 8-MOP plus UVA and have corrected the XPA repair defect (Tsongalis et al., 1990). Both of the normal, but neither of the XPA complexes restored UDS

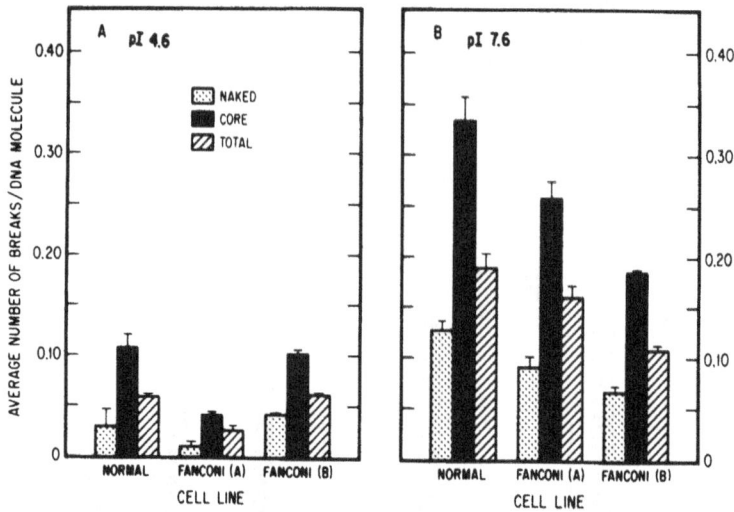

Figure 6. Influence of nucleosome structure on FA endonuclease activity on angelicin-treated DNA. The DNA endonuclease activities, pIs 4.6 and 7.6, from normal human, FA-A and FA-B cells were examined for activity on angelicin plus UVA-treated DNA. Endonuclease activities (A) pI 4.6 and (B) pI 7.6, (0.34 ± 0.04 μg) were incubated with non-nucleosomal and nucleosomal plasmid DNA (0.1 μg) which had been treated with angelicin (25 μg/ml) plus UVA. These values have had subtracted from them the enzyme activity on undamaged DNA. Vertical lines represent ± S.E.M. of 3 or 4 experiments. (Lambert et al., 1992).

in treated XPA cells to higher than normal levels (Figure 7; Tsongalis et al., 1990). In addition, both normal and XPA endonuclease complexes increased UDS in normal cells to higher than normal levels (Tsongalis et al., 1990). Similarly, mixing the normal and XPA endonucleases together and examining their activity on 8-MOP or angelicin plus UVA treated nucleosomal DNA led to complementation of the XPA defect in our cell-free system (Parrish and Lambert, 1990).

These results confirm that the defective protein(s) we have isolated in XPA cell chromatin, which are responsible for normal interaction of the DNA endonucleases with chromatin, are physiologically important in the live cells and are indeed likely to be important in the etiopathogenesis of XP, and, therefore, in the molecular processes by which normal and neoplastic cells cope with psoralen plus UVA damage.

Kinetic Analysis of the Activities of the Normal and FA Endonuclease Complexes

Kinetic analysis of the activities of the endonuclease complexes, pIs 4.6 and 7.6, from normal, FA-A and FA-B cells on DNA treated with 8-MOP plus UVA produced linear, highly reproducible plots using both the Lineweaver and Burke and the Eadie and Hofstee methods, ·

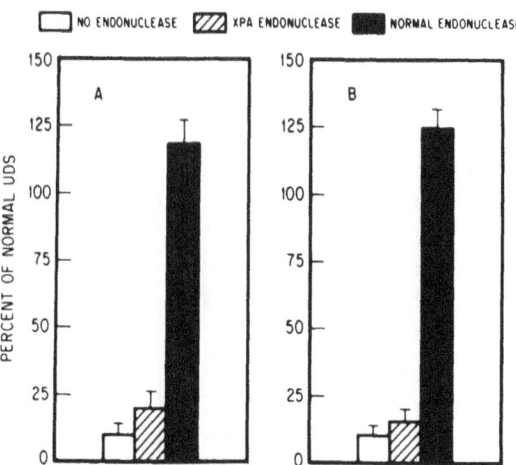

Figure 7. UDS in XPA lymphoblastoid cells in culture treated with 8-MOP plus UVA and electroporated with the normal or XPA DNA endonuclease complexes. Normal or XPA complexes (A) pI 4.6 or (B) pI 7.6 (1.4 µg) were introduced into XPA cells via electroporation. Results are expressed as percent of normal UDS $\pm$ S.E.M. for 4-5 separate experiments with a total of 1.5×10^3 to 2.5×10^3 cells counted. (Tsongalis et al., 1990a)

with coefficients of correlation of at least 0.99 and 0.97, respectively (Figure 8). The turnover number (K_{cat}) of both of the normal, both of the FA-A, and both of the FA-B endonuclease complexes were similar to each other on control DNA (DNA treated with UVA but without 8-MOP) and on DNA treated with 8-MOP plus UVA (Figure 8). All six enzymes showed slightly reduced turnover numbers on the latter substrate, however.

By contrast with these results, reductions were observed in the K_m's of these endonuclease complexes on 8-MOP plus UVA-treated DNA versus control DNA. However, these reductions were not uniform (Figure 9). K_m's of the endonuclease complexes, pI 4.6, from normal, FA-A and FA-B cells on control DNA did not differ significantly (Figure 9). The K_m's of all three endonuclease complexes, pI 4.6, were reduced on 8-MOP plus UVA-treated DNA ($p < 0.001$), but the K_m of the FA-A endonuclease was much higher than that of either the normal endonuclease ($p < 0.001$) or the FA-B endonuclease ($p < 0.001$), which did not differ significantly from each other (Figure 9).

K_m, K_{cat}, and the constants of rate of association, K_1, and of rate of dissociation, K_2, of substrate and enzyme are related in classical enzyme kinetics by the following equation:

$$K_m = \frac{K_2 + K_{cat}}{K_1} \tag{1}$$

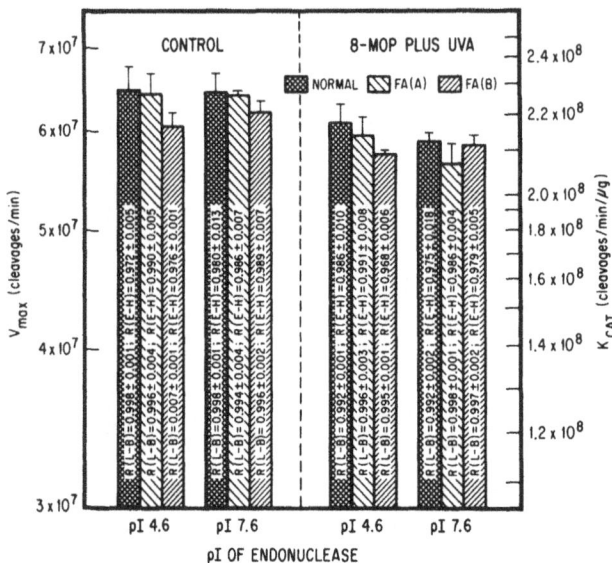

Figure 8. Kinetics (K_{cat}) of the interaction of FA endonuclease activities with 8-MOP plus UVA-treated DNA. Maximum velocities (V_{max}) and turnover numbers (K_{cat}) were determined for the normal human, FA-A and FA-B endonuclease activities, pIs 4.6 and pI 7.6, (0.34 ± 0 04 μg) assayed on non-nucleosomal DNA irradiated with UVA treated either with 8-MOP or without it (control DNA). Graduated reductions in DNA concentration (0.1-0.025 μg) were used. Values shown represent the mean of those obtained from at least 3 experiments. Vertical bars represent ± S.E.M. These values were obtained from linear plots of data producing correlation coefficients, R, as shown (numbers within bars), for Lineweaver and Burke (L-B) and Eadie and Hofstee (E-H) plots. Mean R values of each are shown ± S.E.M. (Lambert et al., 1992).

This follows directly from the definition of K_m. The association constant, K_a, is defined as $K_a = K_1/K_2$ and the dissociation constant, K_d, as $K_d = K_2/K_1$. Under classical kinetic theory, the relative values of K_2 and K_{cat} cannot be determined, and, thus, a value of K_a or K_d separate form K_m cannot be obtained. It is possible, however, using classical kinetic theory, to obtain a meaningful interpretation regarding enzyme-substrate association when K_m changes in significantly greater proportion than does K_{cat}, or changes in the opposite direction. From Equation (1) it is evident that the relatively much larger relative decrease in K_m (Figure 9) with little relative decrease in K_{cat} (Figure 8), for the activities of each of the six endonuclease complexes on 8-MOP plus UVA treated versus undamaged DNA, is necessarily due to an increase in K_1 (rate of association) and/or in K_a (affinity) of the enzyme for this type of damaged DNA.

Thus, since there is little difference in the K_{cat}'s, all three endonuclease complexes, pI 4.6, show greater affinity for, or rate of association with 8-MOP plus UVA-treated DNA than control DNA, but this increase is much less for the FA-A endonuclease than for either the corresponding normal or FA-B endonuclease, as shown by the lesser decrease in K_m for the FA-A endonuclease, pI 4.6.

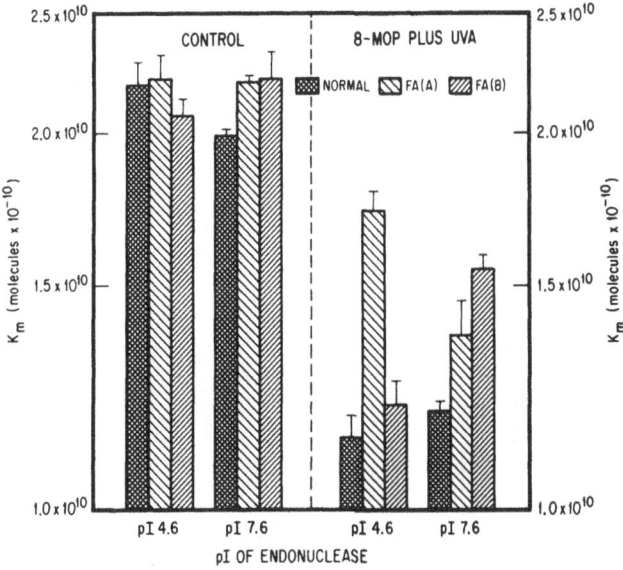

Figure 9. Kinetics (K_m) of the interaction of FA endonuclease activities with 8-MOP plus UVA-treated DNA. Michaelis constants (K_m), expressed as numbers of molecules in the reaction solution (40 μl), were calculated for normal, FA-A and FA-B endonuclease activities, pIs 4.6 and pI 7.6, assayed on non-nucleosomal DNA irradiated with UVA light and treated either with 8-MOP or without it (control DNA). Values shown were obtained from graphic analyses of data based on the Michaelis-Menten equation. Vertical bars represent $\pm$ S.E.M. for at least 3 experiments. (Lambert et al., 1992).

As noted above, the K_m's of the endonuclease complexes 7.6, from normal, FA-A and FA-B cells on control DNA were not significantly different (Figure 9). All three endonuclease complexes, pI 7.6, showed a much lower K_m on 8-MOP plus UVA-damaged DNA than on control DNA. The K_m's of both the FA-A and the FA-B endonucleases, pI 7.6, were less reduced than for the corresponding normal endonuclease, however ($p < 0.01$), with the K_m of the FA-B endonuclease higher than that of the FA-A endonuclease ($p < 0.05$). Since there was little difference in the turnover numbers of either the normal or the FA-A or FA-B endonuclease complexes, pI 7.6, on 8-MOP plus UVA-treated DNA, these decreases in K_m are again due primarily to increases in affinity for or rate of association with the damaged DNA.

Analysis of V_{max} and K_{cat} of normal and XPA endonuclease complexes on psoralen plus UVA-Damaged Non-nucleosomal and Nucleosomal DNA

Both DNA endonuclease complexes from normal and XPA cells were assayed against a range of different substrate concentrations so that kinetic analysis of their activities could be carried out. Kinetic analysis of the activities of both of the normal and both of the XPA endonuclease complexes, pIs 4.6 and 7.6, assayed against untreated, control (with UVA, without psoralen) and psoralen plus UVA damaged DNAs, both naked and reconstituted into nucleosomes (with and without histone H1) all produced linear results on both Lineweaver-Burke and Eadie-Hofstee graphic representations as well as using our more sophisticated methods

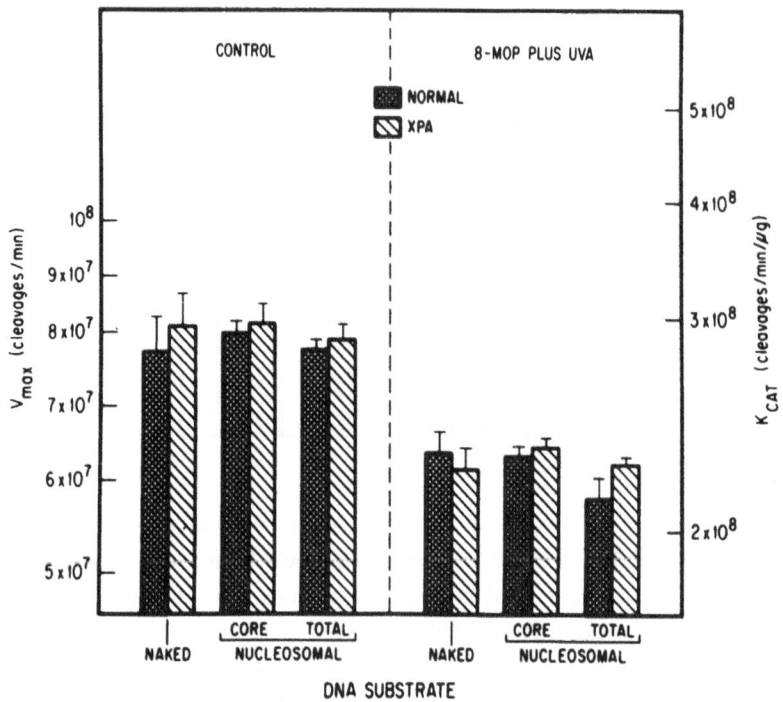

Figure 10. Maximum velocity (V_{max}) (maximum number of cleavages produced per minute per μg endonuclease) of the normal and XPA endonuclease complex, pI 4.6, on naked, core or total nucleosomal DNA treated with 8-MOP (7 μg/ml) plus two doses of UVA 10 W/m^2 for 10 minutes). Control DNA was exposed to two doses of UVA irradiation as above, without treatment with 8-MOP. Vertical bars represent $\pm$ S.E.M. for 5 or more experiments. Assay volume was 40 μl containing 0.34 $\pm$ 0.04 μg endonuclease complex (Parrish et al., 1992).

(Lambert et al., 1993). The coefficient of correlation (R) was at least 0.98, 0.93 and 0.95, respectively, on each of these analyses. The results presented here represent pooled data from two normal or from two XPA cell lines. Values represent the means of 3-5 separate experiments.

Activities of both of the normal and of both of the XPA endonuclease complexes showed a slightly reduced V_{max} and K_{cat} (20-25% reduction) on 8-MOP plus UVA treated DNA compared to their activities on control DNA, but activities of none of these four complexes showed a significant change in these values on damaged or control nucleosomal versus similarly treated non-nucleosomal DNA (Figures 10 and 11). By contrast, the activities of the normal and of the XPA endonuclease complex, pI 7.6, both showed an increase of approximately 80% in V_{max} and K_{cat} on angelian plus UVA damaged DNA compared to control DNA, but again no significant

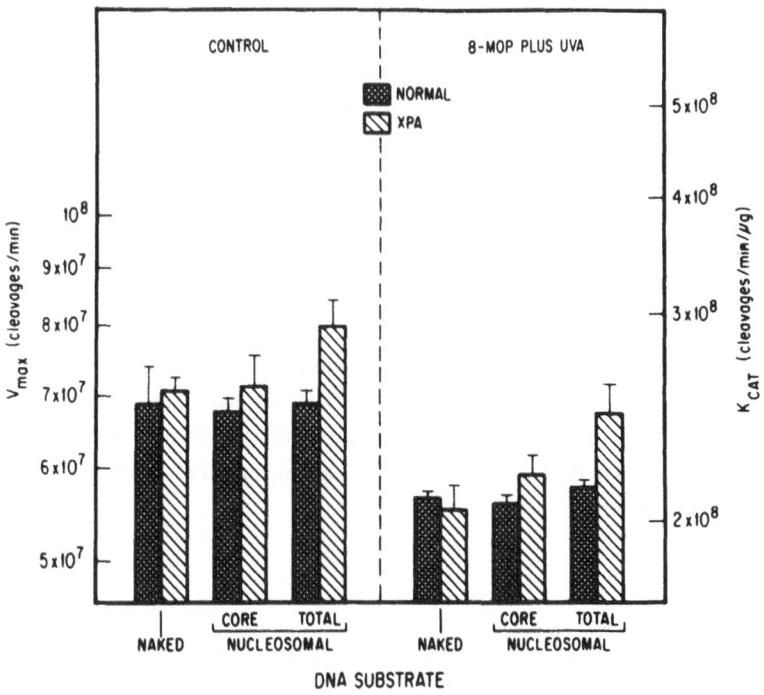

Figure 11. V_{max} and K_{cat} of the normal and XPA endonuclease complex, pI 7.6, on non-nucleosomal or core and total nucleosomal DNA treated with 8-MOP plus two doses of UVA. Control DNA was exposed to two doses of UVA irradiation without treatment with 8-MOP. Reaction conditions and vertical bars are as for Figure 10 (Parrish et al., 1992).

change in these values was noted on damaged or control nucleosomal versus similarly treated non-nucleosomal DNA (Figure 12). Activity of the normal and XPA endonuclease complexes, pI 4.6, on angelicin plus UVA damaged DNA was not examined kinetically since we have found that normal, FA and XP complexes, pI 4.6, have only a low level of activity on this substrate (Lambert et al., 1988; Parrish and Lambert, 1990). All four normal and XP endonuclease complexes showed a V_{max} and K_{cat} approximately 17% higher on control (UVA treated) DNA compared to untreated DNA (data not shown).

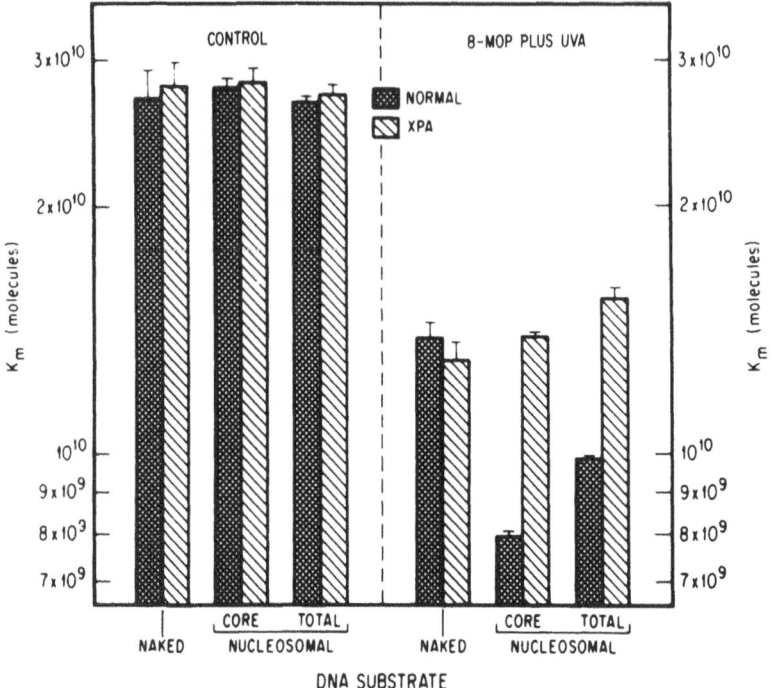

Figure 12. V_{max} and K_{cat} of the normal and XPA endonuclease complex, pI 7.6, on non-nucleosomal or core and total nucleosomal DNA treated with angelicin (25 μg/ml) plus UVA irradiation (10 W/m² for 5 minutes). Control DNA was exposed to UVA, as above, without treatment with angelicin. Assay volume was 40 μl containing 0.34 + 0.04 μg of endonuclease complex. Vertical bars represent ± S.E.M. for 5 or more experiments (Parrish et al., 1992).

The K_m of the Normal and XPA Endonuclease Complexes on Psoralen Plus UVA-Damaged Non-nucleosomal and Nucleosomal DNA

Both normal and both XPA endonuclease complexes showed a reduction in K_m, to approximately 50% of their value on control DNA, on non-nucleosomal DNA treated with 8-MOP plus UVA (Figures 13 and 14). A further decrease was noted in the K_m of both normal complexes on damaged DNA when nucleosomes were present (Figures 13 and 14). This additional decrease was not seen on nucleosomal versus naked DNA treated only with UVA. The K_m of both normal endonuclease complexes on 8-MOP plus UVA damaged core nucleosomal DNA were approximately 60% of those observed for the same enzymes on damaged naked DNA (p < 0.001). This decrease in K_m was also present, but was not as great, with the K_m approximately 80% of that observed on damaged naked DNA, on damaged total nucleosomal (with histone H1) DNA (p < 0.005). Again, no decrease in K_m on total nucleosomal versus naked DNA treated only with UVA was observed.

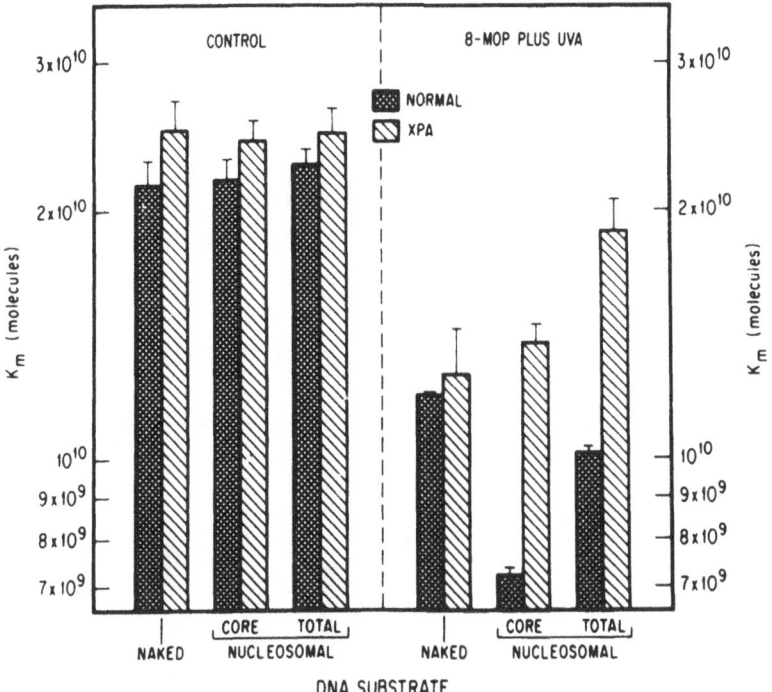

Figure 13. Michaelis constants (K_m), expressed as numbers of substrate molecules within the assay solution (40 μl), of the normal and XPA endonuclease complex, pI 4.6, assayed on naked (non-nucleosomal), core and total nucleosomal DNA treated with 8-MOP plus UVA. Reaction conditions are as for Figure 10. Vertical bars refer to $\pm$ S.E.M. of results obtained graphically for K_m from at least 5 experiments (Parrish et al., 1992).

By contrast, neither XPA endonuclease complex showed these additional decreases, and instead showed increases, in K_m on 8-MOP plus UVA damaged nucleosomal DNA compared with similarly damaged non-nucleosomal DNA (Figures 13 and 14). A significantly greater increase was noted for both XPA complexes against damaged nucleosomal DNA containing histone H1. There was no difference in K_m of either XP endonuclease complex on either type of control nucleosomal DNA compared with that against control naked DNA.

The normal and XPA endonuclease complexes, pI 7.6, showed no change in their K_m on angelicin plus UVA treated naked DNA compared to control naked DNA (Figure 15). However, the normal complex showed a 50% reduction in K_m on similarly damaged core nucleosomal DNA compared to damaged naked DNA. When histone H1 was present this decrease in K_m was not as great; the K_m was 80% of the value on damaged naked DNA. By contrast, activity of the XPA endonuclease complex, pI 7.6, did not show any significant change in K_m on angelicin plus UVA treated nucleosomal DNA compared to its K_m on damaged naked DNA. Activities of each of these four endonuclease complexes showed a reduction of approximately 7% in K_m on DNA irradiated with the dosages of UVA used here (control DNA) versus untreated DNA (data not shown).

DISCUSSION

We have isolated two chromatin-associated DNA endonuclease complexes from normal human lymphoblastoid cells which have specificity for psoralen plus UVA damaged DNA (Lambert et al., 1988; Parrish and Lambert, 1990). These two complexes, pIs 4.6 and 7.6, which recognize psoralen interstrand cross-links and monoadducts, respectively, show increased activity on damaged DNA when nucleosomes are present (Parrish and Lambert, 1990; Lambert

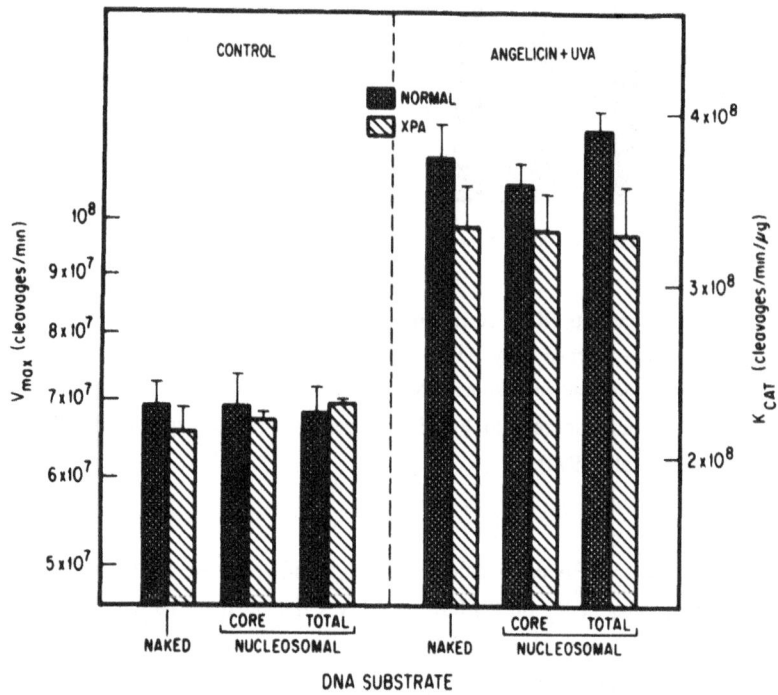

Figure 14. Michaelis constants (K_m) of the normal and XPA endonuclease complex, pI 7.6, on non-nucleosomal and on core and total nucleosomal DNA, treated with 8-MOP plus two doses of UVA. Control DNA was exposed to two doses of UVA without treatment with 8-MOP. Reaction conditions and vertical bars are as for Figure 10 (Parrish et al., 1992).

et al., 1991). These complexes thus perform three functions: damage recognition, endonucleolytic incision and chromatin interaction. Each contains both a DNA endonuclease and a protein needed for endonuclease interaction with damaged nucleosomal DNA (Parrish and Lambert, 1990). Whether damage recognition is associated with a separate protein or is performed by the endonuclease is under investigation. These same two endonuclease complexes are also present in FA-A, FA-B, and XPA cells, but are defective, in different ways, in each diseased cell type. Thus these diseases provide mutants which may be used to facilitate study

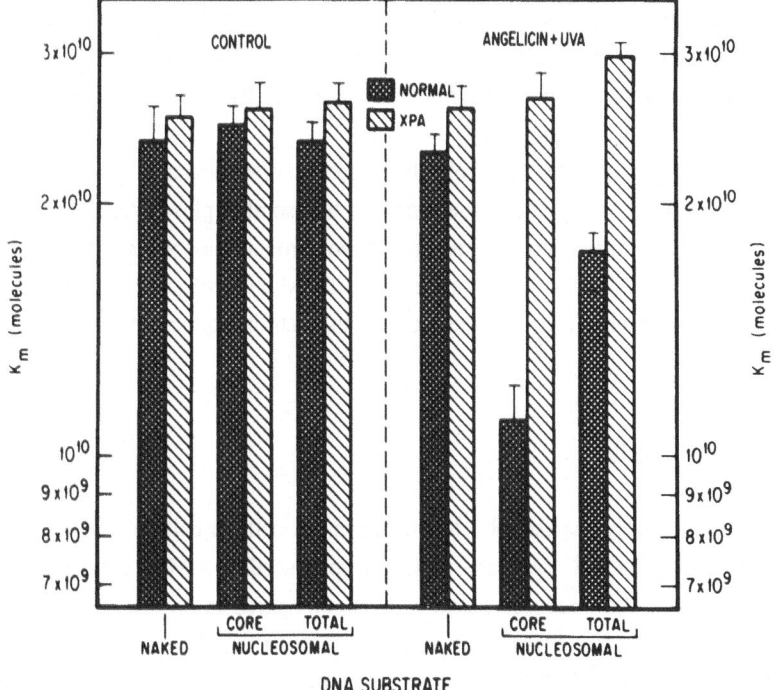

Figure 15. Michaelis constants (K_m) of the normal and XPA endonuclease, pI 7.6, on non-nucleosomal or core and total nucleosomal DNA treated with angelicin plus UVA. Reaction conditions are as for Figure 10. Vertical bars represent $\pm$ S.E.M. of results obtained graphically for K_m from at least 4 experiments (Parrish et al., 1992).

of these endonuclease complexes, and thus of DNA repair mechanisms active on psoralen plus UVA-induced lesions, in normal cells or in cells obtained from patients with other diseases, such as mycosis fungoides, for which psoralen plus UVA is used therapeutically, but for which no deficiency in a DNA repair mechanism is known to exist.

Fanconi Anemia

Several lines of investigation have related the hypersensitivity of FA cells to DNA interstrand cross-linking agents to a defect in repair of DNA damage produced by these agents (Fujiwara et al., 1977; Papadopoulo et al., 1987; Gruenert and Cleaver, 1985; Plooy et al., 1985; Averbeck et al., 1988; Matsumoto et al., 1989). This defect has been proposed to occur in the initial incision step of the repair process in certain FA cell lines (Fujiwara et al., 1977; Fujiwara, 1982; Gruenert and Cleaver, 1985). However, in other studies a defect in repair of interstrand cross-links has not been detected (Fornace et al., 1979; Kaye et al., 1980; Poll et al., 1984). Some of this discrepancy has been attributed to the genetic heterogeneity of the FA cell lines (Duckworth-Rysiecki et al., 1985; Papadopoulo et al., 1987; Moustacchi et al., 1987) and to different culture ages of the cell lines used (Sognier and Hittleman, 1983). The presence of at least four FA complementation groups has been demonstrated (Duckworth-Rysiecki et al., 1985; Moustacchi et al., 1987; Strathdee et al., 1992). Except for the studies reported from our laboratory, however, no defective DNA repair enzyme has been identified in FA cells.

The present study analyzes FA cells from both complementation groups A and B, in culture, for their ability to repair damage produced by psoralen plus UVA light. In addition, it also reports on the identification and isolation of two chromatin-associated DNA endonuclease complexes, pIs 4.6 and 7.6, in FA-A and FA-B cells which recognize adducts produced by psoralen plus UVA light but which are defective in their ability to incise DNA containing these adducts.

Reduced UDS in FA cells

In the present study, analysis of DNA repair in FA cells in culture demonstrates that, in response to monoadducts and interstrand cross-links produced by 8-MOP plus UVA light, both FA-A and FA-B cells show reduced levels of UDS, compared to normal cells, with levels of UDS in FA-A cells slightly lower than those in FA-B cells. In response to monoadducts produced by angelicin plus UVA light, FA-B cells show much lower levels of UDS than either FA-A or normal cells. Plooy et al. (1985) examined UDS in one FA fibroblast cell line exposed to mitomycin C and did not detect any UDS in these cells; however, they also did not detect UDS in similarly damaged normal cells. Fujiwara and Tatsumi (1977) also measured UDS in normal and in FA fibroblasts exposed to mitomycin C; they found similar but extremely low levels of UDS in both groups of cells. However, in both of these studies FA cells showed decreased cell survival and decreased rates of removal of cross-links when exposed to mitomycin C (Fujiwara and Tatsumi, 1977; Plooy et al., 1985). On the other hand, Gruenert and Cleaver (1985) showed decreased repair replication, measured using isopycnic gradient centrifugation, in a SV40 transformed FA cell line containing cross-links produced by 8-MOP plus UVA, compared to SV40 transformed normal cells. This same FA cell line showed levels of repair replication in response to angelicin which were similar to those of normal cells (Greunert and Cleaver, 1985). All of these studies predated the establishment of complementation groups in FA cells. The present results are mainly in agreement with the studies on repair replication carried out by Gruenert and Cleaver (1985). Differences between our results and the above studies could be due to the genetic heterogeneity of the cell lines used or to the different types of DNA interstrand cross-links formed [i.e., pyrimidine-pyrimidine (8-MOP plus UVA) versus purine-purine (mitomycin C)].

Defect in ability of the FA endonuclease complexes to incise psoralen plus UVA-damaged DNA

The present study shows that FA-A cells have an endonuclease complex, pI 4.6, and that

FA-B cells have an endonuclease complex, pI 7.6, which are defective in their ability to incise DNA interstrand cross-links and monoadducts, respectively, produced by 8-MOP or angelicin plus UVA light. These results correlate with our studies showing reduced levels of UDS in FA-A and FA-B cells in culture exposed to these agents. In addition, we have found that the FA-A but not the FA-B endonuclease complex, pI 4.6, has significantly reduced ability, compared to the normal endonuclease, pI 4.6, to incise a shuttle vector containing a single, site-directed nitrogen mustard interstrand cross-link (obtained from Dr. Edward Loechler; unpublished observation). The FA-A, FA-B and normal endonuclease, pI 7.6, had little activity on this cross-linked substrate. This further indicates that FA-A but not FA-B cells have an endonuclease activity which is defective in its ability to incise DNA interstrand cross-links.

These studies are in agreement with those of Papadopoulo et al. (1987) and Averbeck et al. (1988), respectively, which suggest that FA-A cells show a greater reduction in ability to incise DNA-continuing interstrand cross-links and FA-B cells are less efficient at incising DNA containing monoadducts produced by 8-MOP plus UVA. In both of these studies, the FA-B cell line used was derived from the same patient as the one used in the present study. The studies of Papadopoulo et al. (1987) also indicate that the repair defect in FA-A cells appears to be more pronounced than that in FA-B cells, which is in agreement with our findings on endonuclease activity in these cells.

Previous studies examining the viability of FA cells, where the complementation group (A versus B) is known, are also in agreement with our findings. Both Papadopoulo et al. (1987), treating fibroblasts with 8-MOP plus 365-nm UVA light, and Matsumoto et al. (1989), who administered mitomycin C to cells from the same lines examined in the present study, found viability of FA-A and FA-B cells to be approximately 40% and 66%, respectively, of that of similarly treated normal cells. When treated with 4,5',8-trimethylpsoralen plus 405-nm light so as to induce only monoadducts, however, FA-B cells were more sensitive, showing 20% of normal survival versus 33% for FA-A cells (Averbeck et al., 1988). Adjustment of treatment conditions so as to induce both monoadducts and cross-links produced between 17% and 33% of normal survival in the FA cells of the two complementation groups, depending on the ratio of the two types of adducts induced in cellular DNA (Averbeck et al., 1988). The slightly greater reductions in enzyme activity which we have found, compared to the above reductions in cell survival, may be due to the complex mechanisms involved in the latter and the proportion of monoadducts to cross-links present in the DNA.

Dean (1989) reported that a FA-A cell line was able to repair 8-MOP plus UVA-induced cross-links in the dihydrofolate reductase (DHFR) gene. However, he also reported formation of two to three times as many adducts in FA-A cells as in normal cells. Since the number of adducts produced in his system was small, it is possible that significant repair of adducts occurred in normal cells during his treatment protocol with 8-MOP plus UVA, and that this repair was defective in FA-A cells. By contrast, Matsumoto et al. (1989) showed that a FA-A cell line exhibits a deficiency in removal of cross-links induced by mitomycin C in ribosomal RNA genes. Thus, the preponderance of evidence from several laboratories clearly indicates that there is a deficiency in cross-link removal in FA cells.

We have introduced, by electroporation, the normal endonuclease complexes, pIs 4.6 and 7.6, into 8-MOP plus UVA-treated FA-A and FA-B cells, respectively, in culture and have been able to correct the repair defect in these cells (Lambert et al., in preparation). The repair deficiencies in FA cells, therefore, appear to reside in the endonuclease activities we have isolated. The FA repair defect has also been corrected in other laboratories by transfection of FA-A and FA-B cells, exposed to various cross-linking agents, with plasmid and human DNA (Buchwald et al., 1987; Shaham et al., 1987; Moustacchi et al., 1989) and HeLa mRNA (Digweed and Sperling, 1989).

Kinetic Analysis

Decreased affinity, or rate of association, of the FA endonuclease complexes for 8-MOP plus UVA-irradiated DNA

Kinetic analysis indicates that the defect in the FA-A endonuclease complex, pI 4.6, and in the FA-B endonuclease complex, pI 7.6, lies in their ability to associate with damaged substrate. Both normal endonuclease complexes show a decrease in K_m, with little or no change in K_{cat}, indicating an increase in affinity for and/or rate of association with psoralen plus UVA-treated non-nucleosomal DNA. However, the FA-A endonuclease complex, pI 4.6, and the FA-B endonuclease complex, pI 7.6, fail to show as great a decrease in K_m as do the corresponding normal endonucleases, indicating that their affinity for and/or rate of association with this damaged DNA is less than that of the corresponding normal endonuclease complexes. The results correlate with our studies on decreased activity of these endonucleases on 8-MOP plus UVA-treated DNA. The fact that there were decreases in affinity of these FA endonucleases for damaged DNA and that the normal FA-A and FA-B endonuclease samples assayed contained similar amounts of protein further indicates that it is very unlikely that the decreases we observed in the activity of these FA endonucleases were due to quantitative differences in the amount of endonuclease obtained from similar numbers of cells from the respective cell lines in culture.

Recently, our laboratory has identified a protein which selectively binds to cross-linked DNA in normal cells but which is absent or defective in FA-A cells (Hang et al., 1993). The relationship of this defective protein to the biochemical defect described in the present paper is currently under investigation.

Kinetic analysis of the normal and XPA endonuclease complexes on psoralen plus UVA damaged DNA

Kinetic analysis of assays using graduated doses of substrate indicates that the selective activity against 8-MOP plus UVA treated DNA shown by both normal and both XPA endonuclease complexes is associated with increased affinity, or rate of association, of enzyme with the substrate, as indicated by the decreased K_m. In addition, the turnover number is actually slightly decreased on this damaged substrate compared to that on control DNA. The reduced rate of cleavage (K_{cat}), following association of the complex with DNA damaged with 8-MOP plus UVA, may be due to the marked distortion which occurs in DNA following formation of a psoralen DNA cross-link (Vigny et al., 1985; Cimino et al., 1985). By contrast, the increased activity of both the normal and the XPA endonuclease complex, pI 7.6, on angelicin plus UVA treated DNA is associated with an increase in K_{cat}, compared to activity on control DNA, with no decrease in K_m detected. It is possible, however, that an increase in affinity is present which is masked by the increase in K_{cat}, which may, itself, increase K_m (See Equation (1), above).

The increased activity of the normal endonuclease complexes on both 8-MOP (both complexes) and angelicin (the complex, pI 7.6) plus UVA treated DNA when they are reconstituted into nucleosomes is associated only with an increase in affinity, or rate of association, of the complex for the substrate, as indicated by decreases in K_m with no corresponding changes in K_{cat}. This increase in affinity is greatest on damaged core nucleosomal DNA and is diminished but not abolished when histone H1 is present. This increased affinity correlates with a 2.5-fold enhancement of the activity of both normal complexes on 8-MOP or angelicin plus UVA damaged core nucleosomal DNA and only a 1.5 fold increase when histone H1 is present. By contrast, the XPA endonuclease complexes fail to show this decreased K_m (increase in affinity), and actually show an increase in K_m (decrease in affinity) when histone H1 is present, indicating that the XPA endonucleases are defective in their ability to interact with chromatin because of reduced affinity, or rate of association, with damaged nucleosomal substrates. This correlates, in turn, with failure of the XPA endonuclease complexes to show any increase in activity on damaged core nucleosomal DNA and with a reduced activity of these complexes when histone H1 is present.

The increases in affinity and/or rate of association shown by the normal endonuclease complexes are damage-specific, since they are not seen on undamaged nucleosomal versus non-nucleosomal DNA. These increases on damaged nucleosomal DNAs are not due to an increased number of DNA adducts, since we have determined that the number of 8-MOP adducts is reduced approximately 50% on core nucleosomal DNA and 60% when histone H1 is present (Parrish and Lambert, 1990).

Nucleosome Structure

<u>Nucleosome structure enhances FA and normal endonuclease activity on psoralen plus UVA-damaged DNA</u>

Both of the FA-A and FA-B endonuclease activities, pIs 4.6 and 7.6, showed approximately the same 2.5-fold increase in activity on core nucleosomal (minus histone H1) DNA treated with 8-MOP or angelicin plus UVA light as was observed with the two normal endonucleases. The presence of histone H1 reduced this increase, which is consistent with the proposed role of histone H1 in the condensation of chromatin (McGhee and Felsenfeld, 1980; Igo-Kemenes et al., 1982; Klingholz and Stratling, 1982; Watanabe, 1984), making it less accessible to endonucleolytic attack. This increase in endonuclease activity was dependent upon nucleosome assembly, and, as noted above, did not correlate with a change in the number of psoralen adducts. Our studies indicate that associated with each endonuclease complex is a protein which makes the psoralen adducts on the nucleosomal DNA more accessible to endonucleolytic attack (Parrish and Lambert, 1990). Our studies also indicate that the endonuclease and chromatin-interacting protein form part of a complex which is involved in the initial damage recognition/incision step in the repair process (Lambert et al., in preparation). The present results indicate that the FA-A and FA-B endonuclease activities are not defective in their interaction with psoralen plus UVA-damaged nucleosomal DNA but rather are defective in their ability to incise damaged naked DNA. Associated with this defect is a reduced affinity and/or rate of association of these endonuclease complexes with 8-MOP plus UVA-treated naked DNA. The defect in FA-A cells is greatest in the endonuclease complex, pI 4.6, which recognizes DNA interstrand cross-links; in FA-B cells it is greater in the endonuclease complex, pI 7.6, which recognizes the psoralen monoadduct.

<u>The nucleosomal system in relationship to XP endonuclease activities</u>

The enhanced activity of the normal human but not the XPA endonuclease complexes for damaged nucleosomal DNA appears to be related to the presence of histones H3 and H4 (Parrish and Lambert, in preparation). This could either be due to direct interaction of the endonucleases with these histones or due to the fact that these histones can form nucleosome-like structures. The reduced affinity and activity of the normal and XPA endonuclease complexes for damaged nucleosomal DNA when histone H1 is present is in agreement with the proposed role of histone H1 in condensation of chromatin, as noted above. These results are corroborated, in part, by those obtained by Ishimi et al. (1981), who found that histone H1 protected a site in undamaged calf-thymus DNA from micrococcal nuclease.

Enhancement of the affinity of an endonuclease for DNA when it is present in chromatin has also been reported by Sollner-Webb et al. (1986). They found that the apparent affinity of staphylococcal nuclease for chromatin was greater than that for protein-free DNA; however, the activity of the nuclease was less on chromatin than on protein-free DNA. This differs from the present results in which the increased affinities of the endonuclease complexes for damaged nucleosomal DNA correlate with an increase in their activity on this substrate. We have also found that two normal but not XPA chromatin-associated endonuclease complexes, pIs 9.2 and 9.8, which selectively recognize apurinic/apyrimidinic (AP) sites, show increased activity on AP nucleosomal DNA compared to naked AP DNA (Kaysen at al., 1986). It is possible that all of the normal endonuclease complexes have associated with them the same or a similar chromatin protein which makes damage on nucleosomal DNA more accessible to endonucleolytic attack than on naked DNA.

Relationship with Other Cell-Free DNA Repair Systems

Our studies indicate that the defect in XPA cells in the incision step of repair of psoralen plus UVA treated DNA exists in the inability of the XPA endonuclease complex to interact with damaged nucleosomal DNA (Kaysen et al., 1986; Parrish and Lambert, 1990). The studies of Mortelmans et al. (1976), and of Kano and Fujiwara (1983), using crude cell extracts, also suggest that XPA cells are defective in a factor which renders the DNA in UVC-irradiated chromatin accessible to endonucleolytic attack. The work of Hittelman (1986) suggests that XPA cells have a defect in decondensation of chromatin associated with excision repair following UV-irradiation. All of these studies support the concept that a defect related to endonuclease interaction with chromatin is present in XPA cells.

The human endonuclease complex may have some similarities with the UvrABC system in E. coli in which the interaction of different protein subunits is needed for endonucleolytic incision of damaged DNA (Sancar and Sancar, 1988; Grossman, 1988; Orren and Sancar, 1989). In the human endonuclease complex, a chromatin-interacting protein is present which is needed for endonuclease incision of damaged nucleosomal DNA. There is specificity associated with the interaction of each complex with damaged nucleosomal DNA. For example, adding the normal AP endonuclease complex, pI 9.8, does not correct the defect in the ability of the XPA endonuclease complex, pI 7.6, to incise 8-MOP plus UVA damaged nucleosomal DNA (Parrish and Lambert, 1990). It may be that recognition of the specific damaged site by the appropriate endonuclease is needed before the chromatin-interacting protein can exert its effect.

Studies reported by Wood et al. (1988) and by Sibghat-Ullah et al. (1989), appear to contradict the concept that the defect in XPA cells resides at the level of interaction of the endonuclease with damaged chromatin. In those studies soluble cell extracts of normal, but not XPA, cells were reported to be able to remove adducts from exogenous naked DNA irradiated with UVC. Such extracts of mammalian cells, however, have been shown to reconstitute naked plasmid DNA into structures, visualized ultrastructurally, which resemble nucleosomes (Manley et al., 1980; Hough et al., 1982). The defect observed by Wood et al. using these extracts, therefore, may also have been due to an inability of a XPA endonuclease to interact with some type of damaged nucleosome-like structure rather than failure to act on damaged non-nucleosomal DNA.

An XP "correcting factor" has been isolated from calf thymus which, upon microinjection into XPA cells, corrects their repair defect (de Jonge et al, 1983). Correction of the DNA-repair defect after UVC-irradiation has also been reported in XPA cells following microinjection of crude cell extracts from human placenta or HeLa cells (Yamaizumi et al., 1986). Tanaka et al. (1990) have cloned a human XPA cDNA which, when transfected into UVC-irradiated XPA cells, corrects the repair defect. This cDNA encodes a protein with a zinc-finger motif, suggesting that it is a DNA-binding protein (Tanaka et al., 1990; Satokata et al., 1990). This is consistent with our studies, which indicate that the XPA-correcting factor which we have isolated is a protein which makes damaged nucleosomal DNA accessible to damage-specific endonucleases (Lambert and Parrish, 1989; Parrish and Lambert, 1990). Whether the protein in our studies is similar to that encoded by the gene identified by Tanaka and co-workers is under investigation.

XPA is a complex disease, the etiology of which has not yet been worked out (Cleaver, 1990) and it may be associated with more than one defective gene (Lambert and Lambert, 1985; 1989; 1992). Our studies indicate that a defect exists in the interaction of XPA endonuclease complexes with damaged nucleosomal DNA (Lambert and Parrish, 1989; Parrish and Lambert, 1990; Tsongalis, et al 1990a; 1990b); the defect in the ability of the XPA endonuclease complexes to incise damaged nucleosomal DNA correlates with a decreased affinity, or rate of association, of these complexes with this damaged substrate. This defect appears to be related to a protein needed for interaction of the endonucleases with damaged nucleosomal DNA. By contrast, the defect in FA-A and FA-B cells appears to be in the endonucleases themselves, pI 4.6 and pI 7.6, respectively, which are involved in repair of psoralen plus UVA monoadducts and interstrand cross-links. This reduced activity of the FA-A and FA-B endonuclease complexes on their respective substrates also correlates with a reduced affinity, or rate of association, of these complexes with their respective damaged substrates. Taken together, these XP and FA cell lines, therefore, serve as excellent mutants for analysis of DNA endonuclease complexes in human cells responsible for the repair of psoralen plus UVA induced adducts in DNA.

ACKNOWLEDGEMENTS

The Fanconi anemia cell lines were a generous gift of Dr. Manuel Buchwald (Hospital for Sick Children, Toronto, Canada). We would like to thank Robert Lockwood for culturing the human cell lines and for isolating and purifying plasmid DNA. This work was supported by Grant AM 35148 from the National Institutes of Health.

REFERENCES

Amari NMB, WC Lambert and MW Lambert, 1986. Comparison of histones in normal and xeroderma pigmentosum lymphoblastoid cells. **Cell. Biol. Intl. Repts.**, 10:875-880.

Auerbach AD and SK Wolman, 1976. Susceptibility of Fanconi's anemia fibroblasts to chromosome damage by carcinogens. **Nature** (London), 261, 494-496.

Auerbach AD, A Rogatko and TM Schroeder-Kurth, 1989. International Fanconi Anemia Registry: Relation of clinical symptoms to diepoxybutane sensitivity. **Blood**, 73:391-396.

Averbeck D, D Papadopoulo and E Moustacchi, 1988. Repair of 4,5'8-trimethylpsoralen plus light-induced DNA damage in normal and Fanconi's anemia cells. **Cancer Res.**, 48:2015-2020.

Ben-Hur E, and MM Elkind, 1973. Psoralen plus near ultraviolet light inactivation of cultured Chinese hamster cells and its relation to DNA cross-links. **Mutation Res.**, 18:315-324.

Ben-Hur E and P-S Song, 1984. The photochemistry and photobiology of furocoumarins (psoralens). **Adv. Radiat. Biol.**, 11:131-177.

Bohr VA, DH Phillips and PC Hanawalt, 1987. Heterogeneous DNA damage and repair in the mammalian genome. **Cancer Res.**, 47:6426-6436.

Bredberg A, 1982. Genetic toxicity of psoralen and ultraviolet radiation in human cells. **Acta Dermato-Venereol.**, 104:1-4.

Bredberg A, B Lambert and S Soderhall, 1982. Induction and repair of psoralen cross-links in DNA of normal human and xeroderma pigmentosum fibroblasts. **Mutation Res.**, 93:221-234.

Buchwald M, J Ng, C Clarke and G Duckworth-Rysiecki, 1987. Studies of gene transfer and reversion to mitomycin C resistance in Fanconi anemia cells. **Mutation Res.**, 184:153-159.

Cerutti P, M Kaneko and P Beard, 1980. Nucleosomal structure of chromatin: Distribution and excision of DNA damage, In: E. Seeberg and K. Kleepe, Eds., **Chromosome Damage and Repair**, Plenum Press, New York. pp. 49-61.

Cimino GD, HB Gamper, ST Isaacs and JE Hearst, 1985. Psoralens as photoactive probes of nucleic acid structure and function: Organic chemistry, photochemistry. **Annu. Rev. Biochem.**, 54:1151-1193.

Cleaver, J.E., 1990. Do we know the cause of xeroderma pigmentosum? **Carcinogenesis**, 11:875-882.

Cleaver JE, and KH Kraemer, 1989. Xeroderma pigmentosum. In: McKusick, V., Ed. **The Metabolic Basis of Inherited Disease**, 6th ed., McGraw Hill, New York, pp. 2949-2971.

Davie JR, L Numerow and GP Delcuve, 1986. The nonhistone chromosomal protein, H2A-specific protease, is selectively associated with nucleosomes containing histone Hl. **J. Biol. Chem.**, 261:10410-10416.

Dean SW, 1989. Repair of 8-methoxypsoralen + UVA - induced damage in specific sequences in chromosomal and episomal DNA in human cells. **Carcinogenesis**, 10:1253-1256.

de Jonge AJR, W Vermeulen, B Klein and JHJ Hoeijmakers, 1983. Microinjection of human cells extracts corrects xeroderma pigmentosum defect. **EMBO J.**, 2:637-641.

Digweed M and K Sperling, 1989. Identification of a HeLa mRNA fraction which can correct the DNA-repair defect in Fanconi anaemia fibroblasts. **Mutation Res.**, 218:171-177.

Digweed M, S Zakrzewski-Ludcke and K Sperling, 1988. Fanconi's anaemia: Correlation of genetic complementation group with psoralen/UVA response. **Human Genet.**, 78:51-54.

Duckworth-Rysiecki G, K Cornish, CA Clarke and M Buchwald, 1985. Identification of two complementation groups in Fanconi's anemia. **Somatic Cell Mol. Genet.**, 11:35-41.

Elia MC and EN Moudrianakis, 1988. Regulation of H2A-specific proteolysis by histone H3:H4 tetramer. **J. Biol. Chem.**, 263:9958-9964.

Fanconi G, 1967. Familial constitutional panmyelocytopathy, In: Fanconi's anemia I, Clinical Aspects. **Semin. Hematol.**, 4:233-240.

* Fornace AJ, Jr, JB Little and RR Weichselbaum, 1979. DNA repair in Fanconi's anemia fibroblast cell strain. **Biochim. Biophys. Acta**, 561:99-109.

Freifelder D, 1983. In: C.I. Daven, Ed., **Molecular Biology, A Comprehensive Introduction to Procaryotes and Eukaryotes**, Jones and Bartlett, Boston, MA, pp. 132-136.

Fujiwara Y, 1982. Defective repair of mitomycin C cross-links in Fanconi's anemia and loss in confluent normal human and xeroderma pigmentosum cells. **Biochem. Biophys. Acta**, 699:217-225.

Fujiwara Y, M Tatsumi and MS Sasaki, 1977. Cross-link repair in human cells and its possible defect in Fanconi's anemia cells. **J. Mol. Biol.**, 113:635-649.

German J, 1982. Genes which increase chromosomal instability in somatic cells and predispose to cancer. **Prog. Med. Genet.**, 8:61-101.

Gia O, G Palu, M Palumbo, C Antonello and S Marciani-Magno, 1987. Photoreaction of psoralen derivatives with structurally organized DNA. **Photochem. Photobiol.**, 45:87-92.

Glanz A, and FC Fraser, 1982. Spectrum of anomalies in Fanconi anemia. **J. Med. Genet.**, 19:412-416.

Grossman L, PR Caron, SJ Mazur and EY Oh, 1988. Repair of DNA-containing pyrimidine dimers. **FASEB J.**, 2:2696-2701.

Gruenert DC and JE Cleaver, 1985. Repair of psoralen induced cross-links and monoadducts in normal and repair-deficient human fibroblasts. **Cancer Res.**, 45:5399-5404.

Hanawalt P, IM Mellon, D Scicchitano and G Spivak, 1989. Relationships between DNA repair and transcription in defined DNA sequences in mammalian cells, In: M.W. Lambert and J. Laval Eds., **DNA Repair Mechanisms and Their Biological Implications in Mammalian Cells**, Plenum Press, New York, pp. 325-337.

Hang B, Yeung AT and Lambert MW, 1993. A damage-recognition protein which binds to DNA containing interstrand cross-links is absent or defective in Fanconi anemia, complementation group A, cells. **Nucl. Acids Res.**, 21:4187-4192.

Hittelman WN, 1986. Visualization of chromatin events during DNA excision repair in XP cells: Deficiency in localized but not generalized chromatin events. **Carcinogenesis**, 7:1975-1980.

Hough PVC, IA, Mastrangelo, JS Wall, JF Hainfield, MN Simon and JL Manley, 1982. DNA protein complexes spread on N2-discharged carbon film and characterized by molecular weight and its projected distribution. **J. Mol. Biol.**, 160:375-386.

Igo-Kemenes T, W Horz and HG Zachau, 1982. Chromatin. **Annu. Rev. Biochem.**, 51:89-121.

Ishida R and M Buchwald, 1982. Susceptibility of Fanconi's anemia lymphoblasts to DNA-cross-linking and alkylating agents. **Cancer Res.**, 42:4000-4006.

Ishimi Y, Y Ohba, H Yasuda and M Yamada, 1981. The interaction of H1 histone with nucleosome core. **J. Biochem.**, 89:1881-1888.

Kano Y and Y Fujiwara, 1982. Higher inductions of twin and single sister chromatid exchanges by cross-linking agents with Fanconi's anemia cells. **Hum. Genet.**, 60:233-238.

Kano Y and Y Fujiwara, 1983. Defective thymine dimer excision from xeroderma pigmentosum chromatin and its characteristic catalysis by cell-free extracts. **Carcinogenesis**, 4:1419-1424.

Kaye J, CA Smith and PC Hanawalt, 1980. DNA repair in human cells containing photoadducts of 8-methoxypsoralen or angelicin. **Cancer Res.**, 40:696-702.

Kaysen JH, 1984. **The influence of nucleosomes on apurinic/apyrimidinic DNA endonuclease activities from normal human and xeroderma pigmentosum lymphoblastoid cells**, Doctoral Thesis, UMDNJ, Newark, NJ.

Kaysen JH, NMB Amari and MW Lambert, 1986. Enhancement of two apurinic/apyrimidinic endonuclease activities from normal but not xeroderma pigmentosum lymphoblastoid cells by nucleosome structure. **Mutation Res.**, 165:221-231.

Kaysen JH, NMB Amari and MW Lambert, 1987. Positioning of nucleosomes reconstituted with xeroderma pigmentosum and normal histones. **Cell. Biol. Intl. Repts.**, 11:95-101.

Klingholz R and WH Stratling, 1982. Reassociation of histone H1 to H1-depleted polynucleosomes. **J. Biol. Chem.**, 257:13101-13107.

Kraemer KH, MM Lee and J Scotto, 1987. Xeroderma pigmentosum: cutaneous, ocular, and neurologic abnormalities in 830 published cases. **Arch. Dermatol.**, 123:241-250.

Lalt SA, E Stetten, LA Juergens, GR Buchanan and PS Gerald, 1975. Induction by alkylating agents of sister-chromatid exchanges and chromatid breaks in Fanconi's anemia. **Proc. Natl. Acad. Sci. (U.S.A.)**, 72:4066-4070.

Lambert WC and MW Lambert, 1985. Co-recessive inheritance: A model for DNA repair, genetic disease and carcinogenesis. **Mutation Res.**, 145:227-234.

Lambert WC and MW Lambert, 1986. Non-Poisson analysis of DNA endonucleases with sequence substrate specificities. **Gene Anal. Tech.**, 3:75-77.

Lambert WC and MW Lambert, 1987. DNA repair deficiency and cancer in xeroderma pigmentosum. **Cancer Rev.**, 7:56-81.

Lambert WC and MW Lambert, 1989. Co-recessive inheritance: A model for diseases associated with defective DNA repair, In: M.W. Lambert and J. Laval, Eds., **DNA Repair Mechanisms and Their Biological Implications in Mammalian Cells**, Plenum Press, New York, pp., 399-428.

Lambert WC, and MW Lambert, 1992. Co-recessive inheritance: A model for surveillance genes in higher eukaryotes. **Mutation Res.**, 273:179-192.

Lambert MW, D Fenkart and M Clarke, 1988. Two DNA endonuclease activities from normal human and xeroderma pigmentosum chromatin active on psoralen plus ultraviolet light treated DNA. **Mutation Res.**, 193:65-73.

Lambert MW, DE Lee, AO Okorodudu and WC Lambert, 1982. Nuclear deoxyribonuclease activities in human lymphoblastoid and mouse melanoma cells: A comparative study. **Biochim. Biophys. Acta.**, 69:192-203.

Lambert WC, DD Parrish, D Fenkart, H-R Kuo, J Kovacs and MW Lambert, 1993. A new system for analysis of enzyme kinetics data applicable to complex macromolecular interactions. **Clin. Res.**, 41:441A.

Lambert MW, WC Lambert and AO Okorodudu, 1983. Nuclear DNA endonuclease activities on partially apurinic/apyrimidinic DNA in normal human and xeroderma pigmentosum lymphoblastoid cells and mouse melanoma cells. **Chem.-Biol. Interact.**, 46:109-120.

Lambert MW and DD Parrish, 1989. Modulation of activity of human chromatin-associated endonucleases on damaged DNA by nucleosome structure, In: M.W. Lambert and J. Laval, Eds., **DNA Repair Mechanisms and Their Biological Implications in Mammalian Cells**, Plenum Press, New York, pp. 295-324.

Lambert MW, GJ Tsongalis, WC Lambert, B Hang and DD Parrish, 1992. Defective DNA endonuclease activities in Fanconi's anemia cells, complementation groups A and B. **Mutation Res.**, 273:57-71.

Lan SY and MJ Smerdon, 1985. A nonuniform distribution of excision repair synthesis in nucleosome DNA. **Biochemistry**, 24:7771-7783.

Leadon SA and MM Snowden, 1988. Differential repair of DNA damage in human metallothionein gene family. **Mol. Cell. Biol.**, 8:5331-5338.

Manley JL, A Fire, A Cano, PA Sharp and ML Gefter, 1980. DNA-dependent transcription of adenovirus genes in a soluble whole-cell extract. **Proc. Natl. Acad. Sci. (U.S.A.)**, 77:3855-3859.

Matsumoto A, JMH Vos and PC Hanawalt, 1989. Repair analysis of mitomycin C-induced DNA cross-linking in ribosomal RNA genes in lymphoblastoid cells from Fanconi's anemia patients. **Mutation Res.**, 217:185-192.

McGhee JD and G Felsenfeld, 1980. Nucleosome structure. **Annu. Rev. Biochem.**, 49:1115-1156.

Mellon IM, VA Bohr, CA Smith and PC Hanawalt, 1986. Preferential DNA repair of an active gene in human cells. **Proc. Natl. Acad. Sci. (U.S.A.)**, 83:8878-8882.

Mortelmans K, EC Friedberg, H Slor, G Thomas and JE Cleaver, 1976. Defective thymine dimer excision by cell-free extracts of xeroderma pigmentosum cells. **Proc. Natl. Acad. Sci. (U.S.A.)**, 73:2757-2761.

Moustacchi E, D Papadopoulo, C Diatloff-Zito and M Buchwald, 1987. Two complementation groups of Fanconi's anemia differ in their phenotype response to a DNA-crosslinking treatment. **Human Genet.**, 75:45-47.

Moustacchi E, D Papadopoulo, D Averbeck, D Fraser and C Diatloff-Zito, 1989. Processing of photoinduced cross-links and monoadducts in human cell DNA: Genetic and molecular features, In: M.W. Lambert and J. Laval Eds., **DNA Repair Mechanisms and Their Biological Implications in Mammalian Cells**, Plenum Press, New York, pp. 471-482.

Mullenders LHF, AC van Kesteren, CJM Bussmann, AA van Zeeland, and AT Natarajan, 1986. Distribution of U.V.-induced repair events in higher-order chromatin loops in human and hamster fibroblasts. **Carcinogenesis**, 7:995-1002.

Mullenders, LHF, J Venema, L Mayne, A T Natarajan and AA van Zeeland, 1989. Non-random distribution of UV-induced repair in higher-order chromatin loops in human cells and its relationship to preferential repair of active genes, In: M.W. Lambert and J.Laval, Eds., **DNA Repair Mechanisms and Their Biological Implications in Mammalian Cells**, Plenum Press, New York, pp., 339-348.

Okorodudu AO, WC Lambert and MW Lambert, 1982. Nuclear deoxyribonuclease activities in normal and xeroderma pigmentosum lymphoblastoid cells. **Biochem. Biophys. Res. Commun.**, 108:576-584.

Owen DK and A Sancar, 1989. The (A)BC exinuclease of Escherichia coli has only the UvrB and UvrC subunits in the incision complex. **Proc. Natl. Acad. Sci. (U.S.A.)**, 86,5237-5241.

Papadopoulo D, D Averbeck and E Moustacchi, 1987. The fate of 8-methoxypsoralen-photo-induced DNA interstrand crosslinks in Fanconi's anemia cells of defined genetic complementation groups. **Mutation Res.**, 184:271-280.

Parrish DD and MW Lambert, 1990. Chromatin-associated DNA endonucleases from xeroderma pigmentosum cells are defective in interaction with damaged nucleosomal DNA. **Mutation Res.**, 235:65-80.

Parrish DD, WC Lambert and MW Lambert, 1992. Xeroderma pigmentosum endonuclease complexes show reduced activity on and affinity for psoralen cross-linked nucleosomal DNA. **Mutation Res.**, 273:157-170.

Plooy ACM, M van Dijk, F Berends and PHM Lohman, 1985. Formation and repair of DNA interstrand crosslinks in relation to cytotoxicity and unscheduled DNA synthesis induced in control and mutant human cells treated with cis-diamminedichloroplatinum (II). **Cancer Res.**, 45:4178-4184.

Poll EHA, F Arwert, HT Kortbeek and AW Eriksson, 1984. Fanconi anemia cells are not uniformly deficient in unhooking of DNA interstrand crosslink induced by Mitomycin C or 8-methoxypsoralen plus UVA. **Human Genet.**, 68:228-234.

Rinaldy A, T Bellew, T Egli and RS Lloyd, 1990. Increased UV resistance in xeroderma pigmentosum group A cells after transformation with a human genomic DNA clone. **Proc. Natl. Acd. Sci. U.S.A.**, 87:6818-6822.

Sancar A and GB Sancar, 1988. DNA repair enzymes. **Annu. Rev. Biochem.**, 51:29-68.

Santella RM, N Dharmaraja, FP Gasparro and RL Edelson, 1985. Monoclonal antibodies to DNA modified by 8-methoxypsoralen and ultraviolet A light. **Nucl. Acids Res.**, 13:2533-2544.

Sasaki MS, and A Tonomura, 1973. A high susceptibility of Fanconi's anemia to chromosome breakage by DNA cross-linking agent. **Cancer Res.**, 33:1829-1836.

Satokota I, K Tanaka, N Miura, I Miyamoto, Y Satoh, S Kondo and Y Okada, 1990. Characterization of a splicing mutation in group A xeroderma pigmentosum. **Proc. Natl. Acad. Sci. (U.S.A)**, 87:9908-9912.

Schroeder TM, 1982. Genetically determined chromosome instability syndromes. **Cytogenet. Cell Genet.**, 33:129-132.

Shaham M, B Adler, S Ganguly and RSK Chaganti, 1987. Transfection of normal human and Chinese hamster DNA corrects diepoxybutane-induced chromosomal hypersensitivity of Fanconi anemia fibroblasts. **Proc. Natl. Acad. Sci. (U.S.A.)**, 84:5853-5857.

Sibghat-Ullah, I Husain W Carlton and A Sancar, 1989. Human nucleotide excision repair in vitro: Repair of pyrimidine dimers, psoralen and cisplatin adducts by HeLa cell-free extract. **Nucl. Acids Res.**, 17:4471-4484.

Smerdon MJ, 1989. DNA excision repair at the nucleosomal level of chromatin In: M.W. Lambert and J. Laval Eds., **DNA Repair Mechanisms and Their Biological Implications in Mammalian Cells**, Plenum Press, New York, pp., 271-294.

Sognier MA, and WN Hittelman, 1983. Loss of repairability of DNA interstrand crosslinks in Fanconi's anemia cells with culture age. **Mutation Res.**, 108:383-393.

Sollner-Webb B, RD Camerini-Otero and G Felsenfeld, 1976. Chromatin structure as probed by nucleases and proteases: Evidence for the central role of histones H3 and H4. **Cell**, 9:179-193.

Strathdee CA, AMV Duncan and M Buchald, 1992. Evidence for at least four Fanconi anemia genes, including FACC, on chromosome 9. **Nature Genetics**, 1:196-198.

Song PS and KJ Tapley, Jr, 1979. Photochemistry and photobiology of psoralens. **Photochem. Photobiol.**, 29:1177-1197.

Tanaka K, N Miura, I Satokata, I Miyamoto, MC Yoshida, Y Satoh, S Kondo, A Yasui, H Okayama and Y Okada, 1990. Analysis of a human DNA excision repair gene involved in group A xeroderma pigmentosum and containing a zinc-finer domain. **Nature (London)**, 348:73-76.

Tsongalis GJ, WC Lambert and MW Lambert, 1990a. Electroporation of normal human DNA endonucleases into xeroderma pigmentosum cells corrects their DNA repair defect. **Carcinogenesis**, 11:499-503.

Tsongalis GJ, WC Lambert and M W Lambert, 1990b. Correction of the ultraviolet light induced DNA repair defect in xeroderma pigmentosum cells by electroporation of a normal human endonuclease. **Mutation Res.**, 244:257-263.

Uander EE, and B Fleischer-Reischman, 1983. Response of lymphocytes from Fanconi's anemia patients and their heterozygous relatives to 8-methoxypsoralen in a cloning survival test. **Human Genet.**, 64:167-172.

Vigny P, F Gaboriau, L Voituriez and J Cadet, 1985. Chemical structure of psoralen-nucleic acid photoadducts. **Biochimie**, 67:317-325.

Vuillaume M, L Daya-Grosjean, P Vincens, JL Pennetier, P Tarroux, A Baret, R Calvayrac, A Taieb, A Sarasin, 1992. Striking differences in cellular catalase activity between two repair-deficient diseases: Xeroderma pigmentosum and trichothiodystrophy. **Carcinogenesis**, 13:321-328.

Watanabe F, 1984. Condensation of polynucleosomes by histone H1 binding. **FEBS Lett.**, 170:19-22.

Weksberg R, M Buchwald, P Sargent and L Siminovitch, 1979. Specific cellular defects in patients with Fanconi's anemia. **J. Cell. Physiol.**, 101:311-324.

Wood RD, P Robins and T Lindahl, 1988. Complementation of the xeroderma pigmentosum DNA repair defect in cell-free extracts. **Cell**, 53:97-106.

Yamaizumi M, T Sugano, H Asahina, Y Okada and T Uchida, 1986. Microinjection of partially purified protein factor restores DNA damage specifically in group A of xeroderma pigmentosum cells. **Proc. Natl. Acad. Sci. (U.S.A.)**, 83:1476-1479.

INTERFERON MODULATES LYMPHOPROLIFERATION IN THE SKIN

Kristian Thestrup-Pedersen*
Keld Kaltoft†

* Department of Dermatology
† Institute of Human Genetics
University of Aarhus
Aarhus, Denmark

Correspondence to: Prof. Dr. Kristian Thestrup-Pedersen,
Department of Dermatology, University of Aarhus, Marselisorg Hospital,
DK-8000 Aarhus C, Denmark

ABSTRACT/INTRODUCTION

Interferon (IFN) therapy of CTCL patients has proven its efficacy in a number of clinical trials. The pronounced effect in some patients with an apparent cure, and its lack of effect in other cases underscores the fact that we do not know which mechanisms are important for its efficacy, neither do we know the pathophysiological events in CTCL.

This review summarizes the reported clinical experience using interferon therapy in CTCL. It also summarizes how interferon could possibly work in CTCL, based upon present experimental data, and it gives new data on the effect of interferon upon in vitro proliferation of our T cell lines isolated from patients with CTCL (Kaltoft et al., 1994).

CLINICAL EFFICACY OF INTERFERON THERAPY IN CTCL

Table 1 summarizes published trials where INF has been used in CTCL. The different designs and dosages used prevent detailed comparisons. It is thus not possible to see if IFN-alfa

Basic Mechanisms of Physiologic and Aberrant Lymphoproliferation in the Skin
Edited by W.C. Lambert *et al.*, Plenum Press, New York, 1994

535

Table 1. Results from published trials in which interferon (IFN) has been administered for treatment of CTCL.

Reference and IFN Dosage schedule	Route of IFN delivery	Number of patients	of disease	Complete response	Partial response	Not evaluated	Progression of disease
			Stage(s)	Outcome of IFN Treatment:			
a	im*	19	II-IVB	3	6	0	10
b	im	21	II-IVB	0	6	0	10
c	im	20	I-IVA	4	10	0	6
d	sc	10	I-IVA	8	9	0	2
e	im	6	unk.‡	1	3	1	0
f	im	5	II-IV	0	1	4	0
g	im	6	II-III	0	3	3	0
h	iv	6†	II-III	2	1	3	0
	il	10	II-III	5	1	4	0
i	sc	11	II-IVB	2	3	0	0
j	sc	23	II-III	8	9	6	0
k	im	15	unk.	12	2	0	0
l	iv	16	II-IVB	0	5	121	0
m	sc	16	II-III	5	6	5	0
n	sc	45	II-IV+SS	13	15	17	0
Total		212 ✦		58	77	77	28
(Total %)		(100%)		(27%)	(36%)	(36%)	(13%)

* im, intramuscular; sc, subcutaneous; iv, intravenous; il, intralesional

† One patient in the study identified as h received IFN intravenously, 10 intralesionally, and 5 both.

‡ unk.; not stated

✦ of 233 total patients reported, an evaluation was possible on 212 subjects.

a. Bunn et al., 1986; 50 million units per square meter body surface (mU/m^2) three times per week for a total of three months.

b. Ihde et al., 1987; 10 mU/m^2 on day 1, followed by 50 mU/m^2 on days 2-5, repeated every three weeks.

c. Olsen et al., 1987; 3-36 mU/m^2 daily for 1 week, followed by a maintenance regimen of this dose three times per week.

d. Covelli et al., 1987; 3-18 million units (mU) daily for three months, followed by a maintenance regimen of this dose three times per week.

e. De Mel et al., 1990; same schedule as d, above (Covelli et al., 1987) with, in addition, vinblastine, 0.06-0.15 mg per kg body weight administered every third week.

f. Lang et al., 1986; IFN-alfa.

g. Braathen, 1987; IFN-alfa combined with etretinate.

therapy is different in efficacy from IFN-gamma treatment, although Kaplan et al. (1990) suggests that this is so. IFN may be more efficacious when combined with other treatment modalities such as etretinate or psoralen plus ultraviolet A irradiation (PUVA).

It is the impression of the present authors that the early stages benefit most from treatment. A comparable experience comes from IFN usage in various hematological malignancies (Ziegler-Heitbrock et al., 1989). Low dosage IFN should be used in order to avoid intolerable side effects, because it must be realized that most patients have a Karnowsky index above 90. We have obtained a response to IFN in two patients, of twelve who participated in our initial trial on IFN therapy (Thestrup-Pedersen et al., 1988). One went into complete remission when given high-dosage IFN (36 million units three times per week) combined with etretinate, 50 mg daily. He stayed in remission for almost two years before he had a clinical relapse; histology was then non-specific. He was continued on ultraviolet A light (UVA) once weekly with good effect and he is now in complete remission six years following initiation of IFN therapy. The other patient was treated with IFN, alone, and went into complete remission following 18 months of therapy on 6 million units 3 times per week. He relapsed approximately twelve months after stopping therapy, and then was given topical nitrogen mustard with an immediate effect. He developed contact sensitivity, however, and his disease progressed. He was then given IFN-alfa, 3 million units 3 times per week; and he slowly went into remission. The therapy was stopped after nine months of treatment, and he is still in complete remission six years following the start of IFN therapy.

The study by Vegna et al. (1990) included 23 newly diagnosed cases; they experienced an overall response rate of 74% using IFN-alfa, alone.

---

h. Jimbow 1987; IFN-gamma.
i. Thestrup-Pedersen et al., 1988; IFN-alfa, 3-18 mU daily for 3 months, followed by a maintenance regime of this dose once per week; half the patients also received etretinate, 0.5 mg per kg body weight daily.
j. Vegna et al., 1990; 3-18 mU daily for three months, followed by a maintenance regimen of this dose three times per week.
k. Roenigk et al; 1990; 6-30 mU three times per week combined with photochemotherapy (psoralen plus untraviolet A light; PUVA).
l. Kaplan et al., 1990; IFN-gamma.
m. Simoni et al., 1987; IFN-alfa, 3-18 mU daily for 12 weeks, followed by a maintenance regimen of three times per week for six to nine months.
n. Dreno et al., 1991; IFN-alfa, 6 mU daily for two months, followed by 9 mU three times per week for up to 12 months. Etretinate, 0.5 mg per kg body weight per day, was also administered to those patients not showing a response to IFN, alone.

EFFECTS OF INTERFERON

A vast knowledge exists regarding the effects of interferon. We will briefly summarize what we believe may be relevant in order to explain how IFN therapy benefits CTCL patients.

Interferons

IFN consists of at least three different gene products: human interferon-alfa (HuIFN-alfa) is comprised of more than 20 subtypes with 70-80% amino acid homology to each other. Its encoding gene is located on the short arm of chromosome 9 and it is produced by leukocytes or lymphoblastoid cell lines following stimulation by virus or double stranded RNA products. HuIFN-beta is encoded by a different gene, also on chromosome 9; it is released following the same stimulants as IFN-alfa, but is secreted from fibroblasts and epithelial tissue. There exist different subtypes; the previous HuIFN-beta2 is interleukin 6. HuIFN-beta has 29% amino acid homology with HuIFN-alfa. Both INFs bind to the same receptors.

HuIFN-gamma is encoded by a gene on chromosome 12 and is released from activated T lymphocytes, NK cells or T cell lines following stimulation (i.e. exposure to mitogens, antibodies against CD3/Ti, etc.). It binds to a different receptor than does IFN-alfa/beta.

Interferon receptors

The number of IFN receptors varies on different cells, ranging from around 200 - 500 on T cells, to 1,800 on a lymphoma cell line and up to 4,000 on monocytes and Daudi cells (De Maeyer and De Maeyer-Guigard, 1988). Although binding of IFN is a prerequisite for an effect, it may not necessarily lead to one. Receptor expression can vary according to cell activity. Low amounts of interferon may induce an anti-viral effect before an anti-proliferative effect is seen. The availability of T cell clones will improve our knowledge about which mechanisms are important for an effect in CTCL.

HLA expression and adhesion molecules

An important effect of IFN is the up-regulation of class II antigens on cells such as monocytes, endothelial cells, etc. HuIFN-gamma is more potent than HuIFN-alfa in doing so. Besides HLA up-regulation, HuIFN-gamma upregulates adhesion molecules, in particular ICAM-l, in human skin (Griffiths et al., 1989). Some but not all malignant cells can increase their HLA class II antigen expression following IFN. This has been demonstrated in cells from patients with hairy cell leukemia (Baldini et al., 1986).

Phagocytosis and macrophage activation

IFN augments phagocytosis and activates macrophages to increased cytocidal activity. This effect seems partly mediated by the increased release of tumor necrosis factor, TNF (Urban et al., 1986). TNF release is induced by HuIFN-gamma, but not by HuIFN-alfa (Phillip and Epstein, 1986), whereas all INF's can upregulate TNF receptors on some target cells (Tsujimoto et al., 1986).

Natural Killer cell activity

Natural killer (NK) cell activity is boosted by IFN, but, apparently, this is a temporary phenomenon (Golub et al., 1982a;b). Alternatively, NK cell activity may actually become depressed (Greenberg et al., 1984; Spina et al., 1983). Also, high dosages of HuIFN-alfa can reduce NK activity (Edwards et al., 1985).

Interferon and cytokines

IFN affects various cytokines -- and vice versa. Thus, IFN-gamma and TNF-alfa have a synergistic inhibitory effect on cell proliferation (Ruggerio et al., 1986), and IFN-gamma stimulates both IL-1 and TNF-alfa release as well as up-regulates IFN-alfa/beta receptors (Phillips and Epstein, 1986). TNF-alfa can up-regulate IFN receptors (Tsujimoto et al., 1986) and induce IFN-beta expression in fibroblasts, increase 2',5' oligoadenylate synthetase, and mediate an anti-viral effect via IFN-beta (Phillips and Epstein, 1986). Likewise, IL-1 can induce an anti-viral response via IFN-beta (Van Damme et al., 1987). When patients are given IFN a spontaneous production of TNF-alfa and IL-1 beta has been demonstrated (Daniels et al., 1990).

Cellular effects of interferon

Two types of cellular enzyme systems are up-regulated by IFN's and seem to be important for their anti-viral effect:

i) the ribosomal protein kinase Pl and the alfa-subunit of protein synthesis initiation factor, eIF-1alfa

ii) The 2', 5' oligoadenylate synthetase including its activation of endoribonuclease, RNAse L/F.

It is possible to measure the cellular content of 2',5' oligoadenylate synthetase, and it has been found that IFN treated patients who show an up-regulation in vivo of the enzyme show a better clinical response to IFN-treatment (de Mel et al., 1990; Grandér et al., 1990). No data exist so far from CTCL patients treated with IFN.

INTERFERON AND LYMPHOPROLIFERATION

IFN inhibits the transition of cells from G_0/G_1 to S phase (Romeo et al., 1989). Only in a few cases has it been shown that IFN can actually stimulate tumor cells in vitro; this has been documented for cells isolated from patients with chronic lymphocytic leukemia (Roberts et al., 1985).

The Daudi cell line is very sensitive to IFN; one to 10 units/ml leads to almost complete inhibition of proliferation (Nederman et al., 1990). Normally, other cell lines are less sensitive (range 10 to 600 units/ml).

The cellular content of 2',5' oligoadenylate synthetase is up-regulated in IFN-treated cells. A high dosage of murine IFN-beta (MuIFN-beta), 1,800 units/ml, on NIH/3T3 cells leads to a sustained upregulation of the enzyme, despite the withdrawal of IFN, whereas a low dosage of 450 units/ml leads to a temporary upregulation of 2',5' oligoadenylate synthetase (Salzberg et al., 1990).

Interferon inhibits a CTCL cell line

We studied the effect of IFN-alfa2a on the in vitro proliferation of one of our cells lines, My-La. The results are shown in Figure 1. It is clearly seen that the malignant T cell clone CD8[+] phenotype is significantly inhibited by IFN, whereas the reactive T cell clone CD4[+] phenotype is not. Thus, there seems to be a preferential effect of IFN in its capacity to inhibit the malignant clone, which we believe acts as the stimulator in CTCL (Kaltoft et al., 1993). We are now in the process of studying 2',5' oligosynthetase activity, phenotype and cytokine expression in our cell lines.

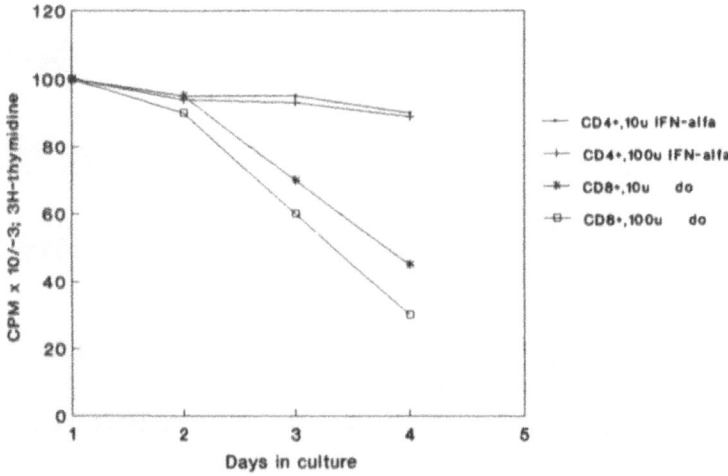

Figure 1. Effect of interferon on cell proliferation in My-La cell lines.

CONCLUSION

IFN seems useful in CTCL and may have a similar degree of efficacy in these disorders as it has in hairy cell leukemia. The effect may be due to a number of immunoregulatory properties of IFN, including its capacity to specifically inhibit malignant T cell clones. It must, however, be realized that not all patients exhibit a favorable response. Future investigations should include determinations of 2',5' oligosynthetase activity in mononuclear cells from blood before and during IFN therapy in order to see if this measurement reflects a better treatment response. Many patients with CTCL have auto-antibodies towards IFN, without prior treatment (Roob, Thingsgaard, and Vejlsgaard, personal communication). This finding indicates that IFN production may already be activated in vivo in these patients.

IFN therapy may, itself, induce neutralizing IFN-antibodies, which may then lead to a relapse of disease (von Wussow et al., 1991). This must also be kept in mind when patients relapse or do not respond to IFN treatment.

Despite these considerations, IFN offers an efficacious therapy for CTCL patients. Future studies are needed in order to increase our knowledge of optimal dosage schedules, choice of IFN, combination therapy, and which stages of disease benefit the most.

REFERENCES

Baldini L, A Cortelezzi, N Polli, A Neri, L Nobili, AT Naiolo, G Lambertenghi-Deliliers and EE Polli, 1986. Human recombinant interferon-alfa2a enhances the expression of class II HLA antigens on hairy cells. **Blood,** 67:458.

Braathen LR, 1987. Interferon alpha-2a combined with etretinate: Effective in the treatment of mycosis fungoides. **Retinoids Today and Tomorrow,** 9:17.

Bunn PA, D Ihde and KA Foon, 1986. The role of recombinant interferon alpha-2a in the therapy of cutaneous T cell lymphomas. **Cancer,** 57:1689.

Covelli A, R Cavalieri and G Coppola, 1987. Recombinant leukocyte A interferon (IFN-rA) as initial therapy in mycosis fungoides and Sézary syndrome. **Proc. Amer., Soc. Clin. Oncol.,** 6:189. (Abstract).

Daniels HM, A Neager, ALWF Eddleston, GJN Alexander and R Williams, 1990. Spontaneous production of tumour necrosis factor alfa and interleukin-1-beta during interferon-alfa treatment of chronic HBV infection. **Lancet,** 335:875.

De Maeyer-Guignard J and E De Mayer, 1986. Immunomodulation by interferons: Recent developments. In: Gresser, Burke, Cantell, et al., Eds: **Interferon.** Academic Press, London.

De Maeyer E and J De Maeyer-Guignard, 1988. **Interferons and other regulatory cytokines (Interferon Receptors).** Wiley Interscience Publications, New York. p. 67.

De Mel WCP, AV Hoffbrand, FJ Giles, AH Goldstone, AB Mehta and K Ganeshaguru, 1990. Alpha interferon therapy for haematological malignancies: Correlation between in vivo induction of the 2',5'oligoadenylate system and clinical response. **Brit. J. Haematol.**, 74:452.

Dean RT and JL Virelizier, 1983. Interferon as a macrophage activating factor. I. Enhance ment of cytotoxicity by fresh and matured human monocytes in absence of other soluble signals. **Clin. Exp. Immunol.**, 51:501.

Dreno B, A Claudy, J Meynadier, JL Verret, P Souteyrand, JP Ortonne, B Kalis, WY Godefroy, K Beerblock and L Thill, 1991. The treatment of 45 patients with cutaneous T-cell lymphoma with low doses of interferon-alfa2a and etretinate. **Brit. J. Dermatol.**, 125:456.

Edwards BS, JA Merrit, RC Fuhlbridg and EC Borden, 1985. Low doses of interferon alpha result in more effective clinical natural killer cell activation. **J. Clin. Invest.**, 75:1908.

Golub SH, P d'Amore and M Rainey, 1982a. Systemic administration of human leukocyte interferon to melanoma patients. II. Cellular events associated with changes in natural killer cytotoxicity. **J. Natl. Cancer. Inst.**, 68:711.

Golub SH, F Dorey, D Hara, DL Morton and MW Burk, 1982b. Systemic administration of human leukocyte interferon to melanoma patients. I. Effects on natural killer function and cell populations. **J. Natl. Cancer. Inst.**, 68:703.

Grandér D, K Oberg, M-L Lundquist, E Tiensuu-Jansson, B Eriksson and S Einhorn, 1990. Interferon-induced enhancement of 2',5'-oligoadenylate synthetase in mid-gut carcinoid tumors. **Lancet**, 336:336.

Greenberg AH, V Miller, T Jablonski and B Pohajdak, 1984. Suppression of NK-mediated natural resistance by interferon-beta treatment of murine lymphomas. **J. Immunol.**, 132:2129.

Griffiths CEM, JJ Voorhees and BJ Nickoloff, 1989. Characterization of intercellular adhesion molecule-1 and HLA-DR expression in normal and inflammed skin: Modulation by recombinant gamma interferon and tumor necrosis factor. **J. Am. Acad. Dermatol.**, 20:617.

Ihde DC, R Stays and EA Sauevllle 1987. Phase II trial of intermittent high-dose recomblnant interferon alpha2a in mycosis fungoides and Sézary syndrome. **Proc. Am. Assn. Cancer Res.**, 208.

Jimbow K, 1987. Clinical effect of gamma-interferon to cutaneous lymphoma and related disordors by systemic and intralesional administration. 17th World Congress of Dermatology, Berlin, 1.

Kaltoft K, S Bisballe, S Dyrberg, E Boel, PB Rasmussen and K Thestrup-Pedersen, 1994. Establishment of two continuous cell strains from a single plaque of a patient with mycosis fungoides. **Cell. Dev. Biol.**, 28A:161.

Kaltoft K, S Bisballe, W Sterry, H Sögaard and K Thestrup-Pedersen, 1993. Cutaneous T-cell lymphoma is defined by a family of genotraumatic T-cell clones. In: Lambert WC, B Giannotti, WA van Vloten, Eds: **Basic mechanisms of physiologic and aberrant lymphoproliferation in the skin**. Plenum Press, New York, This Volume.

Kaplan EH, ST Rosen, DB Norris, HH Roenigk, SR Sake and PA Bunn, 1990. Phase II study of recombinant human interferon gamma for treatment of cutaneous T-cell lymphoma. **J. Natl. Cancer Inst.**, 82:208.

Lang MH, P Altmeyer, E Lodemann and H Holzmann, 1986. Alpha-interferon in the therapy of cutaneous T cell lymphomas. **Z. Hautkr.**, 61:599.

Nederman T, E Karlstrom and B Sodin, 1990. An in vitro bioassay for quantitation of human interferons by measurements of antiproliferative activity on a continuous human lymphoma cell line. **Biologicals**, 18:29.

Olsen E, S Rosen and R Vollmer, 1987. Interferon alpha2a in the treatment of cutaneous T cell lymphoma. **Proc. Amer. Soc. Clin. Oncol.**, 6:189. (Abstract)

Phillip R and LB Epstein, 1986. Tumor necrosis factor as immunomodulator and mediator of monocyte cytotoxicity induced by itself, interferon-gamma and interleukin-1. **Nature**, 323:86.

Robert RH, S Einhorn, G Juliusson, L Ostlund and P Biberfeld, 1985. Interferon produces proliferation and differentiation in primary chronic lymphocytic leukemia cells. **Clin. Exp. Immunol.**, 62:530.

Roenigk HH, TM Kuzel, AP Skoutelis, E Springer, G Yu, W Caro, K Gilyon, D Variakojis, K Kaul and PA Bunn, 1990. Photochemotherapy alone or combined with interferon alpha-2a in the treatment of cutaneous T cell lymphoma. **J. Invest. Dermatol.**, 95:198S.

Romeo G, G Fiorucci and GB Rossi, 1989. **Interferons in cell growth and development**, 5:19.

Ruggerio V, J Tavernier, W Fiers and C Baglioni, 1986. Induction of the synthesis of tumor necrosis factor receptors by interferon-gamma. **J. Immunol.**, 136:2445.

Salzberg S, D Hacohen, S David, S Dovrat, S Ahwan, H Gamliel and M Birnbaum, 1990. Involvement of interferon-system in the regulation of cell growth and differentiation. **Scanning Microscopy**, 4:479.

Simoni R, R Cavalieri, G Coppola, L Ricciotti, O DePita, D Criscuolo, A Covelli, G Pappa and F Mandelli, 1987. Recombinant leukocyte interferon alfa-2a in the treatment of mycosis fungoides. **J. Biol. Regul. Homeost. Agents**, 1:93.

Spina CA, JL Fahey, D Durkos-Smith, F Dorey and G Sarna, 1983. Suppression of natural killer cell cytotoxicity in peripheral blood of patients receiving interferon therapy. **J. Biol. Resp. Modif.**, 2:458.

Thestrup-Pedersen K, R Hammer, K Kaltoft, H Sogaard and H Zachariae H, 1988. Treatment of mycosis fungoides with recombinant interferon-alpha-2a alone and in combination with etretinate. **Br. J. Dermatol.**, 118:811.

Tsujimoto M, YK Yip and J Vilcek, 1986. Interferon-gamma enhances expression of cellular receptors for tumor necrosis factor. **J. Immunol.** 136:2441.

Urban JL, HM Shepard, JL Rothstein, BJ Sugarman and H Schreiber, 1986. Tumor necrosis factor: A potent effector molecule for tumor killing by activated macrophages. **Proc. Natl. Acad. Sci. (USA)**, 83:5233.

Van Damme J, M De Ley, J Van Snick, CA Dinarello and A Billiau, 1987. The role of interferon-beta1 and the 26-Kda protein (interferon-beta2) as mediators of the antiviral effect of interleukin 1 and tumor necrosis factor. **J. Immunol.**, 139:1867.

Vegna ML, G Papa, D Defazio, F Pisani, G Coppola, O De Pita, P Puddu, G Ferranti, R Simoni and F Mandelli, 1990. Interferon alpha-2a in cutaneous T-cell lymphoma. **Eur. J. Haematol.**, 52:32.

Von Wussow P, H Pralle, H-K Hochkeppel, D Jakschies, S Sonnen, H Schmidt, D Müller-Rosenau, HF Haferlach, T Qwingers, U Rapp and H Deicher, 1991. Effective natural interferon-alfa therapy in recombinant interferon-alfa-resistant patients with hairy cell leukemia. **Blood**, 78:38.

USE OF RECOMBINANT INTERFERON-α-2a IN THE TREATMENT OF CUTANEOUS LYMPHOMAS OF T- AND B-CELL LINEAGE

Lorenzo Cerroni
Ketty Peris
Giancarlo Torlone
Sergio Chimenti

Department of Dermatology
University of L'Aquila
Rome, Italy

Correspondence to: Dr. L. Cerroni, Department of Dermatology,
University of Graz, Auenbruggerplatz 8,
A-8036 Graz, Austria

ABSTRACT

Three patients with primary cutaneous B-cell lymphoma (one centroblastic/centrocytic, one centroblastic, one centrocytic; CBCL) and 16 with primary cutaneous T-cell lymphoma (14 mycosis fungoides, one Sézary syndrome and one T-pleomorphic lymphoma; CTCL) were treated with escalating doses (3 to 9-18 million units) of recombinant interferon-α-2a (rIFN-α-2a). Complete response (CR) was obtained in 8 patients (2 CBCL; 6 CTCL), partial response (PR) in 7 CTCL patients, and no response (NR) in 4 patients (1 CBCL; 3 CTCL). Four of 8 patients with CR had recurrent disease under maintenance treatment. Side effects observed in most patients included fever, fatigue, liver alterations, leucocytopenia and thrombocytopenia. All side effects were completely reversible with dose attenuation.

INTRODUCTION

Interferons (IFNs) are members of a large family of regulatory proteins comprised of three main types: IFN-α, IFN-β and IFN-γ. IFN-α is produced by leucocytes, and has been shown to inhibit directly several tumor cell lines in vitro. Fifteen subtypes of IFN-α have been isolated, IFN-α2 being the most predominant subtype in α mixtures (Balkwill, 1989). In recent years, several investigators have used systemically administered IFN-α-2a (Bunn et al., 1986; Dreno et al., 1989; Hagberg et al., 1988; Nicholas et al., 1989; Olsen et al., 1989; Papa et al., 1989; Vegna et al., 1990), IFN-α-2b (Vonderheid et al., 1987), IFN-β (Liberati et al., 1988; Zinzani et al., 1988), and IFN-γ (Kaplan et al., 1990) for treatment of mycosis fungoides (MF) and other cutaneous T-cell lymphomas (CTCL). Complete remissions were reported in about half of patients treated with IFN-α who had not received previous therapy. Discouraging results were obtained with IFN-β and IFN-γ. In addition, IFN-α was also administered intralesionally in early lesions of MF with good responses (Vonderheid et al., 1987; Wolff et al., 1985). In more recent studies, IFN treatment was combined with other therapeutic options, such as retinoids (Knobler et al., 1991; Thestrup-Pedersen et al., 1988; Zachariae and Thestrup-Pedersen, 1990), photochemotherapy (PUVA) (Kuzel et al., 1990a; Otte et al., 1992; Roenigk et al., 1990), and extracorporeal photochemotherapy (Rook et al., 1991). In patients treated with combined therapy, complete response rates were about 80%. In addition to CTCL, IFN-therapy was also used for hairy cell leukemia and low-grade malignancy B-cell lymphomas of lymph nodes (Golomb et al., 1986; O'Connell et al., 1986; Quesada et al., 1984). In this article we will review the therapeutic effect of recombinant IFN-α-2a used alone in the therapy of cutaneous T- and B-cell lymphomas.

PATIENTS

Over the last 6 years, 19 patients (16 males and 3 females; mean age: 58.2 years) with histologically and immunohistochemically confirmed primary cutaneous T-cell (16 cases: 14 patch- and plaque stage MF; 1 Sézary syndrome; 1 T-pleomorphic lymphoma) or B-cell lymphoma (3 cases: 1 centroblastic/centrocytic lymphoma; 1 centroblastic lymphoma; 1 centrocytic lymphoma) were treated with systemically administered rIFN-α-2a. Most of the patients had received previously one or more of various treatment options (PUVA, retinoids, etc.).

TREATMENT PLAN

Subcutaneous injections of rIFN-α-2a were administered daily and escalated from an initial dose of 3 million units (MU) to 9 MU. In patients with minimal or no respone to 9 MU, doses were further escalated up to a maximum of 18 MU. After 8-12 weeks induction with these doses, patients underwent a maintenance phase where the maximal tolerated rIFN-α-2a dose (depending on the patient's response) was administered three times weekly for 6-12 months. In patients showing complete response to treatment, after this period the dose of rIFN-α-2a was reduced to 3 MU three times weekly. All patients with partial or no response at the end of this treatment protocol discontinued IFN-therapy and underwent other therapeutic modalities.

Definition of response: complete response (CR) was defined as disappearance of all clinical manifestations of the disease for a minimum of 4 weeks; partial response (PR) was defined as a minimum of 50% reduction of body involvement by lymphoma lesions; all patients failing to meet one of these two criteria were classified as cases with no response (NR).

RESULTS

Cutaneous B-cell lymphoma. Complete response was achieved in 2 of 3 patients with CBCL. One of these 2 patients (centrocytic lymphoma) had recurrence of cutaneous lesions under maintenance treatment. The other (centroblastic/centrocytic lymphoma) is in complete remission after 2 months maintenance therapy. In one patient (centroblastic lymphoma) the disease remained stationary.

Cutaneous T-cell lymphoma. Complete response was achieved in 6 of 16 patients with CTCL (5 MF, 1 Sézary syndrome). In 7 MF patients a partial remission could be observed, and in 2 the lesions persisted unchanged. The patient with T-pleomorphic lymphoma showed NR and died of systemic disease 9 months after finishing rIFN-α-2a treatment. Three of 6 patients with CR (2 MF, 1 Sézary syndrome) are free of disease after a mean follow-up of 14 months. The other 3 MF-patients had recurrent disease under maintenance treatment (mean interval free of disease: 13 months); one had recurrence of patches of MF, one developed localized nodules and tumors, and one showed lymph node involvement.

SIDE EFFECTS

Most patients experienced pyrexia (fever), headache, fatigue and anorexia at the beginning of rIFN-α-2a treatment. Leukopenia and thrombocytopenia were detected in about two thirds of cases. Liver toxicity was observed in 5 patients. None of the side effects were life-threatening, and all were reversible with dose attenuation. None of the patients had to interrupt the treatment due to toxic effects.

DISCUSSION

Therapy of CTCL, particularly of MF, is not yet standardized (Holloway et al., 1992; Jones, 1990; Kuzel et al., 1990b; Young, 1989). Several new treatments have been proposed for MF during the last few decades. Topical agents (nitrosurea, mechlorethamine (nitrogen mustard)), corticosteroids (both topically and systemically), PUVA, retinoids, extracorporeal photopheresis, total body electron beam radiation therapy, radiotherapy, monoclonal antibodies, and chemotherapy have been used. The role of IFN in MF therapy was recently evaluated by several investigators (Bunn et al., 1987; Bunn et al., 1990; Ziegler-Heitbrock and Thiel, 1990; Zinzani et al., 1991). Complete remissions were reported in 10-27% of previously treated and 50-70% of previously untreated patients. Partial response could be observed in most cases. The majority of patients showed recurrent disease, however, after discontinuing IFN-therapy. In this study, we observed CR in 37.5% of CTCL and 66.7% of CBCL patients. Three patients (15.8%) showed NR to treatment. Although CR and PR rates were 66.7% for CBCL and 81.3% for CTCL, only 4 of 8 patients with CR (21.1% of the total number) are free of disease under maintenance therapy, whereas 4 have had recurrent disease. Thus, combination with other treatment modalities may be necessary to improve the efficacy of therapy.

Various IFN-α doses have been used in different studies for treatment of CTCL. In the first clinical trial, patients received 50 MU/m^2 of rIFN-α-2a three times weekly (Sherwin et al., 1982). In the following years, other investigators used high doses of IFN-α (Bunn et al., 1984; Ihde et al., 1987; Simoni et al., 1987; Thestrup-Pedersen et al., 1988; Tura et al., 1987). Although therapeutic results have been encouraging, toxicity on these regimens has been considerable. Thus, in further studies slightly lower doses of IFN have been used (18-36 MU) (Kohn et al., 1990; Olsen et al., 1989; Hagberg et al., 1988; Vonderheid et al., 1987). To date, the optimal dose of rIFN-γ-2a for treatment of CTCL has not been established; it seems likely that low doses have at least as good clinical activity as do higher doses, with less toxicity, and should therefore be preferred for treatment of patients with cutaneous lymphoma.

Toxic effects due to IFN-α therapy include influenza-like syndrome (fever, headache, chills, malaise, anorexia, myalgia, fatigue and weight loss), increased serum levels of liver enzymes, leukopenia, and thrombocytopenia. Patients usually develop tachyphylaxis for influenza-like symptoms within the first few weeks. Other side effects reported in some cases include gastrointestinal cramps, dizziness, visual blurriness, and painful feet (Vonderheid et al., 1987), reduced libido (Nicolas et al., 1989), cough and hair loss (Olsen et al., 1989), and the nephrotic syndrome (Sherwin et al., 1982). All side effects are reversible with dose attenuation or cessation of the therapy. In one case, multiple basal and squamous cell carcinomas arose during IFN-treatment (Olsen et al., 1989). One patient died of infection during the neutropenic phase (Vegna et al., 1990). Production of anti-IFN antibodies by IFN-α-2a-treated patients has also been reported (Olsen et al., 1989). In this study, side effects were not life-threatening, and usually disappeared after the first few weeks of treatment. Liver toxicity was found in 26.3% of patients. A return to baseline values was observed in all of these patients following IFN dose attenuation.

The mechanism(s) that induces regression of cutaneous lesions in IFN-treated skin lymphomas is still speculative. One possible mechanism may involve augmentation of T-suppressor, natural killer cell, or macrophage activity. IFN-α inhibits T-cell helper lymphocytes by stimulating the activity of T-suppressor lymphocytes in vitro, thus providing a possible explanation for at least one of the effects of the drug in lesions of CTCL. Alteration of antigen expression by malignant cells may also play a role in the IFN-mediated immunologic reactions directed against neoplastic cells. Finally, direct anti-proliferative activity by IFN has been demonstrated in vitro in cell culture (Stadler et al 1989).

In conclusion, IFN-α-2a is a relatively safe therapy for cutaneous lymphoma, and may be considered as a valid alternative to other treatment modalities.

REFERENCES

Balkwill FR, 1989. Interferons. **Lancet** i:1060-1063.

Bunn PA, KA Foon, DC Ihde et al., 1984. Recombinant leukocyte A interferon: An active agent in advanced cutaneous T cell lymphoma. **Ann. Int. Med.**, 101:484-487.

Bunn PA, DC Ihde and KA Foon, 1987. Recombinant interferon alfa-2a: An active agent in advanced cutaneous T-cell lymphomas. **Int. J. Cancer**, Suppl.1:9-13.

Bunn PA, DC Ihde and KA Foon, 1986. The role of recombinant interferon alfa-2a in the therapy of cutaneous T-cell lymphomas. **Cancer**, 57:1689-1695.

Bunn PA and DA Norris, 1990. The therapeutic role of interferons and monoclonal antibodies in cutaneous T-cell lymphomas. **J. Invest. Dermatol.**, 95:209S-212S.

Dreno B, WY Godefroy, M Fleischmann et al., 1989. Low-dose recombinant interferon-alpha in the treatment of cutaneous T-cell lymphoma. **Br. J. Dermatol.**, 121:543-544.

Golomb HM, A Jacobs, A Fefer et al., 1986. Alpha-2 interferon therapy of hairy-cell leukemia: A multicentric study of 64 patients. **J. Clin. Oncol.**, 4:900-905.

Hagberg H, L Juhlin, A Scheynius and U Tjernlund, 1988. Low dosage alpha-interferon treatment in patients with advanced cutaneous T-cell lymphoma. **Eur. J. Haematol.**, 40:31-34.

Halloway KB, FP Flowers and FA Ramos-Caro, 1992. Therapeutic alternatives in cutaneous T-cell lymphoma. **J. Am. Acad. Dermatol.**, 27:367-378.

Ihde DC, R Steis, A Sausviller et al., 1987. Phase II trial of intermittent high dose recombinant interferon-α2a in mycosis fungoides and Sézary syndrome. **Proc. Am. Assoc. Cancer Res.**, 28:208.

Jones SE, 1990. Enigma of therapy for cutaneous T-cell lymphoma. **J. Natl. Cancer Inst.**, 82:169-170.

Kaplan EH, ST Rosen, DB Norris et al., 1990. Phase II study of recombinant human interferon gamma for treatment of cutaneous T-cell lymphoma. **J. Natl. Cancer Inst.**, 82:208-212.

Knobler RM, Trautinger F, Radaszkiewicz T et al., 1991. Treatment of cutaneous T cell lymphoma with a combination of low-dose interferon alfa-2b and retinoids. **J. Am. Acad. Dermatol.**, 24:247-252.

Kohn EC, R Steis, E Sausville et al., 1990. Phase II trial of intermittent high dose recombinant interferon alpha 2a in mycosis fungoides and Sézary syndrome. **J. Clin. Oncol.**, 8:155-160

Kuzel TM, KI Gilyon, E Springer et al., 1990a. Interferon alfa-2a combined with phototherapy in the treatment of cutaneous T-cell lymphoma. **J. Natl. Cancer Inst.**, 82:203-207.

Kuzel TM, E Springer, HH Roenigk Jr. and ST Rosen, 1990b. Mycosis fungoides: Time to define the best therapy. **J. Natl. Cancer Inst.**, 82:200-202.

Liberati AM, B Biscottini, M Fizotti et al., 1988. A phase I study of human natural interferon-β. **J. Interferon Res.**, 8:765-777.

Nicolas JF, JC Balblanc, A Frappaz et al., 1989. Treatment of cutaneous T cell lymphoma with intermediate doses of interferon alpha 2a. **Dermatologica**, 179:34-37.

O'Connell MJ, JP Colgan, MM Oken et al., 1986. Clinical trial of recombinant leukocyte A interferon as initial therapy for favorable histology non-Hodgkin's lymphomas and chronic lymphocytic leukemia. An Eastern cooperative oncology group pilot study. **J. Clin. Oncol.**, 4:128-136.

Olsen EA, ST Rosen, RT Vollmer et al., 1989. Interferon alfa-2a in the treatment of cutaneous T cell lymphoma. **J. Am. Acad. Dermatol.**, 20:395-407.

Otte HG, A Herges and R Stadler, 1992. Kombinationstherapie mit interferon alfa 2a und PUVA bei kutanen T-Zell-Lymphomen. **Hautarzt**, 43:695-699.

Papa G, ML Vegna, D Defazio et al., 1989. Recombinant interferon alpha-2a in untreated cutaneous T-cell lymphomas. **J. Interferon Res.**, 9:Suppl. 2:112.

Quesada JR, J Reuben, JT Manning et al., 1984. Alpha interferon for induction of remission in hairy-cell leukemia. **N. Engl. J. Med.**, 310:15-18.

Roenigk HH Jr., TM Kuzel AP Skoutelis et al., 1990. Photo-chemotherapy alone or combined with interferon alpha-2a in the treatment of cutaneous T-cell lymphoma. **J. Invest. Dermatol.**, 95:198S-205S.

Rook AH, MB Prystowsky, M Cassin et al., 1991. Combined therapy for Sézary syndrome with extracorporeal photochemotherapy and low-dose interferon alfa therapy. **Arch. Dermatol.**, 127:1535-1540.

Sherwin SA, JA Knost, S Fein et al., 1982. A multiple-dose phase I trial of recombinant leukocyte A interferon in cancer patients. **JAMA**, 248:2461-2466.

Simoni R, R Cavalieri, G Coppola et al., 1987. Recombinant leukocyte interferon-γ-2a in the treatment of mycosis fungoides. **J. Biol. Regul. Homeost. Agents**, 1:93-99.

Stadler R, A Mayer-da-Silva, B Bratzke et al., 1989. Interferons in dermatology. **J. Am. Acad. Dermatol.**, 20:650-656.

Thestrup-Pedersen K, R Hammer, K Kaltoft et al., 1988. Treatment of mycosis fungoides with recombinant interferon-2a alone and in combination with etretinate. **Br. J. Dermatol.**, 118:811-818.

Tura S, P Mazza, PL Zinzani et al., 1987. Alpha recombinant interferon in the treatment of mycosis fungoides. **Haematologica**, 72:337-340.

Vegna ML, G Papa, D Defazio et al., 1990. Interferon alpha-2a in cutaneous T-cell lymphoma. **Eur. J. Haematol.**, 45:Suppl. 52:32-35.

Vonderheid EC, R Thompson, KA Smiles and A Lattanand, 1987. Recombinant interferon alfa-2b in plaque-phase mycosis fungoides. Intralesional and low-dose intramuscular therapy. **Arch. Dermatol.**, 123:757-763.

Wolff JM, JA Zitelli, BS Rabin et al., 1985. Intralesional interferon in the treatment of early mycosis fungoides. **J. Am. Acad. Dermatol.**, 13:604-612.

Young RC, 1989. Mycosis fungoides. The therapeutic search continues. **N. Engl. J. Med.**, 321:1822-1823.

Zachariae H and K Thestrup-Pedersen, 1990. Interferon alpha and etretinate combination treatment   of cutaneous T-cell lymphoma. **J. Invest. Dermatol.**, 95:206S-208S.

Ziegler-Heitbrock HWL and E Thiel, 1990. Recombinant IFN-alpha in lymphomas. **J. Invest. Dermatol.**, 95:213S-215S.

Zinzani PL, P Mazza and F Gherlinzoni, 1988. Beta interferon in the treatment of mycosis fungoides. **Haematologica**, 73:545.

Zinzani PL, P Mazza, F Gherlinzoni et al., 1991. Mycosis fungoides: A therapeutical review. **Haematologica**, 76:150-161.

THYMOPENTIN IN SÉZARY SYNDROME:
CLINICAL AND IMMUNOLOGICAL EFFECTS

Maria Grazia Bernengo
Antonella Appino
Mauro Novelli

Clinica Dermatologica
Universita di Torino
Torino, Italy

Correspondence to: Dr. M. G. Bernengo, Clin. Dermatologica,
dell' Univ. di Torino, Via Cheraso 23,
I-10126 Torino, Italy

ABSTRACT

Thymopentin (TP-5) is a synthetic pentapeptide, Arg-Lys-Asp-Val-Tyr, corresponding to the active site of the linear 48-amino acid human hormone, thymopoietin. T helper cell immunostimulation by TP-5 has been demonstrated in a number of animal models and in man. TP-5 restores defective IL-2 levels in aged and thymectomized mice. Increases in cytotoxic/suppressor lymphocytes and in vivo enhancement of NK cell activity have been reported to be induced by this pentapeptide. In this paper, the results of TP-5 treatment in 21 patients with Sézary syndrome (SS), including clinical, immunologic and histologic effects on skin clearing, are examined. No in vitro effect of TP-5, alone, at any concentration, could be demonstrated in Sézary cells; however, the combination of TP-5 and phytohemagglutin (PHA) induced an increment in proliferative response which was only seen in cells from the Sézary syndrome patients. Eight complete remissions and eight partial remissions (76%) were obtained in 21 patients treated by intravenous injection with TP-5, 50 mg three times per week, for a median duration of 15 months of treatment (3-36 months). The response was accompanied by an increase in peripheral blood Sézary cell proliferative activity and an increase in the expression of CD8 and activation antigens, including CD25, and in $CD16^+CD56^+$ cells. By contrast, a significant decrease in CD25 and other activation antigens was found in the skin infiltrate. This reduction paralleled the loss of epidermotropism and the almost complete disappearance of the infiltrate in responsive cases. Circulating levels of soluble interleukin-2 receptor (sIL-2R) were determined before and during TP-5 treatment in 19 of the 21 patients. Pretreatment values were

Basic Mechanisms of Physiologic and Aberrant Lymphoproliferation in the Skin
Edited by W.C. Lambert *et al.*, Plenum Press, New York, 1994

553

900-2,000 U/ml in 4 patients and > 4,000 U/ml (range, 4,519-18,800 U/ml) in the remainder. A decrease was observed during TP-5 treatment in 13 of 19 patients, an increase in four and no change in two. In six of eight patients in whom a complete remission was obtained, sIL-2R levels returned to normal.

INTRODUCTION

Mycosis fungoides (MF) and Sézary syndrome (SS) are part of a spectrum of T-cell proliferative disorders for which the term, cutaneous T-cell lymphoma (CTCL), has been coined (Lutzner et al., 1975; Edelson, 1980). Some therapeutic measures have proved effective in bringing about remissions: topical chemotherapy with mechlorethamine (HN2), photochemotherapy with psoralens and ultraviolet A light (PUVA), radiotherapy, topical, total body electron beam therapy (EBT) and systemic chemotherapy (for review see Wieselthier and Koh, 1990). Topical HN2 is particularly useful in early stage MF and against some tumor lesions, but ineffective in erythrodermic stages, and the duration of response is frequently short. EBT therapy produces durable complete responses with a relatively high frequency and without undue systemic toxicity. Remission periods in patients with extracutaneous disease are short, however, and SS is often unresponsive. Systemic chemotherapy against extracutaneous disease is theoretically the best choice of treatment, as a supplement to skin management, in advanced cases. Since SS involves an elderly population, aggressive chemotherapy is often poorly tolerated, and profound immunodepression often causes death due to opportunistic infection. Objective results have been achieved with lymphokine-activated killer cells in solid neoplasms (Rosenberg et al., 1987). Interferon (IFN) (Bunn et al., 1987) and photopheresis (Edelson et al., 1987) have been reported to induce remissions in CTCL, reinforcing the role of the immune response and of immunomodulatory approaches in these diseases. Thymopentin (TP-5) is a synthetic pentapeptide, Arg-Lys-Asp-Val-Tyr, corresponding to the active site of the linear, 48-amino acid human hormone, thymopoietin (Goldstein et al., 1979). It induces differentiation in immature thymocytes through induction of cyclic-AMP-mediated intracellular events. Furthermore, it modulates intracellular cyclic GMP levels, enhancing helper functions and inducing proliferation in mature T cells. T helper cell immunostimulation by TP-5 has been demonstrated in a number of animal models and in man. TP-5 restores the defective IL-2 population in aged and thymectomized mice. In addition, an increase in cytotoxic/suppressor lymphocytes was observed by Kang et al. (1983), and in vivo enhancement of NK cell activity was found by Hu et al. (1990), in elderly subjects. A double-blind trial with TP-5 versus placebo (Leung et al., 1990) demonstrated a statistically significant reduction in clinical score of severity in atopic dermatitis. Our preliminary results indicated a clinical, histological and immunological activity of TP-5 given to patients with SS (Bernengo et al., 1988). In this paper, we analyze the "in vivo" immunological effects of TP-5 treatment in order to elucidate its mechanism of action.

CLINICAL RESULTS

Eighteen men and 3 women were treated in our department between 1 October, 1985, and

October, 1990, and followed until 30 June, 1991. Their mean age was 67.8 years (range 43 - 88 years) at diagnosis, and 55.7 ± 12.5 years (range 43 - 87 years) at onset of cutaneous manifestations. The median interval from onset to confirmation (skin and peripheral blood involvement) was 9 months (range 1 month in 3 patients to nine years in 1 patient). Frequent biopsies and peripheral blood examinations documented the appearance of Sézary cells (SC) in the peripheral blood, and the changes in chronic cases followed from the onset of the disease. Four cases had a previous history of contact dermatitis with positive patch tests. The allergens were metals, cosmetics and topical medications. Erythroderma was present in 21 of 21 patients, hyperkeratosis of the palms and soles in 18, onychodystrophy in 18, generalized lymphadenopathy in 19 (retroperitoneal enlarged lymph nodes, only, were found with computer assisted tomology (CAT) in 2 patients). Lymph node involvement (LN4, according to Bunn et al., 1979) was found in 18 patients with generalized lymphadenopathy. Hepatosplenomegaly was found in 19. Mean SC in peripheral blood were 26.2% ± 14.2% (range 10 - 60%), the absolute number ranged from 1,032 per mm^3 (in only one patient) to 11,940 per mm^3 (mean 3,181 ± 2,893 per mm^3). SC represented at least 50% of all lymphoid cells. Eight patients had had previous treatment, including chlorambucil, (CHL), cyclophosphamide (COP), vincristine, interferon (IFN), etoposide, and prednisone, without response; 13 patients had not been treated.

Treatment consisted of TP-5, 50 mg, intravenously (IV) three times per week for a median interval of 13 months (3 - 36 months). If complete remission (CR) was obtained, this was reduced to twice per week, and then to once per week for a median interval of six months (range 4 - 25 months). When only partial remission (PR) occurred, the treatment was continued for a median of 7 months, after which it was accompanied by chemotherapy with CHL or COP in 6 patients and with etretinate in one. TP-5 treatment was continued alone in 2 patients, in one for 8 months and in the other one for 36 months. All patients were HIV and HTLV-1 negative. A monoclonal rearrangement of T-cell receptor beta and gamma chain genes was found in each of nine patients tested.

A complete remission (CR) was defined as the complete resolution of all clinical evidence of disease with SC ≤ 2% (< 300/mm^3), lasting at least 1 month. A partial remisison (PR) was defined as at least 50% reduction in the sum of the products of the dimensions of the measurable lesions, reduction of infiltration and erythema, and a greater than 50% decrease in the absolute number of circulating SC. Progression (P) was defined as increase in skin infiltration and a 25% or greater increase in the sum of the perpendicular measurements or the development of any new malignant lesion. Response duration was calculated from the first day of documented CR or PR until relapse.

Objective responses were found in 16 of 21 patients (76%) (95% confidence limits 57.8% - 94.2%): CR in 8 patients and PR in 8. Three patients displayed no substantial response (i.e., decrease in skin infiltration, reduction of itching without reduction of erythema, and a 50% reduction of lymph node size but < 50% reduction of SC percentage in the peripheral blood). Progression was observed in two patients with high peripheral blood SC. Patients who achieved

CR had < 2,600/mm^3 peripheral blood SC at diagnosis. The overall median duration of response was 20 months: CR, 25.5 months (range 14 - 45), and PR, 15.5 months. Regression began after a minimum of 1 month to a maximum of 11 months (median 3.5 months) of treatment. CR was obtained in a median period of 6.1 months (range 2 - 9 months). Five patients died during the follow-up due to progression of the disease and 2 from unrelated causes. One complete responder died 38 months after beginning TP-5 therapy and 14 months after CR. Seven patients are now in CR without therapy.

The fourth-year-survival probability in the 21 patients, after starting TP-5 treatment, is 46.3%. The five-year-survival probability is 49.3% from diagnosis and 67.7% from onset. Four out of six patients previously treated with chemotherapy had had generalized herpesvirus infection before TP-5 treatment. Herpesvirus infection did not recur during TP-5 treatment and the follow-up period. A single herpes simplex episode after treatment with TP-5 was observed in only 2 patients; it was confined to a few vesicles on the upper lip and face.

Three CR and 4 PR (41%) (95% confidence limits: 18.3% - 67.5%) were observed in 17 control patients, selected on basis of their similar clinical histories (13 M, 4 F, aged 49 - 82 years, mean: 64.3, at diagnosis; mean: 62.2, range: 47-81, at onset), treated with a single comparable agent or combination chemotherapy only. In this control group, 14 patients were treated between 1978 and 1986 and 3 patients were treated in 1989. The median duration of CR was 12 months (3 - 96 months) and the median PR duration was 10.5 months (3 - 28 months). Sixteen patients died, 14 due to the disease and 2 from unrelated causes. Severe, generalized herpes simplex with a high temperature and metabolic imbalance, unresponsive to Acyclovir, occurred in 13 patients. Five-year-survival probability in this group is 30.3% from onset and 14.8% from the date of diagnosis. Seven of these control subjects had peripheral blood SC < 2,600/mm^3: 6 of 7 died due to visceral involvement in a median time of 12 months. The five-year-survival probability from diagnosis is 28.6%. By contrast, 13 of 21 patients treated with TP-5 had SC < 2,600/mm^3 and only one patient died. The four-year-survival probability is 66.7% and the median survival is 34 months from the date of diagnosis.

Side effects

No toxicity was observed. The only side-effects observed were episodes of vasovagal syndrome (tachycardia, hypotension and erythematous flush) during the first infusion in 3 cases. These did not require treatment, nor was alteration of the dosage deemed necessary. All patients reported increased sweating during the first month of treatment. Transformation into a high-grade immunoblastic lymphoma was not observed in any case.

IMMUNOLOGICAL FINDINGS

The peripheral blood mononuclear cell (PBMC) immunologic profile was determined before and during TP-5 treatment in 19 patients. Both percentages and absolute numbers of CD4$^+$ cells significantly decreased after treatment and the decrease paralleled the clinical course (Figure 1a). The baseline percentage of CD8$^+$ cells, significantly lower than that of normal controls, increased after therapy, reaching normal values (Figure 1b). The absolute number did not differ from normal controls and the increase was not statistically significant, however, although, if we consider only the responders, the increase in CD8$^+$ cells after therapy was significant (371 $\pm$ 229 versus 604 $\pm$ 369: p = 0.04).

The more relevant finding was an increase in NK cells (CD16$^+$/CD56$^+$ cells), which was confirmed by the appearance of large granular lymphocytes in the peripheral blood (Table 1). Recently, Lynch et al. (1990) identified a subgroup of MF/SS patients with circulating activated granular lymphocytes expressing natural killer cell surface markers (GL/NHK1$^+$). These patients had a longer survival and a slower progression than GL/NHK1 negative patients. In our study, an increase in NK cells was observed in 7 of 8 CR, 5 of 7 PR and 2 stable disease patients. Survival of these patients was significantly higher (p < 0.05) than that of patients with decreasing numbers of NK cells. These data suggest that an anti-tumor cytotoxic immune response is elicited by TP-5.

Activation antigens

Before treatment, less than 5% of unstimulated, freshly isolated PBMC reacted with anti-CD25 antibody in all but one cases. CD71, CD38, HLA-DR, CD69 and TLISA antigens were also found in very low percentages. After a 48 hour culture in medium alone a slight but significant increase in CD25$^+$ cells was observed in comparison to normal controls. A similar increase in CD71$^+$ cells was found. PHA stimulation evoked the appearance of activation antigens in all cases. The percentage of CD25$^+$ cells, although reduced, did not differ significantly from that of normal lymphocytes; on the other hand, CD38 positive and CD69 positive cells were significantly reduced compared to normal lymphocytes. Addition of recombinant IL-2 to PHA did not lead to an increase in expression of activation antigens, which

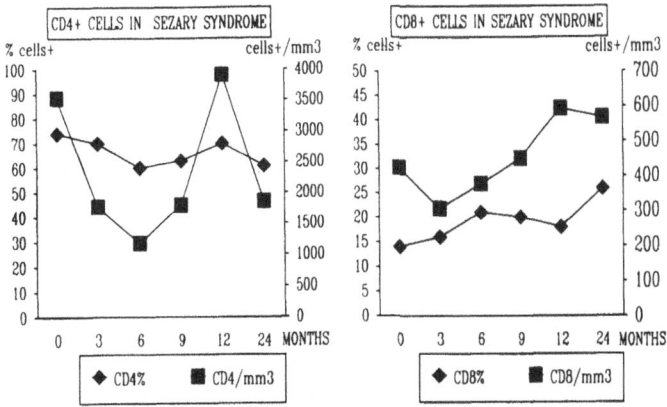

Figure 1. Follow-up analysis of (A) CD4 and (B) CD 8 positive cells in 15 patients.

Table 1. T-cell and NK cell subpopulations before and after TP-5 treatment in SS patients.

	CD4		CD8		CD16-CD56	
	%	mm⁻³	%	mm⁻³	%	mm⁻³
A- Before TP-5 (19)	74.1 ± 15.1	3,536 ± 4,665	14.0 ± 8.8	424 ± 276	7.2 ± 7.5	206 ± 274
B- After TP-5 (19)	61.2 ± 15.6	1,857 ± 2,316	26.1 ± 11.6	568 ± 383	17.8 ± 12.0	504 ± 642
C- Controls (25)	49.0 ± 4.2	1,027 ± 340	25.7 ± 1.0	544 ± 207	20.1 ± 6.2	420 ± 175
A vs B	$p < 0.01$	$p < 0.01$	$p < 0.0001$	N.S.	$p < 0.005$	$p < 0.05$
A vs C	$p < 0.01$	$p < 0.02$	$p < 0.001$	N.S.	$p < 0.001$	$p < 0.005$
B vs C	$p < 0.01$	N.S.	N.S.	N.S.	N.S.	N.S.

remained significantly lower than in normal lymphocytes. SC did not differ from normal lymphocytes when cultured with IL-2, alone.

After TP-5 treatment an increase in all activation antigens was observed; values comparable

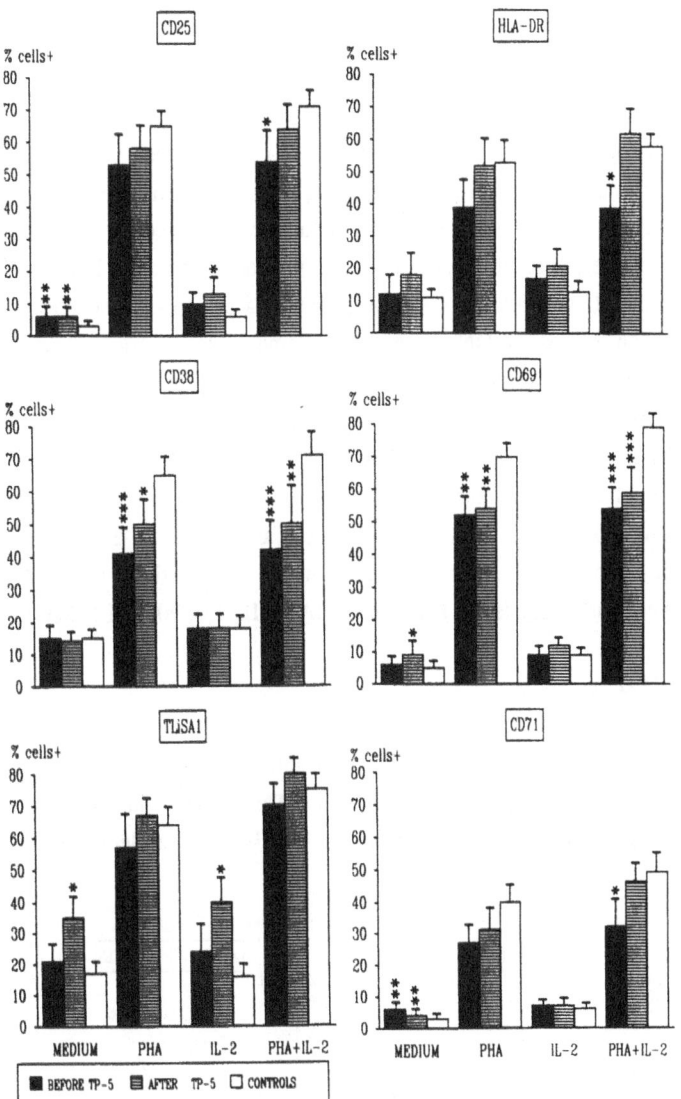

Figure 2. Activation antigens of peripheral blood leukocytes from 15 SS patients cultured for 48 hours before and after TP-5 therapy.

Patients vs normal control: $* = p > 0.05$; $** = p < 0.01$; $*** = p < 0.001$ (Student t test)

to those of normal controls were found, except for CD38 and CD69. An increase in cells bearing CD25, CD71, CD69 and TLISA was found when the lymphoid cells were cultured in medium along with TP-5 (Figure 2). All of these modifications are likely due to the activity of

559

normal cells present in larger numbers after treatment, although the partial acquisition of some functional capacity by the atyical cells cannot be ruled out. In fact, an increase in expression of activation antigens and proliferative activity was found after PHA stimulation in two cases with a pure neoplastic population (SC >95% of lymphoid cells).

Proliferative activity

Before therapy a defective or absent proliferative response to PHA, Conconavalin A (ConA) and pokeweed mitogen (PWM) was observed in 12 of 14 patients tested. The addition of recombinant IL-2 to the culture medium containing PHA led to an increase in the proliferative response in 11 patients. DNA synthesis was not further increased by IL-2 treatment in two patients with normal responses to PHA. Increasing the concentration of PHA (to 5 or 10 μg/ml) did not improve the SC proliferative response, however a prolonged incubation time with PHA and IL-2 induced an increase in DNA synthesis in some cases. SC did not respond directly to IL-2, and their proliferative response was not improved by higher concentrations (250, 500 and 100 U/ml). A prolonged incubation time (72 hours and 7 days) gave a little increase, but in no case did it differ from that of normal lymphocytes. No in vitro effect of TP-5, alone, at any concentration, could be demonstrated in SC; however, the combination of TP-5 (at the optimal dose of 10 μg/ml) and PHA or PHA + IL-2 induced an increase in the proliferative response seen only in the SS patients. After treatment, an "in vivo" activity on DNA synthesis was confirmed by the higher response to PHA and PHA + IL-2 in 90% of patients (Figure 3a).

Serum soluble IL-2 receptors

Another point of clinical interest raised by our study is the utility of the serum sIL-2R test in monitoring of SS clinical course and treatment. This, indeed, has already proved to be a helpful parameter in other hematological disorders, mainly hairy cell leukemia and Hodgkin and

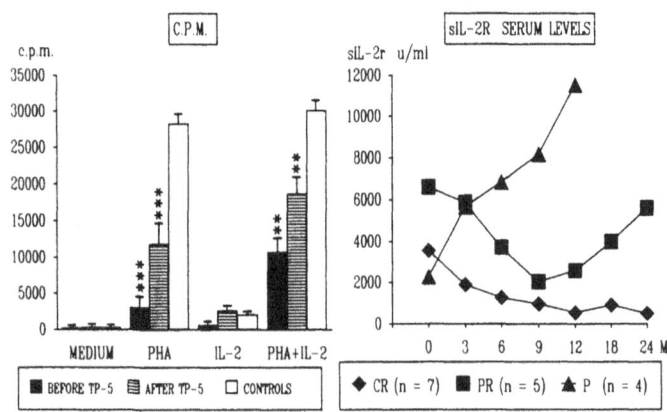

Figure 3. (A) PBL proliferative activity before and after therapy in SS patients compared to normal controls. (B) Follow-up of SS patients with sIL-2R serum levels.

non-Hodgkin lymphomas (Pizzolo et al., 1987; Wagner et al., 1987; Steis et al., 1988). sIL-2R was determined before and during TP-5 therapy in 19 of 21 patients. Pretreatment values were 900 - 2,000 U/ml in 4 patients and >4,000 U/ml (range: 4,519 - 18,800 U/ml) in the remainder. Normalization was observed in 6 CR patients (normal values, 375 $\pm$ 100 U/ml); a > 50% reduction in 5 PR, 1 CR and 1 NC (Figure 3b). Progressively increasing values were obtained in 2 P and in 2 NC. Unchanged values were found in 1 CR and 1 PR.

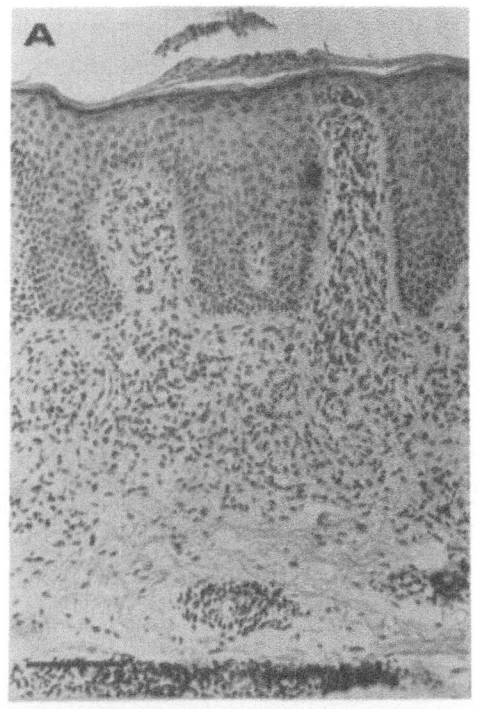

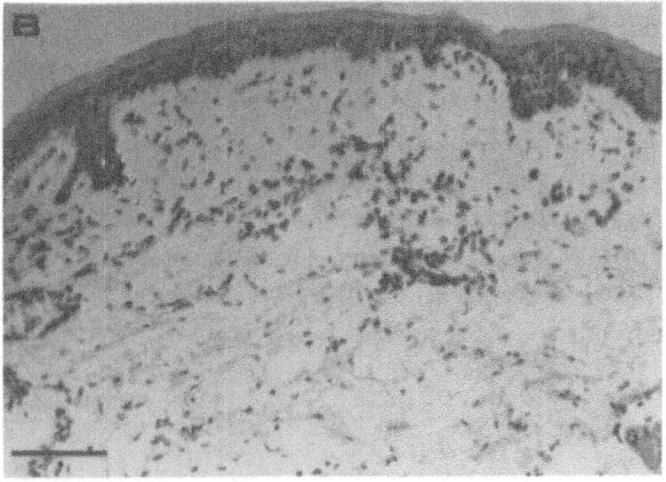

Figure 4. Skin biopsy (A) before treatment and (B) after 5 months of TP-5 therapy. Almost complete disappearance of the infiltrate. Bar: 20 μm.

HISTOLOGY AND IMMUNOHISTOCHEMISTRY

Prior to treatment, a typical band-like infiltrate in the dermis, with epidermotropism of individual cells, was a constant finding. Pautrier abscesses were found in only 4 of 21 cases. The infiltrate reached the deep dermis in three cases and was always composed of small and large cells with hyperchromic cerebriform nuclei; eosinophils were rare. In one case, the infiltrate was very slight. In the upper dermis, the blood vessels were enlarged and the infiltrate was mainly located around them, although single cells infiltrating the epithelium were also noted. Acanthosis was found in all but one patient. To date, biopsies have been repeated at the site of the pretreatment biopsy in 18 of 21 patients: once in 9 patients, twice in 7 patients and three times in two. Virtually complete disappearance of the infiltrate was observed in CR. A few lymphocytes were intermingled with macrophages and epidermotropism was entirely absent (Figures 4a and 4b). Appreciable reduction in the infiltrate and the presence of a spared subepidermal zone were always noted in PR. A marked reduction of acanthosis was found in all patients.

Before treatment, the phenotype of the lymphoid cells in the dermal infiltrate and epidermis was always similar to that in the peripheral blood ($CD3^+$, $CD4^+$, $CD5^+$, $CD8^-$); however, a variable proportion (20-40%) of lymphoid cells expressing CD25 and activation antigens was observed. After treatment, CR was expressed by complete disappearance of CD3 and CD4 positive cells from the epidermis. The rare cells found were $CD8^+$. A reduction in numbers of Langherhans cells, along with a reduction in expression of HLA-DR, in the epidermis and dermis was observed in 12 of 17 cases. A marked reduction of activation antigens (CD25, CD71, CD38) were found in all patients who responded to therapy.

CONCLUSION

These data indicate a restoration of some normal functional properties in peripheral blood lymphocytes in SS patients treated with TP-5, and confirm that an increase in normal cells can exert a control on neoplastic proliferation. When neoplastic cells are present in large numbers, their normal counterparts may not be able to kill or inhibit the expansion of neoplastic clones. Antibiobiotic drugs or anti-CD4 monoclonal antibodies may improve this. Edelson et al. (1987) found, with photopheresis, an increase in $CD8^+$ cells in their responders; furthermore, they observed that CD4/CD8 ratios were lower in responders than in non-responding patients. Combination of TP-5 with photopheresis may offer a way of strengthening the immune response against neoplastic cells in the Sézary syndrome.

REFERENCES

Bernengo MG, GC Doveil, M Meregalli, A Appino and R Massobrio, 1988. Immunomodulation and Sézary syndrome: Experience with thymopentin (TP-5). **Br. J. Dermatol.**, 119:207.

Bunn PA Jr, DC Ihde and KA Foon, 1987. Recombinant interferon alfa-2a, an active agent in advanced cutaneous T-cell lymphomas. **Int. J. Cancer**, Suppl 1:9.

Edelson R, C Berger, F Gasparro, B Jegasothy, P Heald, B Wintroub, E Vonderheid, R Knobler, K Wolff, G Plewig, G McKiernan, I Christiansen, M Oster, H Honigsmann, H Wilford, E Kokoschka, T Rehle, M Perez, G Stingl and L Laroche, 1987. Treatment of cutaneous T-cell lymphoma by extracorporeal photochemotherapy. **N. Engl. J. Med.**, 316: 297.

Edelson RL, MA Lutzner and CH Kirkpatrick, 1974. Morphologic and functional properties of the atypical T lymphocytes of the Sézary Syndrome. **Mayo Clin. Proc.**, 49:558.

Goldstein G, MP Scheid, EA Boyse, DH Schlesinger and J Van Wauwe, 1979. A synthetic pentapeptide with biological characteristic of the thymic hormone thymopoietin. **Science**, 204: 1309.

Hu C, L Radaelli, R Scorza, P Bonara, R Perego and G Fantuzzi, 1990. In vivo enhancement of NK-cell activity by thymopentin. **Int. J. Immunopharmacol.**, 12:193.

Kang K, KD Cooper and JM Hanifin, 1983. Thymopoietin pentapeptide (TP-5) improves clinical parameters and lymphocyte subpopulations in atopic dermatitis. **J. Am. Acad. Dermatol.**, 8:372.

Leung DY, RL Hirsch, L Schneider, C Moody, R Takaoka, SH Li, LA Meyerson, SG Mariam, G Goldstein and JM Hanifin, 1990. Thymopentin therapy reduces the clinical severity of atopic dermatitis. **J. Allergy Clin. Immunol.**, 85:927.

Lutzner M, RL Edelson and P Schein, 1975. Cutaneous T cell lymphomas: The Sézary syndrome, mycosis fungoides and related disorders. **Ann. Intern. Med.**, 83:534.

Lynch J, F Foss, G Schechter, E Sausville, D Ihde and J Trepel, 1990. Prognostic implications of surface immunophenotyping and gene rearrangement studies in mycosis fungoides. **Proc. Am. Assoc. of Cancer Res.**, 31:190.

Pizzolo G, M Chilosi, F Vinante, F Dazzi, M Lestani, G Perona, F. Benedetti, G Todeschini, C Vincenzi, L Trentin and G Semenzato, 1987. Interleukin-2 receptors in the serum of patients with Hodgkin's disease. **Br. J. Cancer**, 55:427.

Rosenberg SA, MT Lotze, LM Muul, AE Chang, FP Auis, S Leitman, WM Lineman, CN Robertson, RE Lee, JT Rubin, CA Seipp, CG Simpson and DE White, 1987. A progress report on the treatment of 157 patients with advanced cancer using lymphocyte-activated killer cells and interleukin-2 or high dose interleukin-2 alone. **N. Engl. J. Med.**, 316:889.

Steis RG, L Marcon, J Clark, W Urba, DL Longo, DL Nelson and AE Maluish, 1988. Serum soluble IL-2 receptor as a tumor marker in patients with hairy cell leukemia. **Blood**, 71:1304.

Wagner DK, J Kiwanuka, BK Edwards, LA Rubin, DL Nelson, IT Magrath and 1987. Soluble interleukin-2 receptor levels in patients with undifferentiated and lymphoblastic lymphomas: Correlation with survival. **J. Clin. Oncol.**, 5:1262.

Wieselthier JS and HK Koh, 1990. Sézary syndrome. Diagnosis, prognosis and critical review of treatment options. **J. Am. Acad. Dermatol.**, 22:381.

WHAT IS MYCOSIS FUNGOIDES? A MODEST PROPOSAL

W. Clark Lambert

Department of Laboratory Medicine and Pathology
Department of Dermatology
UMDNJ-New Jersey Medical School
Newark, New Jersey, U.S.A.

Correspondence to: Dr. W. C. Lambert, Department of Laboratory Medicine and
Pathology, Room C 524, Medical Science Bldg., UMDNJ-New Jersey Medical School,
185 South Orange Avenue,
Newark, NJ 07103-2714, U.S.A.

ABSTRACT

Mycosis fungoides, and related disorders such as Sézary syndrome, which comprise the diseases known collectively as "Cutaneous T Cell Lymphomas" (CTCL), are a heterogeneous group of disorders. Most of these patients experience insidious onset of a cutaneous eruption which shows features difficult or impossible to distinguish from those of a number of inflammatory dermatosis. During a variable, but usually prolonged, course, a cell type appears in the epidermis with a striking morphology, the so-called Sézary or Lutzner cell, depending on its size. In the leukemic forms of these diseases, the Sézary syndrome, these cells are also found in number in the peripheral blood. With further progression, these distinctive cells are found in nests within the epidermis, at which time a definitive diagnosis of mycosis fungoides may be made. These cells have cell markers characteristic of thymus-derived T lymphocytes, and, as the disease progresses, a single T cell clone consisting of these cells often becomes dominant. Further progression of the disease is marked by loss of epidermotrophism, development of tumors comprised of atypical T cells, and visceral involvement by these cells leading eventually to the patient's demise. On the basis of these facts, these disorders have been classified as lymphomas of T lymphocytes.

On further consideration, however, it is clear that these dermatoses have a number of peculiar features. The distinctive Sézary, or Lutzner, cell often does not appear until the eruption has been present for many months, years, or, sometimes, decades. Nor is this cell unique to cases of CTCL; it may be found in a number of inflammatory dermatoses that are clearly not lymphomas, both in lesional skin and circulating in the peripheral blood. Even when this cell is predominant in lesional skin, moreover, it is difficult or impossible to propagate it in culture, even under conditions in which T cell clones reactive to it readily proliferate and form readily identifiable cell lines. Cytogenetic analysis of these cells shows that, unlike a number of cancers, they do not consistently show a distinctive chromosomal abnormality or mutation, but rather show extensive, relatively quite rapid chromosomal changes which occur on a massive scale. Nothing like this has been found in any other type of cancer, with the possible exception of some cases of T cell non-Hodgkin lymphoma and of Hodgkin disease, with which it has been proposed that CTCL may share a common origin. When progression of CTCL to a more aggressive form does occur, it is often accompanied by the appearance and predominance of large, very atypical cells which in general do not resemble Sézary or Lutzner cells. This aggressive stage may occur at any time during the otherwise long course of the disease, and may even be present at the outset.

I believe that the biology of the fascinating array of diseases that comprise the CTCL group should be considered very much an open question, and it is important not to close our minds to any reasonable possibility. In this spirit, I now propose an alternate hypothesis for the etiopathogenesis of some cases of CTCL, which I have termed the **"Thymus Bypass Model"**. It proposes that some cases of CTCL are due not to clonal proliferation and malignant transformation of T lymphocytes, but rather to an error of histogenesis, in which circulating, bone marrow derived precursors of thymocytes home not to the thymus but rather directly to skin, which then acts as an aberrant surrogate thymus. As is thought to occur in thymocytes in the thymus, these cells then proliferate in response to normal human MHC self-antigens, undergoing rapid T cell receptor gene rearrangement as well as rapid chromosomal changes in aberrant attempts to undergo T cell differentiation and apoptosis (in those cells which continue to recognize self antigens following T cell receptor gene rearrangement), respectively. Thus these very atypical appearing cells are seen proliferating in the epidermis and dermis, but they are not T cells, having never been to the thymus, and are not malignant until very late in the course of the disease and even then not in all cases. This simple idea has profound implications for the etiopathogenesis, biology and medical management of CTCL. Thus my "modest proposal" (Swift, 1728, with apologies) is that some Cutaneous T Cell Lymphomas may not be disorders of T cells and, until possibly very late in their course, may not even be lymphomas.

INTRODUCTION

The term, "Cutaneous T Cell Lymphoma" (CTCL) has been applied to a group of diseases which show atypical-appearing cells with morphologic characteristics of thymus-derived T-cells, including cell surface markers and, in many cases, rearrangement of T cell receptor (TCR) genes characteristic of T lymphocytes. This group of disorders is heterogeneous, encompassing mycosis fungoides, Sézary syndrome (which is possibly a leukemic form of mycosis fungoides), pagetoid reticulosis, which may be either localized (the Woringer-Kolopp type) or, less commonly, widespread (the Ketron-Goodman type), T cell chronic lymphocytic leukemia, the rare, non-epidermotrophic T cell lymphomas, and, according to some authors but not to others, large plaque and retiform parapsoriasis (Abel, 1985; Edelson, 1987; Lambert, 1985; 1988; 1993). Even within these different groups, moreover, there is significant heterogeneity, and thus there is general agreement that CTCL is made up of a heterogeneous collection of disorders (Kaudewitz and Braun-Falco, 1991).

Although the justification for classifying these diseases as lymphomas would appear to be ample, on further consideration a number of questions arise. First, although the characteristic atypical T cells that characterize the lesions of CTCL can be identified on basis of their light microscopic and ultrastructural morphology (Lutzner et al., 1968), antigenic determinants detected by monoclonal antibodies (mAb) (Berger et al., 1982; Ralfkiaer et al., 1985; Vonderheid, 1989), and monoclonality detected by molecular T-cell receptor gene rearrangement analysis (Waldmann et al., 1985; Weiss et al., 1985; 1989;), none of these criteria is specific for malignant T cells (Flaxman et al., 1971; Kaudewitz et al., 1993; Kerl et al., 1993; Ralfkiaer et al., 1986; Weiss et al., 1986; Wechsler et al., 1990). Moreover one important alternate hypothesis, that some of the disorders in this group may be due not to malignant transformation of T cells, but rather to their chronic stimulation due to persistence of an antigen (Knobler and Edelson, 1986; Tan et al., 1974), or to a viral infection (D'Incan et al., 1993; Kaudewitz et al., 1993; Meijer et al., 1993), especially a viral infection involving intraepidermal antigen presenting cells (i.e., Langerhans cells), proposed by MacKie (MacKie, 1981; van der Loo et al., 1979), has never been disproven, although no such persistent antigen has ever been found. It has also been hypothesized that atypical T-cells in the skin of patients with mycosis fungoides &undergo proliferation in response to external stimuli provided by the local environment, especially in the epidermis (Nickoloff et al., 1990). At least one case-controlled epidemiologic study has failed to find evidence for exposure to an antigen or other toxic agent as a consistent causative factor in CTCL (Whittemore et al., 1989), however, although several cases of drug-induced CTCL have been reported (Souteyrand et al., 1990).

There is also great variability in the clinical course of CTCL, even within diagnostic groups. Mycosis fungoides often begins very slowly, arising from large plaque parapsoriasis or another inflammatory dermatosis, and proceeds at a very indolent pace, frequently taking years to decades to produce either cutaneous tumors or systemic disease, although it can progress rapidly at any time and may also present initially as tumors (tumeur d'emblée form). Moreover, several investigators have now reported that aggressive behavior of mycosis fungoides is often accompanied by a histological transformation, with emergence of a histologic pattern resembling that of a large cell lymphoma (Buechnert et al., 1979; Catterall et al., 1983; Cerroni et al.,

1992; Dimebrowsky et al., 1987; Greer et al., 1990; Kerl et al., 1991; 1993; Ralfkiaer et al., 1989; Salhany et al., 1988; Scheen et al., 1989; Tykocinsky et al., 1984; van der Putte et al., 1984; Yanagihara et al., 1984). The large cells usually do not resemble Sézary cells. This is consistent with the hypothesis that the atypical cells seen in CTCL are not necessarily malignant, although they may become so after undergoing further transformation. Thus some cases of CTCL may be possible precursors of lymphoma, without, themselves, being a lymphoma.

Considerable research has been conducted, again in a number of different laboratories, on the biology of the "malignant" cell in CTCL lesions. The results strongly indicate that if CTCL is indeed a lymphoma, then it has some very odd characteristics:

First, although transformed (i.e., malignant) cells, are, in general, easier to grow in tissue culture from biopsy tissue or peripheral blood than are non-transformed cells, the opposite is true in cases of CTCL. Even though it is possible to culture reactive T lymphocyte clones from lesions of CTCL (Cooper et al., 1993), it has been repeatedly observed that the "malignant clone" of cells derived from a lesion of CTCL grows poorly in short term culture, and attempts to establish permanent cell lines have generally been unsuccessful from both CTCL lesional tissue and peripheral blood of CTCL patients (Cooper et al., 1993; Goldstein et al., 1986; Kaltoft et al., 1984; 1987; Hansen et al., 1988; Ho et al., 1990; Rheinhold et al., 1990; Abrams et al., 1991b). This is true even when the "malignant clone" is clearly dominant in vivo (Ho et al., 1990). Moreover, when cells are grown from punch biopsies under non-cloning conditions, the "malignant clone" is lost, while, often, reactive T cell clones survive and proliferate (Hansen et al., 1988). Recently, however, these cells have been cultured using IL-7 (Appasamy, 1993; Dalloul et al., 1992; Merle-Béral et al., 1993) which is produced by murine and human keratinocytes (Heufler et al., 1993) and, when overexpressed in transgenic mice, produces a cutaneous T cell lymphoproliferative disorder (Rich et al., 1993).

Second, a very remarkable degree of genetic instability, with numerous chromosomal rearrangements and other abnormalities, has been found by a number of investigators in the atypical cells in lesions of CTCL, particularly in cases of Sézary syndrome (Berger et al., 1987; D'Allesandro et al., 1990; Gamperl et al., 1986; Johnson et al., 1985; Kaltoft et al., 1993; Santos et al., 1990; Shapiro et al., 1987; Sole et al., 1990; Abrams et al., 1991a; 1991b). This is quite different from the chromosomal changes found in most other cancers, where, although aberrations arise and evolve in a clonal manner during tumor progression, the massive numbers and degrees of chromosomal alterations arising in such short periods of time characteristic of CTCL are not seen. Kaltoft et al. (1993) have termed these cells "genotraumatic" T lymphocytes, and have suggested that this extreme chromosomal instability be used as a marker to identify these cells in lesional skin of patients with CTCL, thus aiding in diagnosis. Kaltoft et al. (1993) also noted that clones of T cells with markedly aberrant karyotypes in lesions of CTCL are often not the clone that eventually proliferates as the "malignant" clone.

Kaltoft et al., (1993), noted, in addition, that cells that would fit their definition of "genotraumatic" T cells have also been described in lesional tissue in cases of T cell lymphoma (non-Hodgkin lymphoma of T cell origin) (Fisher et al., 1988; Ohno et al., 1988; Kubonishi et al., 1990; Morikowa et al., 1991) and in Hodgkin diseases (Tilly et al., 1991). It is thus of special interest that it has been proposed that CTCL and Hodgkin disease may arise from a common T cell origin (Davis et al., 1992; Kadin et al., 1990; 1993).

It is important to attempt to carefully analyze precisely what we know, or think we know, versus what we may deduce, both about CTCL and about T lymphocytes, in attempting to formulate a hypothesis regarding the etiopathogenesis of CTCL. T lymphocytes are believed to arise in the bone marrow, as cells already committed to become T cells. These committed cells then circulate into the peripheral blood, sooner or later homing to the thymus, where they undergo several remarkable transformations. These include (i) proliferation, (ii) rearrangement of all four of their TCR domains (α, β, γ and δ), and (iii) extensive cell death, probably via apoptosis, so that only a few of the cells generated actually emerge from the thymus as T cells, the remainder being killed. There is evidence that the cell proliferation, as well as subsequent extensive cell death, is due to recognition of self-antigens by these intrathythmic cells. Thus the cells are first stimulated to undergo proliferation and then those clones which are reactive against self-antigens are eliminated prior to exit of the remaining cells as diverse, but not self-antigen reactive, mature T cells from the thymus. In this way a large pool of T cells, selected for those reactive against a battery of non-self antigens, is generated by a combination of random TCR gene rearrangement, clonal proliferation, and intrathythmic positive and negative selection processes (Adkins et al., 1987; Blackman et al., 1990; Davis and Bjorkman, 1988; Fowlkes and Pardoll, 1989; Kappler et al., 1987; Ransdell and Fowlkes, 1990; Sprent et al., 1990; Strominger, 1989; von Boehmer, 1990; von Boehmer and Kisielow, 1990; Zinkernagel et al., 1980).

The characteristic cells seen in the skin and other tissues in cases of CTCL have unequivocal cell surface markers indicative of the T lymphocyte cell type, as noted above, and they often show a unique, clonal proliferation in vivo, consisting of 5% or more of the cells, showing one particular TCR gene rearrangement. They are thus considered to be thymus-derived T-cells. Despite extensive evidence demonstrating these points, however, <u>there is absolutely no direct evidence that these atypical appearing cells in cases of CTCL ever actually entered the human thymus.</u>

THE THYMUS BYPASS MODEL

As one possible alternate hypothesis for the etiopathogenesis of (some cases of) CTCL, I would like to propose the following, which I have termed the "Thymus Bypass Model":

Definition: The thymus bypass model proposes that some cases of CTCL are due not to malignant clonal proliferation of thymus-derived T lymphocytes, but rather to an error of histogenesis, in which bone marrow-derived precursors of T cells go directly to the skin, where an aberrant proliferation occurs representing an abortive attempt at thymocyte differentiation. This aberrant proliferation is promoted by self-antigens present in the skin, or possibly by influences due to viral infection or to incomplete viral DNA sequences present in cutaneous cells, or to some combination of these. This process is thus not a T-cell disorder and is not a lymphoma, although it may evolve into a lymphoma much later in the course of the disease (probably not until the tumor stage in most cases of mycosis fungoides).

DISCUSSION

The above hypothesis appears to me to fit the available data at least as well as other hypotheses that have been generated. For example, if the "persistent antigen" (Tan et al., 1974) is a self-antigen, then it is not surprising that a foreign antigen has not been identified in cases of CTCL since no such antigen need exist. The "genotraumatic" T lymphocytes appear to be cells undergoing some combination of aberrant proliferation, genetic rearrangement, and/or apoptosis or abortive apoptosis. Therefore, some cases of CTCL, and, by inference, some cases of non-Hodgkin lymphoma and Hodgkin disease, may actually be examples of disorders of apoptosis, rather than lymphomas.

The concept that cells with morphologic features of T lymphocytes may have acquired these features in the skin, or in another site, independently of the thymus, is not without experimental support. Stingl and his colleagues (Stingl et al., 1993; Honjo et al., 1990) found that day 16 murine fetal Thy-1$^+$CD3$^-$ cells, which lack a T cell receptor (TCR; closely related to CD3) can mature into Thy-1$^+$CD3$^+$ cells, independent of the thymus, and that this process probably occurs intraepidermally. Although Nixon-Fulton et al., (1988) failed to find TCR-bearing lymphocytes in congenitally athymic nude mice, Stingl's group found, using a different mouse strain (C57BL/6), that a small minority of Thy-1$^+$ cells in six week old nude (nu/nu) mice had a T cell receptor, and that this percentage, as well as the absolute numbers of these cells, increased with age, so that in 12 week old nu/nu mice 3% of the dendritic Thy-1$^+$ cells in the epidermis were CD3$^+$ and had an intact TCR (Stingl et al., 1993). These findings are consistent with a number of older studies in which T cells, as defined by a variety of phenotypic and functional criteria, were identified in nude (nu/nu) mice (Gillis et al., 1979; Hunig, 1983; Hunig and Bevan, 1980; Ishikawa and Saita, 1980; Klein and Bevan, 1983; MacDonald et al., 1981; 1982; 1984; Maryanski et al., 1981).

Several authors have noted the relative abundance of dendritic cells in the skin of CTCL lesions (Fivenson et al., 1991; 1992; Fivenson and Nickoloff, 1993; Hansen et al., 1990); this has been cited as evidence for a persistent stimulation of cutaneous T cells by antigen or an antigen-like influence, as has expression of Class II MHC antigen by keratinocytes in lesional skin in cases of CTCL (Cooper et al., 1993; Tjernlund, 1978). Just how much contact T cells actually have with these dendritic cells, however, has been questioned (Bani et al., 1990).Whatever direct contact they may or may not have with other cells, these dendritic cells and other active cells, such as keratinocytes, are probably important, and it is also perfectly compatible with the above hypothesis that they play some role in the etiopathogenesis of CTCL, but the nature of that role is unclear. It may or may not be important that the epidermis, like the thymus, has a keratinizing epithelial component, and that this component has antigenic properties similar to those of some keratinocytes (Didierjean and Saurat, 1980).

If it is true that CTCL is not, in many cases, a lymphoma, then it may be possible to control the disease by means that otherwise may not have been considered, such as use of certain lymphokines, or promoters of apoptosis or of cellular differentiation. The possibility that the atypical appearing cells in CTCL may actually be non-transformed, although possibly pre-malignant, cells in a state of abortive or incomplete apoptosis is particularly intriguing, since a number of chemical agents are known to induce apoptosis (Tomei and Cope, 1991). This is the focus of intensive current research (See, for example, Proc. Am. Assoc. Cancer Res, 1993. Vol. 34). Of special interest are studies of apoptosis in non-cancerous, pre-malignant lesions (for one example, see Kamer et al., 1993).

The entire biology of CTCL may now need to be reconsidered. It may well turn out that, like the "Holy Roman Empire", which was neither holy, nor Roman, nor an empire, "cutaneous T cell lymphoma" may in the end prove to be neither a T-cell disorder nor, at least until very late in its course, a lymphoma, although it does appear to be a cutaneous disease.

ACKNOWLEDGEMENTS

The author wishes to thank the participants at the NATO workshop on which this book is based, and, in particular, Dr. Robert E. Tigelaar, for their helpful suggestions and advice.

REFERENCES

Abel EA, 1985. Clinical features of cutaneous T-cell lymphoma. In: BH Thiers and JC Maize, Eds. Cutaneous T-cell lymphomas and related disorders. **Dermatol. Clin.**, 3:647-664.

Abrams JT, S Lessin, SK Ghosh, W Ju, E C Vonderheid, P Nowell, G Murphy, B Elfenbein and E DeFreitas, 1991a. A clonal CD4-positive T cell line established from the blood of a patient with Sézary syndrome. **J. Invest. Dermatol.**, 96:31-37.

Abrams JT, SR Lessin, SK Ghosh, PC Nowell, W Ju, EC Vonderheid, AH Rook and E DeFreitas, 1991b. Malignant and non-malignant T cell lines from human T cell lymphotropic virus type I-negative patients with Sézary syndrome. **J. Immunol.**, 146:1455-1462.

Adkins B, C Mueller, CY Okada, R Reichert, IL Weissman and GJ Spangrude, 1987. Early events in T-cell maturation. **Annu. Rev. Immunol.** 5:325-365.

Appasamy PM, 1993. Interleukin-7: Biology and potential clinical applications. **Cancer Invest.**, 11:487-499.

Bani D, N Pimpinelli, S Moretti and B Giannotti, 1990. Langerhans cells and mycosis fungoides: A critical overview of their pathogenic role in the disease. **Clin. Exp. Dermatol.**, 15:7-12.

Berger CL, S Morrison, A Chu, J Patterson, A Estabrook, S Takezaki, J Sharon, D Warburton, O Irigoyen and RL Edelson, 1982. Diagnosis of cutaneous T cell lymphoma by use of monoclonal antibodies reactive with tumor-associated antigens. **J. Clin. Invest.**, 70:1205-1215.

Berger R and A Bernheim, 1987. Cytogenetic studies of Sézary cells. **Cancer Genet. Cytogenet.**, 27:79-87.

Blackman M, J Kappler and P Marrack, 1990. The role of the T cell receptor in positive and negative selection of developing T cells. **Science**, 248:1335-1341.

Buechner S and T Rufli, 1979. Manifestation eines malignen Lymphoms von hohem Malignitaetsgrad in Spaetstadium der Mycosis fundoides. **Dermatologica**, 159:125-131.

Catterall MD, BJ Addis, JL Smith and PE Coode, 1983. Sézary syndrome: Transformation to a high grade T-cell lymphoma after treatment with cyclosporin A. **Clin. Exp. Dermatol.**, 8:159-169.

Cerroni L, E Rieger, S Hoedl and H Kerl, 1992. Clinicopathologic and immunologic features associated with transformation of mycosis fungoides to large cell lymphoma. **Am. J. Surg. Pathol.**, 16: 543-552.

Cooper KD, L Meunier, V Ho, O Baadsgaard, M-S Lee, E Hansen, S Lisby, D Mehregen, E Allen, GH Vejlsgaard and JT Elder, 1993. Activation of reactive versus malignant T-cells in cutaneous T-cell lymphoma: Role of abnormal antigen presenting cells and T-cell activating molecules. In: WC Lambert, B Giannotti and WA van Vloten, Eds. **Basic Mechanisms of Physiologic and Aberrant Lymphoproliferation in the Skin.** Plenum Press, Inc, New York, This Volume.

D'Allesandro E, P Paterlini, ML Lo Re, M Di Cola, C Ligas, D. Quaglino and G Del Porto, 1990. Cytogenetic Follow-up in a case of Sézary syndrome. **Cancer Genet. Cytogenet.**, 45:231-236.

Dalloul A, L Laroche, M Bagot, MD Mossalayi, C Fourcade, DJ Thacker, DE Hogge, H Merle-Béral, P Debré and C Schmitt, 1992. Interleukin-7 is a growth factor for Sézary lymphoma cells. **J. Clin. Invest.**, 90:1054-1060.

Davis MM and PJ Bjorkman, 1988. T-cell antigen receptor genes and T-cell recognition. **Nature** 334: 395-402.

Davis TH, CC Morton, R Miller-Cassman, SP Balk and ME Kadin, 1992. Hodgkin's disease, lymphomatoid papulosis, and cutaneous T-cell lymphoma derived from a common T-cell clone. **N. Engl. J. Med.**, 326:1115-1122.

Didierjean L and JH Saurat, 1980. Epidermis and thymus: Similar antigenic properties in Hassall's corpuscle and subsets of keratinocytes. **Clin. Exptl. Dermatol.**, 5:395-404.

D'Incan M, P Souteyrand, Y-J Bignon and C Desgranges, 1993. Survey of cutaneous T-cell lymphomas for human T-lymphotropic virus infection. In: WC Lambert, B Giannotti and WA von Vloten, Eds. **Basic Mechanisms of Physiologic and Aberrant Lymphoproliferation in the Skin.** Plenum Press, Inc., New York, This Volume.

Dmitrovsky E, MJ Matthews, PA Bunn, et al., 1987. Cytologic transformation in cutaneous T cell lymphoma: A clinicopathologic entity associated with poor prognosis. **J. Clin. Oncol.**, 5:208-215.

Edelson RL, 1987. Cutaneous T cell lymphoma. **J. Dermatol.**, 14:397-410.

Fischer P, E Nacheva, DY Mason, PD Sherrington, C Hoyle, FGJ Hayhoe and A Karpas, 1988. A Ki-1 (CD30)-positive human cell line (Karpas 299) established from a high-grade non-Hodgkin's lymphoma, showing a 2;5 translocation and rearrangement of the T-cell receptor α-chain gene. **Blood**, 72: 234-240.

Fischmann AB, PA Bunn Jr., JG Guccion, MJ Matthews and JD Minna, 1979. Exposure to chemicals, physical agents, and biologic agents in mycosis fungoides and the Sézary syndrome. **Cancer Treat. Rep.**, 63: 591-596.

Fivenson DP, MC Douglass and BJ Nickoloff, 1992. Cutaneous expression of Thy 1 in mycosis fungoides. **Am. J. Pathol.**, 141:1373-1380.

Fivenson DP and BJ Nickoloff, 1993. Cell trafficing networks in cutaneous T cell lymphoma. In: WC Lambert, B Giannotti and WA van Vloten, Eds. **Basic Mechanisms of Physiologic and Aberrant Lymphoproliferation in the Skin.** Plenum Press, New York, This Volume.

Fivenson DP, RW Dunstan, MC Douglass, BJ Nickoloff and PF Moore, 1991a. Thy-1$^+$ dermal dendrocytes in mycosis fungoides. **J. Invest. Dermatol.**, 96:599A (Abstract).

Fivenson DP, LA Rheins, JJ Nordlund and EA Krull, 1991b. Thy-1 expression and T cell receptor type in mycosis fungoides and benign dermatoses. **J. Natl. Cancer. Inst.**, 83: 1088-1092.

Flaxman, BA, G Zelazny and EJ Van Scott, 1971. Non specificity of characteristic cells in mycosis fungoides. **Arch. Dermatol.**, 104:141-147.

Fowlkes BJ and DM Pardoll, 1989. Molecular and cellular events of T cell development. **Adv. Immunol.**, 44:207-264.

Gamperl R, 1986. Clonal chromosome aberrations in a case of cutaneous T cell lymphoma. **Cancer Genet. Cytogenet.**, 19:341-344.

Gillis S, NA Union, PE Baker and KA Smith, 1979. The in vitro generation and sustained culture of nude mouse cytolytic T-lymphocytes. **J. Exp. Med.**, 149:1460-1476.

Greer JP, KE Salhany, JB Cousar, et al., 1990. Clinical features associated with transformation of cerebriform T cell lymphoma to a large cell process. **Hematol. Oncol.**, 8:215-227.

Hansen ER, O Baadsgaard, S Lisby, KD Cooper, K Thomsen and GL Vejlsgaard, 1990. Cutaneous T cell lymphoma lesional epidermal cells activate autologous CD8$^+$ T lymphocytes: Involvement of both CD1[+], OKM5[+] and CD1[+], OKM5[-] antigen- presenting cells. **J. Invest. Dermatol.**, 94:485-491.

Hansen ER, O Baardsgaard, S Lisby, KD Cooper, K Thomsen and GL Wantzin, 1988. Epidermal cells from mycosis fungoides demonstrate MHC-Class II dependent activation of the CD4[+]CD8[-] lymphocyte subset. **J. Invest. Dermatol.**, 91:386A. (Abstract).

Heufler C, G Topar, A Grasseger, U Stanzl, F Koch, N Romani, AE Namen and G Schuler, 1993. Interleukin 7 is produced by murine and human keratinocytes. **J. Exp Med.**, 178:1109-1114.

Ho VC, O Baardsgaard, JT Elder, et al., 1990a. Genotypic analysis of T-cell clones derived from cutaneous T-cell lymphoma lesions demonstrates selective growth of tumor infiltrating lymphocytes. **J. Invest. Dermatol.**, 95:4-8.

Honjo M, A Elbe, G Steiner, I Assmann, K Wolff and G Stingl, 1990. Thymus-independent generation of Thy-1[+] epidermal cells from a pool of Thy-1[-] bone marrow precursors. **J. Invest. Dermatol.**, 95: 562-567.

Hünig T, 1983. T cell function and specificity in athymic mice. **Immunol. Today**, 4:84.

Hünig T and MJ Bevan, 1980. Specificity of cytotoxic T cells from athymic mice. **J. Exp. Med.**, 152:688-702.

Ishikawa H and K Saito, 1980. Congenitally athymic nude (nu/nu) mice have Thy-1 bearing immunocompetent helper T cells in their peritoneal cavity. **J. Exp. Med.**, 151:965-968.

Johnson GA, GW Dewald, WR Strand and RK Winkelmann, 1985. Chromosome studies in 17 patients with the Sézary syndrome. **Cancer**, 55:2426-2433.

Kadin ME, l990. The spectrum of cutaneous T cell lymphomas. In: WA van Vloten, R Willemze, GL Vejlsgaard and K Thomson, Eds.: Cutaneous Lymphoma, **Curr. Probl. Dermatol.** Basel, Karger, 19:132-143.

Kadin ME, TH Davis, SP Balk, SR Newcom, S Cheifitz and J Massague, 1993. Mechanism for tumor progression in lymphomatoid papulosis: Hypothesis based on studies of tumor cell lines clonally derived from lymphomatoid papulosis. In: WC Lambert, B Giannotti and WA van Vloten, Eds: **Basic Mechanisms of Physiologic and Aberrant Lymphoproliferation in the Skin**. Plenum Press. New York. This Volume.

Kaltoft K, S Bisballe, W Sterry, H Sogaard and K Khestrup-Pedersen, 1993. Sézary syndrome is characterized by genotraumatic T-cells. In: WC Lambert, B Giannotti and WA van Vloten, Eds. **Basic Mechanisms of Physiologic and Aberrant Lymphoproliferation in the Skin**. Plenum Press, New York, This Volume.

Kamer AR, C Liebow, DH Crean, TS Many, K Szepeshanzi, P Bradford and AV Schally, 1993. Somatostatin analogue RC-160 eliminates premalignant lesions induced in the hamster buccal cheek pouch by DXISA. **Proc. Am. Assoc. Cancer Res.**, 34:293 (Abstract).

Kappler JW, N Roehm and P Marrack, 1987. T cell tolerance by clonal elimination in the thymus. **Cell**, 49-273-280.

Kaudewitz P, I Anagnostopoulos, M Hummel and H Stein, 1993. HTLV-1 proviral sequences in cutaneous CD30[+] T large cell lymphomas, 1993. In: WC Lambert, B Grannotti and

WA van Vloten, Eds. **Basic Mechanisms of Physiologic and Aberrant Lymphoproliferation in the Skin**. Plenum Press, New York, This Volume.

Kaudewitz P. and O. Braun-Falco, 1991. Malignant cutaneous lymphomas, In: RH Chamption and RJ Pye, Eds. **Recent Advances in Dermatology**, Churchill Livingstone, Edinburgh, London.

Kerl H, K Cerroni and G Burg, 1991. The morphologic spectrum of T-cell lympomas of the skin: A proposal for a new classification. **Semin. Diagn. Pathol.**, 8:55-61.

Kerl H, L Cerroni and S Hoedl, 1993. Morphologic and prognostic features of advanced mycosis fungoides. In: WC Lambert, B Giannotti, and WA van Vloten, Eds. **Basic Mechanisms of Physiologic and Aberrant Lymphoproliferation in the Skin**. Plenum Press, New York, This Volume.

Klein JR and MJ Bevan, 1983. Secretion of immune interferon and generation of cytotoxic T cell activity in nude mice are dependent on interleukin 2: Age-associated endogeneous production of interleukin 2 in nude mice. **J. Immunol.** 130:1780-1783.

Knobler RM, RL Edelson, 1986. Cutaneous T cell lymphoma. **Med. Clin. N. Am.**, 70:109-13.

Kubonishi I, H Sonobe, T Miyagi, Y Iwahara, JH Ohyashiki, K Ohyasliki, K Toyama, Y Ohtsuki and I Miyoshi, 1990. A Ki-1 (CD30$^+$)-positive T (E$^+$, CD4$^+$, Ia$^+$)-cell line, DL-40, established from aggressive large cell lymphoma. **Cancer Res.**, 50:7682-7685.

Lambert WC, 1993. Inflammatory precursors of mycosis fungoides. In: WC Lambert, B Giannotti, and WA van Vloten, Eds. **Basic Mechanisms of Physiologic and Aberrant Lymphoproliferation in the Skin**. Plenum Press, New York, This Volume.

Lambert WC, 1988. Parapsoriasis. In: TB Fitzpatrick, AZ Eisen, K Wolff, IM Freedberg and KF Ausen, Eds., **Dermatology in General Medicine**, 3rd Ed. McGraw-Hill, New York pp. 991-1008.

Lambert WC, 1985. Premycotic eruptions. In: BH Thiers and JC Maize, Eds., Cutaneous T cell lymphoma and related disorders. **Dermatol. Clinics** 6:629-645.

Lambert WC, 1994. The thymus bypass model: A new hypothesis for the etiopathogenesis of mycosis fungoides and related disorders. In: G Burg, Ed. **Cutaneous Lymphomas, Clinics Dermatol.**, in press.

Lambert WC and RA Schwartz, 1989. Dermatitic precursors of mycosis fungoides. In: RA Schwartz, Ed. **Skin Cancer, Recognition and Management**, Springer-Verlag, New York, pp. 152-161.

Lutzner MA and HW Jordan, 1968. Ultrastructure of an abnormal cell in Sézary's syndrome. **Blood**, 31:719-726.

MacDonald HR and RK Lees, 1984. Frequency and specificity of precursors of interleukin 2-producing cells in nude mice. **J. Immunol.**, 34:605-610.

MacDonald HR, RK Lees, AL Glasebrook and B Sordat, 1982. Interleukin 2 production by lymphoid cells from congenitally athymic (nu/nu) mice. **J. Immunol.** 129:521-525.

MacDonald HR, RK Lees, B Sordat, P Zaech, JL Maryanski and C Bron. 1981. Age-associated increase in expression of the T cell surface markers Thy-1, Lyt-1 and Lyt-2 in congenitally athymic (nu/nu) mice: Analysis by flow microfluorometry. **J. Immunol.**, 126:865-870.

MacKie RM, 1981. Initial event in mycosis fungoides is viral infection of epidermal Langerhans cells. **Lancet**, ii:283-284.

Maryanski JL, HR MacDonald, B Sordat and J-C Cerottini. 1981. Cytolytic T lymphocyte precursor cells in congenitally athymic C57BL/6 nu/nu mice: Quantitation, enrichment and specificity. **J. Immunol.** 126:871-876.

Meijer CJLM, P Kanovaros, N Jiwa, R Willemze, PC de Bruin and JMM Walboomers, 1993. Presence of Epstein-Barr viral DNA and EBV latent gene products in Hodgkin and non-Hodgkin lymphoma: High expression of EBV-DNA sequences in non-Hodgkin lymphoma with variable numbers of CD30 positive cells. In: WC Lambert, B Giannotti and WA van Vloten, Eds. **Basic Mechanisms of Physiologic and Aberrant Lymphoproliferation in the Skin.** Plenum Press, New York, This Volume.

Merle-Béral H, C Schmitt, D Mossalayi, G Bismuth, A Dalloul and F Mentz, 1993. Interleukin-7 and malignant T Cells. **Nouv. Rev. Fr. Hematol.**, 35:231-232.

Morikawa S, K Morikawa, J Hara, M Nagasaki, A Nakano and F Oseko, 1991. Establishment of a novel cell line with T-lineage phenotype (HPB-MLp-W) from a non-Hodgkin's lymphoma patient. **Leukemia Res.**, 15:381-389.

Nickoloff BJ and EM Griffiths, 1990. Intraepidermal but not dermal T lymphocytes are positive for a cell cycle-associated antigen (Ki-67) in mycosis fungoides. **Am. J. Pathol.** 136:261-266.

Nixon-Fulton JL, WA Kuziel, S Santerse, PR Bergstresser, PW Tucker and RE Tigelaar, 1988. Thy-1$^+$ epidermal cells in nude mice are distinct from their counterparts in thymus-bearing mice. A study of morphology, function, and T cell receptor expression. **J. Immunol.** 141:1897-1903.

Ohno H, S Fukuhara, Y Arita, S Doi, R Takahashi, H Fujii, T Honjo, T Sugiyama and H Uchino, 1988. Establishment of a peripheral T cell lymphoma cell line showing amplification of the *c-myc* oncogene. **Cancer Res.**, 48:4959-4963.

Ralfkiaer E, KC Gatter, GL Wantzin, K Thomsen and DY Mason, 1986. Immunohistological reactivity pattern of the anti-cutaneous T-lymphoma antibody BE$_2$. **Br. J. Dermatol.**, 114:677-684.

Ralfkiaer E, G Lange Wantzin, DY Mason, K Hou-Jensen, H Stein and K Thomsen, 1985. Phenotypic characterization of lymphocyte subsets in mycosis fungoides. **Am. J. Clin. Pathol.**, 84:610-619.

Ralfkiaer E, K Thomsen, N Agdal, K Hou-Jensen and G Lange Wantzin, 1989. The development of Ki-1-positive large cell non-Hodgkin's lymphoma in pagetoid reticulosis. **Acta. Derm. Venereol. (Stockh)**, 69:206-211.

Ransdel F and BJ Fowlkes, 1990. Clonal deletion versus clonal anergy: The role of the thymus in inducing self tolerance. **Science**, 248:1342-1348.

Rich BE, J Campos-Torres, RI Tepper, RW Moreadith and P Leder, 1993. Cutaneous lymphoprolieration and lymphomas in interleukin 7 transgenic mice. **J. Exp. Med.**, 177:305-316.

Salhany KE, JS Cousar, JP Greer, TT Casey, JP Eields and RD Colalins, 1985. Transformation of cutaneous T cell lymphoma to large cell lymphoma. A clinicopathologic and immunologic study. **Am. J. Pathol.**, 132:265-277.

Santos M, J Benitez and C Rivas, 1990. Possible correlation between a specific alteration t(7;14) and the rearrangement of TCR observed in a Sézary's syndrome. **Cancer Genet. Cytogenet.**, 46:281-283.

Scheen SR, PM Banks and RK Winkelmann, 1984. Morphologic heterogeneity of malignant lymphomas developing in mycosis fungoides. **Mayo Clin. Proc.**, 59:95-106.

Shapiro PE, D Warburton, CL Berger and RL Edelson, 1987. Clonal chromosomal abnormalities in cutaneous T-cell lymphoma. **Cancer Genet. Cytogenet.**, 28:267-276.

Solé F, N Tarrida, MD Coll, MR Caballin, A De Miguel, S Woessner and J Egozcue, 1990. Cytogenetic study of a patient with the Sézary syndrome. **Cancer Genet. Cytogenet.**, 44:193-196.

Souteyrand P and M D'Incan, 1990. Drug-induced mycosis fungoides-like lesions. In: WA Van Vloten, R Willemze, RG Lang Veilsgaard and Thomsen, Eds. **Cutaneous lymphomas. Curr. Probl. Dermatol.**, 19: Springer Karger, p. 176.

Sprent J, EK Gao and SR Webb, 1990. T cell reactivity to MHC molecules: Immunity versus tolerance. **Science,** 248:1357-1363

Stingl G, R Payert and A Elbe, 1993. Autogeny, features and functions of epidermal T lymphocytes. In: WC Lambert, B Giannotti and WA van Vloten, Eds. **Basic Mechanisms of Physiologic and Aberrant Lymphoproliferation in the Skin.** Plenum Press, New York, This Volume.

Strominger JL, 1989. Developmental biology of T cell receptors. **Science**, 244:943-950.

Swift J. 1728. A modest proposal for preventing the children of the poor people of Ireland from becoming a burden on their parents or country, and for making them beneficial to their public, Dublin.

Tan R, C Butterworth, H McLaughlin, et al., 1974. Mycosis fungoides: A disease of antigen persistence. **Br. J. Dermatol.** 91:607-616.

Tilly H, C Bastard, T Delastre, C Duval, M Bizet, B Lenormand, J-P Daucé, M Monconduit and H Piguet, 1991. Cytogenetic studies in untreated Hodgkin's disease. **Blood**, 77:1298-1304.

Tjernlund UM, 1978. Epidermal expression of HLA-DR antigens in mycosis fungoides. **Arch. Dermatol. Res.**, 261:81-86.

Tomei LD and FO Cope, Eds. 1991. **Apoptosis: The Molecular Basis of Cell Death**. Cold Spring Harbor Laboratory Press, New York.

Tykocinski M, R Schinella and A Greco, 1984. The pleomorphic cells of advanced mycosis fungoides. An ultrastructural study. **Arch. Pathol. Lab. Med.**, 108:387-391.

van der Loo EM, GNP van Muijen, WA van Vloten, W Beens, E Shceffer and CJLM Meijer, 1979. C-type virus-like particles specifically localized in Langerhans cells and related cells of skin and lymph nodes of patients with mycosis fungoides and Sézary's syndrome. **Virchows Arch. B (Cell. Pathol.)**, 31:193-203.

van der Putte SCJ, J Toonstra and DF van Wichen, 1989. B cells and plasma cells in mycosis fungoides. **Am. J. Dermatopathol.**, 11:509-516.

von Boehmer H, 1990. Developmental biology of T cells in T cell-receptor transgenic mice. **Annu. Rev. Immunol.** 8:531-556.

von Boehmer H and P Kisielow. 1990. Self-nonself discrimination by T cells. **Science**, 248:1369-1373.

Vonderheid E, 1989. Diagnostic methods for cutaneous T-cell lymphoma. In: SA Muller, Ed. **Parapsoriasis**, Rochester; Mayo Foundation, 1989, pp. 83-94.

Waldmann TA, MM Davis, KF Bongiovanni and SKJ Korsmeyer, 1985. Rearrangements of genes for the antigen receptor on T cells as markers of lineage and clonality in human lymphoid neoplasms. **N. Engl. J. Med.**, 313:776-783.

Wechsler J, M Bagot, T Henni and P Gaulard, 1990. Cutaneous pseudolymphomas: Immunotypical and immunogenotypical studies In: WA van Vloten, R Willemze, GL Vejlsgaard, and K Thomsen, Eds. **Cutaneous lymphoma. Curr. Probl. Dermatol.**, 19:183.

Weiss LM, E Hu, GS Wood, C Moulds, ML Cleary, E Warnke and J Sklar, 1985. Clonal rearrangements for the T-cell receptor genes in mycosis fungoides and dermatopathic lymphadenopathy. **N. Engl. J. Med.**, 313:539.

Weiss LM, GS Wood, E Hu, EA, Abel, RT, Hoppe and J Sklar, 1989. Detection of clonal T-cell receptor gene rearrangements in the peripheral blood of patients with mycosis fungoides/Sézary syndrome. **J. Invest. Dermatol.**, 92:601-604.

Weiss LM, GS Wood, M Trela, RA Warnke and J Sklar, 1986. Clonal T cell populations in lymphomatoid papulosis. Evidence of a lymphoproliferative origin for a clinically benign disease. **N. Engl. J. Med.**, 315:475-479.

Whittemore AS, EA Holly, I-M Lee, EA Abel, RM Adams, BJ Nickoloff, L Bley, JM Peters and C Gibney, 1989. Mycosis fungoides in relation to environmental exposures and immune response: A case-control study. **J. Natl. Cancer Inst.**, 81:1560-1567.

Yanagihara ET, JW Parker, PR Meyer, JM Cain, F Hofman and RJ Lukes, 1984. Mycosis fungoides/Sézary's syndrome progressing to immunoblastic lymphoma. A T-cell lymphoproliferation with both helper and supressor phenotypes. **Am. J. Clin. Pathol.**, 81:249-257.

Zinkernagel RM, A Althage, E Waterfield, B Kindred, RM Welsh, G Callahan and Pincetl, 1980. Restriction specificites, alloreactivity, and allotolerance expressed by T cells from nude mice reconstituted with H-2 compatible or incompatible thymus grafts. **J. Exp. Med.**, 151:376-399.

TERMS AND ABBREVIATIONS USED IN STUDIES OF CUTANEOUS LYMPHOPROLIFERATIVE PHENOMENA

John L. Bednarczyk *
Bradley W. McIntyre*
Philip J. Cohen‡#
Hon-Reen Kuo ‡
Robert A. Schwartz #
Willem A. van Vloten †
W. Clark Lambert ‡#

* Department of Immunology
  University of Texas M.D. Anderson Cancer Center
  Houston, Texas
  U.S.A.

† Department of Dermatology
  University Hospital
  Utrecht
  The Netherlands

‡ Department of Pathology
# Department of Dermatology
  UMD-New Jersey Medical School
  Newark, New Jersey
  U.S.A.

Correspondence to: W. Clark Lambert, MD, Ph.D., Rm C524 M.S.B.,
UMD-New Jersey Medical School, 185 South Orange Avenue,
Newark, NJ 07103-2714

Basic Mechanisms of Physiologic and Aberrant Lymphoproliferation in the Skin
Edited by W.C. Lambert *et al.*, Plenum Press, New York, 1994

579

This chapter addresses the nomenclature of cutaneous lymphoproliferative phenomena, a subject which is complex, confusing, and constantly evolving. Three tables are provided. The first (Table 1) provides definitions for standard and some not so standard abbreviations in current use. Only the definitions, with limited or no discussion are provided here, since to do more would entail an entire volume on its own. Pages in this book where these terms are used are indicated in the index and from them further references may be obtained. While many of these terms are rather obvious, a number are not so obvious. In some cases an abbreviation or term means one thing in one field, and another in another field, both of which interface with cutaneous lymphoproliferative studies. For example, several very different terms and abbreviations are used to denote allergic contact dermatitis, an entity studied by both clinical dermatologists and clinical and research immunologists for many years. "APC" can denote both "antigen presenting cell", as well as a fluorescent dye.

A second table (Table 2) defines the three different, but mathematically interrelated terms in common use to define morphological (especially nuclear) shape as regards deviation of that shape from a circle. Table 2 also provides conversion formulae so that any of these can be derived from any other. It should be pointed out that these terms reflect the currently embryonic state of histologic morphometry; there are, in fact, not one, but six mathematically independent ways in which a two dimensional shape may deviate from being a circle, only one of which is addressed, and that non-rigorously, by these formulae.

A third table (Table 3) provides definitions for the cellular antigens identified by the CD (Cluster of Differentiation) system. It is important to note that this system has been developed, and is updated and maintained, by and for hematologists. A number of these antigens identify very different structures in the skin than they are used for in bone marrow, blood and lymphoid organs. Thus general tables of CD antigens are often inadequate or inappropriate for studies of cutaneous lymphoproliferative phenomena. For example, CD1, which is used as an identifier of thymocytes, in the skin identifies Langerhans cells (Meunier et al., 1993). The CD system is further discussed below.

A table of Adhesion Molecules and their Ligands has been provided in this volume (pages 122 and 123) by van Dinther-Janssen et al.

Activation antigens may be found under the names of the individual antigens in the folowing Tables (1 and 3) and in the Index: Ber Act8; CD30; T9 (Transferrin receptor, CD71); Tac (α subunit of the IL-2 receptor, CD25); and HLA-DR (for some cell types, including keratinocytes). Proliferation antigens may be similarly found under Ki-67 and PCNA.

Finally, relevant references to this nomenclature are provided at the end of this chapter. These include four recent or forthcoming books (Burg et al., 1994, Lambert, 1995, Luger and

Schwarz, 1994; Nickoloff, 1994) which specifically address cutaneous lymphoproliferative phenomena.

CELL SURFACE ANTIGEN MARKERS

The advent of monoclonal antibody technology in 1975 unfolded a new dimension in the orderly classification of leukocyte cell surface antigens. Previously, the discovery and analysis of these antigens depended on a combination of complex immunogenetic and serological approaches resulting in allo- and xeno-antisera that could be used to monitor antigen expression, to probe antigen function, and for immunoprecipitation for subsequent biochemical studies. Progress utilizing this approach was slow, complicated, and only identified a handful of cell surfce proteins. The development and use of monoclonal antibodies revolutionized protein identification and analysis. Now it became theoretically possible to generate gram quantities of reagents esentially absolutely specific for any given antigen. The fine specificity of monoclonal antibodies became the standard for defining antigens in terms of biochemical structure, tissue expression, and in many cases function. Soon many laboratories were generating monoclonal antibodies and developing their own eccentric terminology for naming proteins. Therefore, it became necessary to devise "official" designations grouping and indicating antibody specificity. Monoclonal antibodies from laboratories worldwide were submitted to the International Workshop on Leukocyte Differentiation. The Workshop distributed panels of antibodies to participating laboratories for screening by whatever method their expertise permitted. This allowed, for example, that the results of a group of antibodies that bound to a particular lymphocyte subpopulation as determined by flow cytometry could be compared with the immunochemical determinations of the relative molecular weights of the antibody reactive antigens, thus providing some initial evidence for molecular identity or distinction among the group. By committee, nomenclature was agreed upon and clearly defined cell surface antigens were assigned a CD or "cluster of differentiation" number.

Currently the CD numbers range from 1 to 130. Many investigators in non-immunological fields are alarmed when they find that their favorite surface antigen that had previously been well-characterized at the biochemical and genetic level is now designated something as nondescript as "CD131". Therefore, understandably, some resistance to the use of the CD nomenclature exists. For others, part of the confusion and dissatisfaction over the CD list is that upon first inspection it is apparent that this is just a running list of molecules without any subgrouping based on tissue expresion, gene family, etc. For example, those investigators studying the family of cell adhesion molecules known as the integrins are at a loss to understand the usefulness of a system that refers to the integrin $\alpha L\beta 2$ (LFA-1) as CD11a/CD18 or the integrin $\alpha 4\beta 1$ (VLA-4) as CD49d/CD29.

Nevertheless the CD system represents the only orderly, widely agreed upon system to catalog the large number of structures found on leukocyte cell surfaces. As such, this system provides international guidelines for standardization of the nomenclature and thus a common forum for the discussion of leukocyte antigen expression, structure, and function. With future development and dissemination of CD data bases, investigators will easily be able to search and cross-reference surface antigens on leukocytes, and, hopefully, with the expansion of the data base to include antigens found on all cell types, a comprehensive list of all known cell surface antigens can be made available.

Table 3 lists the CD designations decided upon at the Fifth International Leukocyte Workshop held in November, 1993 in Boston, MA, USA (Pinto et al., 1994). Although the CD molecule designations arose from analyses of leukocytes, a number of these molecules are also expressed by nonhematopoietic cells. Certain CD molecules are restricted to leukocytes (such as CD45) or to subsets of leukocytes (CD3 on T cells, CD73 on B cells, CD56 on Natural Killer cells) and are therefore useful for identifying functionally or developmentally distinct subsets of leukocytes. To an immunologist, a $CD4^+$ cell represents a T lymphocyte that reacts with antigen in the context of the MHC class II, but a cell that is $CD4^+$ and $CD45RO^+$ indicates a memory T cell (a cell that has already responded to antigen) that is antigen/MHC restricted. As further illustration of the order provided by combining CD information, the CD34 molecule is expressed by both hematopoietic precursors and capillary endothelial cells, but a $CD33^+$ $CD34^+$ cell indicates a hematopoietic precursor of the myeloid lineage. By coupling mAb specific for CD determinants with modern cell sorting and imaging techniques, scientists now have the ability to study the function of different cell populations separately from other cells.

The exact physiologic function of many of the CD molecules is not known. In some cases, such as the enzymes or the adhesion proteins, there are defined ligands and often physiologically relevant functions described. In contrast, what we know about a great many of the CD molecules has come about by use of monoclonal antibodies to either block or induce a functional assay. Thus, even without knowing the physiologic ligand, ligation with monoclonal antibodies has allowed researchers to determine if a particular CD molecule is potentially involved in known cellular functions such as T cell-mediated cytotoxicity, or if it can deliver costimulatory signals for lymphocyte activation and proliferation, or regulate intracellular events such as Ca^{++} flux.

REFERENCES

Barclay AN, ML Birkeland, MH Brown, AD Beyers, SJ Davis, C Somoza, and AF Williams, 1993. **The Leucocyte Antigen Facts Book.** Academic Press, London, England.

Bevilacqua MP and RA Nelson, 1993. Selectins, **J. Clin. Invest.,** 91:379-387.

Burg G, H Kerl and B Thiers Eds., **Cutaneous Lymphomas** In: **Dermatologic Clinics** 12(2):213-460, 1994.

Durum SK and JJ Oppenheim, 1993. Proinflammatory cytokines and immunity. In: Paul WE, Ed. **Fundamental Immunology**, 3rd edition. Raven Press, New York, NY, pp. 801-836.

Gallin JI, 1993. Inflammation. In: Paul WE, Ed., **Fundamental Immunology**, 3rd edition. Raven Press, New York, NY, pp. 1015-1032.

Howard MC, A Miyajima and R Coffman, 1993. T cell derived cytokines and their receptors. In: Paul WE, Ed., **Fundamental Immunology**, 3rd edition. Raven Press, New York, NY, pp. 763-800.

Kincade PW and JM Gimble, 1993. B lymphocytes. In: Paul WE, Ed. **Fundamental Immunology**, 3rd edition., Raven Press, New York, NY, pp. 43-74.

Knapp W, B Dorken, WR Gilks, EP Rioeber, RE Schmidt, H Stein, and AEG von dem Borne, Eds., 1989. **Leukocyte Typing IV**. Oxford University Press, Oxford, England.

Lambert WC: **Dermatopathology, with Cell and Molecular markers.** Harvey Miller Publications, Ltd., London, 1995, in preparation.

Luger TA, T Schwarz, Eds. **Epidermal Growth Factors and Cytokines.** Mariel Decker, Inc., New York, 1994.

Luger TA and T Schwartz, 1991. Therapeutic use of cytokines in dermatology. **J. Am. Acad. Dermatol.**, 24:915-926.

Meunier L, A Gonzalezz-Ramos and KD Cooper, 1993. Heterogeneous populations of class II MHC$^+$ cells in human dermal cell suspensions. **J. Immunol.**, 151:4067-4080.

Nickoloff BJ, Ed. **The Dermal Immune System.** Academic Press, New York, 1994.

Pigott R and C Power, 1993. **The Adhesion Molecule Facts Book**, Acadaemic Press, London, England.

Pinto A, V Gattei, D Soligo, C Parravicini, and L Del Vecchio, 1994. New molecules burst at the leukocyte surface. A comprehensive review based on the 5th international workshop on leukocyte differentiation antigens. Boston, U.S.A., November 3-7, 1993. **Leukemia**, 8:347-358.

Shimizu Y and S Shaw, 1993. Mucins in the mainstream, **Nature**, 366:630-631.

Sonnenberg A, 1993. Integrins and their ligands. In: Dunon D, Mackay CR and Imhof BA, Eds. **Adhesion in Leukocyte Homing and Differentiation**. Current Topics in Microbiology and Immunology, 184:7-35.

Table 1. Commonly used abbreviations

ACD	Allergic Contact Dermatitis (Type IV, cell- mediated hypersensitivity; CHS, DTH) (See also CHS, DTH)	**A-T**	Ataxia-Telangiectasia (Louis-Barr Syndrome) (See also FA, XP)
ACTH	Adenocorticotropin (See also CRH)	**ATL**	Adult T-Cell Lymphoma (ATLL, TCLL) (See also HTLV-1, AIDS)
ADCC	Antibody Dependent Cellular Cytotoxicity	**ATLL**	Adult T-Cell Leukemia/Lymphoma (ATL, TCLL) (See also HTLV-1, AIDS)
aFGF	Acidic Fibroblast Growth Factor (See also bFGF, EGF, FGF, NGF, PDGF, TGFα, TGFβ, IFNα, β,γ, IL-1,-2, etc., TNF-α,-β)	**ATLV**	Adult T-Cell Leukemia Virus (HTLV-1) (See also ATL, ATLL, TCLL, AIDS, HIV)
aGVHD	Acute Graft-Versus-Host Disease (See also GVHD)	**BCC**	Basal Cell Carcinoma (See also NMSC)
AIDS	Acquired Immunodeficiency Syndrome (See also HIV, ATL, ATLL, TCLL)	**bFGF**	Basic Fibroblast Growth Factor (See also aFGF, EGF, FGF, PDGF, NGF, TGFα, TGFβ, IFNα, β, γ, IL1,-2, etc.,TNF-α, -β)
ALC lymphoma	Anaplastic Large Cell lymphoma (ALCL, LCAL) (See also B-LCAL, LCL, T-LCAL)	**B-LCAL**	B Large Cell Anaplastic Lymphoma (See also ALC, LCL, LCAL, T-LCAL)
APAAP	Alkaline Phosphatase-Anti-Alkaline Phosphatase (labelling technique)	**BMT**	Bone Marrow Transplantation
APC	1. Antigen Presenting Cell (See also LC) 2. APC fluorescence label (fluoresces in the far red visible range) (See also LAPC, FITC, PE)	**C3-dR**	Receptor of complement component C3-d
		CAD	Chronic Actinic Dermatitis (See also ACD)
Arg-Gly-Asp	Arginine-Glycine-Aspartate (RGD)	**CALLA**	Common Acute Lymphocytic Leukemia Antigen (CD10)

CAT Computer Assisted Tomography;
Computed Tomography

CBCL Cutaneous B-Cell Lymphoma;
Primary Cutaneous B-Cell
Lymphoma

C-CAM Cell-Cell Adhesion Molecule 105
(See also ELAM-1, ICAM-1,-2,
LECAM-1,-3, LFA-1,-3, N-CAM,
PECAM-1, VCAM-1, VLA-1-5;
also related: E-Cadherin, Integrin
$\alpha V\beta 3$, Integrin $\alpha 6\beta 4$, Mac-1)

CD Cluster of Differentiation
(See also Table 3, this chapter)

CDLE Cutaneous Discoid Lupus
Erythematosus
(See also LE, SCLE, SLE)

cDNA Complementary DNA
(DNA Complementary to cellular
mRNA)

CDR-1,-2,-3 Complementarity-Determining
Region -1,-2,-3

CEA Carcino-Embryonic Antigen

CHL Chlorambucil
(See also CHOP, COP, COP-
BLAM, CVP, CVP-Bleomycin,
VCR)

CHOP Cyclophosphamide, Adriamycin,
Vincristine, Prednisone
(See also CHL, COP, COP-BLAM,
CVP, CVP-Bleomycin, VCR)

CHS Contact Hypersensitivity
(Type IV cell-mediated
hypersensitivity, ACD, DTH)

(See also AD)

CLA Cutaneous Lymphocyte Associated
antigen

CMC Cerebriform Mononuclear Cell
(See also SC)

Con A Conconavalin A
(See also PHA, PWM)

COP Cyclophosphamide
(See also CHL. CHOP,
COP-BLAM, CVP,
CVP-Bleomycin, VCR)

COP-BLAM Cyclophosphamide, Vincris-
tine, Prednisone,
Bleomycin, Adriamycin,
Methotrexate (See also
CHL, CHOP, COP, CVP,
CVP-Bleomycin, VCR)

CRH Corticotropin Releasing Hormone
(See also ACTH)

CS1 Cell attachment domain,
recognized by VLA-4, in
an alternatively spliced
region of fibronectin (See
also FN)

CSF Colony Stimulating Factor
(See also G-CSF, GM-CSF,
M-CSF)

CTC Cytotoxic T Cell (CTL)

CTCL Cutaneous T Cell Lymphoma
(See also ATL, CBCL)

CTL Cytolytic T Lymphocyte (CTC)

CVP Cyclophosphamide, Vincristine, Prednisone
(See also CVP-Bleomycin, CHL, CHOP, COP, COP-BLAM, VCR)

CVP-Bleomycin CVP plus Bleomycin
(See also CVP, CHL, CHOP, COP, COP-BLAM, VCR)

DC Dendritic Cell

DEC Dendritic Epidermal Cell
(See also DETC, Thy1⁺DEC)

DETC Dendritic Epidermal T-Cell
(See also DEC, Thy1⁺DEC)

DISH DNA In Situ Hybridization
(See also FISH, RISH)

DNFB Dinitrofluorobenzene

DRC-1 Dendritic Reticulum Cell-1

DTH Delayed-Type Hypersensitivity
(Type IV, cell-mediated hypersensitivity) (ACD,CHS)
(See also CAD)

EA Early antigen, of EBV
(See also EBER1,2, EBNA, EBV, LMP, VCA, ZEBRA protein)

EBER1,2 Epstein-Barr Encoded RNA probe(s) 1,2
(See also EA, EBNA, EBV, LMP, VCA, ZEBRA protein)

EBNA Epstein-Barr virus Nuclear Antigen
(See also EA, EBER1,2, EBV, LMP, VCA, ZEBRA protein)

EBT Electron Beam Therapy

EBV Epstein-Barr Virus
(See also EA, EBER1,2, EBNA, LMP, VCA, ZEBRA protein)

EC Endothelial Cell (See also HECA)

ECF-A Eosinophil Chemotactic Factor-A

ECM III Extracellular Matrix Protein III
(See also FN, VN)

EGF Epidermal Growth Factor
(See also aFGF, bFGF, FGF, NGF, PDGF, TGFα, TGFβ, IFNα, β, γ, IL-1,-2, etc. TGFα, β, TNFα, β

E-H plot Eadie-Hofstee plot
(See also K_{cat}, K_m, L-B plot, V_{max})

ELAM-1 Endothelial Leukocyte Adhesion Molecule-1 (E-Selectin; LECAM-2)
(See also C-CAM, ICAM-1,-2, LECAM-1,-3, LFA-1,-3, N-CAM, PECAM-1, VCAM-1, VLA-1-5;
also related: E-Cadherin, Integrin αVβ3, Integrin α6β4, Mac-1)

ELISA Enzyme-Linked Immunoabsorbance Assay (See also IRMA)

EMA Epithelial Membrane Antigen

F VIII-RA Factor VIII-RA
(See also Ulex Europaeus lectin)

F XIIIa Factor XIIIa

F XIIIs Factor XIIIs

FA Fanconi Anemia
(See also FA-A,-B,etc., A-T, XP)

FA-A,-B, etc. Fanconi Anemia
Complementation Group
A, B, etc.

FACS Flow Activated Cell Sorting
(<u>See also</u> APC, FITC, L90LS,
LFLS, PE)

FGF Fibroblast Growth Factor(s)
(<u>See also</u> aFGF, bFGF, EGF,
NGF,PDGF, TGFα, TGFβ,
IFNα,β,δ, IL-1,-2, etc., TNFα,β)

FISH Fluorescence In Situ Hybridization
(DNA or RNA)
(<u>See also</u> DISH, RISH)

FITC Fluorescein Isothiocyanate
(<u>See also</u> APC, LAPC, PE)

FN Fibronectin
(<u>See also</u> ECM III, VN)

Form P.E. Form Factor (<u>See also</u> NCI,
RI; Defined in Table 2,
this chapter)

G₀ Non-cycling stage of cell cycle

G₁ Stage of cell cycle following M and
prior to S

G₂ Stage of cell cycle following S and
prior to M

GALT Gut Associated Lymphoid Tissue
(<u>See also</u> MALT, SALT, SIS)

G-CSF Granulocyte Colony Stimulating
Factor
(<u>See also</u> GMCAF, GM-CSF, M-
CSF, MCAF)

GL Granular Lymphocyte
(NK cell surface marker)
(<u>See also</u> NHK1, NK cell)

GMCAF Granulocyte-Macrophage Cell
Activating Factor
(<u>See also</u> G-CSF, GM-CSF,
M-CSF, M-CAF)

GM-CSF Granulocyte/Macrophage
Colony Stimulating Factor
(<u>See also</u> G-CSF, GMCAF, M-CSF,
MCAF)

GVHD Graft-Versus-Host Disease
(<u>See also</u> aGVHD)

H1,H2A,H2B,H3,H4 Histone protein 1, 2A,
2B, 3, 4

H-2 Murine MHC complex (Human
homolog is HLA)

HA Hyaluronan/hyaluronic acid

HAM HTLV-1 Associated Myelopathy
(<u>See also</u> HTLV-1, ATL, ATLL,
TCLL, TSP)

HD Hodgkin Disease

HECA High Endothelial Cell Antigen
(<u>See also</u> EC, HEV)

HEL Hen Egg Lysozyme

HEV High Endothelial Venule
(<u>See also</u> EC, HECA)

HIV I,II Human Immunodeficiency Virus I,II
(<u>See also</u> AIDS, HTLV-1,-2,-5)

HLA Human MHC complex (Mouse homolog is H-2)

HML-1 Human Mucosal Leukocyte Antigen-1 (HMLA-1)

HMLA-1 Human Mucosal Leukocyte Antigen-1 (HML-1)

HN₂ Mechlorethamine Hydrochloride (Nitrogen Mustard).

HNK Human Foreskin Keratinocyte

HPA Hypothalamic-Pituitary-Adrenal axis
(See also Immune HPA)

HSP Heat Shock Protein

HSP65 Mycobacterial Heat Shock Protein 65

³HTdr Tritiated thymidine
(See also Ki-67, PCNA)

HTLV-1,-2-5 Human Lymphotropic Virus-1,-2,-5
(See also ATL, ATLL, HAM, TCLL, TSP, HIV I,II)

HUVEC Human Umbilical Vein Endothelial Cell

ICAM-1 Inter-Cellular Adhesion Molecule-1 (CD54)
(See also C-CAM, ELAM-1, ICAM-2, LECAM-1,-3, LFA-1,-3, N-CAM, PECAM-1, VCAM-1, VLA-1-5; also related: E-Cadherin, Integrin $\alpha\beta3$, Integrin $\alpha6\beta4$, Mac-1)

ICAM-2,-3 Inter-Cellular Adhesion Molecule-2, -3
(See also ICAM-1)

IFNα,β,γ Interferon α, β, γ
(See also aFGF, bFGF, EGF, FGF, IL-1,-2, etc. NGF, PDGF, TGFα, β, TNFα,β)

IFN-αR Interferon-α Receptor

IFN-βR Interferon-β Receptor

IgA,D,E,G,M Immunoglobulin A, Immunoglobulin D, Immunoglobulin E, etc.

IL-1,2, etc. Interleukin-1,2, etc.
(See also aFGF, bFGF, EGF, FGF, NGF, PDGF, TGFα, β, TNFα, β)

IL-1R Interleukin-1 Receptor
(See also sIL-2R)

IL-2R Interleukin-2 Receptor (The α subunit is TAC protein, CD25)
(See also sIL-2R)

IL-4R Interleukin-4 Receptor
(See also sIL-4R)

Immune HPA Immune Hypothalamic-Pituitary-Adrenal axis
(See also HPA)

IP-10 Peptide 10

IRMA Immunoradiometric Assay
(See also ELISA)

K_{cat} Enzyme-Substrate Molecular Turnover Number
(See also K_m, V_{max})

K_m Michaelis Constant (of enzyme kinetics) (See also E-H plot, K_{cat}, L-B plot, V_m)

KC   Keratinocyte

kD   Kilodalton

Klenow pol   Active fragment of E. coli DNA polymerase I

L90LS   Measured side (90˙) Light Scatter (in Flow Cytometry)
(See also LFLS)

LAPC   Label with APC fluorescence dye (i.e., quantitative label)
(See also APC, LFITC, LPE)

LAK cell, or activity   Lymphokine Activated Killer cell, or activity

L-B plot   Lineweaver-Burk plot
(See also E-H plot, K_{cat}, K_m, V_{max})

LC   Langerhans cell
(See also APC)

LCA   Leukocyte Common Antigen (CD45)
(See also CD45 RA, CD45RO)

LCAL   Large Cell Anaplastic Lymphoma (ALCL)
(See also LCL, B-LCAL, T-LCAL)

LCL   Large Cell Lymphoma
(See also ALC, B-LCAL, T-LCAL)

LE   Lupus Erythematosus

(See also CDLE, SCLE, SLE)

LECAM-1   Leukocyte Adhesion Molecule-1 (L-Selectin; LAM-1, Leu-8)
(See also C-CAM, ELAM-1, ICAM-1,-2, LECAM-3, LFA-1,-3, N-CAM, PECAM-1, VCAM-1, VLA-1-5; also related: E-Cadherin, Integrin $\alpha V\beta 3$, Integrin $\alpha 6\beta 4$, Mac-1)

LECAM-3   Leukocyte Adhesion Molecule-3 (GMP-140, PADGEM, CD62)
(See also LECAM-1)

LECCAM   Selectin family of adhesion molecules

LFA-1   Leukocyte Function Associated Antigen-1 (Integrin $\alpha L\beta 2$, CD11a/CD18)
(See also C-CAM, ELAM-1, ICAM-1,-2, LECAM-1,-3, LFA-3, N-CAM, PECAM-1, VCAM-1, VLA-1-5; also related: E-cadherin, Integrin $\alpha V\beta 3$, Integrin $\alpha 6\beta 4$, Mac-1)

LFA-3   Leukocyte Function Associated Molecule-3 (CD58) (See also LFA-1)

LFLS   Measured forward Light Scatter (in Flow Cytometry) (see also L90LS)

LFITC   Label with FITC fluorescence dye (i.e. quantitative label)
(See also FTIC, LAPC, LPE)

LHR   Lymphocyte Homing Receptor

(Lymph Node Homing Receptor)

LMP Latent Membrane Protein, of EBV
(See also EA, EBER1,2, EBNA,
EBV, EB LMP, VCA, ZEBRA
protein

LPAM-2 Mouse homolog of human VLA-4

LPC lymphoma Lymphoplasmocytoid
lymphoma

LPE Label with PE
(i.e., quantitative label)
(See also PE, LAPC, LFTIC)

LPS Lipopolysaccharide

LSA Lichen Sclerosus et Atrophicus
(Lichen Sclerosus et Atrophicans)
(human skin disease)

LyP Lymphomatoid Papulosis

M Mitosis. Stage of cell cycle
following G_2 and prior to G_1
(See also S)

mAb Monoclonal Antibody (mouse
hybridoma generated)

Mad Mucosal Addressin

MALT Mucosa Associated Lymphoid Tissue
(See also GALT, SALT, SIS)

MALT-HEV Mucosa Associated
Lymphoid Tissue High Endothelial
Venule

MBP Myelin Basic Protein

MC Lymphoma Mixed Small and Large

Cell Lymphoma

MCAF Mononuclear Cell Activating Factor
(See also G-CSF,
GMCAF, GM-CSF, M-
CSF)

M-CSF Macrophage Colony Stimulating
Factor
(See also G-CSF, GMCAF,
GM-CSF, MCAF)

MECA-79,-367 Mucosal Endothelial Cell
Antigen-79, -367

MED Minimal Erythema Dose (of UV or
visible light or radiation)

MF Mycosis Fungoides

MF-CTCL Mycosis Fungoides type of
Cutaneous T-Cell Lymphoma

MFCG Mycosis Fungoides Cooperative
Group

MHC Major Histocompatibility Complex
(See also H-2, HLA)

MLC Mixed Leukocyte Culture
(See also MLR)

MLR Mixed Lymphocyte Reaction
(See also MLC)

MM 1. Malignant Melanoma
2. Multiple Myeloma

MMC Mitomycin C

MoMuLV Molony Murine Leukemia
Virus

8-MOP	8-Methoxypsoralen (See also PUVA, TMP)		**NHK1**	Natural Killer Cell surface antigen (see also GL, NK cell)

8-MOP 8-Methoxypsoralen
(See also PUVA, TMP)

mRNA Messenger RNA
(See also cDNA)

MSH Melanocyte Stimulating Hormone
(See also αMSH)

nIFN-α Native Interferon-α
(See also IFNα, β, γ, rIFN-α)

NB Northern Blot (Detects specific RNA sequence)
(See also SB, SWB, WB)

N-CAM Neural Cell Adhesion Molecule (D2-CAM, NKH11, CD56, Leu-19)
(See also C-CAM, ELAM-1, ICAM-1,2, LECAM-1,-3, LFA-1,-3, PECAM-1, VCAM-1, VLA1-5; also related: E-Cadherin, Integrin αVβ3, Integrin α6β4, Mac-1)

NCI 1. Nuclear Contour Index
(See also Form P.E., RI; Defined in Table 2, this chapter).
2. National Cancer Institute (USA).

NDGF Normal Distribution of Goodness Fit (statistical test).

NGF Nerve Growth Factor (See also aFGF, bFGF, FGF, EGF, PDGF, TGFα, TGFβ, IFNα,β,γ,IL-1,-2, etc., TNFα,β)

NGFr Nerve Growth Factor receptor.

NHK1 Natural Killer Cell surface antigen (see also GL, NK cell)

NHL Non-Hodgkin Lymphoma

NMSC Non-Melanoma Skin Cancer

nu/nu mouse Nude mouse (homozygous for the nu gene)

NK cell, or activity Natural Killer cell, or activity (See also GL, NHL-1)

p Prevalence, of a disease or genetic marker (See also PV, Se, Sp)

PAS reaction, or stain Periodic Acid-Schiff reaction, or stain

PBL Peripheral Blood Lymphocyte

PBMC Peripheral Blood Mononuclear Cell (See also PMC)

PCGCC Lymphoma Primary Cutaneous Germinal Center Cell Lymphoma

PCNA Proliferating Cell Nuclear Antigen (Subunit of DNA polymerase δ) (Note: This antigen is also upregulated in cells undergoing DNA repair) (See also [3]HTdr, Ki-67).

PCR	Polymerase Chain Reaction
PDGF	Platelet Derived Growth Factor. (See also aFGF, bFGF, EGF, FGF, NGF, TGFα, TGFβ, IFNα,β,γ, IL-1,-2,etc., TGFα,β,TNFα,β)
PE	Phycoerythrin (See also APC, FITC, LAPC)
PECAM-1	Platelet Endothelial Cell Adhesion Molecule-1 (hec7,endo CAM,CD31) (See also C-CAM, ELAM-1,ICAM-1,-2,LECAM-1,-3,LFA-1,-3, N-CAM, VCAM-1,VLA-1-5; also related: E-Cadherin, Integrin αVβ3,Integrin α6β4, Mac-1)
PgP-1	Phagocytic Protein-1
PHA	Phytohemaglutinin (See also Con A, PWM)
PLC	Pityriasis Lichenoides Chronica (human skin disease) (See also PLEVA,PLVA)
PLEVA	Pityriasis Lichenoides et Varioliformis Acuta (human skin disease) (See also PLVA,PLC)
PLN	Peripheral Lymph Node

PLN-HEV	Peripheral Lymph Node High Endothelial Venule.
PLVA	Pityriasis Lichenoides et Varioliformis Acuta (human skin disease) (See also PLEVA, PLC)
PMA	Phorbol Myristate Acetate
PMC	Peripheral (blood) Mononuclear Cell (PBMC).
PML	Polymorphonuclear Leukocyte; Neutrophil (PMN)
PMN	Polymorphonuclear leukocyte; Neutrophil (PML)
PNad	Peripheral Lymph Node Addressin
pol	Polymerase (DNA or RNA) (See also Klenow pol)
POMC	Proopiomelanocortin
PPD	Tuberculin Purified Protein Derivative
PUVA	Psoralen plus Ultraviolet A light (radiation); Photochemotherapy (See also 8-MOP, TMP)
PV (+ or -)	Predictive Value (positive or negative), of a diagnostic test or criterion (See also p, Se, Sp)
PWM	Pokeweed Mitogen (See also Con A, PHA).

rIFN-α Recombinant Interferon-α
(See also IFN-α,β,γ,
nIFN-α).

R Receptor (suffix)

Ra Receptor Antagonist
(suffix)

RGD Arginine-Glycine-Aspartate
(Arg-Gly-Asp)

RISH RNA In Situ
Hybridization (See also
DISH, FISH).

R-S cell Reed-Sternberg Cell

RI Roundness Index (See also
Form P.E., NCI; Defined
in Table 2, this chapter).

RT Reverse Transcriptase
(retroviral enzyme) (See
also HIV, HTLV-1,-2).

S Synthesis, of DNA, stage
of cell cycle following G_1
and prior to G_2.

S1 Nuclease Nuclease which selectively
digests single stranded
DNA

SALT Skin Associated Lymphoid
Tissue (See also SIS,
GALT, MALT)
(See also M)

SB Southern Blot (Detects
specific DNA sequences)
(See also NB, SWB, WB).

SC 1. Sézary Cell (See also
CMC).
2. Sunburn Cell

SCC 1. Small Cleaved Cell
(lymphoma)
2. Squamous Cell Carcinoma

SCLE Subacute Cutaneous Lupus
Eythematosus (See also
CDLE, LE, SLE)

Se Sensitivity, of a diagnostic
test or criterion. (See also
p,PV,Sp)

SF Superfamily

SIg Surface (cell surface)
Immunoglobulin

sIL-1R Soluble Interleukin-1
Receptor (See also IL-1R)

sIL-2R Soluble Interleukin-2
Receptor (The α subunit is
the TAC protein, CD25)
(See also IL-2R)

sIL-4R Soluble Interferon-4
Receptor (See also IL-4R)

SIS Skin Immune System (See
also SALT, GALT,
MALT)

SL Specific Lysis

SLE Systemic Lupus
Erythematosus (See also CDLE, LE,
SCLE

SLEX	Sialyted Lewis X Antigen	**TGFα**	Transforming Growth Factor α (See also aFGF, bFGF, EGF, FGF, NGF, PDGF, TGFα, TGFβ, IFNα, β,γ,IL-1,-2,etc., TNF-α,-β)
Sp	Specificity, of a diagnostic test or criterion (See also p,PV,Se)		
SS	Sézary Syndrome	**TGFβ**	Transforming Growth Factor β (See also TGFα)
SS-CTCL	Sezary Syndrome type of Cutaneous T Cell Lymphoma.	**T$_H$0 cell**	T helper 0 (T helper zero) cell (This cell type secretes most or all of the cytokines secreted by both T$_H$1 and T$_H$2 cells).
sTNFαR	Soluble Tumor Necrosis Factor α Receptor. See also TNFα,TNFαR, TNFβ)		
SWB	South-Western Blot (Detects specific DNA sequences cross-linked to specific proteins) (See also NB, SB, WB)	**T$_H$1 cell**	T helper 1 (T helper one) cell (This cell type secretes IL-2, IFN-γ, and TNF-β, and is associated with cell-mediated immune responses such as DTH (type IV allergic hypersensitivity).
TAC protein	α subunit of IL-2 receptor (CD25)		
TCLL	Adult T Cell Leukemia Lymphoma ATL, ATLL). See also AIDS, HTLV-1)	**T$_H$2 cell**	T helper 2 (T helper two) cell. (This cell type secretes IL-4 and IL-5, and is associated with antibody mediated responses and type I allergic hypersensitivity)
TCR	T Cell Receptor		
TCRGR	T Cell Receptor Gene Rearrangement		
TCT.1	T Cell Target 1	**Thy1$^+$DEC**	Thy1$^+$ Dendritic Epidermal Cell (See also DEC, DETC)
TdT	Terminal Deoxyribonucleotidyl Transferase	**TIL**	Tumor Infiltrating Lymphocyte
		T-LCAL	T Large Cell Anaplastic Lymphoma (See also ALCL, B-LCAL,LCAL)

TMP   4,5',8-Trimethylpsoralen (See also 8-MOP,PUVA)

TNF-α   Tumor Necrosis Factor-α (Cahectin) (See also aFGF,bFGF,EGF,FGF, IL-1,-2,etc., NGF,PDGF, TGFα,β,TNF-β)

TNF-β   Tumor Necrosis Factor-β (Lymphotoxin) (See also TNF-α).

TNFαR   Tumor Necrosis Factor α Receptor (See also TNFα,TNFRI, sTNFαR,TNFβ)

TNFRI   Tumor Necrosis Factor Receptor I (See also TNFα,TNFβ,TNFαR, sTNFαR)

T-NHL   T Cell Non-Hodgkin Lymphoma

TNM stage   Tumor/Node/Metastasis system stage

TP-5   Thymopentin

TSP   Tropical Spastic Paralysis (See also HTLV-1 ATL,ATLL,HAM,TCLL)

UV light, or radiation   Ultraviolet light, or radiation

UV-A   Long wavelength ultraviolet (320 to 400nm wavelength)

UV-B   Short wavelength ultraviolet (found in sunlight; 292 to 320nm wavelength)

UV-C   Short wavelength ultraviolet (not found in sunlight; 200 to 292nm wavelength)

UIP   Usual Interstitial Pneumonitis

V_{max}   Theoretical Maximum Velocity, of an enzymatic reaction (with substrate concentration extrapolated to infinite) (See also E-H plot, K_{cat},K_m,L-B plot)

VCA   Viral Capsid Antigen, of Epstein-Barr virus (EBV) (See also EA,EBER1,2,EBNA, EBV, LMP, ZEBRA protein)

VCAM-1   Vascular Cell Adhesion Molecule-1 (INCAM-110). (See also C-CAM,ELAM-1,ICAM-1,-2,LECAM-1,-3,LFA-1,-3,N-CAM,VLA-1-5; also related: E-Cadherin, Integrin αVβ3, Integrin α6β4, Mac-1)

VCR   Vincristine (See also CHL, CHOP, COP, COP-BLAM,CVP,CVP-Bleomycin)

VLA-1   Very Late Antigen-1 (Integrin $\alpha1\beta1$,CD49a/CD29). (See also C-CAM,ELAM-1,ICAM-1,-2,LECAM-1,-3,LFA-1,-3,N-CAM,VCAM-1, VLA-2-5; Also related: E-Cadherin, Integrin $\alpha V\beta3$, Integrin $\alpha6\beta4$, Mac-1)

VLA-2   Very Late Antigen-2 (Integrin $\alpha2\beta1$, ECMRI, Platelet glycoprotein Ia-IIa, Collagen receptor, CD49b/CD29) (See also VLA-1)

VLA-3   Very Late Antigen-3 (Integrin $\alpha3\beta1$,ECMRII,CD49c/CD29) (See also LPAM-2, VLA-1)

VLA-4   Very Late Antigen-4 (Integrin $\alpha4\beta1$,LPAM-2,CD49d/CD29). See also VLA-1)

VLA-5   Very Late Antigen-5 (Integrin αF,GPIc-IIa, Fibronectin receptor, CD49e/CD29) (See also VLA-1)

VLA-6   Very Late Antigen-6 (Integrin $\alpha6\beta1$, IcIIa, Laminin Receptor,CD49f/CD29) (See also VLA-1)

VN   Vitronectin (See also ECM III,FN)

WB   Western Blot (Detects specific proteins) (See also NB,SB,SWB)

XP   Xeroderma Pigmentosum (See also XP-A,-B, etc., A-T,FA).

XP-A,-B,etc.   Xeroderma Pigmentosum, Complementation Group A,B,etc.

ZEBRA protein Switch protein, of Epstein-Barr virus (EBV). (See also EA,EBER1, 2,EBNA,EBVLMP,VCA).

Table 2. Indices of nuclear and morphologic shape.

Index	Restriction	Definition Verbal	Definition Mathematical	Range	Relationship to other indices	Page citations
Nuclear Contour Index (NCI)[1]	Cell nuclei	Ratio of perimeter to square root of area[1]	$NCI = P/\sqrt{A}$	3.544908 to infinity[1] (3.544908 is a circle)	NCI $= 2\sqrt{\pi}\,/\sqrt{FPE}$ $= 3.544908/\sqrt{FPE}$ $= 2\sqrt{\pi}\,RI$ $= 3.544908RI$	291-299, 325-332, 364
Form factor or Form P.E. (FPE)[2,3]	Any morphologic structure	Fractional (proportional) extent to which shape is a circle[2]	$FPE = 4\pi A/P^2$ $= 12.56637A/P^2$	0 to 1.0[2] (1.0 is a circle)	FPE $= 4\pi\,/NCI^2$ $= 12.56637/NCI^2$ $= 1/RI^2$	333-342
Roundness Index (RI)[1,4]	Any morphologic structure	Ratio of perimeter to the circumference of a circle of equal area[1]	$RI = P/2\sqrt{\pi}\,\sqrt{A}$ $= 0.2820947P/\sqrt{A}$	1.0 to infinity[1] (1.0 is a circle)	RI $= NCI/2\sqrt{\pi}$ $= 0.2820947NCI$ $= 1/\sqrt{FPE}$	

1. Not mathematically defined at NCI or RI = infinity

2. Not mathematically defined at FPE = 0

3. Incorporated into some manufacturers' image analysis softwear, including Zeiss Kontron IBAS 2000

4. Incorporated into some manufacturers' image analysis softwear, including Leitz (Leica) Quantimet 500 and Quantimet 600 series

Table 3. The CD System

CD Designation	Synonym	Distribution	Postulated Function
CD1a	T6, Leu-6	Cortical thymocytes, epidermal Langerhans cells, B-cell subset, dendritic cells.	Antigen presentation (?)
CD1b		Dermal Langerhans cell subset, cortical thymocytes, epidermal Langerhans cells in certain inflammatory conditions	Antigen presentation (?)
CD1c		Epidermal Langerhans cells, dermal Langerhans cells, cortical thymocytes, B-cells	Antigen presentation (?)
CD1d		Intestinal epithelium	antigen presentation (?)
CD2	T11, lymphocyte function associated antigen-2 (LFA-2), E-rosette receptor, Leu-5	T-cells, thymocytes, NK cells	Binds CD58 (LFA-3) and CD16a (FCγ receptor). Cell adhesion. Signal transduction. T-cell and NK cell activation
CD3	T3, T-cell receptor associated complex, Leu 4	Thymocytes, mature T-cells	Complex of 5 proteins associated with T-cell receptor. Signal transduction. T-cell activation.
CD4	T4, Leu-3	Thymocytes, T-cell subset (MHC class II reactive cells), monocytes, macrophages (histiocytes and microglial cells)	Binds MHC class II antigen. Signal transduction. T-cell activation.
CD5	T1, Leu-1	Thymocytes, T-cell subset, B-cell subset	Binds CD72. Signal transduction. T- and B-cell activation
CD6	T12	Thymocytes, T-cell subset, B-cell subset, brain	Signal transduction. T-cell activation.
CD7	gp40, Leu-9	Majority of T-cells, thymocytes, hematopoietic precursors	Unknown. T-cell activation.
CD8	T8, Leu-2	Thymocytes, T-cell subset (MHC class I reactive cells), NK subset	Binds MHC class I antigen. T-cell costimulation
CD9	p24 (tetraspans family member)	Pre-B-cells, monocytes, platelets, activated T-cells	Platelet activation and aggregation. Pre-B-cell adhesion.

CD	Other names	Distribution	Function/Comments
CD10	Common acute lymphoblastic leukemia antigen (CALLA), neutral endopeptidase, metalloendopeptidase, enkephalinase, gp100, J5	T and B lymphoid precursors, B-cell blasts, granulocytes, bone marrow stromal cells, smooth muscle subset, cultured fibroblasts, brain tissue.	Protease. Cleaves biologically active peptides.
CD11a	Integrin α^L subunit, alpha subunit of LFA-1	Leukocytes	CD11a/CD18 complex (LFA-1) binds ICAM-1 (CD54),-2 (CD102), and -3 (CD50). Cell-cell adhesion. Signal transduction. Lymphocyte activation.
CD11b	Integrin α^M subunit complement receptor type 3 (CR3), Mac-1, Mo1, OKM-1, Leu 15	Granulocytes, monocytes, NK-cells	CD11b/CD18 complex (Mac-1) binds CD50, CD54 and iC3b. Cell-cell adhesion. Phagocytosis
CD11c	Leukocyte adhesion receptor p150,95 Integrin α^X subunit, complement receptor type 4 (CR4), Leu-M5	Granulocytes, monocytes, tissue macrophages (histiocytes), NK cells, B-cell subset, T-cell subset, hairy cell leukemia, B-cell chronic lymphocytic leukemias	CD11c/CD18 complex (p150,95) binds fibrinogen and possibly iC3b
CDw12		Monocytes, granulocytes, and platelets	Unknown
CD13	gp150, aminopeptidase N, Leu-M7, MY7	Monocytes, granulocytes, small intestine, renal tuble epithelial cells, central nervous system, fibroblasts, osteoclasts	Protease. Cleaves NH_2-terminal amino acids from small peptides
CD14	gp55, Mo2, MY4, Leu M3	Monocytes, some granulocytes and macrophages	Binds complex consisting of LPS and LPS-binding proteins. Signal transduction. Ligation induces $TNF\alpha$ synthesis and increases CD11b/CD18 activity.
CD15	Lewis X (Le^x), lacto-N-fucopentaeose III, 3-fucosyl-N-acetyl-lactosamine, Leu-M1	Neutrophils, eosinophils, monocytes	
CD15s	Sialyl-Lewis X (sLe^x)	Granulocytes, monocytes, macrophages, B-cells	Binds CD62E (ELAM-1) and CD62P proteins
CD16	$Fc\gamma RIIIA$ and B	Macrophages, NK cells, neutrophils	Receptor for aggregated IgG
CD16b	$Fc\gamma RIIIB$	Granulocyte form only	GPI-linked form of CD16

CD	Alternative names	Cellular distribution	Function
CDw17	Lactosylceramide (LacCer)	Granulocytes, monocytes, platelets, follicular dendritic cells, histiocytes	Packaging/exocytosis of neutrophil granules
CD18	Integrin β_2 subunit, β subunit of LFA-1, Mac-1, and p150,95	Leukocytes (platelets negative)	Associates with CD11a, CD11b & CD11c to form adhesion receptors
CD19	B4, Leu-12	Pan B-cell, follicular dendritic cells	Signal transduction. Costimulation of B cell activation. See CD81
CD20	B1, Bp35, Leu-16	Pan-B-cell (plasma cells negative), follicular dendritic cells	Signal transduction. B-cell activation. Possible calcium channel
CD21	C3d receptor, Complement receptor 2 (CR_2), EBV receptor, B2	Mature B-cells, follicular dendritic cells, thymocyte subset	Binds C3d, Epstein Barr Virus & possibly interferon α. B-cell activation and proliferation. Signal transduction. See CD81
CD22	B-lymphocyte cell adhesion molecule (BL-CAM), Bgp135, B3, Leu-14	Mature B-cells (lost after activation), hairy cell leukemia cells	Binds CD45RO and CD75. Signal transduction
CD23	FcϵRII, low affinity IgE receptor, Blast-2, B6, Leu-20	Activated B-cells, activated macrophages, eosinophils, platelets, dendritic cells	Binds IgE
CD24		B-cells, granulocytes, thymocyte subset, neuroblastomas	Signal transduction in B-cells and granulocytes
CD25	Interleukin-2 Receptor (IL-2R), TAC antigen	Activated T-cells, B-cells and monocytes; NK cells	Binds IL-2. Activation and proliferation of lymphocytes
CD26	Dipeptidyl Peptidase IV (DPP IV), gp120, Ta1	T-cells and B-cells, macrophages (increased with activation); kidney and intestinal brush border, liver bile canaliculi, spleen sinus	Protease. Cleaves NH_2-terminal X-Pro dipeptides. Binds collagen. Signal transduction. Costimulation of T-cells.
CD27		Thymocyte subset, mature T-cells, EBV transformed B-cells, plasma cells	Binds CD70
CD28	Tp44, Leu-28	Thymocytes, T-cell subset, activated B-cells, plasma cells	Binds CD80 (B7). Costimulation of T cell activation. Signal transduction

CD	Other names	Cellular distribution	Function / Comments
CD29	Integrin β_1 subunit, 4B4, very late antigen (VLA) β subunit	Ubiquitous (but not on erythrocytes)	Forms heterodimers with CD49-a–f, CD51 and integrin $\alpha7$ and $\alpha8$ subunits to form adhesion receptors
CD30	Ki-1, Ber-H2	Activated T- and B-cells, Reed-Sternberg cells	Unknown
CD31	Platelet endothelial cell adhesion molecule-1 (PECAM-1), GPIIa, hec7, endoCAM	Platelets, monocytes, macrophages, granulocytes, B-cells, endothelial cells	Cell-cell adhesion
CD32	FcγRII, Fc receptor for aggregated IgG	Monocytes, granulocytes, B-cells eosinophils, endothelial cells	Binds aggregated IgG. IgG-mediated phagocytosis. Signal transduction
CD33	gp67, MY9, Leu-M9	Myeloid progenitor cells, monocytes, histiocytes and granulocytes	Unknown
CD34	HPCA-1, HPCA-2	Hematopoietic precursor cells, capillary endothelial cells	Binds CD62L (L-Selectin). Cell-cell adhesion
CD35	Complement receptor type 1 (CR1), C3b/C4b receptor	T-cell subset, granulocytes (basophils negative), monocytes, histiocytes, follicular dendritic cells, B-cells, erythrocytes, some NK-cells	Binds C3b and C4b. Phagocytosis of immune complexes
CD36	OKM5, platelet glycoprotein IV, GPIIIb, PAS IV	Monocytes, macrophages, platelets, B-cells (weakly) perivascular dermal cells, some of which are dendritic	Binds thrombospondin, collagen and Plasmodium falciparum
CD37	gp52-40, Tetraspans family member	Mature B-cells, T-cells and myeloid cells (weakly)	See CD81. May form receptor linked ion-channel with CD53, CD81 and CD82. See CD81
CD38	T10, Leu-17	Thymocytes, pre-B-cells, activated T-cells, plasma cells	Lymphocyte activation
CD39	gp80	Activated T-, B- and NK cells; monocytes, some macrophages, Langerhans cells, vascular endothelium	Homotypic adhesion of B-cells

CD	Alternative names	Cellular expression	Function
CD40	gp50	B-cells, monocytes (weakly), carcinoma cells, follicular dendritic cells	B-cell/T-cell adhesion. B cell activation and proliferation. Binds gp39
CD41a	Integrin α^{IIb} subunit, platelet glycoprotein IIb/IIIa, Plt-1	Platelets, megakaryocytes	The CD41/CD61 complex binds fibrinogen, von Willebrand factor, fibronectin, vitronectin, and thrombospondin. Platelet adhesion
CD42a	Platelet glycoprotein X, GPIX	Platelets, megakaryocytes	See CD42d
CD42b	Platelet glycoprotein Ibα, GPIB-α	Platelets, megakaryocytes	See CD42d
CD42c	Platelet glycoprotein Ibβ, GPIB-β	Platelets, megakaryocytes	See CD42d
CD42d	Platelet glycoprotein V, GPV	Platelets, megakaryocytes	The CD42 complex mediates platelet binding to von Willebrand factor on endothelium at sites of injury
CD43	Leukosialin, sialophorin, Leu-22	Thymocytes, T-cells, granulocytes, monocytes, macrophages, NK cells, activated B-cells, plasma cells, bone marrow hematopoietic precursors	Binds CD54. Induces CD11a/CD18 function. T-cell costimulation
CD44	Phagocytic glycoprotein 1 (Pgp-1), Hermes, Hutch-1, extracellular matrix receptor type III (ECMR III), HCAM, p85, Leu-44	Medullary thymocytes, T- and B-cells, granulocytes, erythrocytes, epithelial cells, central nervous system tissue, fibroblasts, skeletal muscle, many types of tumor cells	Binds hyaluronate. Helps mediate lymphocyte binding to endothelial cells in the high endothelial venules and inflamed vascular endothelium. Tumor metastasis
CD44R	Restricted epitope on CD44		Alternatively spliced form of CD44
CD45	Leukocyte common antigen, L-CA, B220, T-200, HLe-1	Pan leukocyte. Isoforms (CD45RA, CD45RB and CD45RO) generated by alternative exon splicing	Signal transduction. Two phospho-tyrosine phosphatase domains in cytoplasmic tail
CD45RA	2H4, Leu-18	B-cells, naive T-cell subset, monocytes	domain)
CD45RB		B-cells, T-cell subset, monocytes, macrophages, granulocytes (weakly)	

CD45RO	Leu-45RO	Thymocytes, activated and memory subset of T-cells, B-cell subset, monocytes, macrophages	Binds CD22
CD46	Membrane cofactor protein (MCP), HuLy-m5, trophoblast leucocyte-common antigen	Haematopoietic and non-haematopoietic cells, (erythrocytes negative)	Binds C3b or C4b. Complexed C3b/C4b degraded by factor I. Protects tissue from complement-mediated lysis
CD47		All cell types	Unknown
CD48	Blast-1, HuLy-m3, BCM-1	Leukocytes, bone marrow precursor subset, bronchial and salivary epithelium	Signal transduction
CD49a	Integrin α1 subunit, very late antigen (VLA)-1 α subunit	Activated T-cells, activated B-cells, monocytes, melanomas, cultured nerve cells, smooth muscle	CD49a/CD29 complex binds collagen and laminin
CD49b	Integrin α2 subunit, VLA-2 α subunit; ECMR I	T-cells, B-cells, monocytes, platelets, fibroblasts, endothelial cells, melanomas	CD49b/CD29 complex binds collagen and laminin
CD49c	Integrin α3 subunit, VLA-3 α subunit; ECMR II	B-cells, kidney glomerulus, thyroid, many non-hematopoietic cell lines	CD49c/CD29 complex binds collagen, laminin, fibronectin, epiligrin and bacterial invasin
CD49d	Integrin α4, subunit, VLA-4 α subunit	Thymocytes, T- and B-cells, NK cells, eosinophils, basophils, hematopoietic precursors, developing muscle, certain melanoma, neural and sarcoma lines	CD49d/CD29 complex (LPAM-2) binds CD106 (VCAM-1), fibronectin, bacterial invasin, and upon activation thrombospondin. The related complex CD49d/β7 binds the mucosal addressin cell adhesion molecule-1 (MAdCAM-1) Cell adhesion, lymphocyte recirculation, homotypic aggregation. Signal transduction. Lymphocyte activation and proliferation
CD49e	Integrin α5 subunit, VLA-5 α subunit	Broadly expressed	CD49e/CD29 complex is the classically defined receptor for fibronectin. Signal transduction. Lymphocyte activation and proliferation. Gene transcription in non-lymphoid cells
CD49f	Integrin α6 subunit, VLA-6 α subunit	Thymocytes, T- and B-cells monocytes and granulocytes	The CD49f/CD29 complex binds laminin and bacterial invasin. Embryonic development, polarity determination in kidney mesenchyme

CD	Name	Cellular distribution	Function
CD50	ICAM-3	Thymocytes, T- and B-cells, monocytes and granulocytes	Binds CD11a/CD18 and CD11b/CD18. Cell-cell adhesion
CD51	Integrin α^v subunit, vitronectin receptor α subunit	Platelets, endothelial cells, smooth muscle cells, fibroblasts, osteoclasts, melanoma cells	CD51 forms adhesion receptor complexes with at least five different β subunits (β1 [CD29], β3 [CD61], β5, β6, and β8). Mediates adhesion of cells to extracellular matrix proteins such as fibronectin (CD51/CD29, CD51/CD61 and CD51/β6) or vitronectin (CD51/CD61, CD51/β5)
CD52	CAMPATH-1	Thymocytes, T- and B-cells, subsets of granulocytes and eosinophils	Unknown
CD53	Tetraspans family member	Thymocytes, pan-leukocyte, osteoclasts and osteoblasts	May form receptor linked ion-channel with CD37, CD81 and CD82. See CD81.
CD54	Intercellular adhesion molecule-1 (ICAM-1), Leu-54	Induced or upregulated on a range of activated cell types, including T- and B-cells, thymocytes, monocytes, dendritic cells, endothelial cells, fibroblasts, keratinocytes, chondrocytes, and epithelial cells	Binds CD11a/CD18, CD11b/CD18, CD43 and rhinovirus. Cell-cell adhesion mediating lymphocyte recirculation, antigen presentation, cellular cytotoxicity, adhesion of leukocytes to inflammatory endothelium
CD55	Decay accelerating factor (DAF)	Widely expressed on hematopoietic and nonhematopoietic cells	Blocks C3 convertase formation and enhances convertase decay. Protects tissue from damage after complement activation
CD56	Neural cell adhesion molecule (M-CAM), NKH-1, Leu-19	At least three isoforms found on NK cells, neurons, astrocytes, Schwann cells, and developing muscle	Binds homophilically and mediates cell-cell adhesion. Signal transduction
CD57	HNK-1, Leu-7	NK cells, monocyte subset, T- cells, B-cells	Unknown
CD58	LFA-3	Broad expression	Binds CD2. T-cell adhesion to cells expressing CD58. Signal transduction
CD59	Protectin, P-18, MAC inhibitor, H19, MIRL, HRF20	Broad expression, but low levels on B-cells	Binds C8 and C9 complement components. Blocks assembly of the membrane attack complex protecting cells from damage after complement activation

CDw60		T-cell subset, monocytes, platelets	Signal transduction. T-cell activation
CD61	Integrin β_3 subunit of the platelet glycoprotein IIIa, vitronectin receptor β subunit	Platelets, megakaryocytes	Forms adhesion receptors with either CD41 (αIIb) or CD51 (αV). CD41/CD61 binds fibrinogen, fibronectin, von Willebrand factor, and vitronectin. CD51/CD61 binds fibrinogen, fibronectin, von Willebrand factor, victronectin, thrombospondin, osteospondin and bone sialoprotein-1
CD62E	E-selectin, ELAM-1, LECAM-2	Endothelium	Binds sialylated Lewis^x (CD15s) and Lewis^a antigens and the P selectin glycoprotein ligand (PSGL-1). Mediates binding of leukocytes to vascular endothelial during inflammation
CD62L	L-selectin, LAM-1, LECAM-1, TQ-1, Leu-8	B-and T-cells, monocytes, NK cells, neutrophils, eosinophils, hematopoietic precursors and thymocyte subsets	Binds glycosylation-dependent cell adhesion molecule (GlyCAM-1), CD34 and mucosal addressin cell adhesion molecule (MAdCAM-1). Lymphocyte entry into peripheral lymph nodes. Helps mediate the initial adhesion of leukocytes to inflamed vascular endothelium
CD62P	P-selectin, PADGEM, GMP-140, LECAM-3	Platelets, endothelial cells, megakaryocytes	Binds sialylated Lewis^x and PSGL-1. Leukocyte binding to activated platelets and inflamed endothelium
CD63	Platelet activation antigen, ME491, MLA1, PTLGP40	Activated platelets, monocytes, macrophages, weakly on granulocytes, T-cells and B-cells	Cell adhesion. Signal transduction
CD64	FcγRI	Monocytes, histiocytes	Binds monomeric IgG. Phagocytosis of immune complexes and antibody-dependent cellular cytotoxicity
CD65	Ceramide dodeasaccharide 4c, VIM-2	Granulocytes, monocytes	Signal transduction
CD66a	Biliary glycoprotein-1 (BGP-1)	Neutrophils, granulocytes, colon carcinoma	Cell adhesion. Hematopoietic differentiation
CD66b	Carcinoembryonic antigen (CEA) gene member 6 (old CD67), CGM6, p100	Granulocytes	Signal transduction

CD66c	Non cross-reacting antigen (NCA)		
CD66d	Carcinoembryonic antigen (CEA) gene member 1, CGM1		
CD66e	Carcinoembryonic antigen (CEA)		
CD68	Macrosialin	Primarily in cytoplasmic granules of monocytes, macrophages, neutrophils, basophils, large lymphocytes, liver cells, kidney tubules and glomeruli	Unknown
CD69	AIM, EA-1, MLR-3, Leu-23	Platelets, thymocytes, NK cells, activated T- and B-cells, activated macrophages	Very early marker of lymphocyte activation. Signal transduction. Lymphocyte activation, proliferation and induction of function
CD70	CD27-ligand	Subsets of activated T- and B-cells	Binds CD27. Signal transduction. T-cell proliferation
CD71	T9, transferrin receptor	Activated T- and B-cells macrophages, proliferating and dividing cells in other tissue	Uptake of iron
CD72		B-cells (except plasma cells) and some histiocytes	Binds CD5. Signal transduction. B-cell activation and proliferation
CD73	Ecto-5'-nucleotidase	Thymocytes, B- and T-cell subsets, some endothelial and epithelial cells	Dephosphorylation of deoxyribonucleoside monophosphates to nucleosides that are then taken up into the cell
CD74	MHC class II invariant chain (Ii)	B-cells, macrophages, monocytes	Associates with α and β subunits of MHC class II during biosynthesis. Blocks binding of endogenous peptide to nascent complex. Released in acidic environment
CDw75	neuraminidase sensitive epitope on glycosphingolipids and proteins arising from activity of a 2,6-sialyltransferase	Mature B-cells, T-cell subset	Binds CD22. B-cell/B-cell adhesion
CDw76	Previously CD76. Neuraminidase sensitive epitopes (76.1 and 76.2) on glycosphingolipids and proteins arising from activity of a 2,6-sialyltransferase	Mature B-cells, T-cell subset	Unknown

Marker	Other names / antigen	Cellular expression	Function
CD77	Globotriaclyceramide (Gb₃), Pᵏ blood group antigen, Burkitt's lymphoma associated antigen	Subset of germinal center B-cells, follicular dendritic cells, endothelial cells and some epithelial cells, Burkitt's lymphoma	Unknown. Binds bacterial lectins. Expressed by germinal center B-cells undergoing apoptosis
CDw78	B₄, Leu-21	B-cell subset, increased upon activation. Histiocytes and epithelial cells	Unknown
CD79a	mb-1, surface Ig receptor complex α subunit (Igα)	B-cells and plasma cells	Complexes in the plasma membrane with the transmembrane receptor forms of IgM and IgD. Signal transduction. B cell activation and proliferation
CD79b	B29, Igβ	B-cells and plasma cells	Complexes in the plasma membrane with the transmembrane receptor forms of IgM and IgD. Signal transduction. B-cell activation and proliferation
CD80	B7, BB1	B- and T-cell subsets, macrophage subsets, dendritic cells, germinal center cells	Binds CD28 and CTLA-4. B cell activation and differentiation
CD81	Target of antiproliferative antibody (TAPA-1). Tetraspans family member	B- and T-cells, plasma cells, monocyte subset, endothelial and epithelial cells	Homotypic B cell adhesion. Lymphocyte proliferation. Forms possible transporter/ion channel complex on B cell with CD19, CD21, CD37, CD53, CD82, HLA-DR and Leu-13)
CD82	R2, IA4, 4F9	Broad expression on leukocytes, endothelial and epithelial cells	Signal transduction. See CD81. May form receptor-linked ion channel with CD37, CD53 and CD81
CD83	HB15	Interdigitating dendritic reticulum cells and circulating dendritic cells (but not follicular dendritic cells), Langerhans cells, germinal center lymphocytes	Unknown
CDw84	2G7	Platelets, monocytes, T-cell subset, B-cells	Unknown
CD85	VMP-55, GH1/75	B-cells, plasma cells and monocytes	Unknown
CD86	FUN-1, BU63	Germinal center cells, activated B- cells, monocytes	Unknown
CD87	Urokinase plasminogen activator receptor, UPA-R	Granulocytes, monocytes, eosinophils, activated T-cells	Binds urokinase plasminogen activator. Enhances fibrinolysis

CD	Name/Alternative	Cellular expression	Function
CD88	C5a receptor, C5aR, anaphylatoxin receptor	Polymorphonuclear leukocytes, mast cells, monocytes, macrophages, smooth muscle	Smooth muscle contraction. Leukocyte chemotaxis
CD89	IgA receptor, IgaR, FcαR	Neutrophils, monocytes, macrophages, eosinophils, T- and B-cell subsets	Binds IgA. Endocytosis. Signal transduction
CDw90	Thy-1 (mouse)	Subset of CD34$^+$ cells, most primitive hematopoietic precursors, fibroblasts, stromal cells	Hematopoietic precursor differentiation and proliferation
CD91	α2-macroglobulin receptor, α^{2}M-R	Monocytes, macrophages, hepatocytes, fibroblasts, smooth muscle cells	Binds α2-macroglobulin
CDw92	VIM15	Neutrophils, monocytes, endothelial cells, platelets	Unknown
CD93	VIMD2	Neutrophils, monocytes, endothelial cells	Unknown
CD94	KP43	NK cells, α/β and γ/δ T-cell subsets	Regulation of LFA-1 dependent adhesion and cell-mediated cytolysis
CD95	APO-1, FAS	Broadly expressed on many hematopoietic and nonhematopoietic cell lines and tumor lines	Apoptotic death
CD96	T-cell activation increased late expression (TACTILE) antigen	Activated T-cells	Unknown
CD97	GR1, BL-KDD/12	T-cell subset, NK subset, eosinophils	Unknown
CD98	4F2, 2F3	Thymocytes, activated T-cells, activated NK cells, monocytes, heart and skeletal muscle, basal layer keratinocytes, dividing cells	Signal transduction. Cellular activation and proliferation
CD99	MIC2, E2, 12E7, Huly-m6, FMC29, Ewing's sarcoma marker	Peripheral blood lymphocytes, T- and B-cell dependent areas of lymph nodes, CD34$^+$ hematopoietic precursors, endothelial cells	Rosette formation between T-cells and erythrocytes. Signal transduction
CD99R	CD99 mAb restricted		
CD100	BD16, BB18, A8	Resting and activated T-cells	Signal transduction. T-cell activation and proliferation

CD	Name / synonyms	Cellular expression	Function / comments
CDw101	BB27, BA27	Granulocytes, monocytes, T-cell subset	Only those CD28$^+$ T-cells that are CDw101$^+$ will be activated by anti-CD28 mAb ligation
CD102	ICAM-2	Resting lymphocytes, monocytes, endothelial cells, platelets	Binds CD11a/CD18 complex. Cell-cell adhesion
CD103	HML-1, Integrin αE subunit, Integrin αEL subunit	Intraepithelial lymphocytes, 2-6% of lymphocytes in the peripheral blood, subset of memory T-cells	The αEβ7 complex mediates T-cell interaction with epithelial cells
CD104	Integrin β4 subunit	Thymocytes, epithelial cells, keratinocytes, Schwann cells, some neuronal, endothelial and tumor cells	The α6β4 complex binds laminin. Found in hemidesmosomes
CD105	Endoglin	Endothelial cells, activated monocytes, subset of CD34$^+$ precursors, osteoclast cell lines, erythroid progenitor cells	Binds transforming growth factor β1 and β3
CD106	Vascular cell adhesion molecule-1 (VCAM-1), intercellular adhesion molecule-110 (INCAM-110)	Endothelial cells, monocytes, bone marrow stromal cells, follicular dendritic cells	Binds CD49d/CD29 and CD49d/β7 complexes. Cell-cell adhesion
CD107a	Lysosomal associated membrane protein-1 (LAMP-1)	Platelets	Unknown
CD107b	LAMP-2	Platelets	Unknown
CDw108	MEM-150, MEM-121	Activated T-cells, some stromal cells	Cellular activation
CDw109	GR-56, platelet activation factor, 8A3, 7D1	Endothelial cells, activated T-cells, activated platelets	Signal transduction. Cellular activation and proliferation
CD115	Macrophage-colony stimulating factor receptor (M-CSFR), CSF-1R	Monocytes, macrophages, bone marrow progenitors, placenta	Binds M-CSF. Signal transduction. hematopoietic development. Adhesion of progenitors to stromal cells through membrane associated M-CSF
CDw116	Granulocyte, macrophage-colony stimulating factor receptor (GM-CSFR) α chain, HGM-CSFR	Monocytes, macrophages, neutrophils, eosinophils, fibroblasts, endothelial cells, bone marrow progenitors	Shares β subunit with CD123 (IL-3R) and CD125 (IL-5R) signal transduction. Hematopoietic cell development. Cellular activation (mature leukocytes)

CD	Name	Cellular expression	Function
CD117	c-Kit receptor, stem cell factor receptor, SCFR	Bone marrow progenitors, Langerhans cells, mast cells, melanocytes, endothelial cells, osteoclasts	Binds stem cell factor. Signal transduction. Development of hematopoietic, gonad and pigment cells. Adhesion of progenitors to stromal cells through membrane associated stem cell factor
CD118	Interferon α, β receptor (IFN-α, βR)	Broad cellular expression	Signal transduction. B-cell differentiation and macrophage activation
CDw119	IFN-γR	Macrophage, monocyte, T- and B-cells, epithelial cells, fibroblasts	Signal transduction. Activation of monocytes and macrophages. Up regulates MHC class I and II. Regulates B-cell and helper T-cell activation
CD120a	Tumor necrosis factor receptor (TNFR) type 1	Broadly expressed	See CD120b
CD120b	TNFR type 2	Broadly expressed	Signal transduction. TNF mediates cellular cytotoxicity (tumor necrosis), has antiviral activity, induces lymphocyte proliferation and is an important mediator of inflammation. Regulates adhesion molecule expression
CDw121a	Interleukin-1 receptor (IL-1R) type 1	T-cells, thymocytes, fibroblasts, endothelial cells	See CD121b
CDw121b	IL-1R type 2	B-cells, macrophages, monocytes	Signal transduction. IL-1 is an important early mediator of inflammation. Increases lymphocyte proliferation, induces production of other cytokines as well as prostaglandins from monocytes and macrophages. Regulates adhesion molecule expression. Induces sleep and, by acting on hypothalamus, fever
CD122	IL-2Rβ	NK cells, B- and T-cell subsets	Forms high affinity IL-2R complex with CD25 and IL-2Rγ. Activation and proliferation of macrophages, T- cells, B-cells, and NK cells
CD123	IL-3R	Bone marrow stem cells, granulocytes, monocytes, megakaryocytes	Shares β subunit with CD116 (GM-CSFR) and CD125 (IL-5R). Signal transduction. Development of multipotent hematopoietic precursors. Enhances phagocytosis and antibody-dependent cytotoxicity of mature myeloid cells

CDw124	IL-4R	Mature B- and T-cells, monocytes and macrophages, hematopoietic precursor cells, fibroblasts, epithelial cells	Growth and development factor for hematopoietic cells in general. Important in the activation and differentiation of B-cells
CD125	IL-5R	Eosinophils and basophils, eosinophil/basophil precursors	Shares β subunit with CD116 (GM-CSFR) and CD123 (IL-3R). Signal transduction. Development of eosinophil precursors
CD126	IL-6R	Activated B-cells and plasma cells, thymocytes and T-cells, hepatocytes, osteoclasts	Forms receptor complex with CDw130. Signal transduction. Cellular activation and proliferation
CDw127	IL-7R	Bone marrow lymphoid precursors, pre-B-cells, mature T-cells, monocytes	Cellular proliferation
CDw128	IL-8R	Neutrophils, basophils, T-cell subset	Chemoattraction/chemotaxis of neutrophils, basophils and T-cells
CDw130	IL-6R-gp130SIG	Most leukocytes (strongly on activated B-cells and plasma cells), endothelial cells	β subunit of the receptors for IL-6, IL-11, leukemia inhibitory factor, oncostatin M, and G-CSF

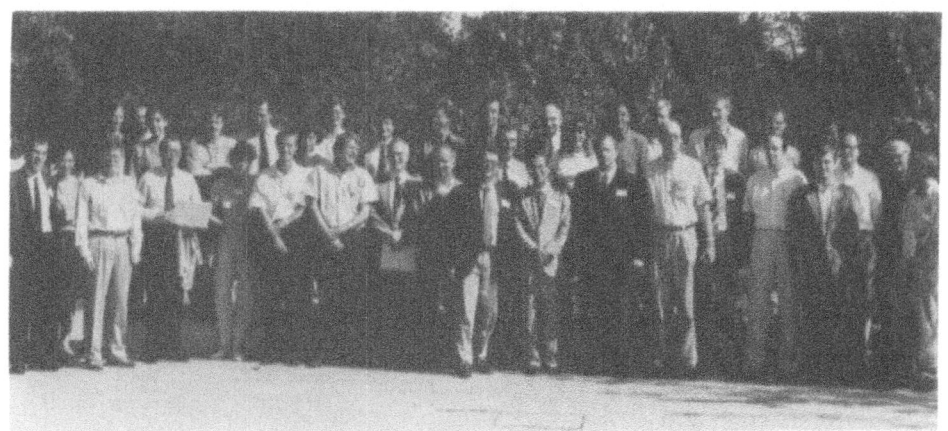

Participants at the NATO Advanced Research Workshop, "Basic Mechanisms of Physiologic and Aberrant Lymphoproliferation in the Skin", San Mineato, Italy, October 1-6, 1991.

Back row

Muriel Lambert, Vittorio Manzari, Marie Louise Geerts, Hans van Oostveen, Volker Mielke, Martine Bagot, Sean Whittaker, Michel D'Incan, Reinhard Dummer, Lorenzo Cerroni, Neil Smith, Raphaella Gianotti, Sergio Chimenti, Peter Hartfield, Udo Rijlaarsdam, Heinrich Veelken, Emilio Berti.

Front row

Bram Preesman, Pierre Souteyrand, Anne Marie Busschots, Richard Edelson, Helmut Kerl, Jannie Borst, Frank Nestlé, Chris Meijer, Eric Vonderheid, David Ramsey, Nicolo Pimpinelli, Benvenuto Giannotti, W. Clark Lambert, Willem van Vloten, Peter Kaudewitz, Rein Willemze, Kevin Cooper, Robert Tigelaar, Tom Lawley, Keld Kaltoft.

INDEX OF AUTHORS AND CONFERENCE PARTICIPANTS

(Conference participants in **boldface type**; group photograph on page 613)

MCAF (Mononuclear Cell Activating
    Factor), 77-91,590
MECA-367, 119,124,590
MECA-79, 119,590
Mechlorethamine hydrochloride (nitrogen
    mustard, HN_2), 284,470-
    477,499,537,547,554
    contact hypersensitivity, 471
MED (minimal erythema dose), 473
Medication, topical, as allergen, 555
    MEL-14, 115-129,158-174
    see also LECAM-1
Melanocyte stimulating hormone, see
MSH
Melanocyte, 96,104
Melanocytic disorder, 235
Melanoma, 225,451-457,459-466
    metastatic, 459,460
    precursor lesion, 225
Melanophagocytosis, 30
Mendelian inheritance, 500
Metal allergen, 555
Metastatic melanoma, 459,460
Methotrexate, 284
Methoxsalen, see 8-Methoxypsoralen
8-Methoxypsoralen (8-MOP),
    104,108,109,284,483,497-526
Methycellulose colony forming ability,
428
MF-CTCL (mycosis fungoides),
    30,62,63,141-153,159-
    174,179,186,187,195-
    202,217,226,255-262,291-297,317-
    323,363-367,370-
    376,379,382,395,409-
    415,498,519,545,553,554,565-
    571,590
    classical, 161-163,590
    erythrodermic (E-MF),
        159,161,163,173,198,199,276-
        287,367
        see also CTCL, SS-CTCL
    large cell lymphoma type, 260-262
    leukemic, 363-367
        see also SS-CTCL
    patch stage, 370-376
        see also parapsoriasis
    plaque stage, 367,370
    tumor stage, 163,173,198,199,367,370-
        376
    see also ATL

see also CTCL
see also lymphoma
see also SS-CTCL
MF3 patient, 403
MFCG stage, 285,590
MHC (major histocompatibility complex),
    394
Mg^{+2} dependent reverse transcriptase, 178
MH6 hybridization, 372
    MHC, 5,41
    MHC class I, 2,9-11,95-100,119,437
    MHC Class I^k molecule, 493
    MHC class II, 2,9-11,58,61,95-
        100,199-129,437
    MHC self-antigen, 566,569
Mice, see mouse
Michaelis constant (K_m), 498,504,505,511-
    526,588
Michaelis-Menten equation, 504
Microglobulin, 47
Microorganism, pathogenic, 99
Microscopy, 217-226,231-240,243-
    253,255-2662,265-271,275-288,291-
    298,301-314,328,364,370-
    376,379,451-457,567
Migration, lymphocyte, 113-129
Mimicry, molecular, 447
Minimal erythema dose (MED), 473
Mink lung epithelial cell line, 429,430
Minocycline-induced hyperpigmentation,
    84
Mitomycin C (MMC),
    179,485,486,488,499,520
Mitosis, 87,318,590
Mixed small and large cell (MC)
    lymphoma, 308
Mixed leukocyte culture (MLC), 486
MLC (mixed leukocyte culture), 486,590
MMC (mitomycin C),
    179,485,486,488,499,520,590
Model, Cox, 276,279
Model, genetic, for carcinogenesis,
    218,219,500
Model, thymus bypass, 566,569,570
Model, for tumor progression, 425-432
"Modest Proposal" (Swift), 566
Molecular genetics, 185,195-
    202,231,232,243,244,364,370-
    376,379,383,395,421,440
    molecular hybridization, see
        hybridization, nucleic acid

Molecular mimicry, 447
Molony Murine Leukemia Virus
     (MoMuLV), 180
MoMuLV (Molony Murine Leukemia
     Virus), 180,590
Monoadduct, psoralen, 497
Monoclonal T cell population, 379
Monoclonal T cell proliferation, 198
Monoclonality, 567,569
Monocyte, 59,118,120,121,381,385,435-
     447,538
Monomyelocytic cell, 95-100
Mononuclear cell, 234-235,328,439-447
     cerebriform (CMC), 328
     peripheral, see PBMC
     see also cerebriform nucleus
Mononuclear Cell Activating Factor
     (MCAF), 77-91
Mononucleosis infectiosa, 206,209
8-MOP(8-methoxypsoralen; Methoxalen),
     104,108,109,284,483,590
Morbus Crosti, 344
Morbus Hodgkin, see Hodgkin disease
Morphometry, 334,364
Mouse, 1-12,17-
     23,104,118,119,121,143,158-
     1714,462,483-494,540,553,570
     aged, 553
     AKR/J, 41
     AKR/OLa, 18-23
     athymic, 17-19
     B10.A, 484,485
     BALB/c, 20
          BALB/c nude, 490
     BGPL-Thy-1a, 18-23
     C3H/HeN, 107
     C57/BL/6, 18-23,45,570
          C57/BL/6 vit/vit, 39,40,47,48
     CDH/He/Han, 18-23
     knockout, 12
     nude, 17-19,484,490
          nu/nu, 42,43
     scid, 40
     T cell, see T cell
     thymectomized, 553
     transgenic, 7
mRNA, 95-100,104,105,590
MSH, see also αMSH, 95,591
MT1 (anti CD43), 305,311-313
MT2 (anti CD45RA), 305,311-313
Mucha-Habermann disease (PLEVA), 222
Mucinosis, follicular, 278

Mucosa, oral, 61
Mucosa, respiratory tract, 455
Mucosa-associated lymphoid tissue
     (MALT), 65,313,334
Mucosal addressin (Mad), 119
Mucosal HEV, 121
Mucous membrane, 57
MuIFN-β, 540
Multilobulated lymphoma, 240
Multiple myeloma, 225
Multivariant analysis, 276,279
Murine TCR genes, see TCR
Murine experimental encephalomyelitis,
     394,395
Mutant cell lines, human, see FA and XP
Mutation, 202
My-La cell line, 540
My-Ta cell line, 403
Myalgia, 548
Mycobacterial heat shock protein 65
     (HSP65), 10,11,65
Mycobacterium tuberculosis, 10
Mycosis fungoides form of cutaneous T
     cell lymphoma, see MF-CTCL
Mycosis cell, 244
     see also cerebriform nucleus
Myelin basic protein (MBP), 485,486
Myelocytic leukemia, 413
Myeloma, multiple, 225
Myelopathy, HTLV-1 associated (HAM),
     186

N nucleotide, 4,41
N-CAM (CD56), 88,119-129
     see also CD56
Nae I (RE), 440
Nails, 221
Naive T cell, see CD45RA
Nasal T cell lymphoma, 211
Nasopharangeal carcinoma, 206
Nasopharynx, 303
NCI (nuclear contour index), 291-
     297,325-331,364,580,591,597
NDGF (normal distribution of goodness
     fit), 335-341
Neoplasm, 99,436,554
     secondary, in CTCL, 436
     solid, 554
Nephrotic syndrome, 548
Nerve Growth Factor receptor (NGFr), 65
     antibody against, 305,311-313
Neurodermatitis, 244

The manufacturer's authorised representative in the EU is Springer
Nature Customer Service Centre GmbH, Europaplatz 3, 69115 Heidelberg,
Germany. If you have any concerns regarding our products, please
contact ProductSafety@springernature.com

Printed and bound by CPI Group (UK) Ltd, Croydon, CR0 4YY
26/04/2026
02097340-0003